Ninth Edition

SAUER'S MANUAL OF SKIN DISEASES

Ninth Edition

SAUER'S MANUAL OF SKIN DISEASES

John C. Hall, MD

Primary Staff
St. Luke's Hospital
Lecturer of Medicine
University of Missouri-Kansas City School of Medicine
Clinician
Kansas City Free Health Clinic
Kansas City, Missouri

With 35 Contributing Authors

. Lippincott Williams & Wilkins
a Wolters Kluwer business

Philadelphia · Baltimore · New York · London
Buenos Aires · Hong Kong · Sydney · Tokyo

Acquisitions Editor: Sonya Seigafuse
Developmental Editor: Annette Ferran
Managing Editor: Nancy Winter
Manufacturing Manager: Kathleen Brown
Project Manager: Bridgett Dougherty
Design Coordinator: Risa Clow
Compositor: TechBooks
Printer: Quebecor World Kingsport

© 2006 by LIPPINCOTT WILLIAMS & WILKINS
530 Walnut Street
Philadelphia, PA 19106 USA
LWW.com

Printed in the USA

Library of Congress Cataloging-in-Publication Data

Hall, John C., 1947–
   Sauer's manual of skin diseases / John C. Hall ; with 35 contributing authors.—9th ed.
     p. ; cm.
  Includes bibliographical references and index.
  ISBN 0-7817-2947-5 (alk. paper)
  1. Skin—Diseases—Handbooks, manuals, etc.   I. Sauer, Gordon C. (Gordon Chenoweth), 1921– Manual of skin diseases. II. Title.   III. Title: Manual of skin diseases.
  [DNLM: 1. Skin Diseases. WR 140 H177s 2006]
RL74.S25 2006
616.5—dc22

                                                2006000878

10 9 8 7 6 5 4 3 2 1

CONTENTS

CONTRIBUTORS

Rodney S. W. Basler, MD
Founding Chair, Taskforce on Sportsmedicine
American Academy of Dermatology
Clinical Assistant Professor, Department Internal Medicine
* (Dermatology)*
University of Nebraska Medical Center
Omaha, Nebraska
Chapter 40: Sports Medicine Dermatology

Francisco G. Bravo, MD
Assistant Professor
Department of Dermatology
Univesidad Peruana Cayetano Heredia
Attending Physician
Dermatology Service
Instituto de Enfermedades Infecciosas y Tropicales Alexander
* von Humboldt*
Hospital Nacional Cayetano Heredia
Lima, Peru
Chapter 38: Tropical Diseases of the Skin

Robin Buchholz, MD
Attending
St. Luke's-Roosevelt Hospital Center and
* Beth Israel Medical Center*
Assistant Clinical Professor of Dermatology
Columbia University College of Physicians and Surgeons
New York, New York
Chapter 14: Psoriasis

Clay J. Cockerell, MD
Clinical Professor
Dermatology and Pathology Departments
Director
Dermatopathology Department
University of Texas Southwestern Medical Center at Dallas
Dallas, Texas
Chapter 24: Cutaneous Diseases Associated with Human
Immunodeficiency Virus

Ellen de Coninck
Stanford University School of Medicine
Stanford, California
Chapter 20: Psychodermatology

Jon A. Dyer, MD
Assistant Professor of Dermatology and Child Health
Department of Dermatology
University of Missouri—Columbia
Columbia, Missouri
Chapter 10: Dermatologic Immunology

Mary M. Feldman, MD
Fellow at Dermatopathology
University of Texas Southwestern Medical Center at Dallas
Dallas, Texas
Chapter 24: Cutaneous Diseases Associated With
Human Immunodeficiency Virus

Gary Goldenberg, MD
Resident
Department of Dermatology
Wake Forest University School of Medicine
Winston-Salem, North Carolina
Chapter 32: Collagen Vascular Diseases

Warren R. Heymann, MD
Head, Division of Dermatology
Department of Clinical Medicine
UMDNJ-Robert Wood Johnson Medical School at Camden
Cooper Hospital/University Medical Center
Camden, New Jersey
Chapter 33: The Skin and Internal Disease

Kimberley A. Horii, MD
Assistant Professor of Pediatrics
Department of Pediatrics, Section of Dermatology
University of Missouri, Kansas City School of Medicine
Children's Mercy Hospital
Kansas City, Missouri
Chapter 36: Pediatric Dermatology

David B. Huang, MD, MPH
Division of Infectious Diseases
Department of Medicine
Baylor College of Medicine
University of Texas at Houston School of Public Health
Division of Infectious Diseases, Department of Medicine
University of Texas Health Science Center at Houston
Houston, Texas
Chapter 23: Dermatologic Virology

Amy Y. Jan, MD, PhD
Resident
Division of Dermatology
Department of Medicine
University of Washington School of Medicine
Seattle, Washington
Staff Dermatologist
Kaiser Permanente
Baldwin Park, California
Chapter 35: Genodermatoses

Joseph L. Jorizzo, MD
Professor, Former and Founding Chair
Department of Dermatology
Wake Forest University School of Medicine
Winston-Salem, North Carolina
Chapter 32: Collagen Vascular Diseases

Thelda M. Kestenbaum, MD
Associate Professor of Medicine
University of Kansas Medical Center
Kansas City, Kansas
Chapter 28: Diseases Affecting the Hair

Christopher J. Kligora, MD
Department of Pathology
St. Luke's Hospital
Kansas City, Missouri
Chapters 1 and 2: Structure of the Skin and Laboratory Procedures and Tests

John Koo, MD
Director, Psoriasis Treatment Center
Vice Chairman
Department of Dermatology
University of California-San Francisco
San Francisco, California
Chapter 20: Psychodermatology

Frank Custer Koranda, MD, MBA
Associate Clinical Professor
*Department of Otolaryngology-Head and Neck
   Surgery*
Division of Dermatology
University of Kansas Medical Center
Kansas City, Kansas
Staff Surgeon
Department of Otolaryngology-Head and Neck Surgery
St. Luke's Shawnee Mission
Shawnee Mission, Kansas
Chapters 6 and 7: Physical Dermatologic Therapy and Fundamentals of Cutaneous Surgery

Laurie Linden, MD
Resident, Department of Dermatology
Henry Ford Hospital
Detroit, Michigan
Chapter 34: Dermatologic Reactions to Ultraviolet Radiation and Visible Light

Henry W. Lim, MD
Department of Dermatology
Henry Ford Hospital
Detroit, Michigan
Chapter 34: Dermatologic Reactions to Ultraviolet Radiation and Visible Light

Alejandro Morales, MD
Associate Professor
Department of Dermatology
Universidad Peruana Caayetano Heredia
Chief, Instituto Dermatologica
Lima, Peru
Chapter 38: Tropical Diseases of the Skin

Scott A. Norton, MD, MPH
Dermatology Service
Walter Reed Army Medical Center
Washington, DC
Chapter 39: Cutaneous Signs of Bioterrorism

Marianne O'Donoghue, MD
Associate Professor
Department of Dermatology
Rush Presbyterian-St. Luke's Medical Center
Chicago, Illinois
Chapter 8: Cosmetics for the Physician

Larisa Ravitskiy, MD
Chief Resident
Division of Dermatology
Robert Wood Johnson
UMDNJ
Cooper University Hospital
Camden, New Jersey
Chapter 33: The Skin and Internal Disease

Adam I. Rubin, MD
Resident in Dermatology
Department of Dermatology
Columbia University College of Physicians and Surgeons
Columbia University Medical Center
New York, New York
Chapter 29: Diseases Affecting the Nail

Richard K. Scher, MD
Professor of Clinical Dermatology
Department of Dermatology
Columbia University College of Physicians and Surgeons
Columbia University Medical Center
New York, New York
Chapter 29: Diseases Affecting the Nail

Vidya Sharma, MBBS, MPH
Professor of Pediatrics
Department of Pediatrics, Section of Dermatology
University of Missouri, Kansas City School of Medicine
Children's Mercy Hospital
Kansas City, Missouri
Chapter 36: Pediatric Dermatology

J. K. Shornick, MD, MHA
Private Practice
Groton, Connecticut
Chapter 41: Dermatoses of Pregnancy

Virginia P. Sybert, MD
Staff Dermatologist
Health Group Permanente
Clinical Professor
Division of Medical Genetics
Department of Medicine
University of Washington School of Medicine
Seattle, Washington
Chapter 35: Genodermatoses

Micole Tuchman, MS
Third-Year Medical Student
New York Medical College
New York, New York
Chapter 14: Psoriasis

Stephen K. Tyring, MD, PhD, MBA
Department of Dermatology
University of Texas Health Science Center at Houston
Center for Clinical Studies
Houston, Texas
Chapter 23: Dermatologic Virology

Kenneth R. Watson, DO
Department of Pathology
St. Luke's Hospital
Kansas City, Missouri
Chapters 1 and 2: Structure of the Skin and Laboratory Procedures and Tests

Jeffrey M. Weinberg, MD
Director, Clinical Research Center
St. Luke's-Roosevelt Hospital Center
 and Beth Israel Medical Center
Assistant Columbia University College of
 Physicians and Surgeons
New York, New York
Chapter 14: Psoriasis

Robin S. Weiner, MD
Chief Resident
Department of Dermatology
University of Missouri-Columbia
Columbia, Missouri
Chapter 27: Malignant Melanoma

Jashin J. Wu, MD
Department of Dermatology
University of California, Irvine
Irvine, California
Chapter 23: Dermatologic Virology

Jaeyoung Yoon, MD, PhD
Mohs Dermatologic Surgeon
Department of Dermatology
University of Missouri-Columbia
Columbia, Missouri
Chapter 27: Malignant Melanoma

Preface to the First Edition (Abridged)

Approximately 15 percent of all patients who walk into the general practitioner's office do so for care of some skin disease or skin lesion. It may be for such a simple treatment as the removal of a wart, for the treatment of athlete's foot or for something as complicated as severe cystic acne. There have been so many recent advances in the various fields of medicine that the medical school instructor can expect his students to learn and retain only a small percentage of the material that is taught them. I believe that the courses in all phases of medicine, and particularly the courses of the various specialties, should be made as simple, basic and concise as possible. If the student retains only a small percentage of what is presented to him, he will be able to handle an amazing number of his walk-in patients. I am presenting in this book only the material that medical students and general practitioners must know for the diagnosis and the treatment of patients with common skin diseases. In condensing the material many generalities are stated, and the reader must remember that there are exceptions to every rule. The inclusion of these exceptions would defeat the intended purpose of this book. More complicated diagnostic procedures or treatments for interesting problem cases are merely frosting on the cake. This information can be obtained by the interested student from any of several more comprehensive dermatologic texts.

This book consists of two distinct but complementary parts: The first part contains the chapters devoted to the diagnosis and the management of the important common skin diseases. In discussing the common skin diseases, a short introductory sentence is followed by a listing of the salient points of each disease in outline form. All diseases of the skin have primary lesions, secondary lesions, a rather specific distribution, a general course which includes the prognosis and the recurrence rate of the diseases, varying subjective complaints, and a known or unknown cause. Where indicated, a statement follows concerning seasonal incidence, age groups affected, family and sex incidence, contagiousness, relationship to employment and laboratory findings. The discussion ends with a paragraph on differential diagnosis and treatment. Treatment, to be effective, has to be thought of as a chain of events. The therapy outlined on the first visit is usually different from the one given on subsequent visits or for cases that are very severe. The treatment is discussed with these variations in mind.

The second part consists of a very complete Dictionary–Index to the entire field of dermatology, defining the majority of rare diseases and the unusual dermatologic terms. The inclusion of this Dictionary–Index has a dual purpose. First, it enables me to present a concise first section on common skin diseases unencumbered by the inclusion of the rare diseases. Second, the Dictionary–Index provides rather complete coverage of all of dermatology for the more interested student. In reality, two books are contained in one.

Dermatologic nomenclature has always been a bugaboo for the new student. I heartily agree with many dermatologists that we should simplify the terminology, and that has been attempted in this text. Some of the changes are mine, but many have been suggested by others. However, after a diligent effort to simplify the names of skin diseases, one is left with the appalling fact that some of the complicated terms defy change. One of the main reasons for this is that all of our field, the skin, is visible to the naked eye. As a result, any minor alteration from normal has been scrutinized by countless physicians through the years and given countless names. The liver or heart counterpart of folliculitis ulerythematosa reticulata (ulerythema acneiform, atrophoderma reticulatum symmetricum faciei, atrophoderma vermiculatum) is yet to be discovered.

What I am presenting in this book is not specialty dermatology but general practice dermatology. Some of my medical educator friends say that only internal medicine, pediatrics, and obstetrics should be taught to medical students. They state that the specialized fields of medicine should be taught only at the internship, residency, or postgraduate level. That idea misses the very important fact that cases from all of the so-called specialty fields wander in to the general practitioner's office. The general practitioner must have some basic knowledge of the varied aspects of all of medicine so that he can properly take care of his general everyday practice. This basic knowledge must be taught in the undergraduate years. The purpose of this book is to complement such teaching.

Gordon C. Sauer, MD

PREFACE

Some important changes have been made to this 9th edition of *Sauer's Manual of Skin Diseases*.

Many more expert authors have contributed to this edition—almost three times as many as contributed to the last edition. The book has been redesigned to enhance its usefulness. And the Dictionary–Index now also lists the many drugs mentioned in the treatment sections of the book, which makes the book useful to pharmacists as well as dermatologists and general practitioners. The new relevant topic unique to this edition is Cutaneous Manifestations of Bioterrorism, once again improving the currency and completeness of the text.

All chapters have been updated and new authors, who are experts in their field, have written the chapters on immunodermatology, psoriasis, psychodermatology, malignant melanoma, diseases of the nails, collagen diseases, reactions to ultraviolet radiation, nail disease, bioterrorism and skin disease, sports medicine dermatology, and dermatoses in pregnancy.

Updates of chapters from outstanding authors who have written previous chapters include dermatology cosmetics, fundamentals of cutaneous surgery, and conditions of the hair.

Numerous new color photographs have been added to the text, which greatly enhance the dermatology diagnosis. It is often said that "a picture is worth a thousand words" and in no specialty is this more true than in dermatology.

I have kept most chapters in the basic proven structure that Dr. Sauer has been recognized for worldwide during his outstanding dermatology teaching career.

John C. Hall, MD

ACKNOWLEDGMENTS

I have never enjoyed a task more than spending time with and learning from Dr. Sauer. From my earlier training days, I am forever indebted to Drs. Richard Q. Crotty and Clarence S. Livingood for the opportunity of a dermatology residency. I had the unique honor of having trained under Dr. Livingood and Edward A. Krull. Dr. Livingood taught me much about the science and the art of medicine. I feel that I have stood in the shadow of giants.

As brevity is the soul of wit, it is also the soul of the early understanding of a complex subject. An overview is more priceless at the onset of learning than a mountain of detail. To stir one's interest and curiosity about a field of scientific endeavor, one needs to see that field as a whole. Therein lies the true genius of Gordon Sauer.

Thanks to pathologist Kenneth R. Watson and to pharmacist Doug Albers, both of whom have been of invaluable help both in producing this book and throughout my career. My family—Charlotte, Shelly, Kim, Brian, and Sam—and my office staff—Yolanda, Brandy, Christa, Pam, and Fran—have been unwavering in their support and patience. My parents, the late William E. Hall and Susan R. Hall, and my wife's parents, Arnold W. Peterson and the late Fern Marie Peterson, have given me endless encouragement.

I would like to acknowledge the diligent work of Yolanda Payton, who was instrumental in the revision and typing of the text. She was assisted by Brandy Del Debbio. My office manager Christa Czysz and nurse Pam Skripsky also made the publication a reality.

In the eight previous editions, further acknowledgments were made, but it would be redundant to repeat them here. Finally, a great deal of credit again goes to Lippincott Williams & Wilkins, especially to Annette Ferran, Developmental Editor. The book profited by my association with them.

For the most realistic presentation of skin diseases, color photography is essential. However, the cost of color reproduction is so great that it is almost impossible to enjoy the advantages of color figures and still keep the price of the book within the range where it will have the broadest appeal. This problem has been solved for the ninth edition of this book through the generosity of several pharmaceutical companies, which contributed the cost of the color figures credited to them. For this edition, the drug companies Intendis and 3M contributed money for additional new color figures.

Chapters have been revised for this edition by Marianne O'Donoghue, MD, Frank Custer Koranda, MD, Thelda M. Kestenbaum, MD, Kenneth R. Watson, DO, Warren R. Heymann, MD, Francisco G. Bravo, MD, Alejandro Morales, MD, Virginia P. Sybert, MD, and Vidya Sharma, MBBS, MPH. All of these authors have contributed to other editions and I feel fortunate to have their expertise displayed again in this edition.

I also feel very fortunate to have added new chapter authors to this edition. They are Christopher J. Kligora, MD, Jon A. Dyer, MD, Jeffrey M. Weinberg, MD, Robin Buchholz, MD, Micole Tuchman, MS, Stephen K. Tyring, MD, PHD, MBA, David B. Huang, MD, MPH, Jashin J. Wu, MD, Larisa Ravitskiy, MD, Mary M. Feldman, MD, Clay J. Cockerell, MD, Robin S. Weiner, MD, Jaeyoung Yoon, MD, PHD, Richard K. Scher, MD, Adam I. Rubin, MD, Amy Y. Jan, MD, PHD, Kimberly A. Horii, MD, Rodney S.W. Basler, MD, Henry W. Lim, MD, Laurie Linden, MD, J. K. Shornick, MD, MHA, Gary Goldenberg, MD, Joseph L. Jorrizzo, MD, and Scott A. Norton, MD, MPH. Seldom has such an army of talented clinicians and authors been displayed in a text of this type and I am honored by their efforts. The labor and input of these knowledgeable contributors are greatly appreciated.

I frequently hear from dermatologists and nondermatologists alike that this book is their first exposure to the study of skin diseases. The ninth edition and all preceding editions are a tribute to Dr. Sauer's ability to open up the specialty of dermatology to those who wish to use its magic to help in the care of their patients.

FUNDAMENTALS OF DERMATOLOGY

CHAPTER 1

Structure of the Skin

Kenneth R. Watson, DO, and Christopher J. Kligora, MD

The skin is the largest organ of the human body. It is composed of tissue that grows, differentiates, and renews itself constantly. Because the skin is a barrier between the internal organs and the external environment, it is uniquely subjected to noxious external agents and is also a sensitive reflection of internal disease. An understanding of the cause and the effect of this complex interplay in the skin begins with a thorough understanding of the basic structure of this organ.

Layers of the Skin

The skin is divided into three rather distinct layers. From the inside out, they are the subcutaneous tissue, the dermis, and the epidermis (Fig. 1-1).

Subcutaneous Tissue

The subcutaneous tissue constitutes the largest volume of adipose tissue in the body. The thickness of the subcutaneous fat varies from one area of the body to another. It is especially thick in the abdominal region and thin in the eyelids. Fat cells are derived from mesenchymal cells, as are fibroblasts. They are organized into lobules by fibrous septae, which contain most of the blood vessels, nerves, and lymphatics that nourish the skin. The subcutaneous tissue serves as a receptacle for the formation and the storage of fat as well as a site of highly dynamic lipid metabolism for nutrition. It also provides protection from physical trauma and insulation to temperature changes.

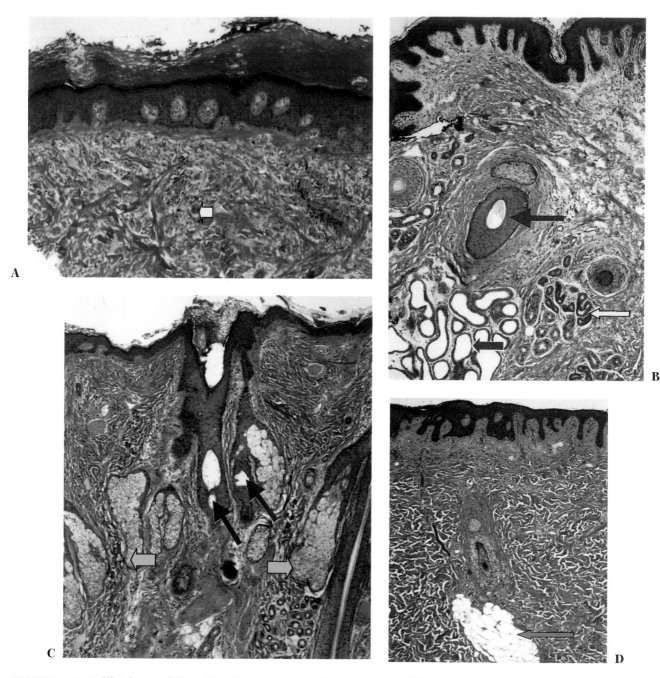

FIGURE 1-1 ■ Histology of the skin. Photomicrographs from four different areas of the body: palm (**A**), axilla (**B**), face (**C**), and trunk (**D**). Note the variations in the histologic features: thickened keratin layer from the palm (*arrowhead*), multiple glandular elements from the axilla (hair follicle, *thin arrow*; apocrine gland, *thick arrow*; eccrine gland, *yellow arrow*), numerous pilosebaceous units from the face (hair follicle, *thin arrow*; sebaceous gland, *thick arrow*), and thick dermis from the trunk (subcutaneous fat, *arrow*). *(Courtesy of Dr. K. Watson.)*

Dermis

The dermis consists of connective tissue, cellular elements, and ground substance. It has a rich blood and nerve supply and contains pilosebaceous, apocrine, and eccrine structures. Anatomically, it is divided into two compartments. The first consists of thin collagen fibers, which are located beneath the epidermis (papillary dermis) and surrounding adnexal structures (periadnexal dermis). Together, the collagen fibers are regarded as a single unit called the *adventitial dermis.* This is an important unit because it is altered together with the adjacent epithelium in many inflammatory diseases. The second compartment, known as the *reticular* or *deep dermis,* is composed of thick collagen bundles and comprises the bulk of the dermis.

The *connective tissue* component of the dermis consists of collagen fibers, including reticulin fibers, and elastic fibers. These fibers contribute to the support and elasticity of the skin.

Two different types of collagen predominate in the dermis. Type I collagen is predominantly found within the thick fibers of the reticular dermis. Type III collagen, also known as *reticulin,* is largely found within the thin fibers of the papillary and periadnexal dermis. These reticulin fibers are not visible in hematoxylin and eosin–stained sections, but can be identified with silver stains. They are abundant in certain pathologic conditions such as tuberculous granulomas, syphilis, sarcoidosis, and some mesenchymal tumors. The proteins present in collagen fibers are responsible for nearly one fourth of a person's overall protein mass. If tannic acid or the salts of heavy metals, such as dichromates, are combined with collagen, the result is leather.

Elastic fibers are thinner than most collagen fibers and are entwined among them. They are composed of the protein elastin. Elastic fibers do not readily take up acidic or basic stains, such as hematoxylin and eosin, but they can be identified with the Verhoeff–Van Gieson stain.

Cellular elements of the dermis include fibroblasts, endothelial cells, mast cells, and a variety of miscellaneous cells, including smooth muscle, nerve, and hematopoietic cells. The hematopoietic cells include lymphocytes, histiocytes (macrophages), eosinophils, neutrophils, and plasma cells. They are present in various pathologic conditions in varying amounts.

Fibroblasts form collagen and produce ground substance. They are involved in immunologic and reparative processes, and are increased in numerous skin disorders.

Mast cells arise from undifferentiated mesenchymal cells. They have intracytoplasmic basophilic metachromatic granules containing heparin and histamine. The normal skin contains relatively few mast cells, but their number is increased in many different skin conditions, particularly the itching dermatoses, such as atopic eczema, contact dermatitis, and lichen planus. In *urticaria pigmentosa,* the mast cells may occur in tumorlike masses.

Histiocytes (macrophages) are present in only small numbers in the normal skin. However, in pathologic conditions, they migrate to the dermis as tissue monocytes. They play a predominant role in the phagocytosis of particulate matter and bacteria. Under special pathologic conditions they may form giant cells. They are also involved in the immune system by phagocytizing antigens.

Lymphocytes and plasma cells are found in only small numbers in normal skin, but are significantly increased in pathologic conditions such as increased plasma cells in syphilis.

The *ground substance* of the dermis is a gel-like amorphous matrix not easily seen in routine sections, but it may be identified with colloidal iron and Alcian blue stains. It is of tremendous importance because it contains proteins, mucopolysaccharides, soluble collagens, enzymes, immune bodies, metabolites, and many other substances.

Epidermis

The epidermis is the most superficial of the three layers of the skin and averages in thickness about the width of the mark of a sharp pencil (<1 mm). It contains several types of cells including keratinocytes, dendritic cells (melanocytes and Langerhans cells), and Merkel cells.

The keratinocytes, or keratin-forming cells, are by far the most common and develop into four identifiable layers of the epidermis (Fig. 1-2). From inside out, they are as follows:

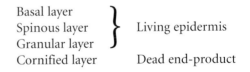

Basal layer	
Spinous layer	} Living epidermis
Granular layer	
Cornified layer	Dead end-product

The basal layer lies next to the dermis. This layer can be thought of as stem cells, which are capable of progressive maturation into cell forms higher in the epidermis. It normally requires 3 or 4 weeks for the epidermis to replicate itself by the process of division and differentiation. This cell turnover is greatly accelerated in such diseases as psoriasis and ichthyosiform erythroderma. In these diseases, the turnover rate may be as short as 2 to 3 days.

The spinous layer, or stratum malpighii, is made up of several layers of epidermal cells, chiefly of polyhedral shape. The cells of this layer are connected by intercellular bridges, which may be seen in routine sections.

The granular layer is composed of flatter cells containing protein granules called *keratohyalin granules.* In lichen planus, the granular cell layer is focally increased.

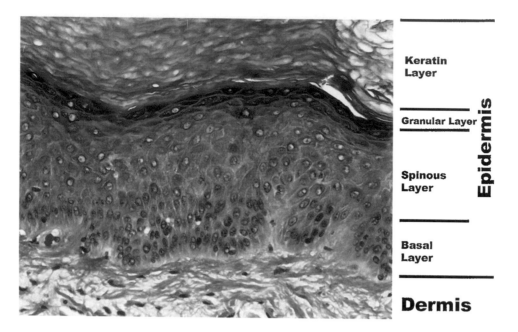

Keratin
Layer

Granular Layer

Spinous
Layer

Basal
Layer

Epidermis

Dermis

FIGURE 1-2 ■ Histology of the epidermis. A photomicrograph from the palm. *(Dr. K. Watson.)*

The outermost layer of the epidermis is the *cornified (horny) layer*. It is made up of stratified layers of dead keratinized cells that are constantly shedding (Fig. 1-3). The chemical protein in these cells is called *keratin* and is capable of absorbing vast amounts of water. This is readily seen during bathing, when the skin of the palms and the soles becomes white, swollen, and wrinkled. The cornified layer provides a major barrier of protection for the body. The normal oral mucous membrane does not have granular or cornified layers.

The *melanin-forming cells,* or *melanocytes,* are sandwiched between the more numerous keratin-forming cells in the basal layer. These melanocytes are dopa-positive because they stain darkly after contact with a solution of levorotatory 3,4-dihydroxyphenylalanine, or *dopa.* This laboratory reaction closely simulates physiologic melanin formation, in which the amino acid tyrosine is oxidized by the enzyme tyrosinase to form dopa. Dopa is then further changed, through a series of complex metabolic processes, to melanin.

Melanin pigmentation of the skin, whether increased or decreased, is influenced by many local and systemic factors (see Chap. 31). Melanocyte-stimulating hormone from the pituitary is the most potent melanizing agent. Melanin is transferred from melanocytes to basal keratinocytes. Skin color is largely related to the amount of melanin present in basal cells.

Langerhans cells are found scattered evenly throughout the epidermis. They are bone marrow–derived mononuclear cells. They are involved in cell-mediated hypersensitivity, antigen processing and recognition, stimulation of immune-competent cells, and graft rejection. Sunlight suppresses their immune function. Their number is decreased in certain skin diseases, such as psoriasis. Staining with membrane adenosine triphosphatase and monoclonal antibodies such as S-100 protein and CD-1 can be done for identification. By electron microscopy, they contain characteristic racquet-shaped Birbeck granules.

Merkel cells are normally located in the basal layer, although they are inconspicuous in routine sections. Ultrastructurally, they contain dense core neurosecretory granules. They are assumed to function as a touch receptor. They give rise to primary neuroendocrine carcinoma of the skin (Merkel cell tumor).

Vasculature

A continuous arteriovenous meshwork perforates the subcutaneous tissues and extends into the dermis. Blood vessels of varying sizes are present in most levels and planes of the skin. In fact, the vascularization is so extensive that it has been postulated that its main function is to regulate heat and blood pressure of the body, with providing

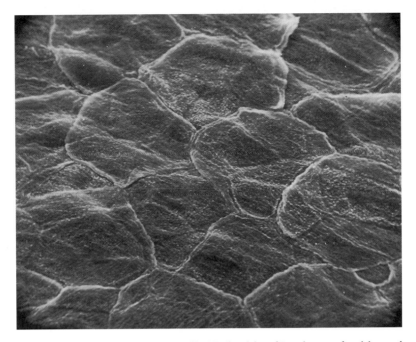

FIGURE 1-3 ■ Keratin-layer cells. Underside of top layer of epidermal keratin layer cells on Scotch tape stripping is seen with Cambridge Mark II Stereoscan at 1000×. *(Courtesy of Drs. J. Arnold, W. Barnes, and G. Sauer.)*

nutrition to the skin a secondary function. No blood vessels are present within the epidermis.

A special vascular body, the glomus, deserves mention. The glomus body is most commonly seen on the tips of the fingers and the toes, and under the nails. Each glomus body consists of a venous and arterial segment, called the *Sucquet-Hoyer canal*. This canal represents a short-circuit device that connects an arteriole with a venule directly, without intervening capillaries. The result is a marked increase in the blood flow through the skin. If this body grows abnormally, it forms an often painful, red, benign glomus tumor, commonly beneath the nail.

Nerve Supply

The nerve supply of the skin consists of sensory nerves and motor nerves.

Sensory Nerves

The sensory nerves mediate the sensations of touch, temperature, and pain. The millions of terminal nerve endings, or Merkel cell–neurite complexes, have more to do with the specificity of skin sensation than the better known, highly specialized nerve endings, such as the Vater–Pacini and Wagner–Meissner tactile corpuscles.

Itching is the most important presenting symptom of an unhappy patient. It may be defined simply as the desire to scratch. Itching apparently is a mildly painful sensation that differs from pain in having a lower frequency of impulse stimuli. The release of proteinases (such as follows itch-powder application) may be responsible for the itch sensation. The pruritus may be of a pricking or burning type and can vary greatly from one person to another. Sulzberger called those abnormally sensitive people *itchish*, analogous to *ticklish*. Itching can occur without any clinical signs of skin disease or from circulating allergens or local superficial contactants. The skin of atopic or eczema patients tends to be more itchy. Scratching makes the itching worse. This results in a perpetual itch–scratch cycle.

Motor Nerves

The involuntary sympathetic motor nerves control the sweat glands, arterioles, and smooth muscle of the skin. Adrenergic fibers carry impulses to the arrector pili muscles, which produce gooseflesh if they are stimulated. This is caused by traction of the muscle on the hair follicles to which it is attached. Cholinergic fibers, if stimulated, increase sweating and may cause a specific type of hives called *cholinergic urticaria* (see Chap. 12).

Appendages

The appendages of the skin include both the cornified appendages (hairs and nails) and the glandular appendages.

Hairs

Hairs are produced by the hair follicles, which develop from germinative cells of the fetal epidermis. Because no new hair follicles are formed after birth, the different types of body hairs are manifestations of the effect of location as well as external and internal stimuli. Hormones are the most important internal stimuli influencing the various types of hair growth. This growth is cyclic, with a growing (anagen) phase and a resting (telogen) phase. The *catagen cycle* is the transition phase between the growing and resting stages and lasts only a few days. Ninety percent of the normal scalp hairs are in the growing (anagen) stage, and 10% are in the resting (telogen) stage, which lasts from 60 to 90 days. The average period of scalp hair growth ranges from 2 to 6 years. However, systemic stresses, such as childbirth, or systemic anesthesia may cause hairs to enter a resting stage prematurely. This *postpartum effect* or *postanesthetic effect* is noticed most commonly in the scalp when these resting hairs are depilated during combing or washing, and the thought of approaching baldness causes sudden alarm.

Types

The adult has two main types of hairs: (1) the vellus hairs (lanugo hairs of the fetus) and (2) the terminal hairs. The vellus hairs ("peach fuzz") are the fine, short hairs of the body, whereas the terminal hairs are coarse, thick, and pigmented. Terminal hairs are developed almost extensively on the scalp, brow, and extremities.

Hair Follicles

Hair follicle may be thought of as an invagination of the epidermis, with its different layers of cells. These cells make up the matrix of the hair follicle and produce the keratin of the mature hair. The protein-synthesizing capacity of this tissue is enormous. At the rate of scalp hair growth of 0.35 mm per day, more than 100 linear feet of scalp hair is produced daily. The density of hairs in the scalp varies from 175 to 300 hairs per square centimeter. Up to 100 hairs may be normally lost daily.

Nails

The second cornified appendage, the nail, consists of a nail plate and the tissue that surrounds it. This plate lies in a nail groove that, like the hair follicle, is an invagination of the epidermis. Unlike hair growth, which is periodic, nail growth is continuous. Nail growth proceeds at about one third of the rate of hair growth, or about 0.1 mm per day. It takes about 3 months to restore a removed fingernail and about three times that long for the regrowth of a new toenail. Nail growth can be inhibited during serious illnesses or in old age, increased through nail biting or occupational trauma, and altered because of hand dermatitis or systemic disease. Topical treatment of nail disturbances is unsatisfactory, owing to the inaccessibility of the growth-producing areas.

Glandular Appendages

The three types of glandular appendages of the skin are the sebaceous glands, apocrine glands, and eccrine glands (Fig. 1-4).

The *sebaceous glands* are present everywhere on the skin, except the palms and the soles. In most areas they are associated with hair follicles. There are sebaceous glands that are not associated with hair follicles, such as the buccal mucosa and vermillion border of the lip, nipple, and areola of the breast, labia minora, and eyelids (Meibomian glands). The sebaceous glands are holocrine glands,

---

SAUER'S NOTES

1. Shaving of excess hair, as women do on their legs and thighs, does not promote more rapid growth of coarse hair. The shaved stubs appear more coarse, but if allowed to grow normally, the hairs appear and feel no different than before shaving.
2. The value of intermittent massage to stimulate scalp hair growth has not been proved.
3. Hair cannot turn gray overnight. The melanin pigmentation, which is distributed throughout the length of the nonvital hair shaft, takes weeks to be shed through the slow process of hair growth.
4. Heredity is the greatest factor predisposing to baldness, and an excess of male hormone may contribute to hair loss. Male castrates do not become bald.
5. Common male pattern baldness cannot be reversed by over-the-counter "hair restorers." Minoxidil solution (Rogaine), which is sold over the counter, is beneficial for a limited percentage of patients, and finasteride (Propecia) pills, available by prescription, are helpful in most patients.

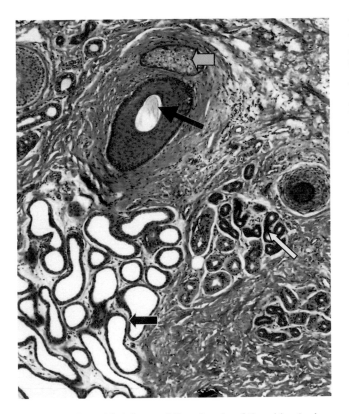

FIGURE 1-4 ■ Histology of the glands of the skin. A photomicrograph from the axilla. (sebaceous gland, long black arrow; apocrine sweat glands, short black arrow; sebaceous gland, short blue arrow; eccrine sweat glands, yellow arrow) *(Courtesy of Dr. K. Watson.)*

forming their secretions through the disintegration of the entire glandular cell. The secretion from these glands is evacuated through the sebaceous duct to a follicle that may contain either a large terminal hair or vellus hair. This secretion, known as *sebum,* is not under any neurologic control but is a continuous outflowing of the material of cell breakdown. The sebum covers the skin with a thin lipoidal film that is mildly bacteriostatic and fungistatic and retards water evaporation. The scalp and the face may contain as many as 1000 sebaceous glands per square centimeter. The activity of the gland increases markedly at the age of puberty, and, in certain people, it becomes plugged with sebum, debris, and bacteria to form the blackheads and the pimples of acne.

Apocrine glands are found in the axillae, genital region, breast, external ear canal (ceruminous glands), and eyelid (Moll's glands). They do not develop until the time of puberty. They consist of a coiled secretory gland located in the deep dermis or subcutaneous fat and a straight duct that usually empties into a hair follicle. The function of the secretions is unknown; however, they may act as pheromones. They are responsible for the production of body odor (the infamous "BO"). Any emotional stresses that cause adrenergic sympathetic discharge produce apocrine secretion. This secretion is sterile when excreted but undergoes decomposition when contaminated by bacteria from the skin surface, resulting in a strong and characteristic odor. The purpose of the many cosmetic underarm preparations is to remove these bacteria or block the gland excretion. The apocrine glands are involved in *hidradenitis suppurativa,* an inflammatory process that results from follicular obstruction and retention of follicular products, which usually occurs in patients with the acne–seborrhea complex.

Eccrine sweat glands are distributed everywhere on the skin surface, with the greatest concentration on the palms, soles, and forehead. They develop as a downgrowth from the primitive epidermis. They are composed of coiled secretory glands, a coiled duct, a straight duct, an intraepidermal coil, and an eccrine pore. The eccrine sweat glands and the vasculature of the skin serve in the maintenance of the stable internal body temperature, despite marked environmental temperature changes. They flood the skin surface with water for cooling, and the blood vessels dilate or constrict to dissipate or conserve body heat. Their prime stimulus is heat and their activity is under the control of the nervous system, usually through the hypothalamus. Both adrenergic and cholinergic fibers innervate the glands. Blockage of the eccrine ducts results in the disease known as *miliaria* (*prickly heat*). If eccrine glands are congenitally absent, as in *anhidrotic ectodermal dysplasia,* a life-threatening hyperpyrexia may develop.

Acknowledgments

We acknowledge the valuable assistance of Dean Shepard, from St. Lukes Hospital Photographic services.

Suggested Reading

Ackerman BA. Histologic diagnosis of inflammatory skin diseases. Philadelphia, WB Saunders, 1978.

Barnhill RL. Textbook of dermatopathology. New York, McGraw-Hill, 1997.

Briggaman RA. Epidermal-dermal junction structure, composition, function and disease relationships. Prog Dermatol 1990;24(2):1.

Farmer RE, Hood AF. Pathology of the skin. Norwalk, CT, Appleton & Lange, 1990.

Fleischer AB. The clinical management of itching, therapeutic protocols for pruritis. London, Parthenon Publishing Group, 1998.

Goldsmith L. Physiology, biochemistry, and molecular biology of the skin. New York, Oxford University Press, 1991.

Hurwitz RM, Hood AF. Pathology of the skin, atlas of clinical-pathological correlation. Stamford, CT, Appleton & Lange, 1997.

Lever WE, Schaumburg-Lever G. Histopathology of the skin, ed 7. Philadelphia, JB Lippincott, 1990.

Murphy GF, Elder EE. Atlas of tumor pathology, nonmelanocytic tumors of the skin. Washington, DC, Armed Forces Institute of Pathology, 1991.

Nickolof BJ. Dermal immune system. Boca Raton, FL, CRC Press, 1993.

Rosen T, Martin S. Atlas of black dermatology. Boston, Little, Brown and Company, 1981.

CHAPTER 2

Laboratory Procedures and Tests

Christopher J. Kligora, MD and Kenneth R. Watson, DO

In addition to the usual laboratory procedures used in the workup of medical patients, certain special tests are of importance in the field of dermatology. These include skin tests, fungus examinations, biopsies, and immunologic diagnosis. For special problems, additional testing methods are suggested in the sections on the various diseases.

Skin Tests

There are three types of skin tests:

- Intracutaneous
- Scratch
- Patch

The intracutaneous tests and the scratch tests can have two types of reactions, either an immediate wheal reaction or a delayed reaction. The immediate wheal reaction develops to a maximum in 5 to 20 minutes and is elicited in testing for the cause of urticaria, atopic dermatitis, and inhalant allergies. This immediate wheal reaction test is seldom used for determining the cause of skin diseases.

The delayed reaction to intracutaneous skin testing is exemplified best by the tuberculin skin test. Tuberculin is available in two forms, as purified protein derivative and as a tuberculin tine test. The purified protein derivative test is performed by using tablets that come in two strengths and by injecting a solution of either one intracutaneously. If there is no reaction after the test with the first strength, then the second strength may be employed.

The tuberculin tine test (Mantoux) is a simple and rapid procedure using OTK. Nine prongs, or tines, covered with OTK are pressed into the skin. If at the end of 48 or 72 hours there is more than 2 mm of induration at the site of any prong insertion, the test is positive.

Patch tests are used commonly in dermatology and offer a simple and accurate method of determining whether a patient is allergic to any of the testing agents. There are two different reactions to this type of test: a primary irritant reaction and an allergic reaction. The primary irritant reaction occurs in most of the population if they are exposed to agents (in appropriate concentrations) that have skin-destroying properties. Examples of these agents include soaps, cleaning fluids, bleaches, "corn" removers, and counterirritants. The allergic reaction indicates that the patient is more sensitive than normal to the agent being tested. This test reaction is idiosyncratic and not necessarily related to concentration or dose. It also shows that the patient has had a previous exposure to that agent or a cross-sensitizing agent.

The technique of the patch test is simple, but the interpretation of the test is not. For example, consider a patient presenting with dermatitis on top of the feet. It is possible that shoe leather or some chemical used in the manufacture of the leather is causing the reaction. The procedure for a patch test is to cut out a 1/2-inch-square piece of the material from the inside of the shoe, moisten the material with distilled water, place it on the skin surface, and cover it with an adhesive band or some patch-test dressing. The patch test is left on for 48 hours. When the patch test is removed, the patient is considered to have a positive patch test if there is any redness, papules, or vesiculation under the site of the testing agent. Delayed reactions to allergens can occur, and, ideally, a final reading should be made after 96 hours (4 days), that is, 2 days after the patch is removed.

The patch test can be used to make or confirm a diagnosis of poison ivy dermatitis, ragweed dermatitis, or contact dermatitis caused by medications, cosmetics, or industrial chemicals. Fisher (1995) and Adams (1990) compiled lists of chemicals, concentrations, and vehicles to be used for eliciting the allergic type of patch test reaction. Most tests can be performed very simply, however, as in the case of the shoe-leather dermatitis. One precaution is that the patch must not be allowed to become wet in the 48-hour period. A patch test kit, T.R.U.E. Test (Glaxo), includes ready-to-apply self-adhesive allergen tapes.

A method of testing for food allergy is to use the Rowe elimination diet. The procedure is to limit the diet to the following basic foods, which are known to be hypoallergenic: lamb, lemon, grapefruit, pears, lettuce, spinach, carrots, sweet potato, tapioca, rice and rice bread, corn sugar, maple syrup, sesame oil, gelatin, and salt. The patient is to remain on this basic diet for 5 to 7 days. At the end of that time, one new food can be added every 2 days. The following foods can be added early: beef, white potatoes, green beans, milk (along with butter and American cheese), and white bread with puffed wheat. If there is a flare-up of the dermatitis, which should occur within 2 to 8 hours after ingestion of an offending food, the new food should be discontinued for the present. More new foods are added until the normal diet, minus the allergenic foods, is regained.

Keeping a "diet diary" of all foods, medicines, oral hygiene items, or anything injected or inhaled can sometimes be a retrospective way of identifying an allergen. The skin reaction usually occurs less than 8 hours after ingestion.

Fungus Examinations

The KOH preparation is a simple office laboratory procedure for the detection of fungal organisms present in skin and nails. It is accomplished by scraping the diseased skin and examining the material with the microscope. The skin scrapings are obtained by abrading a scaly diseased area with a scalpel. If a blister is present, the underside of the blister is examined. The material is deposited on a glass slide and then covered with 20% aqueous potassium hydroxide solution and a coverslip. The preparation can be gently heated or allowed to stand at room temperature for 15 to 60 minutes. The addition of dimethyl sulfoxide to the KOH preparation eliminates the need to heat the specimen. A diagnostically helpful pale violet stain can be imparted to the fungi if the 20% KOH solution is mixed with an equal amount of Parker's Super Quik permanent blue-black ink. The slide is then examined microscopically for fungal organisms (Fig. 2-1).

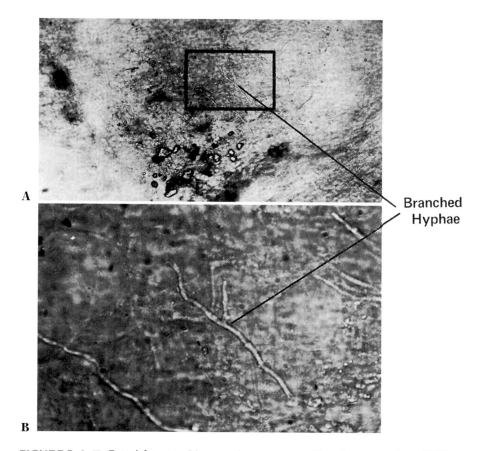

Branched Hyphae

FIGURE 2-1 ■ Fungi from a skin scraping as seen with microscope in a KOH preparation. (**A**) Low-power lens (100×) view. (**B**) High-power lens (450×) view of area outlined above. *(Courtesy of Dr. D. Gibson.)*

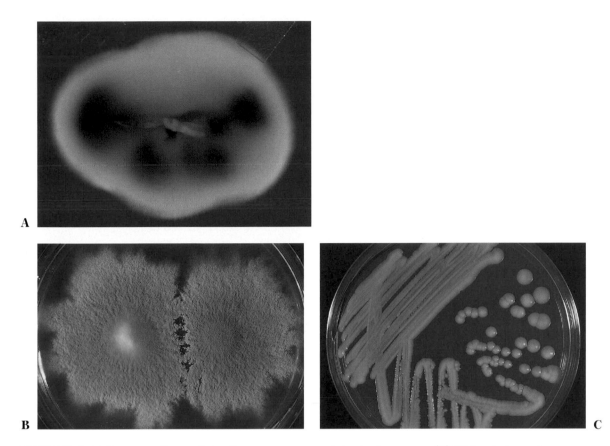

FIGURE 2-2 ■ Fungus cultures: Subcultures grown on potato dextrose agar. (**A**) Trichophyton rubrum; (**B**) Microsporum gypseum; (**C**) *Candida albicans. (Courtesy of Dr. K. Watson.)*

For culture preparation, a portion of the material from the scraping can be implanted on several different types of agar, including mycobiotic agar, IMA inhibitory mold agar, BHI with blood, chloramphenicol, gentamicin agar, and Sabouraud's glucose agar. A white or variously colored growth is noted in approximately 1 to 3 weeks (Fig. 2-2).

The species of fungus can be identified by morphology on the culture plate, biochemical characteristics, and microscopic morphology with a lacto-phenol cotton blue stain of a smear from the fungal colony.

Biopsies

The biopsy and microscopic examination of a questionable skin lesion may be invaluable. A definitive diagnosis is nearly always rendered with most pigmented lesions and other cutaneous tumors. In the case of inflammatory lesions, histologic findings may or may not be diagnostic, depending on the disease process, the age of the lesion, clinical description of the lesion(s) including extent of involvement, other symptoms and/or medical conditions,

and a differential diagnosis. In cases where histologic findings are not diagnostic, at the very least many pertinent diagnoses on the clinical differential can be excluded. In addition to diagnosis, other useful parameters can be obtained with cutaneous lesions, such as depth of invasion, lymphovascular space invasion, perineural involvement, and adequacy of surgical margins. The quintessential example is malignant melanoma, where most of these factors plus several others may only be assessed histologically and are essential for staging and prognosis.

SAUER'S NOTES

1. The skin biopsy specimen must include adequate tissue for proper interpretation by the pathologist.
2. Communication between a pathologist knowledgeable in this disease and the clinician is mandatory for accurate tissue diagnosis.

There are four principal techniques for performing skin biopsies:

1. surgical excision with suturing,
2. punch biopsy,
3. excision with scissors, and
4. shave biopsy.

The decision in favor of one method depends on such factors as location of the biopsy, cosmetic result desired, depth of the disease being looked for, type of lesion to be removed (flat or elevated), and simplicity of technique. For example, vesicles should be completely excised in an attempt to keep the roof intact; scalp biopsy specimens should extend into the subcutis to include the bulbs of terminal follicles. The instruments and materials needed to perform a skin biopsy are discussed in Chapter 7.

Surgical Excision

The technique of performing surgical excision biopsies with suturing of the skin is well known. In general, this type of biopsy is performed if a good cosmetic result is desired and if the entire lesion is to be removed. The disadvantage is that this procedure is the most time consuming of the three techniques, and it is necessary for the patient to return for removal of the sutures. Absorbable sutures can eliminate the need for a return visit. It is important that a sharp scalpel be used to reduce compression artifact, and that care is taken not to crush the specimen with the forceps.

Punch Biopsy

Punch biopsies can be done rather rapidly, with or without suturing of the wound. A punch-biopsy instrument of appropriate size is needed. Disposable biopsy punches are available. A local anesthetic is usually injected at the site. The operator rotates the instrument until it penetrates to the subcutaneous level. The circle of tissue is then removed. Bleeding can be stopped with pressure or by the use of one or two sutures. An elliptical wound instead of a circular wound can be produced by stretching the skin perpendicular to the desired suture line before the punch is rotated. The resultant scar, after suturing, is neater. Punch biopsies may be inadequate for evaluation of vesiculobullous diseases and must be deep enough to include subcutaneous fat if used for diagnosis of panniculitis or tumors in a subcutaneous location. In most instances, pigmented lesions should not be punched unless they can be completely excised.

Scissors Biopsy

The third way to remove skin tissue for a biopsy specimen is to excise the piece with sharp pointed scissors and stop the bleeding with light electrosurgery, Monsel solution, or aluminum chloride solution. This procedure is useful for certain types of elevated lesions and in areas in which the cosmetic result is not too important. The greatest advantage of this procedure is the speed and the simplicity with which it can be done.

Shave Biopsy

A scalpel or razor blade can be used to slice off a lesion. This can be performed superficially or deeply. Hemostasis can be accomplished by pressure, light electrosurgery, Monsel solution, or aluminum chloride solution. This method is generally not recommended for excision of melanocytic lesions or other potentially malignant tumor where margin assessment is required.

Biopsy Handling

The biopsy specimen must be placed in an appropriate fixture, usually 10% formalin. If the specimen tends to curl, it can be stretched out on a piece of paper or cardboard before fixing. Mailing specimens in formalin during winter may result in freezing artifact. This can be avoided by the addition of 95% ethyl alcohol, 10% by volume.

Cytodiagnosis

The Tzanck test is useful in identifying bullous diseases such as pemphigus and vesicular virus eruptions (herpes simplex and herpes zoster). The technique and choice of lesions are important. For best results, select an early lesion. In the case of a blister, remove the top with a scalpel or sharp scissors. Blot the excess fluid with a gauze pad, then gently scrape the floor of the blister with a scalpel blade. Try not to cause bleeding. Make a thin smear of the cells on a clean glass slide. If you are dealing with a solid lesion, squeeze the material between two slides. The slide may be air dried, but it can also be fixed by placing it in 95% ethanol for 15 seconds. Stain the slide with Wright-Giemsa stain or hematoxylin and eosin.

In addition to skin testing, fungus examination, biopsies, and cytodiagnosis, there are certain tests for specific skin conditions that are discussed in connection with the respective diseases.

Additional Studies

The deposition of immunoglobulin and complement may be detected by direct immunofluorescence. This is an extremely valuable technique for the diagnosis of lupus erythematosus and autoimmune bullous diseases. It is performed on a frozen section; therefore, the biopsy specimen must be received fresh or in Michel's solution.

Immunohistology is particularly helpful in the accurate diagnosis and classification of neoplasms. It is possible to identify specific antigens in a routinely processed tissue section by attaching a labeled antibody. For example, malignant melanoma may be identified using antibodies directed against S-100 protein as well as other more sensitive melanoma specific antigens, such as MART-1 and tyrosinase (Fig. 2-3). Epithelial tumors label with antibodies for cytokeratins. Different cytokeratin subtypes may be used to help differentiate certain epithelial tumors that are histologically similar. For example, cytokeratin 7 helps to differentiate metastatic small cell carcinoma of the lung from primary Merkel cell carcinoma of the skin, as well as both mammary and extramammary Paget's disease from squamous cell carcinoma in situ (Bowen's disease). Mesenchymal tumors, such as dermatofibroma, are generally immunoreactive for the intermediate filament vimentin, as well as a host of other markers, depending on the tumor type and cell origin. Leukocyte common antigen labels most lymphomas and leukemias. Multiple other antibodies can be used to distinguish the cell line, diagnosis, and prognosis. CD3, CD4, CD8, CD5, and CD7 are all T-cell markers that can be used to distinguish patch stage MF

from benign mimics, such as small plaque parapsoriasis and other forms of eczema.

DNA technology may be very useful. In situ hybridization allows recognition of specific DNA or RNA sequences using a gene probe in frozen or paraffin tissue sections. For example, a variety of different viruses, including herpes simplex, cytomegalovirus, and a human papillomavirus, can be identified using this technique.

Flow cytometry is another method of identifying specific cell antigens, and is generally only useful with lymphomas and leukemias. This test is most commonly performed on lymph nodes, peripheral blood, and bone marrow, but may also be performed on solid organs, such as skin, provided the abnormal cell population is of sufficient quantity. A fresh specimen is needed. Following manipulation of the tissue to tease out the abnormal cells into a liquid media, the individual cells are labeled with antibodies (up to four at once) and passed through a light-scattering source that is able to measure cell size as well as antigen expression. The main advantage that flow cytometry has over tissue immunohistochemistry is the ability to characterize small populations of abnormal cells and to establish monoclonality via the analysis of immunoglobulin light chain expression. Polymerase chain reaction (PCR) may now also be used to establish monoclonality in both fresh and paraffin-embedded tissue. Disadvantages include lengthy time to diagnosis, cost, and extreme sensitivity with DNA carryover/contamination problems from other specimens. PCR is able to pick up very small populations of clonal cells that may not be truly neoplastic or malignant.

Acknowledgment

We acknowledge the assistance of Dr. Cindy Essmeyer and members of her staff, Marcella Godinez, M.T., Katrin Boese, M.T., and Tammy Thorne, M.T., in preparation of the section on fungus examination. We also acknowledge the valuable assistance of Dean Shepard, from St. Lukes Hospital Photographic services.

Suggested Reading

Ackerman AB. Histopathologic diagnosis of inflammatory skin diseases. Philadelphia, Lea & Febiger, 1978, p. 149.

Adams RM. Occupational skin disease. Orlando, FL, Grune & Stratton, 1990.

Beare JM, Bingham EA. The influence of the results of laboratory and ancillary investigations in the management of skin disease. Int J Dermatol 1981;20:653.

Epstein E, Epstein E Jr. Skin surgery, ed 6. Philadelphia, WB Saunders, 1987.

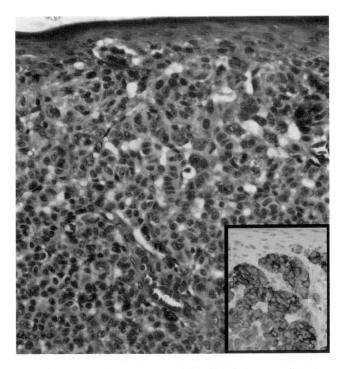

FIGURE 2-3 ■ Photomicrograph of malignant melanoma with positive immunoreactivity for Mart-1 (*inset*). *(Courtesy of Dr. K. Watson.)*

Fisher AA. Contact dermatitis, ed 4. Philadelphia, Lea & Febiger, 1995.

Hurwitz RM, Hood AF. Pathology of the skin: Atlas of clinical–pathological correlation. Stamford, CT, Appleton & Lange, 1998.

Isenberg HD, ed. Essential procedures for clinical microbiology. ASM Press, 1998.

Koneman EW, Roberts GD. Practical laboratory mycology, ed 3. Baltimore, Williams & Wilkins, 1985.

Lever WF, Schaumburg-Lever G. Histopathology of the skin, ed 7. Philadelphia, JB Lippincott, 1990.

Vassileva S. Immunofluorescence in dermatology. Int J Dermatol 1990;332:153.

CHAPTER 3

Dermatologic Diagnosis

John C. Hall

To aid in determining the diagnosis of a presenting skin problem, this chapter contains discussions of primary and secondary lesions and also of diagnosis by location. Included are lists of seasonal skin diseases, military dermatoses, and dermatoses of African Americans.

Primary and Secondary Lesions

Most skin diseases have some characteristic primary lesions and it is important to examine the patient closely to find them. Commonly, however, the primary lesions have been obliterated by the secondary lesions of overtreatment, excessive scratching, or infection. Even in these cases, it is usually possible, by careful examination, to find some primary lesions at the edge of the eruption or on other, less irritated areas of the body (Fig. 3-1). Combinations of primary and secondary lesions frequently occur as part of the clinical picture.

Primary Lesions

- *Macules* are up to 1 cm and are circumscribed, flat discolorations of the skin (Fig. 3-2A). Examples include freckles, flat nevi, and some drug eruptions.

SAUER'S NOTES

1. One of the dermatologist's tools of the trade is a magnifying lens. *Use it.*
2. A complete examination of the entire body is a necessity when confronted with a diffuse skin eruption or an unusual localized eruption.
3. Touch the skin and skin lesions. You learn a lot by palpating and patients appreciate that you are not afraid of "catching" the problem. (For the uncommon contagious problem, use precaution).
4. When in doubt of the diagnosis, verify your clinical impression with a biopsy. The most frequent reason for a successful malpractice suit in dermatology is failure to diagnose.

- *Patches* are larger than 1 cm and are circumscribed, flat discolorations of the skin. Examples include vitiligo, some drug eruptions, senile freckles, melasma and measles rash.
- *Papules* are up to 1 cm and are circumscribed, elevated, superficial, solid lesions (Fig. 3-2B). Examples include elevated nevi, some drug eruptions, warts, and lichen planus. A *wheal* is a type of papule that is edematous and transitory (present less than 24 hours). Examples include hives, drug eruptions, food allergies, numerous underlying illnesses, and sometimes insect bites.
- *Plaques* are larger than 1 cm and are circumscribed, elevated, superficial, solid lesions. Examples include mycosis fungoides and lichen simplex chronicus.
- *Nodules* range to 1 cm and are solid lesions with depth; they may be above, level with, or beneath the skin surface (Fig. 3-2C,D). Examples are nodular secondary or tertiary syphilis, basal cell cancers, dermatofibromas and xanthomas.
- *Tumors* are larger than 1 cm and are solid lesions with depth; they may be above, level with, or beneath the skin surface (Fig. 3-2E). Examples include tumor stage of mycosis fungoides and larger basal cell cancers.
- *Vesicles* are up to 1 cm in size and are circumscribed elevations of the skin containing serous fluid (Fig. 3-2F). Examples include early chickenpox, zoster, herpes simplex and contact dermatitis.
- *Bullae* are larger than 1 cm and are circumscribed elevations containing serous fluid. Examples include pemphigus, bullous pemphigoid, and second-degree burns.
- *Pustules* vary in size and are circumscribed elevations of the skin containing purulent fluid (Fig. 3-2G). Examples include acne and impetigo.
- *Petechiae* range in size to 1 cm and are circumscribed deposits of blood or blood pigments. Examples are thrombocytopenia, vasculitis and drug eruptions.

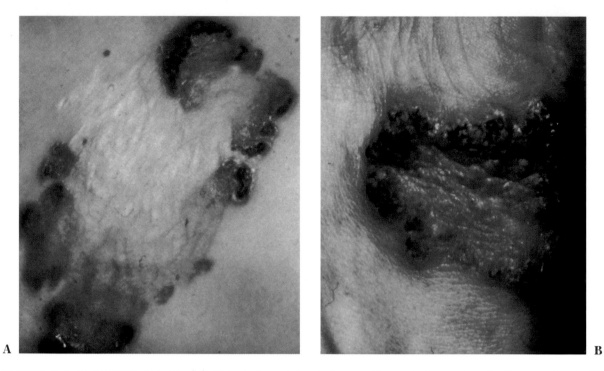

FIGURE 3-1 ■ Nodular lesions. **(A)** Grouped nodular lesions with central scarring (tertiary syphilis). **(B)** Grouped warty, nodular lesions with central scarring (tuberculosis verrucosa cutis). *(Courtesy of Marion B. Sulzberger, Folia Dermatologica, No. 1, Geigy Pharmaceuticals.)*

■ *Purpura* is a circumscribed deposit of blood or blood pigment that is larger than 1 cm in the skin. Examples include senile purpura and vasculitis.

Secondary Lesions

■ *Scales* are shedding, dead epidermal cells that may be dry or greasy. Examples are dandruff (greasy) and psoriasis (dry).

■ *Crusts* are variously colored masses of skin exudates of blood, serum, pus or a combination of these (Fig. 3-3A). Examples include impetigo, infected dermatitis or any area of excoriation.

■ *Excoriations* are abrasions of the skin, usually superficial and traumatic. Examples are scratched insect bites, scabies, eczema, and dermatitis herpetiformis.

■ *Fissures* are linear breaks in the skin, sharply defined with abrupt walls. Examples include congenital syphilis, athlete's foot, and hand eczema.

■ *Ulcers* are irregularly sized and shaped excavations in the skin extending into the dermis or deeper that usually heal with a scar. Examples include stasis ulcers of legs, pyoderma gangrenosum, and tertiary syphilis.

■ *Scars* are formations of connective tissue replacing tissue lost through injury or disease. Examples are

discoid lupus, lichen planus in the scalp, and third-degree burns.

■ *Keloids* are hypertrophic scars beyond the borders of the original injury (Fig. 3-3B). They are elevated, can be progressive, and usually are the result of some sort of trauma in the skin. Keloids are common in dark-skinned people. They are common on the upper torso and with body piercing, particularly piercing of the earlobe. Rarely, keloid can occur spontaneously. Any kind of full-thickness trauma can heal with a keloidal scar. They are unsightly and can be numb, pruritic, or painful.

■ *Lichenification* is a diffuse area of thickening and scaling with a resultant increase in the skin lines and markings (Fig. 3-3C). It is often seen in atopic dermatitis.

Several combinations of primary and secondary lesions commonly exist on the same patient. Examples are *papulosquamous lesions* of psoriasis, *vesiculopustular lesions* in contact dermatitis, and *crusted excoriations* in scabies.

Special Lesions

Some primary lesions, limited to a few skin diseases, can be called *specialized lesions.*

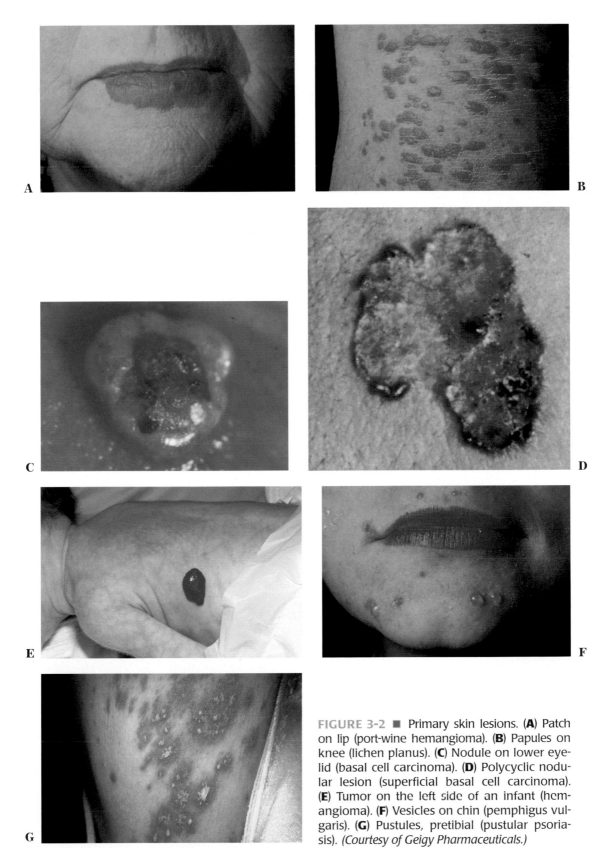

FIGURE 3-2 ■ Primary skin lesions. (**A**) Patch on lip (port-wine hemangioma). (**B**) Papules on knee (lichen planus). (**C**) Nodule on lower eyelid (basal cell carcinoma). (**D**) Polycyclic nodular lesion (superficial basal cell carcinoma). (**E**) Tumor on the left side of an infant (hemangioma). (**F**) Vesicles on chin (pemphigus vulgaris). (**G**) Pustules, pretibial (pustular psoriasis). *(Courtesy of Geigy Pharmaceuticals.)*

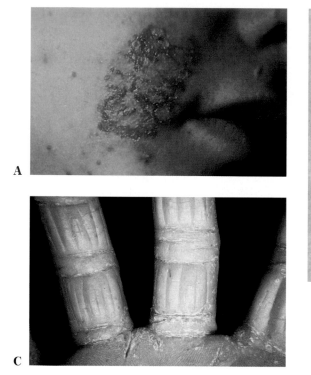

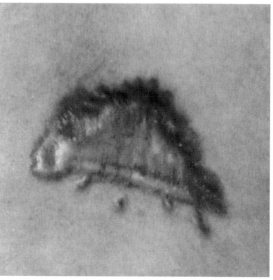

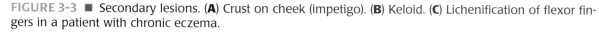

FIGURE 3-3 ■ Secondary lesions. (**A**) Crust on cheek (impetigo). (**B**) Keloid. (**C**) Lichenification of flexor fingers in a patient with chronic eczema.

- *Burrows* are very small and short (in scabies) or tortuous and long (in creeping eruption) tunnels in the epidermis.
- *Comedones* or *blackheads* are plugs of whitish or blackish sebaceous and keratinous material lodged in the pilosebaceous follicle, usually seen on the face, chest, or back and, rarely, on the upper part of the arms. Examples include acne and Favre-Racouchot on sun-damaged skin on the temporal areas. These are a hallmark of chloracne.
- *Cutaneous horn* is a localized spike-shaped area of marked overgrowth of keratin that can stick above the skin half an inch or more. It is quite localized usually 0.5 to 1 cm in width or less. It most commonly overlies actinic keratoses, but can overlie seborrheic keratoses, squamous cell carcinomas, warts, porokeratosis, or, less likely, hyperkeratotic basal cell cancers.
- *Follicular plugs* are keratin plugs in the hair follicle that are 1 to 3 mm in size and most characteristically seen in lupus erythematosus and lichen planus.

- *Malperforans ulcer* is seen in diabetics and leprosy patients. There is an associated neuropathy, so the ulcers are painless although deep and destructive. Ulcers associated with vasculitis and factitial ulcers can also have the same appearance.
- *Milia* are whitish papules, 1 to 2 mm in diameter, that have no visible opening onto the skin surface. Examples are found in healed burn or superficial traumatic sites, healed bullous disease sites, or newborns. They are not uncommon on the face in adults or more widespread in newborns.
- *Striae cutis distensae* are red, resolving to white, linear areas of atrophy that maybe indented. They are seen on the thighs, buttocks, and breasts mainly, in rapid weight loss, prolonged use of topical or systemic corticosteroids, body building (especially with androgen ingestion), and pregnancy, where it is most pronounced over the abdomen.
- *Telangiectasias* are dilated superficial blood vessels. Examples include spider hemangiomas, chronic radiodermatitis, basal cell cancer, sebaceous hyperplasia, prolonged chronic sun exposure, and rosacea.

In addition, distinct and often diagnostic changes can occur in the nail plates and the hairs. These are discussed in the chapters relating to these appendages.

Diagnosis by Location

A physician is often confronted with a patient with skin trouble localized to one part of the body (Figs. 3-4, 3-5, 3-6, and 3-7). The following list of diseases with special locations is meant to aid in the diagnosis of such conditions, but this list must not be considered inclusive. Generalizations are the rule and many of the rare diseases are omitted. For further information concerning the particular diseases, consult the Dictionary–Index.

- *Scalp:* Seborrheic dermatitis, contact dermatitis, psoriasis, folliculitis, pediculosis, and hair loss due to the following: male or female pattern, alopecia areata, tinea, chronic discoid lupus erythematosus, postpregnancy alopecia, or trichotillomania.
- *Ears:* Seborrheic dermatitis, psoriasis, atopic eczema, lichen simplex chronicus, actinic keratoses, melanoma, varix, seborrheic keratoses, and squamous cell carcinomas.
- *Face:* Acne, rosacea, impetigo, contact dermatitis, seborrheic dermatitis, folliculitis, herpes simplex, lupus erythematosus, and dermatomyositis, nevi, melanoma (especially lentigo maligna melanoma), basal cell cancer, actinic keratosis, squamous cell carcinoma, seborrheic keratosis, milia, and sebaceous hyperplasia.
- *Eyelids:* Contact dermatitis due to cosmetics, especially fingernail polish or hair sprays, seborrheic dermatitis, atopic eczema, skin tags, syringomas and basal cell cancer.
- *Posterior neck:* Neurodermatitis (lichen simplex chronicus), seborrheic dermatitis, psoriasis, folliculitis or contact dermatitis, and acne keloidalis in dark-skinned people.

- *Mouth:* Aphthae, herpes simplex, geographic tongue, syphilis, lichen planus, traumatic fibromas, oral hairy leukoplakia, squamous cell cancer, candidiasis, and pemphigus.
- *Axillae:* Contact dermatitis, seborrheic dermatitis, hidradenitis suppurativa, erythrasma, acanthosis nigricans, and Fox–Fordyce disease.
- *Chest and back:* Tinea versicolor, pityriasis rosea, acne, seborrheic dermatitis, psoriasis, and secondary syphilis, epidermoid cyst on back; seborrheic keratoses, senile or cherry angiomas, nevi, and melanomas especially on the back in men.
- *Groin and crural areas:* Tinea infection, candida infection, bacterial intertrigo, scabies, pediculosis, granuloma inguinale, warts and skin tags, hidradenitis suppurativa, folliculitis, seborrhea, and inverse psoriasis.
- *Penis:* Contact dermatitis, fixed drug eruption, condyloma acuminata, candida balanitis, chancroid, herpes simplex, primary and secondary syphilis, scabies, balanitis xerotica obliterans, warts, psoriasis, seborrhea, and pearly penile papules.
- *Hands:* Contact dermatitis, id reaction to fungal infection of the feet, atopic eczema, psoriasis, verrucae, pustular psoriasis, nummular eczema, erythema multiforme, secondary syphilis (palms), fungal infection, dyshidrotic eczema, warts, and squamous cell carcinoma on the dorsal hands.
- *Cubital fossae and popliteal fossae:* Atopic eczema, contact dermatitis, and prickly heat.
- *Elbows and knees:* Psoriasis, xanthomas, dermatomyositis, granuloma annulare, and atopic eczema.
- *Feet:* Fungal infection, primary or secondary bacterial infection, contact dermatitis from footwear or foot care, atopic eczema, verrucae, psoriasis, erythema multiforme, dyshidrotic eczema, and secondary syphilis (soles of feet).

SAUER'S NOTES

In diagnosing a rather generalized skin eruption, the following three mimicking conditions must be considered first and ruled in or out by appropriate history or examination:

1. drug eruption,
2. contact dermatitis, and
3. infectious diseases, such as acquired immunodeficiency syndrome, other viral exanthems and secondary syphilis.

Seasonal Skin Diseases

Certain dermatoses have an increased incidence in various seasons of the year. In a busy dermatologist's office, one sees "epidemics" of atopic eczema, pityriasis rosea, psoriasis, and winter itch, to mention only a few. Knowledge of this seasonal incidence is helpful from a diagnostic standpoint. It is sufficient simply to list these seasonal diseases here, because more specific information concerning them can be found elsewhere in this text. Remember that there are exceptions to every rule.

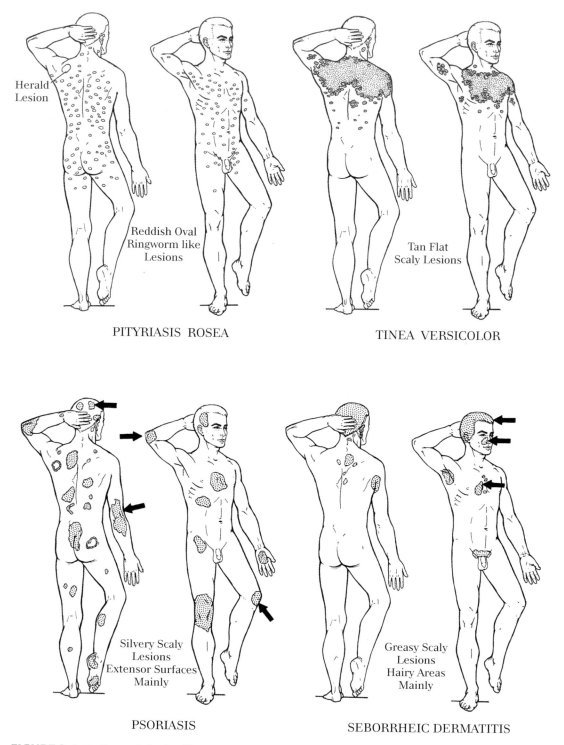

Herald
Lesion

Reddish Oval
Ringworm like
Lesions

PITYRIASIS ROSEA

Tan Flat
Scaly Lesions

TINEA VERSICOLOR

Silvery Scaly
Lesions
Extensor Surfaces
Mainly

PSORIASIS

Greasy Scaly
Lesions
Hairy Areas
Mainly

SEBORRHEIC DERMATITIS

FIGURE 3-4 ■ Dermatologic silhouettes. Diagnosis by location.

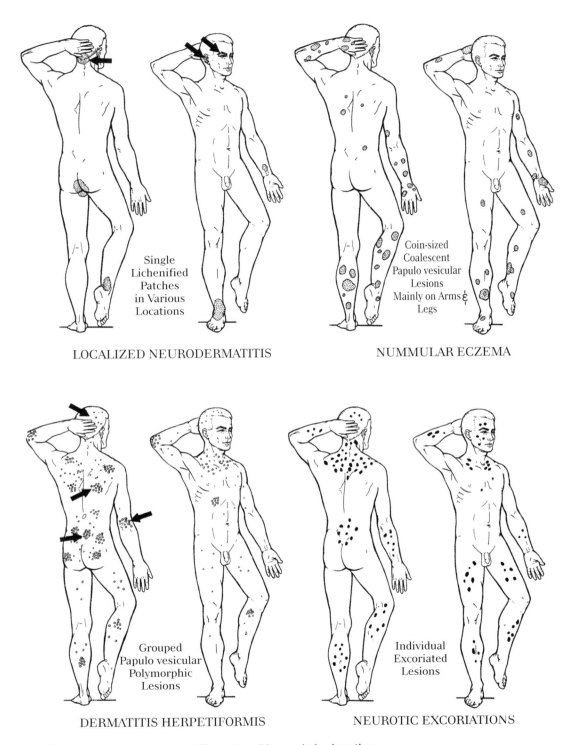

FIGURE 3-5 ■ Dermatologic silhouettes. Diagnosis by location.

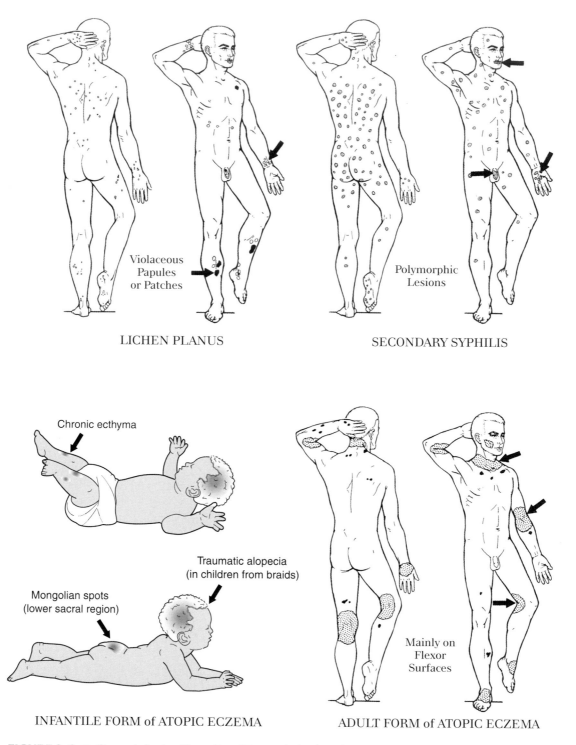

Violaceous
Papules
or Patches

LICHEN PLANUS

Polymorphic
Lesions

SECONDARY SYPHILIS

Chronic ecthyma

Traumatic alopecia
(in children from braids)

Mongolian spots
(lower sacral region)

INFANTILE FORM of ATOPIC ECZEMA

Mainly on
Flexor
Surfaces

ADULT FORM of ATOPIC ECZEMA

FIGURE 3-6 ■ Dermatologic silhouettes. Diagnosis by location.

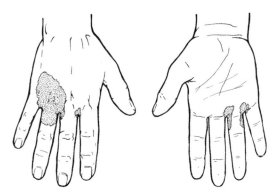

CONTACT DERMATITIS ("Housewife")

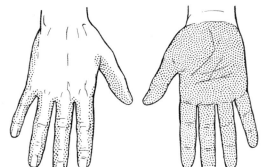

DYSHIDROSIS or ID (Due to Tinea of Feet)

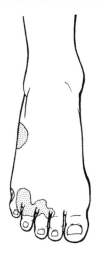

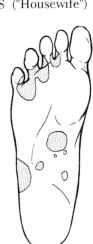

FUNGUS INFECTION

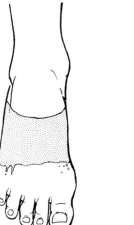

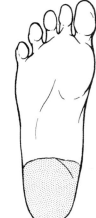

CONTACT DERMATITIS (Shoes)

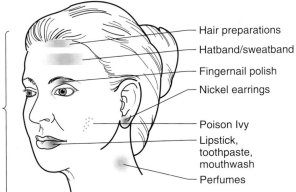

Cosmetics & airborne allergens

Hair preparations
Hatband/sweatband
Fingernail polish
Nickel earrings
Poison Ivy
Lipstick, toothpaste, mouthwash
Perfumes

CONTACT DERMATITIS

FIGURE 3-7 ■ Dermatologic silhouettes. Diagnosis by location.

Winter

- Atopic eczema
- Contact dermatitis of hands
- Psoriasis
- Seborrheic dermatitis
- Nummular eczema
- Winter itch and dry skin (xerosis)
- Ichthyosis

Spring

- Pityriasis rosea
- Erythema multiforme
- Acne (flares)
- Viral exanthems

Summer

- Contact dermatitis due to poison ivy
- Tinea of the feet and the groin
- Candida intertrigo
- Miliaria or prickly heat
- Impetigo and other pyodermas
- Polymorphous light eruption
- Insect bites
- Tinea versicolor (noticed after suntan)
- Darier's disease (uncommon)
- Epidermolysis bullosa (uncommon)

Fall

- Winter itch
- Senile pruritus
- Atopic eczema
- Acne (less sun, more stress with school starting)
- Pityriasis rosea
- Contact dermatitis due to ragweed
- Tinea of the scalp (schoolchildren)
- Viral exanthems

Military Dermatoses

Certain parts of the world continue to be at war, and under its ravages the lack of good personal hygiene, the lack of adequate food, and the presence of overcrowding, injuries, and pestilence can result in the aggravation of any existing skin disease and an increased incidence of the following skin diseases:

- Scabies
- Pediculosis
- Syphilis and other sexually transmitted diseases
- Bacterial dermatoses
- Tinea of the feet and the groin
- Pyoderma
- Miliaria
- Leishmaniasis

Dermatoses of Dark-Skinned People

The following skin diseases are seen with greater frequency among dark-skinned people than in light-skinned people (Figs. 3-8 and 3-9):

- Keloids
- Dermatosis papulosa nigra (variant of seborrheic keratoses that are dark, small, multiple, facial, and more common in women)
- Pyodermas of legs in children
- Pigmentary disturbances from many causes, both hypopigmented and hyperpigmented
- Traumatic marginal alopecia (from braids and from heated irons used in hair straightening)
- Seborrheic dermatitis of scalp, aggravated by grease on hair
- Ingrown hairs of beard (pseudofolliculitis barbae)
- Acne keloidalis nuchae
- Annular form of secondary syphilis
- Granuloma inguinale
- Mongolian spots
- Acral lentiginous melanomas
- Tinea capitas (in children who braid their hair)

On the other hand, certain skin conditions are rarely seen in dark-skinned people:

- Squamous cell or basal cell carcinomas
- Actinic keratoses
- Psoriasis
- Superficial spreading, nodular, and lentigo maligna melanoma
- Scabies

Descriptive Terms Often Used in Dermatology

- *Acneiform* refers to a resemblance of acne as seen in acne, folliculitis, rosacea, some drug eruptions such as topical, and systemic corticosteroids.
- *Annulare* or *arciform lesions* refer to a peripheral circular curving of the lesions seen in such diseases as erythema annulare centrifugum; erythema chronica nigrans of Lyme disease; erythema marginatum of Scarlet fever; erythema gyratum perstans, which can be associated with underlying malignancy; tinea; impetigo; and psoriasis.
- *Atrophic* thinning of the skin as in mycosis fungoides with fine superficial "cigarette-paper" wrinkling atrophy or deep with result in scar formation as in discoid lupus erythematosus or third degree burns.

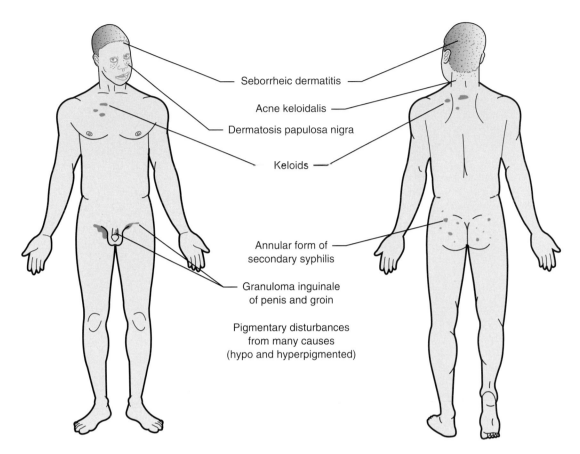

Seborrheic dermatitis

Acne keloidalis

Dermatosis papulosa nigra

Keloids

Annular form of
secondary syphilis

Granuloma inguinale
of penis and groin

Pigmentary disturbances
from many causes
(hypo and hyperpigmented)

FIGURE 3-8 ■ Dermatologic silhouettes. Conditions more common among dark-skinned patients.

■ *Changes of color*
Hyperpigmented, with increased pigment as seen in postinflammatory hyperpigmentation and residual lesions of lichen planus or dermatitis herpetiformis.

Hypopigmented, decreased pigment as seen in pityriasis alba and postinflammatory hypopigmentation.

Depigmented, loss of pigment as in vitiligo or scar.

Violaceous reddish purple discoloration, as seen in vasculitis and the tumors of mycosis fungoides.

Apple-jelly colored, reddish-brown color, seen most often in sarcoidosis particularly upon pressing the skin with a clear glass slide called diascopy.

Porcelain-white color, stark white color, which can be seen in morphea, generalized cutaneous scleroderma, Degos disease, and atrophie blanche type of vasculitis.

Heliotrope, which refers to violaceous color as seen on upper eyelids in dermatomyositis.

Cayenne pepper, which are tiny reddish-brown spots due to hemosiderin staining of the skin seen most in the pigmented purpuric dermatoses.

■ *Cushingoid* appearance is seen in patients on high-dose, long-term systemic corticosteroids in which the face has a round or moonlike appearance and there is increased central body fat particularly over the back with a "buffalo hump." Acne striae, rosacea, and hirsutism are also often seen.

■ *En crurasse* refers to a shieldlike induration usually at the chest wall as seen in scleroderma and infiltrated malignancy, particularly breast cancer.

■ *Exophytic* means protruding from the skin such as in some squamous cell carcinomas, warts, and advanced cutaneous lymphoma.

■ *Filiform* refers to tiny filamentous projections that come from a tumor usually indicative of a filiform wart.

■ *Form fruste* refers to an atypical or partial example of a skin disease.

■ *Herpetiform* means "in a group" and is seen in the blisters of herpes simplex, herpes zoster varicella, and the autoimmune blistering disease dermatitis herpetiformis.

■ *In cognito* refers to a hidden skin disease such as in scabies patients who frequently bathe or dermatitis

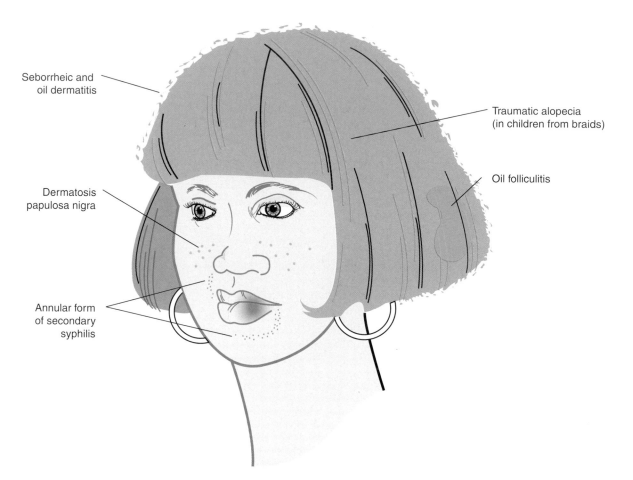

Seborrheic and oil dermatitis

Traumatic alopecia (in children from braids)

Oil folliculitis

Dermatosis papulosa nigra

Annular form of secondary syphilis

FIGURE 3-9 ■ Dermatologic silhouette. Conditions more common among dark-skinned patients.

herpetiformis that is so excoriated that no primary skin lesions can be seen.

■ *Keratotic* refers to thickening of the horny layer of skin such as in some squamous cell carcinomas, chronic palm and sole psoriasis, or eczema.

■ *Leonine facies* is a lion-like look to the face with thickening of the normal furrows over the entire face most often described with cutaneous T-cell lymphoma, leprosy, or tertiary syphilis.

■ *Morbilliform* is usually used to refer to a measles-like eruption that is symmetric, macular, and consists of 1 cm or smaller, usually red, macules that can become confluent. This is seen most often in morbilliform drug eruptions and viral exanthems, including measles, rubella, and HIV exanthem, as some examples.

■ *Peau de orange* refers to bulging of the skin with an orange-peel look that has a mottled texture and is seen in cutaneous mucinosis such as myxedema; lymphoma of the skin such as T-helper cell lym-phoma; other cutaneous malignancies such as breast cancer; and elephantiasis nostra verrucosa such as seen in chronic lymphedema of the lower extremities with repeated episodes of cellulitis.

■ *Pedunculated* refers to a stalklike attachment to the skin as in skin tags.

■ *Perifollicular* refers to eruptions that seem to be around the hair follicle. This term is often used to describe folliculitis, keratosis pilaris, and follicular eczema.

■ *Poikiloderma* has three components that consist of fine "cigarette paper" wrinkling atrophy, alternating hyper- and hypopigmentation, and telangiectasias. This is seen as a result of radiation dermatitis, chronic corticosteroid use topically, and, systemi-cally, chronic sun exposure most often seen as poikiloderma of Civatte on the sides of the neck. It is also found in collagen vascular disease (most commonly lupus erythematosus) as well as in der-matomyositis. It can be a generalized eruption, in which case it is called *poikiloderma atrophicans vasculare* and is considered by most authorities to be a cutaneous T-cell lymphoma.

- *Psoriasiform* means resembling psoriasis, as in psoriasis or some cases of cutaneous T-cell lymphoma.
- *Punched out* is most often used in relationship to an arterial ischemic ulcer, vasculitic ulcer, or mal perforans ulcer.
- *Reticulate* means a lacy distribution of skin lesions as seen in oral lichen planus. The pigmentation of poikiloderma, the pigmentation seen in erythema ab igne, and can also be referred to as weblike.
- *Sclerodermoid* refers to indurated skin, often with loss of pigment, and is characteristic of scleroderma, bleomycin injection sites, pentazocine (TALWIN) injection sites, and chronic cutaneous graft-versus-host disease.
- *Telangiectatic* means covered with telangiectasias as in rosacea.
- *Umbilicated* is a tumor or plaque that has a central indentation or dell. This is often used to describe molluscum contagiosum and can also be seen in sebaceous hyperplasia, basal cell carcinoma, and sometimes in viral blisters such as in herpes simplex or herpes zoster varicella virus.
- *Varicelliform* means to resemble smallpox such as in smallpox, chickenpox, herpes zoster, or pityriasis lichenoides et varioliformis of Muccha and Habermann.
- *Verrucous* means wartlike appearance.
- *Zosteriform* refers to the distribution cutaneous disease in a nerve root distribution. This is seen in herpes zoster, some epidermal and other hamartomatous nevi, and occasionally vitiligo, among others.

Descriptive Terms Often Used in Dermatology

Exophytic: protruding from the skin, as in an exophytic squamous cell carcinoma, lymphoma or keloid.

Keratotic: thickening of the horny layer of the skin causing dry, heaped up, hard skin such as in a keratotic actinic keratosis.

Pedunculated: a narrow, stalk-like attachment to the skin as often seen in skin tags.

Psoriasiform: resembling psoriasis as in a psoriasiform plaque of mycosis fungoides.

Varioliformis: to resemble small pox as in pityriasis lichenoides et varioliformis acuta.

Varicelliform: to resemble chicken pox as in Kaposi's varicelliform eruption.

Verrucous: wartlike in appearance such as in a verrucous keratoacanthoma.

Suggested Reading

Archer CB. Black and white skin diseases: An atlas and text. Oxford, UK, Blackwell Science, 1995.

Bouchier IAD, Ellis H, Fleming PR. French's index of differential diagnosis, ed 13. London, Butterworth-Heinemann, 1996.

Callen JP. Color atlas of dermatology, 2 ed. Philadelphia, W.B. Saunders, 1999.

Du Vivier A. Atlas of clinical dermatology, 3 ed. Philadelphia, W.B. Saunders, 2002.

Eliot H, Ghatan Y. Dermatological differential diagnosis and pearls. London, Parthenon, 1998.

Goodheart HP. Goodheart's photoguide of common skin disorders, 2 ed. Philadelphia, Lippincott Williams & Wilkins, 2003.

Habif TP. Clinical dermatology, 4 ed. St. Louis, Mosby, 2004.

Habif TP, Campbell JL Jr., Chapman MS, et al. Skin disease: Diagnosis and treatment. St. Louis, Mosby, 2001.

Helm KF, Marks JG. Atlas of differential diagnosis in dermatology. Philadelphia, W.B. Saunders 1998.

Holloway V, ed. Ethnic hair & skin: What is the state of the science? J Am Acad Dermatol 2003;48(6 Suppl):XX

Hunter J, Savin J, Dahl M. Clinical dermatology, 3 ed. Oxford, UK: Blackwell Publishing Ltd, 2003.

Jackon R. Morphological diagnosis of skin disease. Lewiston, NY, Manticore, 1999.

Johnson BL, Moy RL, White GM. Ethnic skin: Medical and surgical. St. Louise, C.V. Mosby, 1998.

Kerdel FA, Jimenez-Acosta, F. Dermatology: Just the facts. New York, McGraw-Hill, 2003.

Lawrence CM, Cox NH. Physical signs in dermatology, 2 ed. St. Louis, Mosby, 2001.

Provost TT, Flynn JA. Cutaneous medicine: Cutaneous manifestations of systemic disease. Hamilton, Ontario, BC Decker, 2001.

Poyner TF. Common skin diseases. Oxford, UK, Blackwell Science, 1999.

Rotstein H. Principles and practice of dermatology, ed 3. Newton, MA, Boston Publishing Co, 1993.

Rycroft RJG, Robertson SJ. A color handbook of dermatology. London, Manson, 1999.

Steigleder GK. Pocket atlas of dermatology, ed 2. New York, Theime, 1993.

Sybert VP. Skin manifestations in individuals of African or Asian descent. Pediatr Derm 1996;13:2.

White GM, Cox NH. Diseases of the skin: A color atlas and text. St. Louis, Mosby, 2000.

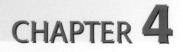

Introduction to the Patient

John C. Hall

When a patient visits your office for the first time, after the usual conversation in which you introduce yourself, the following type of exchange may transpire:

PHYSICIAN: What can I do for you, Mrs. Jones?

MRS. JONES: I have a bad breaking out on my hands.

PHYSICIAN: (*Writes on his chart under* Present Complaint, *"hand dermatitis"*) How long have you had this breaking out?

MRS. JONES: Well, I've had this before, but what I have now has been here for only 3 weeks.

PHYSICIAN: (*Writes, "duration, 3 weeks"*) When did you have this before, Mrs. Jones?

MRS. JONES: Let me see. I think this happened twice before. The first time was shortly after I got married, and I thought that it had to do with the fact that I had my hands in soap and water more than before. It took about a month to heal up. I treated it with salves that I had at home. It wasn't bad that time. The next time I broke out it was a little bit worse. This was after my first child was born. Johnny is 3 years old now. I guess I should have expected my hands to break out again now because I just had my second baby 3 months ago.

PHYSICIAN: (*Finishes writing, "The patient states that she has had this eruption on two previous occasions. Home treatment only. Both eruptions lasted about 1 month. Present eruption attributed to care of baby born 3 months ago."*) Mrs. Jones, what have you been putting on your hands for this breaking out?

MRS. JONES: Let me take off my bandages, and I'll show you how my hands look.

PHYSICIAN: Let me help you with those bandages. However, I want to ask you a few more questions before I look at your hands.

MRS. JONES: Well, first I used a salve that I got at the drugstore that said on the label it was good for athlete's foot. One of my neighbors told me that she used it for her hand trouble, and it had cured her hands. I don't think that her hands looked like mine, though, and I sort of feel that the salve made my hands worse. Then I decided I would burn out the infection, so I soaked my hands in some bleaching solution. This helped some with the itching, but it made the skin too dry. Then I remembered that you had given me some salve for Johnny's "infantigo," so I put some of that on. That softened up my hands but didn't seem to help with the itching. So here I am, Doctor.

PHYSICIAN: (*Writes, "Treated with athlete's foot Rx, bleach soaks, Johnny's impetigo Rx"*) How much itching are you having?

MRS. JONES: Well, my hands sting and burn when I get any soap and water on them, but I can sleep without them bothering me.

PHYSICIAN: (*Notes, "Mild itching"*) Are you taking any medicine by mouth now for anything? I even want to know about laxatives, vitamins, or aspirin. Have you had any shots recently?

MRS. JONES: No, I'm not taking any medicine.

PHYSICIAN: Now, are you sure?

MRS. JONES: Well, I do take sleeping medicine at night occasionally, and, oh yes, I'm taking some diet pills that Dr. Smith gave me about 2 months ago.

PHYSICIAN: (*Writes, "Drugs—takes sleeping medicine h.s. and diet pills"*) Mrs. Jones, does anyone in your family have any allergies? Does anyone have any asthma, hay fever, or eczema? Your parents, brothers, sisters, children, other family members?

MRS. JONES: No, not that I know of, Doctor.

PHYSICIAN: Have you ever had any of those conditions? Any asthma, hay fever, or eczema?

MRS. JONES: No, I haven't had any of those. Sometimes I have a little sinus trouble though.

PHYSICIAN: (*Writes, "No atopy in patient or family"*) Now, let me have a good look at those hands. I also want you to remove your shoes and socks so that I can get a good look at your feet. (*Examines the patient's hands and feet carefully*) Now, are you sure that you don't have this anywhere else, Mrs. Jones?

MRS. JONES: No, I am positive I don't, because I looked all over my skin this morning when I took a shower. However, I do have a mole on my back that I want you to look at, Doctor.

PHYSICIAN: Has it been bothering you recently?

MRS. JONES: Well, no, but my bra strap rubs it sometimes.

PHYSICIAN: (*Examines the mole on her back*) That is a small mole, Mrs. Jones. It doesn't have any unusual color, and I see no reason for having it removed. It could be removed if you wish, but I don't think it is necessary.

MRS. JONES: Well, I don't want it removed if you don't think it is necessary. Now, what do you think about my hands?

PHYSICIAN: Let me make a few notes about what I saw and then I'll tell you about your hands and the treatment. (*Writes, "Physical exam: (1) A crusting, vesicular dermatitis is seen mainly in the webs of the fingers of both hands, worse on the right hand. There is no sharp border to the eruption. The nail of the right ring finger has several transverse furrows. The feet are clear. (2) In the midline of the upper back is a 3- × 3-mm flat, faintly brownish lesion. Diagnosis: (1) Contact dermatitis, probably due to excess soap and water. (2) Pigmented compound nevus."*)

PHYSICIAN: Mrs. Jones, you have a very common skin condition, commonly called *housewives' eczema* or *housewives' dermatitis*. I feel sure that it is aggravated by having your hands in soap and water so many times a day. Most busy mothers don't even have enough time to dry their hands

carefully every time they are wet. Some people appear to be more sensitive to soaps than others. It isn't a real allergy, just a sensitivity because the soap and the water have a tendency to remove the normal skin's protective oils and fats. Some of those blisters are infected, and we will have to take care of that infection along with the other irritation. Here is what we will do to treat your hands. (*Gives careful instructions to Mrs. Jones, particularly with regard to the hand soaks, the way the salve is to be applied, advice concerning avoidance of excess soap and water, the use of rubber and cotton gloves, and so on.*)

History Taking

This play-by-play description, a type of conversation that is repeated many times a month in any busy practitioner's office, illustrates some of the basic points in history taking.

A careful history is followed by a complete examination of the skin problem, and this, in turn, is followed by therapy, or what I prefer to call *management*. For good management of the patient, I have found it helpful to write out the diagnosis, other information, and instructions. Advantages to the patient and physician are multiple. The patient has an individualized short note about the diagnosis, cause (if known), what the physician can or cannot do (if there is no cure, as for atopic eczema or psoriasis, say so), and instructions about diet, bathing, therapy, and so on. For the physician, the advantage is that a copy can be kept in the patient's chart and used later to help refresh the patient's memory about instructions, or it could even be used advantageously in a medicolegal problem regarding information given to the patient.

Patient information pamphlets available from the American Academy of Dermatology, drug companies, and various disease-specific organizations are helpful, especially when handed to the patient by the physician. Note in the chart that this was done.

Charting the History

A common way of arranging a medical record is called "SOAP." This stands for *Subjective, Objective, Assessment,* and *Plan*. Each chart should indicate a presenting complaint, a history of the present illness, a review of systems, past medical history, physical examination, a diagnosis with pertinent differential diagnoses, and a proposed plan of action. As part of a good examination record, the dermatologist should place in the patient's chart simple diagrams appropriately marked with the site, size, and configuration of growths, scars, rashes, and so on. You need not

---

SAUER'S NOTES

A complete skin exam should be done at the initial visit if appropriate rapport has been established with the patient. This is especially important in light-skinned, blonde- or red-haired, blue-eyed individuals. It is mandatory in a patient with a personal or family history of skin cancer or many moles, marked sun exposure, immunosuppression, or when requested by patient, family member, or referring physician.

> ### SAUER'S NOTES
>
> A careful, thorough medical history from your patient is very important.
>
> #### LOCAL TREATMENT HISTORY
>
> Find out how much treatment and what kind of local treatment has been administered by the patient or by physicians. Many over-the-counter medications can aggravate a dermatosis.
>
> #### SYSTEMIC DRUG HISTORY
>
> Don't just ask, "Are you taking any medicines?" Ask, "Are you taking any medicine for *any* reason? Are you on birth control pills (if appropriate), are you on vitamins or sleeping pills, do you take aspirin or Tylenol, do you get any shots?" This history is important for two reasons. First, something about the patient can be learned from the drugs taken. For example, it is important to know if a person is taking insulin for diabetes or corticosteroids for arthritis. This information can well influence your treatment of the patient. Second, drugs can cause many skin eruptions, and your index of suspicion of a drug eruption will be higher if that information is consistently requested.
>
> #### ALLERGY HISTORY
>
> "Do you or did you ever have any asthma, hay fever, eczema, or migraine headaches?" A positive allergy history is important for two reasons. First, a family or a patient history of allergies can aid in making a diagnosis of atopic dermatitis. Second, if there is a positive allergy history, usually it can be predicted that the patient's skin disorder will respond more slowly to treatment than a similar dermatitis in a nonallergic patient. Patients with atopy are more "itchish."

be an artist to draw a face, back, chest, or hand. You can also use a printed sticker or stamp of the site. Mark in the lesions or configurations on the drawing and note the size. The value of these simple annotations is multiple. They benefit you, your patient, and, if necessary, your lawyer.

Regardless of what method of patient chart organization is used, a uniform complete medical record is mandatory in today's environment of managed care, medicolegal hazards, insurance industry reimbursement issues, and Medicare and Medicaid mandates. Use of a computer can make some of these tasks faster, easier, and more accurate. Patient confidentiality is always to be kept in mind. Medical records need to be legible.

> ### SAUER'S NOTES
>
> When a patient is in the hospital, many people in white coats or with stethoscopes around their necks come and go. The visit of the dermatologic consultant (or others) may be forgotten in the confusion and misery of the hospital confinement.

Hospitalized Patient Visits

As a dermatologist, you will sometimes be asked to examine the skin condition of a hospitalized patient. In these situations, you may be one of several doctors to visit the patient. There is a simple measure that should help the patient to remember the dermatologist's visit: Leave your calling card or an instruction sheet where you write down your diagnosis and instructions. This card, or instruction sheet, has your name, address, and phone number. You can even write on the reverse some information you may wish to convey about the skin problem you were asked to see. And when your bill comes, the patient and family will have it as a reminder of your visit.

> ### SAUER'S NOTES
>
> The specialty of dermatology, like any medical field, needs good public relations efforts. Most important, we need to promote better public relations in our own sphere of influence.
>
> 1. We need to provide correct diagnoses, correct therapy, and proper management for the patient. This should be our most tangible public relations effort.
> 2. It is important to be a visible dermatologist. This can be accomplished by attending medical meetings and assuming offices in medical societies. There are also medical societies in surrounding communities that need speakers. When you begin practice, it helps to go from door to door, at least in your own office building, to meet the possible referring physicians face to face.
> 3. After you get a patient referred from another physician, do not fail to thank the physician. Write a note and include the diagnosis with a short description of your treatment. With new federal guidelines in place you need to ask the patient for permission to do this and record this permission in the chart.
> 4. A physician should provide services to the community. One can give medical talks to lay groups and serve on civic committees.
> 5. Physicians should have courteous and competent personnel in the office. Pay attention to what goes on at your front desk.

CHAPTER 5

Dermatologic Therapy

John C. Hall

Many hundreds of medications are available for use in treating skin diseases. Most physicians, however, have a few favorite prescriptions that they prescribe day in and day out. These few prescriptions may then be altered slightly to suit an individual patient or disease. For commonly used preparations, pretyped prescriptions save time and are legible.

Treatment of most of the common skin conditions is simpler to understand when the physician is aware of three basic principles:

1. The *type of skin lesion,* more than the cause, influences the kind of local medication used. The old adage, "If it's wet, dry it with a wet dressing, and if it's dry, wet it with an ointment," is true in most cases. For example, to treat a patient with an acute oozing, crusting dermatitis of the dorsum of the hand, whether due to poison ivy or soap, the physician should prescribe wet soaks. For a chronic-looking, dry, scaly patch of psoriasis on the elbow, an ointment is indicated because it holds moisture in the skin; an aqueous lotion or a wet dressing is more drying. Bear in mind, however, that the type of skin lesion can change rapidly under treatment. The patient must be followed closely after beginning therapy. An acute oozing dermatitis treated with water soaks can change, in 2 or 3 days, to a dry, scaly lesion that requires an ointment. Conversely, a chronic dry patch may become irritated with greasy ointment and begin to ooze.

2. The second basic principle in treatment is *first do no harm* and never overtreat. It is important for the physician to know which of the chemicals prescribed for local use on the skin are the greatest irritants and sensitizers. It is no exaggeration to say that a commonly seen dermatitis is *overtreatment contact dermatitis.* The overtreatment is often performed by the patient, who has gone to the neighborhood drugstore, or to a friend, and used any, and many, of the medications available for the treatment of skin diseases. It is

certainly not unusual to hear the patient tell of using an athlete's foot salve for the treatment of the lesions of pityriasis rosea.

3. The third principle is to *instruct the patient adequately regarding the application of the medicine prescribed.* The patient does not have to be told how to swallow a pill, but does have to be told how to put on a wet dressing. Most patients with skin disorders are ambulatory, so there is no nurse to help them; they are their own nurses. The success or the failure of therapy rests on adequate instruction of the patient or person responsible for the care. Even in hospitals, particularly when wet dressings or aqueous lotions are prescribed, it is wise for the physician to instruct the nurse regarding the procedure.

With these principles of management in mind, let us now turn to the medicine used. It is important to stress that we are endeavoring to present here only the most basic material necessary to treat most skin diseases. For instance, there are many solutions for wet dressings, but Domeboro solution is our preference. Other physicians have preferences different from the drugs listed, and their choices are respected, but to list all of them does not serve the purpose of this book.

Two factors have guided us in the selection of medications presented in this formulary. First, the medication must be readily available in most drugstores; second, it must be a very effective medication for one or several skin conditions. The medications listed in this formulary also are listed in a complete way in the treatment section concerning the particular disease. Instructions for more complete use of the medications, however, are as follow in this formulary.

Formulary

A particular topical medication is prescribed to produce a specific beneficial effect.

Effects of Locally Applied Drugs

Anesthetic agents are used in the skin to decrease pain when injections, laser, cryotherapy, electrolysis, excisions, or other procedures are performed. These include lidocaine hydrochloride 3% cream (LidaMantle), 30% to 40% lidocaine compounded in velvachol or acid mantle cream, EMLA cream or disc (2.5% lidocaine and 2.5% prilocaine), and ethyl chloride spray. Anesthetic agents for mucous membranes are used to temporarily ameliorate discomfort from mucous membrane diseases. They include viscous solution of lidocaine (2%), Hurricaine liquid or gel spray (20% benzocaine); for ophthalmic use, Alcaine solution (0.5% proparacaine) and Pontocaine (0.5% tetracaine).

Antipruritic agents relieve itching in various ways. Commonly used chemicals include menthol (0.25%), phenol (0.5%), camphor (2%), pramoxine hydrochloride (1%), and coal tar solution (liquor carbonis detergens [LCD]) (2% to 10%). These chemicals are added to various bases for the desired effect. Numerous safe and unsafe proprietary preparations for relief of itching are also available. The unsafe preparations are those that contain sensitizing antihistamines, benzocaine, and related -*caine* derivatives.

Keratoplastic agents tend to increase the thickness of the horny layer. Salicylic acid (1% to 2%) is an example of a keratoplastic or thicken the horny layer.

Keratolytics remove or soften the horny layer. Commonly used agents of this type include salicylic acid (4% [Salex Lotion and Cream] to 10%), resorcinol (2% to 4%), urea (20% to 50%), and sulfur (4% to 10%). A strong destructive agent is trichloroacetic acid. Urea in 5% to 10% concentration (Eucerin Plus Lotion and Carmol) is moisturizing, whereas in 20% to 50% (Vanamide, Keralac, Carmol) concentration, it is keratolytic. Alpha hydroxy acids (lactic acid [Lac-Hydrin 5% or 12% Cream and Lotion or Amlactin and Amlactin XL 12% Cream or Lotion]), which is sold over the counter, glycolic acid (Aqua Glycol is sold over the counter in various concentrations) in 5% to 12% concentrations are moisturizers, whereas in higher concentrations up to 80%, they are keratolytic and can be used in the office for facial peeling, with caution.

Antieczematous agents remove oozing and vesicular excretions by various actions. The common antieczematous agents include Domeboro solution packets or dissolvable tablets that are nonprescription, coal tar solution (2% to 5%), hydrocortisone 0.5% to 2% (0.5% and 1% are available without a prescription), and more potent corticosteroid derivatives incorporated in solutions, foams, and creams.

Antiparasitic agents destroy or inhibit living infestations. Examples include permethrin (Elimite or Actin) cream for scabies, γ-benzene hexachloride (Kwell) cream and lotion for scabies and pediculosis, crotamiton (Eurax) for scabies, and permethrin (Nix) for pediculosis. For scabies and lice, 10% sulfur can be mixed in petrolatum and is effective and very safe, even in infants and pregnant women, but is malodorous and stains.

Antiseptics destroy or inhibit bacteria, fungi, and viruses.

Antibacterial topical medications include gentamicin (Garamycin), mupirocin (Bactroban), bacitracin (recently found to cause a significant number of cases of contact dermatitis), Polysporin, and neomycin (Neosporin), which causes an appreciable (at least 1%) incidence of allergic contact sensitivity. Soaps can have extra antibacterial additives such as Lever 2000 and Cetaphil Antibacterial Soap.

Antifungal and *anticandidal topical agents* include miconazole (Micatin, Monistat-Derm), clotrimazole (Lotrimin, Mycelex), ciclopirox (Loprox), econazole (Spectazole), oxiconazole (Oxistat), naftifine (Naftin), ketoconazole (Nizoral), butenafine HCl (Mentax, Lotrimin Ultra), and terbinafine (Lamisil). Sulfur (3% to 10%) is an older but effective antifungal and anticandida agent (see Table 19-3). Nystatin is anticandida but not antifungal.

Antiviral topical agents are acyclovir (Zovirax) ointment or cream and penciclovir (Denavir).

Emollients soften and moisturize the skin surface. Nivea oil, mineral oil, and white petrolatum are good examples. Newer emollients are more cosmetically elegant and effective.

Ointments moisturize the skin. Examples include Vaseline Petroleum Jelly, Lanolin, Aquaphor, Cetaphil, and Eucerin.

Creams dry the skin but are more cosmetically acceptable than ointments because they do not feel greasy and do not leave oil marks on paper products. Examples are Dermovan and Acid Mantle Cream.

Types of Topical Dermatologic Medications

Baths

1. Tar bath

    Coal tar solution (USP, LCD)   120.0
    Or Cutar bath oil

    Sig: Add 2 tbsp to a tub of lukewarm water, 6 to 8 inches deep.
    Actions: Antipruritic and antieczematous

2. Starch bath

    Limit or Argo starch, small box
    Sig: Add half box of starch to tub of cool water, 6 to 8 inches deep.
    Actions: Soothing; antieczematous and antipruritic
    Indications: Generalized itching and urticaria

3. Aveeno (regular and oilated) colloidal oatmeal bath

    Sig: Add 1 cup to the tub of water.
    Actions: Soothing and cleansing
    Indications: Oilated for generalized itching and dryness of skin, winter and senile itch. The regular is for oozing draining wet dermatitis.

4. Oil baths (see section on oils and emulsions) for dry skin.

5. Bleach baths and compresses. For baths add 1 cup of bleach to full tub of water to soak for several minutes and as compresses 1 tablespoonful to 1 quart of water to use as compresses for several minutes b.i.d. to treat recurrent recalcitrant *Staphylococcus aureus* folliculitis.

Soaps and Shampoos

1. Dove soaps, Neutrogena soaps, Cetaphil, Basis

    Action: Mild cleansing agents
    Indications: Reduces dry skin or winter itch when substituted for irritating soaps

2. Dial soap, Lever 2000, Cetaphil Antibacterial Soap

    Actions: Cleansing and antibacterial
    Indications: Acne, pyodermas

3. Capex shampoo 120.0

    Sig: Shampoo as needed.
    Actions: Anti-inflammatory, antipruritic, and cleansing
    Indications: Dandruff, psoriasis of scalp
    Comment: Contains fluocinolone acetonide, 0.01%

4. Selsun Suspension or Head and Shoulders Intensive Treatment shampoo 120.0

    Sig: Shampoo hair with three separate applications and rinses. You can leave the last application on the scalp for 5 minutes before rinsing off. Do not use another shampoo as a final cleanser. Contains selenium sulfide.
    Actions: Cleansing and antiseborrheic
    Indications: Dandruff, itching scalp (not toxic if used as directed but poisonous if swallowed, so keep out of reach of small children).

SAUER'S NOTES

LOCALLY APPLIED GENERIC PRODUCTS

Advantages: Lower cost—you can prescribe a larger quantity at relatively less expense and patients appreciate your sharing their concern regarding cost.
Disadvantages: With a proprietary product, you are quite sure of the correct potency and bioavailability of the agent, you know the delivery system, and you know the ingredients in the base.

If you prescribe a proprietary medication when a less expensive generic is available, explain to the patient your reason for doing this.

5. Tar shampoos: Tarsum (can be applied overnight or for several hours as a scalp oil and then shampooed out), Polytar, T/Gel Regular and Maximum Strength, Pentrax, Ionil T, and so on

   Sig: Shampoo as necessary, even daily.
   Actions: Cleansing and antiseborrheic
   Indications: Dandruff, psoriasis, atopic eczema of scalp

6. Nizoral shampoo 120.0 or Loprox shampoo

   Sig: Shampoo two or three times a week.
   Actions: Anticandidal, antiseborrheic
   Indication: Dandruff, tinea versicolor, and to decrease spread of tinea capitis
   Comment: Nizoril is available as 1% over the counter or 2% as a prescription.

7. T-Sal and other salicylic acid shampoos.

   Indications: Treatment for psoriasis and seborrheic dermatitis

Wet Dressings or Soaks

1. Burow's solution, 1:20

   Sig: Add 1 Domeboro tablet or packet to 1 pint of tap water. Cover affected area with sheeting wet with solution and tie on with gauze bandage or string. Do not allow any wet dressing to dry out. It can also be used as a solution for soaks.
   Actions: Acidifying, antieczematous, and antiseptic
   Indications: Oozing, vesicular skin conditions

2. Vinegar solution

   Sig: Add ½ cup of white vinegar to 1 quart of water for wet dressings or soaks, as above.
   Indications: Antieczematous, anti-yeast, antifungal, antibacterial including antipseudomonas

3. Salt solution

   Sig: Add 1 tbsp of salt to 1 quart of water for wet dressings or soaks, as above.
   Indications: Antieczematous, cleansing

Powders

1. Purified talc (USP) or Zeasorb-AF powder 60 (contains miconazole)

   Sig: Dust on locally b.i.d. (supply in a powder can)
   Actions: Absorbent, protective, and cooling
   Indications: Intertrigo, diaper dermatitis

2. Tinactin powder, Micatin powder, Zeasorb-AF powder, or Desenex powder

   Sig: Dust on feet in morning
   Actions: Absorbent antifungal and anti-yeast

   Indications: Prevention and treatment of tinea pedis and tinea cruris as well as candida intertrigo
   Comment: These powders are available over the counter.

3. Mycostatin powder 15.0

   Sig: Dust on locally b.i.d.
   Action: Anticandida
   Indication: Candida intertrigo

Shake Lotions

1. Calamine lotion (USP) 120

   Sig: Apply locally to affected area t.i.d. with fingers or brush.
   Actions: Antipruritic, antieczematous
   Indications: Widespread, mildly oozing, inflamed dermatoses

2. Nonalcoholic white shake lotion

   a. Zinc oxide 24.0
   b. Talc 24.0
   c. Glycerin 12.0
   d. Distilled water q.s. ad 120.0

3. Alcoholic white shake lotion

   a. Zinc oxide 24.0
   b. Talc 24.0
   c. Glycerin 12.0
   d. Distilled water q.s. ad 120.0

4. Proprietary lotions

   a. Sarna lotion (with menthol and camphor)
   b. Cetaphil lotion
   c. Aveeno Anti-itch lotion (contains pramoxine)

Oils and Emulsions

1. Zinc oxide, 40%

   Olive oil q.s. 120.0

   Sig: Apply locally to affected area by hand or brush t.i.d.
   Actions: Soothing, antipruritic, astringent
   Indications: Acute and subacute eczematous eruptions

SAUER'S NOTES

1. Shake lotions 2, 3, and 4 are listed for physicians who desire specially compounded lotions. One or two pharmacists near your office will be glad to compound them and keep them on hand.
2. To these lotions you can add sulfur, resorcinol, menthol, phenol, and so on, as indicated.

2. *Bath oils*

Nivea skin oil, Alpha-Keri, Cutar Bath Oil (contains tar)
Sig: Add 1 to 2 tbsp to a tub of water. *Caution:* Avoid slipping in tub.
Actions: Emollient, lubricant
Indications: Winter itch, dry skin, atopic eczema

3. *Hand and body emulsions:* A multitude of products are available over the counter. Some have petrolatum or phospholipids (Moisturel), some have urea or alpha hydroxy acids (Curel), and some are lanolin free. Examples are Curel, Nivea, Eucerin, Cetaphil, Neutrogena Norwegian Hand Formula, SBR Lipocream, Lac-Hydrin Lotion 5% and 12% Cream and Lotion (the 12% is a prescription), and Amlactin 12% Cream and Lotion.

Sig: Apply locally as necessary.
Actions: Emollient, lubricant
Indications: Dry skin, winter itch, atopic eczema

4. *Scalp oil*

Derma-Smoothe FS oil (fluocinolone acetonide 0.01%) 120.0
Sig: Moisten scalp hair and apply lotion overnight; wear a plastic cap
Indications: Scalp psoriasis, lichen simplex chronicus, severe seborrheic dermatitis

Tinctures and Aqueous Solutions

1. Povidone–iodine (Betadine) solution (also in skin cleanser, shampoo, and ointment) 15

Sig: Apply with swab t.i.d.
Actions: Antibacterial, antifungal, antiviral
Indication: General antisepsis

2. *Gentian violet solution*

Gentian violet, 1%
Distilled water q.s. 30.0
Sig: Apply with swab b.i.d.
Actions: Antifungal, antibacterial
Indications: Candidiasis, leg ulcers

3. *Antifungal solutions*

a. Lotrimin, Mycelex, Loprox, Tinactin, Micatin, Monistat-Derm, and Lamisil spray, among others 30.0

Sig: Apply locally b.i.d.
b. Fungi-Nail 30.0

Sig: Apply locally b.i.d.
Comment: Contains resorcinol, salicylic acid, parachlorometaxylenol, and benzocaine in a base with acetic acid and alcohol

c. Penlac nail lacquer

Sig: Apply thin coat two times a week; contains ciclopirox

d. Castellanti's paint (can get as uncolored): Used for intertrigo

Pastes

1. Zinc oxide paste (USP)

Sig: Apply locally b.i.d.
Actions: Protective, absorbent, astringent
Indications: Localized crusted or scaly dermatoses

Creams and Ointments

A physician can write prescriptions for creams and ointments in two ways: (1) by prescribing proprietary creams and ointments already compounded by pharmaceutical companies or (2) by formulating one's own prescriptions by adding medications to certain bases, as indicated for the particular patient being treated. For the physician who uses the second method, two different types of bases are used:

1. *Water-washable cream bases:* These bases are pleasant for the patient to use, nongreasy, and almost always indicated when treating intertriginous and hairy areas. Their disadvantage is that they can be too drying. A number of medications, as specifically indicated, can be added to these bases (i.e., menthol, sulfur, tars, hydrocortisone, and triamcinolone).

a. Unibase
b. Vanicream
c. Acid Mantle Creme
d. Dermovan
e. Unscented cold cream (not water washable)

2. *Ointment bases:* These petroleum jelly–type bases are, and should be, the most useful in dermatology. Although not as pleasant for the patient to use as the

---

SAUER'S NOTES

1. Over-the-counter 0.5% or 1.0% Cortaid has proved effective and well tolerated as an emergency nonprescription treatment.

2. Do not use group I topical agents for longer than 2 weeks, or more than a 45-g tube per week. A rest period must follow for 2 weeks.

3. Do not overuse the more potent topical steroids because of possible side effects.

SAUER'S NOTES

COMPOUND PREPARATIONS

Compound proprietary preparations are frequently prescribed, particularly by family practice physicians and nondermatologic specialists. Physicians should know the ingredients in these compound preparations and should know the side effects. Here are some popular compounds:

Mycolog II cream: Contains Nystatin and triamcinolone. *Beware:* It is not beneficial for fungus (tinea) infections; the triamcinolone after long-term use can cause atrophy, striae, and telangiectasia of the skin, especially in intertriginous areas and on the face.

Lotrisone cream: Contains clotrimazole and betamethasone dipropionate. *Beware:* The betamethasone with long-term use can cause atrophy, striae, and dilated vessels especially in intertriginous areas and on the face. It also can have significant enough absorption to cause systemic corticosteroid side effects.

Iodoquinol–hydrocortisone cream (Vytone): Contains iodoquin plus 1% hydrocortisone. *Beware:* The iodoquin causes a moderate yellow stain on skin and clothing.

Cortisporin ointment: Contains 1% hydrocortisone with Neosporin, Polysporin, and bacitracin. *Beware:* Neomycin allergies can occur infrequently and bacitracin has now also become a significant allergen.

---

cream bases, their greasy quality alleviates dryness, removes scales, and enables the medicaments to better penetrate skin lesions. Disadvantages are that it can flare or cause folliculitis, acne, or rosacea and it is less cosmetically acceptable because of the greasy feel. Any local medicine can be incorporated into these bases.

a. White petrolatum (USP)
b. Zinc oxide ointment (USP)
c. Aquaphor (contains lanolin)
d. Eucerin (contains lanolin)

For the physician who wishes to prescribe ready-made, proprietary preparations, these are listed in groups:

3. *Antifungal ointments and creams:* Lotrimin cream, Lotrimin Ultra Cream, Mycelex cream, Spectazole cream, Loprox cream, Tinactin cream, Lamisil cream, Oxistat cream, Naftin cream, Nizoral cream, Mentax cream, and others (see Table 25-3)

   Action: Antifungal

4. *Antibiotic ointments and creams:* Bactroban ointment (can get a generic) and cream, gentamicin ointment and cream, Neosporin ointment, Mycitracin ointment,

Polysporin ointment (antibiotic solutions are discussed in Chapter 13 under Acne Therapy)

5. *Antiviral ointments for herpes simplex virus infections:* acyclovir ointment and penciclovir cream

6. *Corticosteroid ointments and creams* (Table 5-1)

   a. Hydrocortisone preparations (0.5% and 1% hydrocortisone creams and ointments are available over the counter and generically)

      ■ Hytone 1% and 2.5% cream and ointment

   b. Desonide preparations (can be written generically)

      ■ Tridesilon cream and ointment
      ■ DesOwen cream and ointment

   c. Triamcinolone preparations (0.5%, 0.1%, 0.025%, 0.01%)

      ■ Kenalog ointment and cream
      ■ Aristocort ointment and creams
      ■ Also available generically

   d. Other fluorinated corticosteroid preparations (see Table 5-1 for a listing of these preparations, which are ranked according to potency)

7. *Corticosteroid antibiotic ointments and creams:* Cortisporin ointment

8. *Corticosteroid antifungal–antiyeast preparations*

   a. Lotrisone (anticandidal and antifungal), contains betamethasone and clotrimazole
   b. Mycolog II cream and ointment (anticandida), contains triamcinolone and nystatin; generic unavailable

9. *Antipruritic creams and lotions*

   a. Eurax cream
   b. Sarna lotion
   c. Prax lotion
   d. PramaGel
   e. Doxepin (Zonalon) cream (may cause drowsiness)
   f. Aveeno Anti-itch Lotion
   g. Eucerin Calming Cream
   h. Eucerin anti-itch spray

10. *Retinoic acid products*

    a. Retin-A cream (0.025%, 0.05%, 0.1%) and Retin-A gel (0.01% and 0.025%), Retin-A Micro (0.04% and 0.1%) and Renova (0.02% and 0.05%)

       Actions: Antiacne comedones and small pustules (especially the gel) and antiphotoaging

       Indications: Acne of comedonal and small pustular type; aging wrinkles on face; removal of mild actinic keratoses and prevention of actinic keratoses, and treatment of freckles, molluscum contagiosum, and flat warts

TABLE 5-1 ■ Potency Ranking of Some Commonly Used Topical Corticosteroids*

Group I

Cordran tape
Diprolene AF cream 0.05%
Diprolene ointment 0.05%
Diprolene gel 0.05%
Psorcon cream 0.05%
Psorcon ointment 0.05%
Temovate cream 0.05%
Temovate ointment 0.05%
Temovate gel 0.05%
Temovate emollient 0.05%
Temovate solution 0.05%
Ultravate cream 0.05%
Ultravate ointment 0.05%

Group II

Cyclocort ointment 0.1%
Diprolene AF cream 0.05%
Diprosone ointment 0.05%
Halog cream 0.1%
Halog ointment 0.1%
Halog solution 0.1%
Halog-E cream 0.1%
Lidex cream 0.05%
Lidex gel 0.05%
Lidex ointment 0.05%
Lidex solution 0.05%
Maxiflor ointment 0.05%
Topicort cream 0.25%
Topicort gel 0.05%
Topicort ointment 0.25%

Group III

Aristocort cream 0.5%
Aristocort ointment 0.5%
Aristocort A cream 0.5%
Aristocort A ointment 0.5%
Betamethasone ointment 0.1%
Cutivate ointment 0.005%
Cyclocort lotion 0.1%
Diprosone cream 0.05%
Elocon ointment 0.1%
Kenalog cream 0.5%
Kenalog ointment 0.5%
Maxiflor cream 0.05%
Topicort LP cream 0.5%

Group IV

Aristocort ointment 0.1%
Cordran ointment 0.05%
Cyclocort cream 0.1%
Desonide ointment 0.2%
Elocon cream 0.1%
Elocon lotion 0.1%
Fluocinolone ointment 0.025%
Fluocinolone cream 0.2%
Halog cream 0.025%
Halog ointment 0.025%
Kenalog cream 0.1%
Kenalog ointment 0.1%

Group V

Aristocort cream 0.1%
Betamethasone valerate cream 0.1%
Betamethasone valerate lotion 0.1%
Cloderm cream 0.1%
Cordran cream 0.05%
Cordran lotion 0.5%
Cordran ointment 0.025%
Cutivate cream 0.1%
Dermatop cream 0.1%
DesOwen ointment 0.05%
Fluocinolone cream 0.025%
Kenalog cream 0.1%
Kenalog lotion 0.1%
Kenalog ointment 0.025%
Locoid cream 0.1%
Locoid ointment 0.1%
Tridesilon ointment 0.05%

Group VI

Aclovate cream 0.05%
Aclovate ointment 0.05%
Aristocort cream 0.1%
Betamethasone valerate 0.1%
DesOwen cream 0.05%
DesOwen ointment 0.05%
DesOwen lotion 0.05%
Fluocinolone cream 0.01%
Fluocinolone solution 0.01%
Kenalog cream 0.025%
Kenalog lotion 0.025%
Locoid solution 0.1%
Tridesilon cream 0.05%

Group VII

Epifoam 1.0%
Fluocinolone cream 1.0%, 2.5%
Hydrocortisone cream 1.0%, 2.5%
Hydrocortisone lotion 1.0%, 2.5%

*Group I is the superpotency category. Potency descends with each group, to group VII, which is the least potent (groups II and III are potent corticosteroids; IV and V are midstrength corticosteroids; VI and VII are mild corticosteroids). There is no significant difference between agents within groups II through VII. The compounds are arranged alphabetically within the groups. In group I, Temovate cream or ointment is most potent. *(Courtesy of the late Dr. Richard B. Stoughton and Dr. Roger C. Cornell.)*

b. Differin (Adapalene gel and cream 0.1%)

Action: Retinoic acid receptor binder
Indications: Acne of comedonal and small pustular type.

c. Avita (tretinoin 0.025%) cream

Action: Antiacne
Indications: Acne of comedonal and small pustular type.

11. *Miscellaneous creams, ointments, and gels*

a. MetroGel (metronidazole 0.75%) 15.0

Noritate Cream (metronidazole 1%) 30.0
Indications: Rosacea, perioral dermatitis

b. Dovonex ointment (also comes as cream and scalp solution) 30.0 or 100.0

Action: Antipsoriatic
Comment: Moderately expensive

c. Tazorac gel or cream (tazarotene) 0.05% and 0.1%

Action: Antipsoriatic, antiacne, antiphotoaging; actinic keratosis and skin cancer preventative
Comment: Very expensive; may be irritating; contraindicated in women with childbearing potential

12. *Scabicidal and pediculicidal preparations*

a. Eurax cream and lotion

Action: Scabicidal

b. Kwell (lindane) lotion and cream

Actions: Scabicidal and pediculicidal

c. Elimite or Actin cream

Action: Scabicidal

d. Nix creme rinse

Indications: Head lice, nits

e. Ovide (malathion) topical

Action: Pediculicidal
Indications: Head lice, nits

f. Ivermectin oral

Action: Scabicidal
Indications: Scabies

13. *Sunscreen creams and lotions:* Para-aminobenzoic acid (and the esters of PABA), octyl dimethyl PABA (padimate O), octocrylene, octyl salicylate, methylanthranilate, avobenzone (Parsol 1789), cinnamates (octylmethoxycinnamate), oxybenzone (benzophenone-3) are effective ultraviolet light absorbers. Zinc oxide and titanium oxide are light blockers. There are many products on the market. Any sunscreen with a sun protective factor (SPF) of 30 or above offers effective sun-damage protection against short wavelength ultraviolet light or UVB (290 to 310 nm), if used correctly. There is no equivalent sun protective factor number in the United States for long wavelength ultraviolet light or UVA, which is also important in photoaging, development of skin precancers and skin cancers, lupus erythematosus, porphyrias, and usually the most important wavelength for photoallergic reactions. Therefore, titanium dioxide, zinc oxide or avobenzone needs to be present to appropriately block out UVA. Outside of the United States many authorities think that Mexoryl XL is the best and most complete sunscreen for protection from UVA.

Sig: Apply to exposed areas before going outside. This should be done at least ½ hour in advance for the best effect. Reapplication is important if exposure to water or significant sweating occurs. After 1 hour reapplication is advisable. Too thin of an application is a common mistake.

Action: Screening out ultraviolet rays
Indications: Polymorphous light eruption, photoaging, systemic and chronic lupus erythematosus, some cases of dermatomyositis, photoallergy from systemic or topical medications, some types of porphyria and prevention of skin precancers and skin cancers especially in light-complexioned people

Aerosols and Foams

Various local medications have been incorporated in aerosol and foam-producing containers. These include corticosteroids (Olux Foam, Luxiq Foam), antibiotics (Evoclin Foam), antiacne agents (Ovace Foam), antirosacea agents (Ovace Foam), antifungal agents (Lamisil Spray), antipruritic medicines (Eucerin Spray), and so on.

Kenalog spray (63-g can) and Diprosone aerosol are effective corticosteroid preparations for scalp psoriasis and seborrhea.

Triamcinolone (Luxiq) and clobetasol (Olux) are corticosteroid foams and Ovace foam is sodium sulfacetamide foam used for seborrhea, acne, and rosacea. Evoclin is erythromycin foam used to treat acne.

Corticosteroid Medicated Tape

1. Cordran tape (also comes as a patch)

Indications: Small areas of psoriasis, neurodermatitis, lichen planus

Medicated Skin Patches

Several are available for transdermal delivery of such agents as nitroglycerin, EMLA patch, and lidocaine patch for topical anesthesia, nicotine antismoking patches, and hormones.

Fluorouracil Preparations and Imiquimod

Imiquimod (Aldara) is used topically for superficial basal cell cancers, actinic keratoses, molluscum contagiosum, genital warts, and other warts under occlusion. It is being used experimentally for other skin diseases such as Bowen's disease and lentigo maligna melanoma. Other indications may well become approved with more experience with this topical medication. See section on actinic keratosis therapy in Chapter 26 and wart therapy.

Local Agents for Office Use

1. Podophyllum in cpd. tincture benzoin

   Podophyllum resin (USP) 25%
   Cpd. tct. benzoin q.s. ad 30.0
   Sig: Apply small amount to warts with cotton-tipped applicator every 4 or 5 days until warts are gone. Excess amount may be washed off in 3 to 6 hours after application to prevent irritation.
   Action: Removal of venereal warts
   Comment: Other podophyllum proprietary preparations such as podofilox (Condylox) are marketed.

2. Trichloroacetic acid solution (saturated) or bichloracetic acid

   Sig: Apply with caution with cotton-tipped applicator (have water handy to neutralize within a few seconds).
   Indications: Warts on children, seborrheic keratoses, xanthelasma, sebaceous hyperplasia

3. Modified Unna's boot

   a. Dome-Paste Bandage
   b. Gelocast
   c. Compression gelatin bandage with zinc oxide and glycerin then wrapped with Coflex flexible wrap
      Indications: Stasis ulcers, localized neurodermatitis (lichen simplex)

4. Ace bandage, 3 or 4 inches wide

   Indications: Stasis dermatitis, leg edema

Local Therapy Rules of Thumb

Students and general practitioners state that they are especially confused by dermatologists' reasons for using one

---

SAUER'S NOTES

1. You can compound preparations with LCD, sulfur, resorcinol, and salicylic acid.
2. These chemicals can be used to complement the corticosteroids in a mixture.
3. When prescribing one of these chemicals, always begin with the lower percentage of the drug. Increase the percentage only when a stronger action is desired and no irritation has occurred with the concentration already tried.
4. I am quite aware of the arguments against the use of pharmacy-compounded prescriptions. They have worked exceptionally well for me and for my patients.

---

chemical for one skin lesion and not another or one chemical for unrelated skin diseases. The answer to this dilemma is not easily given. More often than not, the major reason for our preference is that experience has taught us and those before us that the particular drug works. Some drugs do have definite chemical actions, such as anti-inflammatory, antipruritic, antifungal, or keratolytic actions, and these have been listed in the formulary. But there is no definite scientific explanation for the beneficial effect of some of the other drugs, such as tar or sulfur on cases of psoriasis.

In an attempt to solve this apparent confusion, here are some generalizations summarizing our experience.

Tars (coal tar solution [LCD], 3% to 10%; crude coal tar, 1% to 5%; anthralin, 0.1% to 1%).

Consider for use in cases of:

  Atopic eczema
  Psoriasis
  Seborrheic dermatitis
  Lichen simplex chronicus
  Avoid in intertriginous areas (can cause a folliculitis and irritation).

Sulfur (sulfur, precipitated, 3% to 10%)

Consider for use in cases of:

  Tinea of any area of body
  Acne vulgaris and rosacea
  Seborrheic dermatitis
  Pyodermas (combine with antibiotic salves)
  Psoriasis
  Insect bites in children

Resorcinol (Resorcinol Monoacetate, 1% to 5%)

Consider for use in cases of:

> Acne vulgaris and rosacea (usually with sulfur)
> Seborrheic dermatitis
> Psoriasis

Salicylic Acid (1% to 5%, Higher with Caution)

Consider for use in cases of:

> Psoriasis
> Lichen simplex chronicus, localized thick form
> Tinea of feet or palms (when peeling is desired)
> Seborrheic dermatitis

Avoid use in intertriginous areas.

Menthol (.25%); Phenol (.5% to 2%); Camphor (1% to 2%)

Consider for use in any pruritic dermatoses. Avoid use over large areas of body.

Hydrocortisone and Related Corticosteroids (Hydrocortisone Powder) (0.5% to 2%) and Triamcinolone (0.1%, 0.025% and 0.01%)

Consider for use in cases of:

> Contact dermatitis of any area
> Seborrheic dermatitis
> Intertrigo of axillary, crural, or inframammary regions
> Atopic eczema
> Lichen simplex chronicus

Avoid use over large areas of body and for prolonged periods.

Fluorinated Corticosteroids Locally

These chemicals are not readily available as powders for personal compounding, but triamcinolone, fluocinolone, and others are available as generic creams and ointments. Consider for use with or without occlusive dressings, in cases of:

> Psoriasis, localized to small area (see Chap. 14)
> Lichen simplex chronicus (see Chap. 11)
> Lichen planus, especially hypertrophic type

Also anywhere that hydrocortisone is indicated but limit duration of therapy. Avoid use over large areas of the body. Class I topical corticosteroids should be used for no more than 14 consecutive days.

SAUER'S NOTES

LOCAL CORTICOSTEROID THERAPY

1. Avoid prescribing strong local corticosteroid preparations for generalized body use.
2. Do not prescribe the most potent ("biggest-gun") corticosteroid therapy on the initial visit.
3. The fluorinated corticosteroids should not be used on the face and intertriginous areas, where long-term use can result in atrophy and telangiectasia of the skin. There are exceptions.
4. The potent corticosteroids can have a definite systemic effect.
5. Fluorinated corticosteroid prescriptions rarely should be written for p.r.n. refills.
6. Continued long-term use of a local corticosteroid can result in a diminished effectiveness (tachyphylaxis).
7. The pros and cons of prescribing generic corticosteroids are discussed early in this chapter.

Quantity of Cream or Ointment to Prescribe

Several factors influence any general statements about dosage: the severity of the dermatosis, whether it is acute or chronic dermatosis, the base of the product (a petrolatum-based ointment spreads over the skin farther than a cream and is more moisturizing), whether it is dispensed in a tube or jar (patients use less from tubes), and the intelligence of the patient.

- 15 g of a cream used b.i.d. treats a mild hand dermatosis for 10 to 14 days.
- 30 g of a cream used b.i.d. treats an arm for 14 days.
- 60 g of a cream used b.i.d. treats a leg for 14 days.
- 480 to 960 g or 1 to 2 lb of a cream used b.i.d. treats the entire body for 14 days. This is seldom a practical prescription, but unmedicated white petrolatum or a cream base is economical to use over a large surface area. Other therapeutic agents should be used to make the dermatoses less extensive (i.e., internal corticosteroids).

Specific Internal Drugs for Specific Diseases

As in all fields of medicine, certain diseases can be treated best by certain specific systemic drugs. These drugs may not be curative, but they should be considered when beginning to outline a course of management for a particular patient. Many factors influence the decision to use or not

SAUER'S NOTES

1. There are potential side effects from any systemic therapy. Be aware of these possible reactions by being knowledgeable concerning every drug you prescribe.
2. The risk/benefit ratio for your patient must always be considered.
3. Be aware of cross-reactions with a patient on multiple medications.

use such a specific drug. Here follows a list of skin diseases and some systemic medicines considered specific (or as specific as possible) for the disease. For proper dosage and contraindications, check the appropriate sections in this book or in current books on therapy.

- *Acne vulgaris or rosacea in the scarring or severe stage:* antibiotics, Nicomide and in women spironolactone and birth control pills. For severe cases of cystic acne in men or women without indication of or risk of pregnancy, isotretinoin (Accutane) is indicated.
- *Acquired immunodeficiency syndrome (AIDS):* Many systemic drugs are used, directed as specifically as possible against opportunistic organisms, tumors, and the human immunodeficiency virus. Highly active antiretroviral therapy (HAART) is the most effective therapeutic regimen for AIDS. Because of its expense, only 10% of HIV-infected patients worldwide are treated with HAART. This is a critical problem on the African continent.
- *Alopecia areata:* corticosteroids in any of four forms—topical, intralesional, or rarely parenteral or oral. Topical dinitrochlorobenzene (DNCB) sensitization.
- *Atrophie blanche vasculitis:* pentoxifylline (Trental), anticoagulants such as aspirin, clopidogrel (Plavix), dipyridamole (Persantine), and less commonly warfarin (Coumadin).
- *Bullous pemphigoid:* systemic and group I topical corticosteroids, tetracycline in combination with niacinamide, dapsone, methotrexate, azathioprine, intravenous immunglobulin, other immunosuppressives.
- *Creeping eruption:* thiabendazole, topical or oral.
- *Darier's disease:* vitamin A, for controlled periods of time, and possibly isotretinoin, acitretin.
- *Dermatitis herpetiformis:* dapsone and sulfapyridine.
- *Granuloma annulare:* intralesional corticosteroids.

- *Herpes simplex:* acyclovir (Zovirax) topical, oral, or intravenous; famciclovir oral (Famvir), valacyclovir oral (Valtrex), foscarnet sodium intravenous (Foscavir). Suppressive therapy for 1 year is advocated by some to reduce diseases severity and transmission. Foscarnet can be used intravenously for resistant cases.
- *Herpes zoster:* acyclovir oral or intravenous, famciclovir oral, and valacyclovir oral.
- *Kawasaki's syndrome:* intravenous γ-globulin and aspirin.
- *Keloids:* intralesional corticosteroids, 585-nm pulsed dye laser, 30-second liquid nitrogen cryosurgery and silicon gel sheets for 12 to 24 hours each day for at least 2 months.
- *Lichen simplex chronicus:* intralesional corticosteroids, topical corticosteroids with or without occlusion.
- *Lupus erythematosus:* for systemic lupus erythematosus, use corticosteroids or immunosuppressive agents with care; for discoid form, use topical and intralesional corticosteroids and hydroxychloroquine or related antimalarials (beware of eye damage).
- *Mycosis fungoides* (T-helper–cell lymphoma or cutaneous T-cell lymphoma): psoralens and ultraviolet light (PUVA), narrow band UVB, corticosteroids, antimetabolites, retinoids (bexarotene [Targretin]), denileukin deftitox (for CD25-positive tumors), topical nitrogen mustard, topical bischloroethylnitrosourea (BCNU), electron beam, extracorporeal photophoresis, bone marrow transplant (for end-stage disease when all other therapy has failed), and α_{2b}-interferon.
- *Necrobiosis lipoidica diabeticorum:* topical and intralesional corticosteroids.
- *Pemphigus:* corticosteroids systemically, cyclosporine, intravenous immunoglobulin, and antimetabolites.
- *Pruritus from many causes:* antihistamines (topical and oral) and tranquilizer-like drugs. Doxepin (Zonalon) cream may be beneficial, but can cause drowsiness when used over large areas. Selected cases can be treated with oral corticosteroids.
- *Psoriasis, localized:* intralesional and topical corticosteroids, tar, dovonex (Calcipotriene) especially in combination with topical corticosteroids. Occasionally oral antibiotics such as sulfasalazine or tetracycline, or oral antiyeast medications such as ketoconazole.

- *Psoriasis, severe:* corticosteroids topically, PUVA, methotrexate, cyclosporine (Neoral), and, in men or postmenopausal or sterile women acitretin (Soriatane). A whole new class of drugs called *biologicals* is now available. These include infliximab (Remicade) intravenously, etanercept (Enbrel) subcutaneously, efalizumab (Raptiva) subcutaneously, and alefacept (Amevive) intramuscularly. Etanercept and infliximab are especially helpful in patients with accompanying psoriatic arthritis. Humira subcutaneously is approved for psoriatic arthritis and is expected to be approved for psoriasis.
- *Pyodermas of skin:* systemic antibiotics are valuable, when indicated.
- *Sarcoidosis:* topical, intralesional and systemic corticosteroids; antimalarials; and, when severe and recalcitrant, methotrexate. Early reports with infliximab and related tumor necrosis factor-α blockers have been promising.
- *Sporotrichosis:* saturated aqueous solution of potassium iodide orally and ketoconazole orally.
- *Syphilis:* penicillin or other antibiotics.
- *Tinea of scalp, body, crural area, nails:* topical imidazole, ciclopirox or allylamine; or orally griseofulvin and, for selected cases orally, ketoconazole, itraconazole (Sporanox) or terbinafine hydrochloride (Lamisil).
- *Tuberculosis of the skin:* dihydrostreptomycin, isoniazid, *p*-aminosalicylic acid, and rifampin.
- *Urticaria:* oral antihistamines, oral corticosteroids and, when severe, intramuscular and intravenous corticosteroids. When associated with other signs of anaphylaxis, such as shortness of breath, subcutaneous epinephrine (this can be used by patients in an emergency as EpiPen).

Suggested Reading

Arndt KA, Bowers KE. Manual of dermatologic therapeutics, ed 6. Philadelphia, Lippincott Williams & Wilkins, 2002.

Bronaugh RL, Maibach HI. Topical absorption of dermatological products. New York, Marcel Dekker, 2002.

Drake LA, Dinehart SM, Farmer ER, et al. Guidelines of care for the use of topical glucocorticosteroids. J Am Acad Dermatol 1996;35:615.

el-Azhary RA. Azathioprine: Current status and future considerations. Int J Dermatol 2003;42,335–341.

Katz HI. Dermatologist's guide to adverse therapeutic interactions. Philadelphia, Lippincott–Raven, 1997.

Lebwohl MG, Heymann WR, et al. Treatment of skin disease: Comprehensive Therapeutic Strategies. St. Louis, Mosby, 2002.

Levine N, Levin CC. Dermatology therapy: A to Z essentials. New York, Springer, 2004.

Olsen EA. A double-blind controlled comparison of generic and trade-name topical steroids using the vasoconstriction assay. Arch Dermatol 1991;127:197.

Physician's Desk Reference. Oradell, NJ, Medical Economics, 2005.

Scheman AJ, Severson DL. Pocket guide to medications used in dermatology, ed 8. Philadelphia, Lippincott Williams & Wilkins, 2003.

Shelley WB, Shelley ED. Advanced dermatologic therapy II. Philadelphia, WB Saunders, 2001.

Wakelin SH. Handbook of systemic drug treatment in dermatology. London, Manson Publishing, 2002.

Wolverton SE. Comprehensive dermatologic drug therapy. Philadelphia, WB Saunders, 2001.

CHAPTER 6

Physical Dermatologic Therapy

Frank Custer Koranda, MD, MBA

The therapeutic options of dermatologists have widely expanded with advances in technology. Most of these technologies can be employed in an office setting. Some of the more common technologic applications include lasers, intense pulsed light (IPL), photodynamic therapy (PDT), radiofrequency devices, liposuction, lipotransfer, fat autograft muscle injection (FAMI), Botox, tissue fillers, and augmentation.

Lasers

Laser is an acronym for light (L) amplification (A) by the stimulated (S) emission (E) of radiation (R). The characteristics of laser light are that the light is monochromatic (a single wavelength), it is collimated (the rays are parallel or nondivergent), and it is coherent (the rays are in phase so that they can pass over distances without loss of energy).

Carbon Dioxide Laser

When laser light contacts the skin, the light energy is absorbed. The energy causes thermal coagulation or with greater energy, tissue vaporization. The carbon dioxide (CO_2) laser has a wavelength of 1600 nm in the midinfrared spectrum, which is invisible. The CO_2 laser light is absorbed by the water in the tissue. It is an ablative laser causing damage to all tissue because the water content is the laser target. When the CO_2 laser is used in a focused mode, it can be used as a cutting instrument with a width of 0.2 mm as compared with the 0.25 mm width of a #15 scalpel blade. As the CO_2 laser cuts, it vaporizes the tissue. In a defocused mode, the CO_2 laser effect is that of tissue coagulation and in this mode it can seal blood vessels 0.5 mm or smaller in diameter. The CO_2 laser produces thermal damage, which can spread beyond the target tissue.

The depth of penetration of the CO_2 laser is controlled by the power output measured in watts and by the time on target. *Fluence* is the measurement of the energy density to the target and is expressed as joules per square centimeter.

Because the CO_2 laser is invisible, it is coupled and coaxially aligned with a low-power laser in the visible spectrum that serves as the aiming device. The helium neon aiming laser usually produces a red light.

The initial CO_2 lasers were of a continuous wave output unless deactivated by the foot control. In the early 1990s, pulsed focused CO_2 lasers were introduced. The concept of pulsing the laser was to decrease thermal damage to surrounding, nontarget skin. The initial pulsed CO_2 lasers were of 0.1 to 1.0 second in duration. To further reduce thermal transfer, ultrapulsed CO_2 lasers were developed to deliver high-energy output over a very short duration. The Coherent Ultrapulsed CO_2 laser can deliver 250 to 500 watts of power over a less than 1 millisecond pulse.

The ultrapulsed laser reduces tissue damage by timing the pulse duration to approximate the tissues' thermal relaxation time, that is, the time for a tissue to significantly cool by heat conduction. The principles of selective photothermolysis apply to most lasers: first, there is selective absorption of the laser energy or light by the target tissue; second, by the use of a brief pulse at high enough power, effective energy may be transmitted to the target with limited heat dispersal beyond the target. The CO_2 laser is used for a wide variety of treatments and conditions:

- resurfacing of the face for rejuvenation of the skin and reduction of wrinkles;
- vaporization of actinic cheilitis;
- planing for rhinophyma (Figure 6-1), angiofibromas of tuberous sclerosis, sebaceous hyperplasia;
- removal of common warts and condylomata accuminatum;
- removal of keloids and hypertrophic scars (Figure 6-2); and
- incisional surgery requiring more precision and when hemostasis by methods other than electrocoagulation is needed.

These examples are a limited list of the applications of the CO_2 laser.

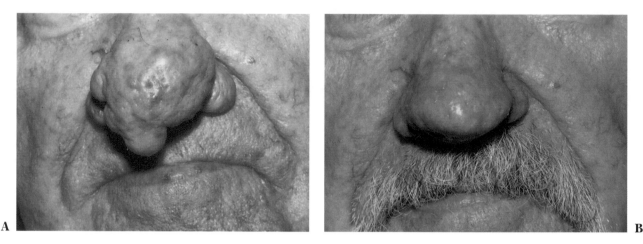

FIGURE 6-1. ■ Rhinophyma before (**A**) and after (**B**) nasal planing with the Coherent CO_2 Ultrapulsed laser.

The CO_2 laser was one of the first lasers to have been widely employed for a variety of cutaneous conditions. Today there are hosts of other lasers with different wavelength outputs and other varied characteristics such as pulsed modes, pulse durations, and pulsed repetitions power. These lasers have different uses depending on the absorption spectrum of the target tissues. The wavelength of the laser is matched to the absorption peaks of the target tissues.

These lasers have wavelengths in the visible (400 to 700 nm) to the near infrared (700 to 1200 nm) spectrums. In general, as the wavelength of the light increases, the depth of penetration into the skin increases and so does the depth at which the energy is absorbed. In addition to identifying the absorption spectrum of the targeted structure, the depth of the structure in the skin also influences the selection of a laser with the appropriate wavelength output. The wavelength must also be different from the absorption peaks of any intervening tissue, which could absorb the laser light before it reaches its target tissue.

Visible light is the spectrum in which lies the absorption of melanin, hemoglobin, oxyhemoglobin, and tattoo inks. Beside utilizing the principles of selective photothermolysis, the tissue overlying the target is often additionally protected with cooling cryogen sprays or other cooling devices just prior to firing the laser.

Pulsed Dye, Nd:Yag, Q-Switched, and Diode Lasers

The pulsed dye laser usually with a 585-nm wavelength and a 450-microsecond or 0.45-millisecond pulse has been used extensively for congenital hemangiomas, particularly port wine stains (Figure 6-3). Multiple treatments, sometimes more than 20, are required. The necessity for retreatment 5 to 8 years after apparently successful treatment is not unusual. Recurrence may be due to contributing

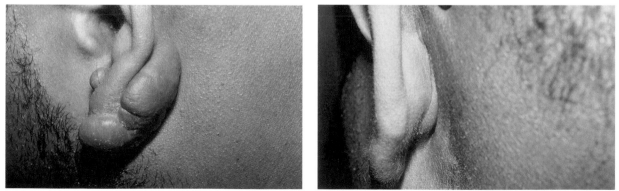

FIGURE 6-2. ■ Keloid of ear before (**A**) and after (**B**) removal with the Coherent CO_2 Ultrapulsed laser.

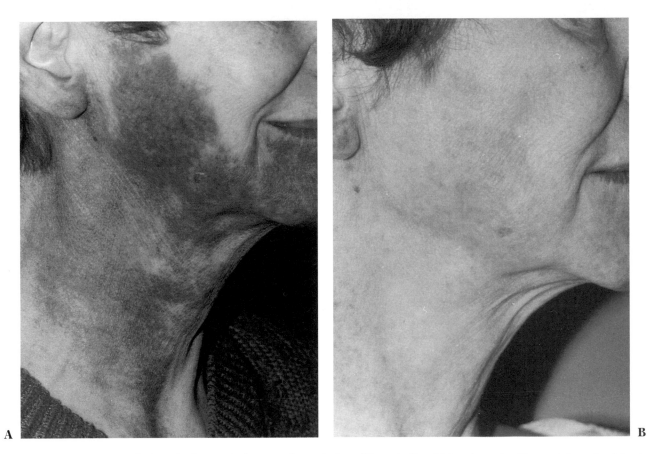

FIGURE 6-3. ■ Congenital port wine stain hemangioma before (**A**) and after (**B**) treatment with candela pulsed tuneable 585-nm dye laser.

vessels at a depth beyond the reach of the 585-nm wavelength laser.

For deeper penetration, a neodymium:yttrium aluminum garnet (Nd:Yag) laser at 1064 nm can be directed toward deeper vasculature while sparing the overlying melanin. This type of laser has also been used for deeper and larger leg vein treatments (Figure 6-4).

Q-switched (QS) lasers have a pulse duration of 10 to 20 nanoseconds. QS lasers are most frequently used for tattoo removal by heating and fracturing the ink pigment

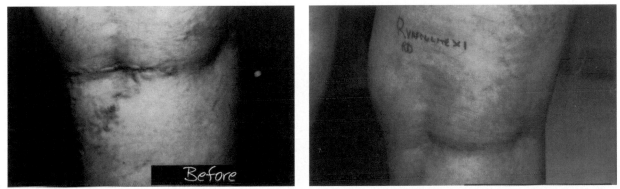

FIGURE 6-4. ■ Varicose veins of the leg before (**A**) and after (**B**) treatment with Lumenis Vasculite laser.

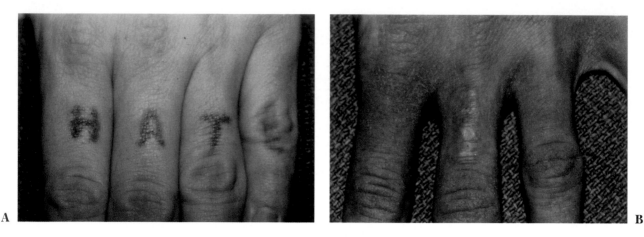

FIGURE 6-5. ■ Homemade tattoo before (**A**) and after (**B**) laser removal.

particles. The fragmented particles are extruded through the epidermis and cleared by the lymphatic system. Usually six or more treatments are required and often all the remnants of the tattoo cannot be removed. Some residual scarring or pigmentary changes in the skin are not uncommon. The selection of the proper laser depends on the color of the tattoos. Green pigment is best removed by a red light laser; red pigment, by a green light; and yellow pigment is poorly removed by all lasers. The QS-Ruby (694 nm) and QS Alexandrite (755 nm) lasers are used for blue and green inks, the QS Nd:YAG (1064) for black ink, and the QS Nd:YAG/2 (532 nm) for red inks. Most professional tattoos require the use of different lasers for effective treatment of multicolored tattoos. Homemade tattoos with India ink are easier to remove than professional tattoos (Figure 6-5).

Hair removal lasers are usually in the 694- to 1064-nm wavelengths, so that there is sufficient depth of penetration for absorption by the melanin in the hair follicle. The 800-nm diode laser is effective for hair removal. This laser also contains a cooling system to afford additional protection against injury to the overlying skin. Although the lasers have been touted for permanent removal of hair, more truly this is a process for the progressive reduction of hairs. The process requires several treatments and often follow-on treatments in ensuing years. Usually, laser treatment is only effective for pigmented hairs. The most common side effects are hyper- or hypopigmentation. The darker the skin and the higher the fluences applied to the tissue, the most apt this is to develop.

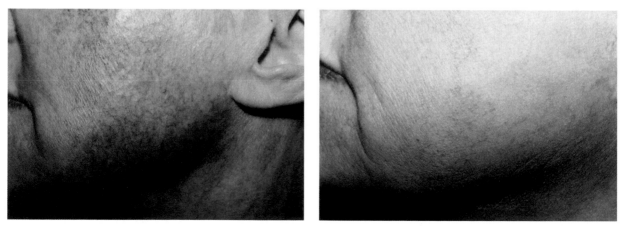

FIGURE 6-6. ■ Facial telangiectasias before (**A**) and after (**B**) treatment with Lumenis Photoderm IPL.

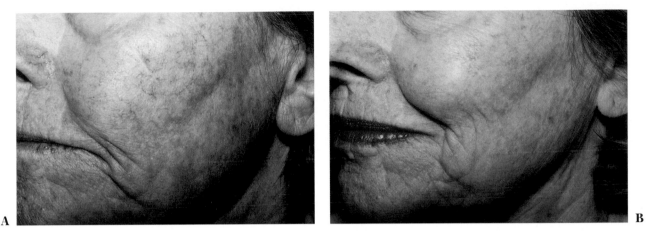

FIGURE 6-7. ■ Actinically damaged facial skin before (**A**) and after (**B**) treatment with Lumenis Photoderm IPL.

Intense Pulsed Light

IPL is a noncoherent, broad band of wavelengths from 515 to 1200 nm generated by a high-energy flash lamp. Wavelengths of light for treatment are selected by the use of optical cutoff filters that eliminate wavelengths of light less than the filter. The various cutoffs of the filters are 515, 550, 560, 570, 590, 615, 645, 690, and 755 nm. Presently, there are several companies that produce IPL devices. The first IPL device and the one that I have used extensively is the Photoderm system by Lumenis of Santa Clara, California. Initially, in the mid-1990s, the IPL was promoted for the treatment of leg veins, but the indications for IPL have greatly expanded and leg veins are the least indication. IPL is very effective for

- facial telangiectasias (Figure 6-6),
- the vascular component of rosacea,
- poikiloderma of Civatte, and
- mottled facial pigmentation from actinic damage (Figure 6-7).

In treating these conditions, it was observed that there was also an improvement in skin tone and decrease in fine wrinkling (Figure 6-8). Now a major indication is for facial

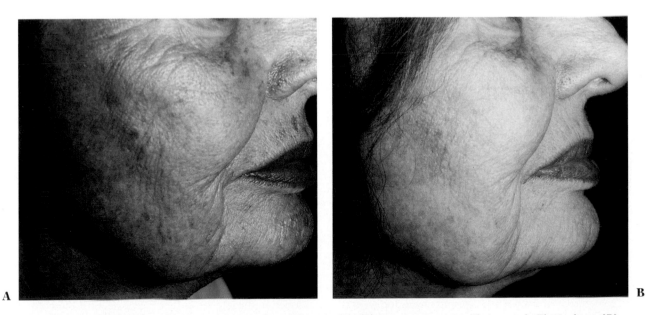

FIGURE 6-8. ■ Photoaged skin of face before (**A**) and after (**B**) one treatment with Lumenis Photoderm IPL.

rejuvenation. This photorejuvenation process is done as a series of three to four IPL treatments at 3- to 4-week intervals.

Photodynamic Therapy

The basis of PDT is that a photosensitizing drug is taken up by tissue that is then exposed to light sources whose wavelength matches the absorption spectrum of the photosensitizing drug. The photosensitized tissue is excited by the light and destroyed. This phenomenon was first observed in 1900 when *Paramecium caudatum* in acridine orange solution were exposed to light and then died quickly. Starting 30 years ago, extensive experimentation was carried out with the intravenous administration of hematoporphyrin derivative (HpD) to patients with various types of cancers. The cancer cells tend to take up the HpD more selectively than the normal cells. The cancers were exposed to appropriate wavelength light sources. The photoreaction in theory destroys the cancer cells. Results were variable.

In 1999 the U.S. Food and Drug Administration (FDA) approved the use of a topical photosensitizer, delta-aminolevulenic acid (ALA), for the treatment of actinic keratoses on the head and scalp. ALA is a precursor to protoporphyrin IX (PpIX), which is formed when ALA is absorbed into the skin. Because cancerous and precancerous cells have a higher turnover rate than normal cells, they have lower iron stores, which leads to enhanced absorption of ALA over normal cells.

The epidermis of dysplastic tissue is also a less effective barrier to penetration. PpIX peak absorption band is at 409 nm (the Soret band). PpIX also has markedly lesser absorption peaks at 509, 544, 584, and 635 nm. When the PpIX laden cells are exposed to the appropriate light source, singlet oxygen phototoxic reaction occurs leading to cell death. The Blu-U light, with a peak output at about 417 nm but with a range of 410 to 440 nm, is often used for treatment of actinic keratoses.

It has been observed that moderately severe acne responds well to PDT with Blu-U light. IPL with output above 560 nm and lasers with 585- or 595-nm output provide for deeper penetration and might provide an even more enhanced effect on the sebaceous gland, the focus of acne development.

Following PDT, the skin is red and peels, and may crust in some areas depending on the intensity of the reaction. Because ALA is a photosensitizing drug and there will be some residual amount in the skin after treatment, it is imperative that the patient avoid direct exposure to outside light. The patient must be instructed to stay indoors for the first 36 hours, continue to stay out of direct sunlight for the next 2 weeks, and remain indoors as much as possible. When outdoors, a wide-brimmed hat should be worn for the next week. Daily sunscreen application with an effective UVA block is required. A micronized zinc oxide sunscreen provides the best UVA block.

IPL has been used for photorejuvenation of the face resulting in a decrease in fine wrinkling, smoothing of texture, decrease in telangiectasias, and evenness of coloration. IPL photorejuvenation may be further enhanced by combining it with the application of ALA. Enhanced IPL photorejuvenation is usually done as a series of three treatments separated by 3 to 4 weeks. After treatment, the same precautions against sun exposure as with other PDT are mandatory.

Radiofrequency Devices

The radiofrequency device is an attempt to nonablatively (cause no damage to the skin surface) rejuvenate the facial skin. The Thermage ThermaCool TC or Thermalift system was granted FDA clearance in 2002. With this method, the epidermis is protected by cryogen cooling as the radiofrequency is delivered into the dermis. As the radiofrequency energy is absorbed, the collagen fibers contract. Later and ongoing for 4 to 6 months, collagen synthesis occurs in response to the thermal energy. Although some patients have achieved significant improvement, overall success is disappointing. At best, the improvement was subtle (Figure 6-9). Approximately 20% of patients were reported not to respond to this treatment. This is probably due to individual healing responses.

High energy levels of radiofrequency were used, which could be quite uncomfortable despite topical anesthetic creams. The most severe side effect, which was not common, was waffling or an unevenness of the skin surface after treatment, probably owing to loss of fat.

Although Thermage Inc. has never suggested that the Thermacool technique was equivalent to a facelift without surgery, there are physicians and spas advertising the procedure as such. The Thermacool technique is not a replacement for facelifts, chemical peels, or laser resurfacing.

Conceptually, radiofrequency devices have great potential, but that potential has not been achieved with the present technology.

Liposuction

Liposuction is a technique for recontouring or sculpturing various body areas by fat extraction through various sized cannulas to which suction is applied. The technique was developed in the late 1970s by Dr. Yves-Gerard Illouz of Paris, France, and then introduced into the United States. The

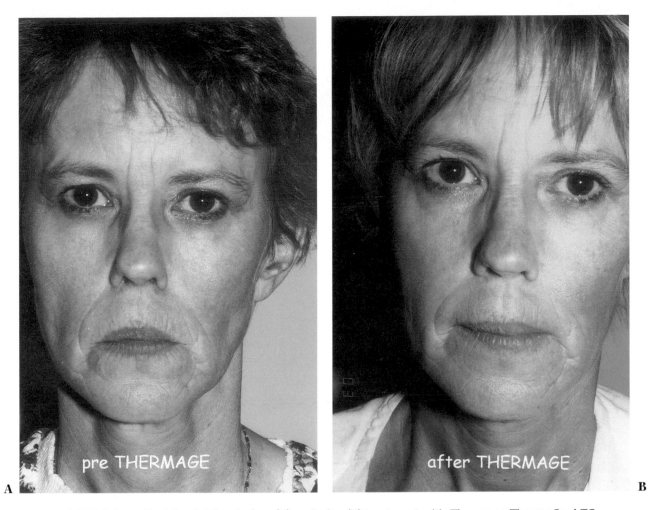

A   **B**

FIGURE 6-9. ■ Facial wrinkling before (**A**) and after (**B**) treatment with Thermage ThermaCool TC.

early methods of doing liposuction were the "dry method" carried out under general anesthesia. With large volumes of fat removal (greater than 1500 mL), these procedures were associated with fluid balance problems necessitating fluid replacement and the need initially for homologous blood transfusions and then modified by using autologous blood transfusions. Dr. Eugene Courtiss in *Plastic and Reconstructive Surgery*, in 1992, noted that 44% of 108 patients undergoing large-volume liposuction required hospitalization after the procedure.

In 1986, dermatologist Dr. Jeffrey Klein revolutionized the technique and the safety of liposuction with his work on tumescent liposuction with the infiltration of a large volume of dilute epinephrine and lidocaine in saline into the areas of liposuction. With this tumescent technique, blood loss is minimal and it is possible to perform liposuction without

general anesthesia. Another dermatologist, Dr. Patrick Lillis, advanced the tumescent technique by demonstrating the safety of using greater concentrations of lidocaine.

Although liposuction is most commonly done on the abdomen, thighs, and arms, it is a significant adjunct in the rejuvenation of the jowls (Figure 6-10) and the neck (Figure 6-11). The procedure is performed on an outpatient basis with tumescent anesthesia. Intravenous sedation or general anesthesia may also be employed if the patient desires.

Lipotransfer and Fat Autograft Muscle Injection

The transfer of autologous fat or fat grafting was first reported in 1893 to fill out scars. Since then, it has gone in and out of popularity because of problems with viability

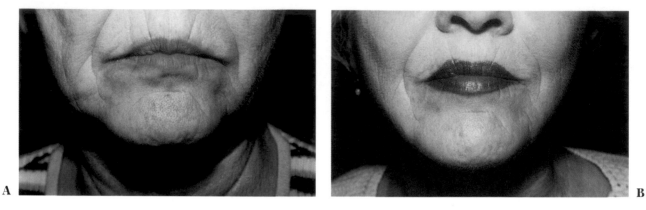

A   B

FIGURE 6-10. ■ Jowling of the face and neck fullness before (**A**) and after (**B**) liposuction.

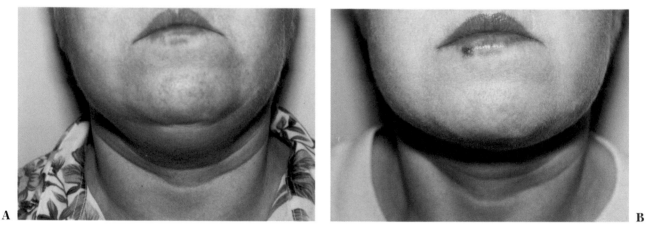

A   B

FIGURE 6-11. ■ Neck fullness and lipomatosus before (**A**) and after (**B**) liposuction.

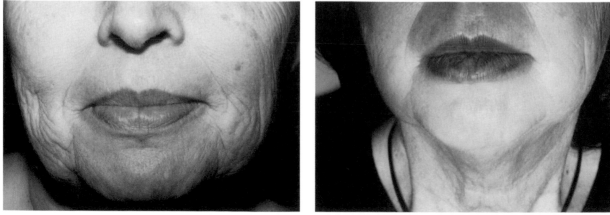

A   B

FIGURE 6-12. ■ Aging face before (**A**) and after (**B**) FAMI.

and survival of the grafts. Traumatic harvesting of the fat is most important and this is usually accomplished by low-pressure aspiration of the fat into a blunt cannula attached to a 10-mL syringe. The plunger is gradually pulled back in a slow, deliberate maneuver. The fat should also be injected at low pressure to further avoid trauma. Dr. Roger Amar has refined lipotransfer with the technique of injecting the fat into the facial musculature; muscle tissue is an ideal recipient site because it is well vascularized. He has coined the term, *fat autograft muscle injection* (FAMI).

Part of the aging process is tissue atrophy, not only of the subcutaneous soft tissue, but also of the facial musculature. The FAMI technique addresses the muscle atrophy (Figure 6-12).

Botulinum Toxin Type A

Botulinum toxin (BT) type A is a neurotoxin from the organism *Clostridium botulinum,* which is the causative agent of botulism. Botulism is associated with food poisoning from improperly sterilized canned goods. BT acts at the presynaptic terminal of motor nerves to block the release of acetylcholine. Death from botulism is caused by paralysis of the diaphragmatic muscles.

In 1980, minute doses of BT injected into eye muscles were reported to correct strabismus. Soon BT was used for other neurologic conditions. A husband and wife, Dr. Alastair Carruthers, a dermatologist, and Dr. Jean Carruthers, an ophthalmologist, first used BT for cosmetic purposes in 1988. Dr. Jean Carruthers observed a loss of wrinkles in patients she was treating with BT for blepharospasm.

The cosmetic use of BT is better known by its registered name, Botox. BT injections are one of the most common cosmetic procedures performed. The cosmetic use of BT is best indicated for the upper third of the face to erase horizontal forehead folds, smooth out the vertical and horizontal furrows of the glabella, ablate the "crow's feet" of the lateral orbit, and lift the eyebrows by blocking the depressor muscles (Figure 6-13). The effect of BT usually lasts about 4 months and then needs to be repeated if the

individual wishes to maintain the effect. BT has also been used to efface the vertical rhytides of the upper lip, weaken platysmal neck bands, and blunt the marionette line effect of the depressor labii muscle. Some patients being treated cosmetically with BT have also noticed improvement and lessening of migraine headaches.

Engineered Materials for Soft Tissue Fillers and Augmentation

Injectable Bovine Collagen

Since 1979, injectable bovine collagen from Zyderm has been the main stay of injectable soft tissue fillers. It has been used for

- filling of wrinkles and rhytides,
- filling of depressed scars,
- accentuation of nasolabial folds, and
- augmentation of the lip.

Modifications in the collagen have been Zyderm II, which contains nearly double the weight of collagen that was in Zyderm I, and Zyplast, which contains cross-linked collagen. Zyplast is intended for deeper placement into the mid and deep dermis to fill out deeper contours such as the nasolabial folds and in the lips.

Zyplast is contraindicated in the glabellar folds because of an associated case of blindness, which may have been caused by the material entering a blood vessel because of the deeper placement. Zyderm may be used in the glabellar furrows.

Injectable bovine collagen has an allergic potential; skin testing is required prior to use. Immunologic response can still occur and include swelling or edema, erythema, and firmness in the area of injection. The incidence is about 2%. A rarer response is that of an abscess-type response, which can cause scarring.

The collagen is usually injected through a 30-gauge needle. Overall injectable collagen has been a reliable product with predictable results. The collagen is not permanent.

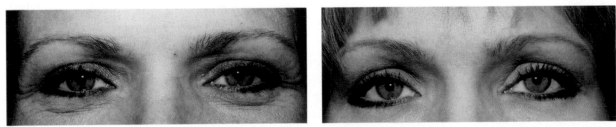

FIGURE 6-13. ■ Periorbital area before (**A**) and after (**B**) BT injection.

The average duration is about 4 to 6 months. To maintain the effect, repeated injections of the collagen are necessary. This deficiency at times is also an asset in that a patient may not like the new appearance such as fuller lips.

Injectable Collagen From Human Fibrocyte Cell Cultures

CosmoDerm I and II and CosmoPlast are human collagen injectable fillers. The cell line is from the foreskin of newborns. No skin testing is required because the antigenic potential has been removed.

Injection is with a 30-gauge needle. CosmoDerm I and II are for more superficial placement in the dermis and CosmoPlast for deeper placement and filling. Duration is about 4 to 6 months. Occasionally, the product may trigger transient flulike symptoms.

Injectable Hyaluronic Acid

The Restylane lines of injectable hyaluronic acid are from nonanimal material. It is produced from streptococcal bacteria and does not have an allergic potential because there is no protein. Hyaluronic acid is a polysaccharide and is part of the ground substance of connective tissues. Hyaluronic acid is hydrophilic and there may be some increased edema about the injection sites in the immediate posttreatment days. Restylane comes in three forms:

- Restylane Fine Lines for superficial wrinkles,
- Restylane for all-purpose use, and
- Perlane for filling of deeper contours, nasolabial folds and marionette lines, and for augmentation of the lips.

The difference in the three is in molecular size; Fine Lines has the smallest molecules and Perlane, the largest. The hyaluronic acid is injected through a 27-gauge needle. Injection into the lips and perioral areas is painful. It is best to regionally anesthetize these areas with infraorbital and mental nerve blocks. Although swelling, erythema, bruising, and mild discomfort may occur at the sites of injection, they only last a few days. Longer term difficulties, namely, edema, erythema, acneiform eruption, and induration, are rare. The longer maintenance of effect of hyaluronic acid, 6 to 9 months on average, and its nonallergenic nature have made it one of the more popular options for a soft tissue filler.

Injectable Soft Tissue Fillers With Microparticles

The microparticles in some injectables are to give a permanent effect. In Artecoll, there are polymethylmethacrylate microspheres. With any foreign body, there is always a potential for foreign body reaction, which can occur years after injection. Because of the microsize of the particles, they cannot simply be removed. Acrylomas or granulomas have occurred after Artecoll injection. Treatment of these reactions is difficult and may have limited success.

Radiance is another injectable with microparticles, calcium hydroxyapatite. Although some physicians have been using it off label for facial fillers, it has not been FDA approved for use on the face. The microspheres of hydroxyapatite are radiopaque and are therefore visible on x-rays. With any procedure or medical material, the risk to benefit must be considered.

Expanded Polytetrafluoroethylene Facial Implants

Expanded polytetrafluoroethylene (e-PTFE), better known as Gore-Tex, is a permanent substance that has been used in abdominal and vascular surgery for over 25 years. For more than 10 years, it has been used to augment soft tissue.

e-PTFE is nonallergenic, biocompatible, and reported to not incite tissue reaction. e-PTFE has micropores that allow for the ingrowth of some tissue, which serves to anchor it. This ingrowth may make e-PTFE more difficult to remove. Capsule formation about the implant has usually not been a problem. e-PTFE is supplied in sheets of various sizes, in oval and circular hollow tubes, in multistrands, and in implants shaped for the chin, nose, and malar areas.

Softform and UltraSoft tubular e-PTFE implants are innovative methods of coupling the e-PTFE hollow tube to an insertion trocar. This system is usually used for augmentation of the nasolabial folds and the upper and the lower lips.

The procedure is done under local anesthesia or with nerve block. A small stab incision is made at both ends of the site where the tube will be placed. The trocar is inserted into one of the incisions. Usually, it is the inferior incision for nasolabial fold augmentation and the lateral incision for upper lip augmentation. The trocar is tunneled under the dermis and passed out the incision at the other end. The attached e-PTFE tube is pulled through the tunnel. Using a scissors, the e-PTFE tube is cut with a downward bevel. The total length of the e-PTFE tube is left slightly longer than the distance between the incisions. A small pocket is formed with the scissors below the inferior incision and above the superior incision so that the ends of the tube can be buried away from the incision. The incision sites are closed with one or two stitches of 6-0 nylon (Figure 6-14).

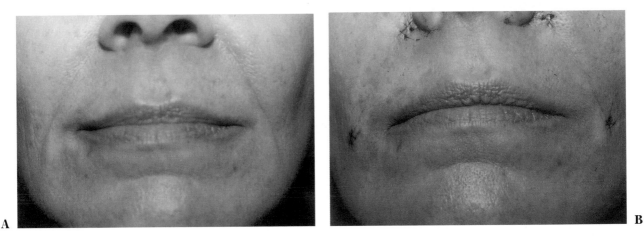

FIGURE 6-14. ■ Nasolabial folds before (**A**) and after (**B**) insertion of UltraSoft Tubular e-PTFE Implant.

When the tubular system is used to augment the lip, a single tube is run along the entire length of the lower lip. However, two tubes are used for the upper lip in order not to efface the "cupid's bow" of the philtrum and to accentuate it.

In the upper lip, the e-PTFE tube is placed from the corner of the mouth to the high point of the cupid's bow on each side (Figure 6-15). Although the e-PTFE tubes can nicely fill out the nasolabial folds and augment the lips, the tubes are palpable. Infection has not been a problem. Because of their superficial, subdermal placement, the e-PTFE tubes may excite some reactivity at the incision site with drainage and tissue inflammation. This reaction may necessitate removal of the tube. For the most part, I have discontinued the use of these implants for the nasolabial folds and the lips because of shrinkage of the length of the tube by a third or more in a significant number of patients.

Tempered Optimism

We physicians have the opportunity and the ability to improve the human condition. Technologic advances continue to enhance this capability. But medical treatments have potential risks as well as benefits. With any treatment or procedure or material used, there will always be some patients who have unanticipated and untoward sequelae and difficulties despite the best of evaluation, precautions, equipment, and technique. Biologic systems have an inherent unpredictability.

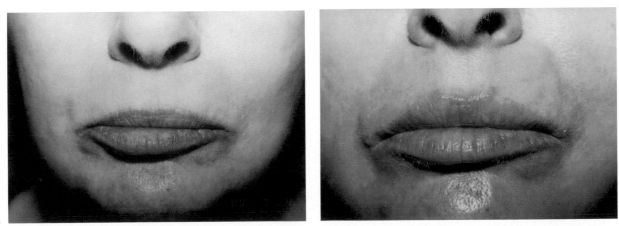

FIGURE 6-15. ■ Upper lip before (**A**) and after (**B**) insertion of UltraSoft Tubular e-PTFE Implant.

Suggested Reading

Coven TR, Burack LH, Gilleaudeau R, et al. Narrowband UV-B produces superior clinical and histopathological resolution of moderate-to-severe psoriasis in patients compared with broadband UV-B. Arch Dermatol 1997;133:1514.

Goldschmidt H, Panizzon RG. Modern dermatologic radiation therapy. New York, Springer-Verlag, 1991.

Kalka K, Merk H, Mukhtar H. Photodynamic therapy in dermatology. J Am Acad Dermatol 2000;42:389–413.

Sebben JE. Cutaneous electrosurgery. Chicago, Year Book Medical Publishers, 1989.

Spicer MS, Goldberg DJ. Lasers in dermatology. J Am Acad Dermatol 1996;34:1.

Zanolli MD, Feldman SR. Phototherapy treatment protocols for psoriasis & other phototherapy responsive dermatoses. London, Parthenon Publishing Group, 2000.

CHAPTER 7

Fundamentals of Cutaneous Surgery

Frank Custer Koranda, MD, MBA

Attention to detail is the essence of surgical perfection. Disregard or ignorance of any of the fundamentals of surgery is often the difference between the optimal and the merely acceptable healed wound.

Instrument Selection

If an instrument facilitates one's surgery, it is usually worth its cost. Quality instruments are expensive. For most types of cutaneous surgery, the Webster needle holder, the neurosurgery needle holder, and the Halsey needle holder are well designed (Figure 7-1A). Because of the smaller size of suture and the finer, precise needles that are generally best suited for cutaneous surgery, the needle holders should have smooth jaws. Serrated jaws can cut fine sutures and damage precision needles. For very delicate surgery and for very fine sutures, the Castroviejo needle holder is preferred (Figure 7-1B). The amount of motion necessary to lock and unlock the Castroviejo is less than that required for the standard type of needle holder.

To lessen tissue damage, the skin should be handled in the least traumatic manner. Gentle handling requires the use of skin hooks such as the single-hook Frazier or the fine double-hook Tyrell. When using forceps, usually finer types such as the Bishop-Harmon ophthalmic forceps are advantageous (Figure 7-1C).

The No. 3 scalpel handle is used with the Nos. 10, 11, and 15 blades. For very precise incisions, the 15C blade should be used. This blade was originally designed for periodontal surgery. For scissors dissection, the Metzenbaum, Malis, or Ragnell scissors may be used (Figure 7-1D). For finer work, a Stevens scissors is well suited (Figure 7-1E). A Littler scissors is also well designed for this function. For cutting sutures precisely and for suture removal, the pointed, delicately curved Gradle scissors are ideal (Figure 7-1F).

A basic cutaneous surgical pack may include the following:

- Webster or neurosurgery smooth-jawed needle holder
- Adson delicate forceps with teeth or Micro-Adson forceps with teeth
- Dissecting scissors
- Utility scissors
- Halsted mosquito hemostats
- Backhaus towel clips, 3$1/2$ inch
- Round toothpicks for skin marking (toothpicks dipped in methylene blue make a finer line than the standard marking pen and are less expensive)
- Gauze sponges
- Cotton tipped applicators as an option for point control of bleeding

Suture Selection

Sutures may be divided into two general groups, absorbable and nonabsorbable. The absorbable sutures are

- plain gut,
- chromic gut,
- polyglycolic acid (Dexon),
- polyglactin 910 (Vicryl),
- polydioxanone (PDS),
- polyglyconate (Maxon),
- poliglecaprone (Monocryl), and
- braid synthetic absorbable (Panacryl).

Gut sutures, which are made from the small intestine submucosal layer of sheep and the small intestine serosal layer of cattle, undergo degradation by phagocytosis by eliciting a foreign body response. Plain gut gradually

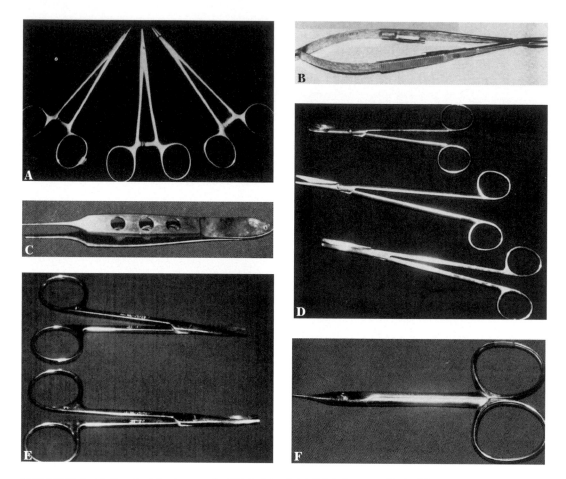

FIGURE 7-1. ■ Surgical instruments. (**A**) *Left to right:* Webster needle holder, neurosurgery needle holder, and Halsey needle holder. (**B**) Castroviejo needle holder. (**C**) Bishop-Harman ophthalmic forceps. (**D**) Metzenbaum, Malis, and Ragnell scissors. (**E**) Stevens scissors. (**F**) Gradle scissors.

loses its tensile strength over 2 weeks. Chromic suture is gut suture that has been coated with chromic salts to delay its degradation. It has a slightly prolonged tensile strength over that of plain gut. Another modification of gut suture is the fast-absorbing plain gut, which breaks down in 4 to 7 days and can be used for the skin stitch. After 4 to 7 days, the fast-absorbing suture can be wiped out of the wound with a moistened, cotton-tipped applicator. In small children and for individuals who cannot return for suture removal, this is another option. The disadvantage is that there is more of an inflammatory response to this material than to nylon.

Synthetic absorbable sutures undergo degradation by hydrolysis. The synthetic sutures usually produce less of an inflammatory response in the subcutaneous tissue than do the gut sutures. Although Vicryl and Dexon are somewhat similar in their tensile strength properties, Vicryl has a better tensile strength profile maintaining 75% at 2 weeks and 50% at 3 weeks. The hydrolysis and absorption of Vicryl is also significantly faster than that of Dexon. PDS and Maxon both maintain their tensile strength longer, 70% at 3 weeks, 50% at 4 weeks, and 25% at 6 weeks. Hydrolysis occurs between 180 and 210 days.

Undyed Monocryl maintains 50% to 60% of its tensile strength at 1 week and 20% to 30% at 2 weeks. Panacryl, a braided synthetic absorbable suture, retains 80% of its strength at 3 months.

The frequently used nonabsorbable sutures are silk, nylon, and polypropylene. Silks sutures are frequently used for eyelids and lips so that there are no sharp, irritating ends. The monofilament nylons such as Ethilon are general purpose sutures. Prolene and Surgilene, a polypropylene type of monofilament suture, have the characteristics of an increased memory and high tensile strength.

For subcutaneous sutures on the face, usually a 4-0 or 5-0 size suture is used. For skin sutures on the face usually a 5-0 or 6-0 size suture is used. For delicate work 7-0 size suture may be indicated. It is easier to handle the 7-0 size with a Castroviejo needle holder.

For skin and fascia, one uses a reverse cutting needle. With the reverse cutting needle, the cutting edge is on the outside. For facial surgery and for other fine cutaneous surgery, precision point needles should be used. There is reduced tissue drag and trauma with these supersmooth finished, highly honed needles. In the Ethicon system, these needles have the code prefix *P* or *PS* (*plastic* or *plastic surgery*) and in the Davis and Geck system *PR* or *PRE* (*plastic reconstructive*). The P3 or PS 3 size needles have good utility for facial surgery. For general cutaneous surgery, an FS (for skin) reverse cutting needle may be used, but there is an appreciable drag as compared with the precision needles.

Types of Stitches

Buried Subcutaneous

The buried subcutaneous stitch (Figure 7-2) is used to close the dead space to prevent hematoma and a nidus for infection. It also reduces the tension on the incision line. Burying the knot decreases the amount of tissue reaction in the more superficial part of the wound so that the major part of the inflammatory response is away from the surface of the incision line and less apt to disrupt it.

To bury the knot, the needle is first inserted through the deeper tissue and exits more superficially on the same side of the wound and then enters superficially on the other side of the wound and exits through the deeper tissue on that side of the wound. Absorbable suture is usually used.

Simple Stitch

The simple stitch (Figure 7-3) is made through the epidermis and dermis from one side to the other. The entry and the exit points should be about 2 to 3 mm from the wound edge. For proper entry of the needle, a greater "bite" of tis-

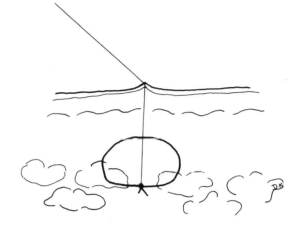

FIGURE 7-2. ■ Buried subcutaneous stitch.

sue is taken more deeply than superficially. This helps to evert the wound edges.

The simple stitch is an approximating and everting stitch that is also used to adjust the height of wound edges so that they are even. If one side of the wound is lower than the other, a slightly deeper bite should be taken on the lower side for coarse adjustment of the wound edges. The knot is then placed on the lower side of the wound to further finely adjust the height of the wound edges.

Vertical Mattress Stitch

The vertical mattress stitch (Figure 7-4) tents up the skin edges. This eversion provides for good epidermal apposition and compensates for contracture that later occurs in the wound and may cause a linear depression in the wound.

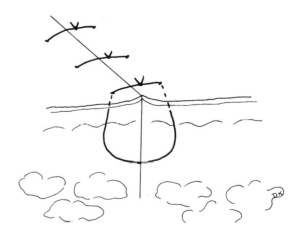

FIGURE 7-3. ■ Simple stitch.

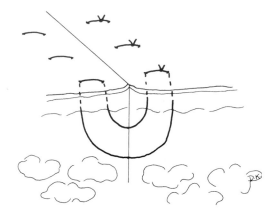

FIGURE 7-4. ■ Vertical mattress stitch.

If the edges of the wound are not everted sufficiently by the simple stitches, using a vertical mattress for every two or three simple sutures usually provides good eversion.

Horizontal Mattress Stitch

The horizontal mattress stitch (Figure 7-5) is used for the closure of a wound under tension. It can cause strangulation of the skin. Because of this it is often used with a bolster such as a piece of a red Robinson catheter slipped over the part of the suture in contact with the skin to reduce pressure on the skin. In general it is not a suitable stitch for facial surgery.

Corner Stitch (Tip Stitch, Half-Buried Mattress)

The corner stitch (Figure 7-6) is used for V-shaped corners to prevent necrosis of the skin tip. It is inserted vertically down through the main segment of tissue and out through

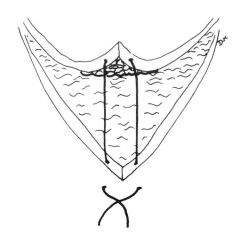

FIGURE 7-6. ■ Corner stitch (tip stitch, half-buried mattress stitch).

the dermis. It then enters horizontally through the dermal tissue in the tip of the flap and then back up through the main segment of tissue. The suture must enter and leave the flap tip in the same dermal plane that it exits and reenters the dermis of the main body of tissue.

Running Intradermal Stitch

The running intradermal stitch (Figure 7-7) is placed in the dermis and may be left in for an extended period without causing cross-hatching. The suture used may be a permanent type such as Prolene or an absorbable such as PDS. The stitch enters the skin at a point 4 to 5 mm beyond the end of the incision. From this point it is brought into the wound and then is placed through the dermis on one side and crosses to the other side. The stitch is continued in a

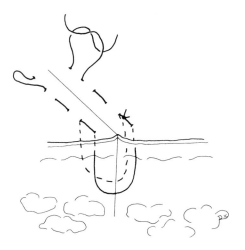

FIGURE 7-5. ■ Horizontal mattress stitch.

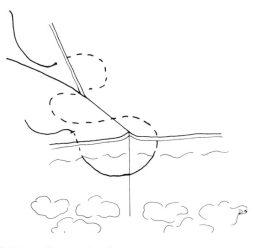

FIGURE 7-7. ■ Running intradermal stitch.

running "S" pattern, staying in the same plane of the dermis on both sides of the wound. In a long-running intradermal stitch that is to be removed, it is wise to have it go out through the skin and then back down through the skin at the midpoint and then proceed intradermally. This facilitates later removal; this midpoint of the suture may be cut and only half the amount of suture needs to be pulled out from each end. By using a PDS suture or Monocryl for an intradermal stitch, the need for removal can be avoided.

Although the intradermal stitch nicely coapts the wound, at times it may be wise to also use a few simple stitches for the first 3 days for wound edge eversion and additional support. Another method of wound support is the use of Mastisol and Steri-strips.

Running Simple Stitch

The running simple stitch (Figure 7-8) is a repeated, continuous over-and-over simple stitch that is a rapid method of closure. This type of stitch can evenly distribute tension along the wound, and it is easier and less traumatic to remove than multiple interrupted stitches. By adjusting the depth of bite of tissue with each placement of the suture, the height of the wound edges may also be adjusted.

Suture Tying

Sutures should be tied so that they lay down as square knots. The sutures should be tied to coapt the wound edges but not to strangulate. Most err by tying too tightly. One way of avoiding too tightly tied knots is to not snug down the second throw of the suture. By leaving this throw slightly loose, it also compensates for the tissue edema that develops in wounds. Tying too tightly is a major cause of suture track marks on the skin. Leaving sutures in too long is another factor.

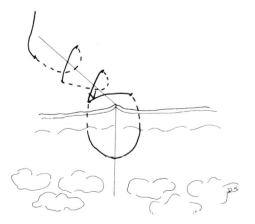

FIGURE 7-8. ■ Running simple stitch.

Hemostasis

Meticulous hemostasis is essential to good wound healing. A rule of thumb on controlling bleeders is that named vessels should be clamped and ligated and unnamed vessels may be electrocoagulated. In tying vessels, use the smallest size suture that is practical. The suture should be cut on the knot to leave the least amount of foreign material in the wound that might cause foreign body reaction.

For electrocoagulation, a biterminal device may be used. With the biterminal unit, current enters the patient through an active or coagulating electrode. When tissue contact is made, heat is generated and coagulation occurs. The current passes through the patient and out via the dispersing electrode, the grounding pad. The patient usually becomes part of the current circuit.

The grounding pad should be placed as close as possible to the surgical site. If possible, the heart should not be in between the active electrode and the grounding pad because it then becomes part of the current pathway. The area of coagulation should be kept dry with sponging or with suction; bleeding into the surrounding area disperses the current and diminishes the coagulation effect.

Biterminal coagulation is not bipolar coagulation. *Bipolar coagulation* refers to the system where a single electrode has both terminals contained in it. With bipolar coagulation forceps, the current passes between the tines of the forceps coagulating the tissue between the tines. Bipolar coagulation is more precise, produces less tissue damage, and does not involve current transmission through the patient.

Electrocautery is essentially a red-hot branding iron that seals blood vessels by the direct application of heat. Electrocautery systems use either low-frequency alternating current or direct current. The current remains in the electrode tip and does not pass into the patient. Electrocautery provides better hemostasis in a very wet field than does electrocoagulation. There are a variety of disposable, battery-powered cautery pens.

In the preoperative history, it is important to ask whether the patient has any implanted electrical devices such as a pacemaker or neurostimulator. With the defibrillating pacemakers, electrocoagulation should not be used until the proper protective measures have been undertaken. The manufacturers have toll-free numbers to call for the precautions with the different electrical implants. In the event there is a question, the cautery pens should be safe because they seal blood vessels by heat and not by electricity.

Patient Preparation

Written instructions to the patient before surgery helps to prevent misunderstandings.

1. The patient should take no aspirin, aspirin-containing products, or nonsteroidal anti-inflammatories for 2 weeks before surgery because they interfere with platelet aggregation and prolong the bleeding time.
2. Shampoo the hair the night before or morning of surgery.
3. Apply no creams or makeup to face after washing the morning of surgery.
4. No smoking for 72 hours prior to surgery.
5. Take regularly prescribed medicines the morning of surgery.
6. Do not wear clothing that pulls over the head.
7. Wear loose, comfortable clothing.
8. Bring a companion to drive home.

Skin Preparation

It is best to shave as little hair as possible; do not shave the eyebrows because they grow very slowly. Cleanse the skin with Betadine or Hibiclens; do not use Hibiclens around the eye. Use Betadine or Shur-Clens (Poloxaner 188) about the eye. Prepare a large enough surgical area so that one may see not only the immediate surgical site but also the relationship to the surrounding anatomic landmarks to be sure that closure of the wound is not distorting some other structure such as the nose, lip, and eyelid.

Incision lines are marked out before any distortion by infiltrative anesthesia. Round toothpicks dipped in methylene blue or Bonney's blue make a more exact line than most skin-marking pens.

Anesthesia

Most cutaneous surgery requires only local infiltrative or regional block anesthesia. The standard agent, 1% lidocaine, is an effective, safe, short-acting local anesthetic to which allergic reactions are exceedingly rare. By the addition of epinephrine, systemic absorption of lidocaine is lessened, the duration of action is markedly prolonged, and a local hemostatic effect is achieved. It usually takes 15 minutes to achieve optimal vasoconstriction. The available commercial preparations usually combine lidocaine with 1:100,000 epinephrine. Some patients react to epinephrine with apprehension, body tremors, diaphoresis, palpitations, tachycardia, and increased blood pressure. These side effects can be decreased or eliminated by increasing the dilution of epinephrine to 1:200,000 or even to 1:400,000 without significantly changing its efficacy.

The maximum recommended dosage of lidocaine is 500 mg, the equivalent of 50 mL of a 1% solution. The earliest sign of toxicity is on the central nervous system (CNS)

with mild sedation, which may proceed to seizure activity. Cardiac toxicity usually occurs at twice the level.

The injection of lidocaine, especially with epinephrine, is uncomfortable. This discomfort may be obviated by applying a topical lidocaine type anesthetic agent to the skin under occlusion for 45 minutes prior to the injection. This is particularly useful for young children and very apprehensive adults.

Warming the anesthetic agent to room temperature and buffering the agent decreases the discomfort of the injection. Lidocaine is buffered by diluting it 10% with 8.4% sodium bicarbonate.

At the end of the procedure, a longer acting anesthetic, 0.25% bipuvicaine with 1:200,000 epinephrine, can be injected for a more prolonged anesthesia of 3 to 6 hours. Even after sensation returns, there is still an analgesia that will persist for some time. Toxic limit for bipuvicaine is 3 mg/kg. Bipuvicaine can cause cardiac toxicity at the same levels needed to cause CNS toxicity. Bipuvicaine binds tightly to myocardial tissue and may trigger dysrhythmias.

Ropivacaine is a newer, long-acting local anesthetic with a lesser potential for cardiac toxicity than bipuvicaine. Ropivacaine has a toxic limit of 3 mg/kg. Epinephrine does not decrease its systemic absorption as with lidocaine and bipuvicaine.

Placement of Incisions

Incisions should be planned so that they are parallel to or within wrinkle and smile lines. When there is lack of definite wrinkles, place incisions in the direction of relaxed skin tension lines. These lines run at right angles to the contraction vectors of the underlying muscle.

Another guide for camouflaging scars is to place incision lines at the boundaries of aesthetic and anatomic units. Examples are the vermilion junction, the paranasal fold (the junction of the nose and the cheek), the submandibular area (the junction of the cheek and the neck), the submental area (the junction of the chin and neck), the preauricular area, and along the eyebrow or in the hair.

Incisions

Incisions should be made vertical to the skin surface. Obliquely angled incisions do not coapt as well. An exception to the rule of vertical incisions is in the area adjacent to the eyebrows or in the hair. Incisions placed here should be at an angle that parallels the angle of the hair shaft as it emerges from the skin to avoid transection of the hair follicle.

Wounds, even small, should be undermined to reduce tension. Undermining may be done with a scissors or scalpel. On the face, the level of undermining is usually just under the dermal plexus. On the scalp, the level is between the aponeurosis and the periosteum, which is a relatively blood-free plane.

Excisions

The standard excision is fusiform in shape. If the length-to-width ratio of the fusiform is less than 4:1 or if one side is longer than the other, redundant tissue will develop at the corners of the closure. These so-called dog ears or standing cones of tissue, if small, level out and flatten as the wound undergoes contracture. If large, they should be removed by tenting up the corner of the wound with a skin hook to define the extent of the dog ear. The dog ear is incised along its base on one side or the other. The final wound curves toward the side on which the incision is placed. After making the incision along one side of the base of the dog ear, the flap of tissue that is created is pulled across the incision. Where the base of the redundant tissue crosses the incision, it is transected. The dog ear is thus eliminated and the wound is closed (Figure 7-9).

Wound Dressings

In the first hours after the incision, a coagulum forms over the wound. Between 12 and 72 hours, there are two spurts of mitotic activity and epidermal cells begin migrating across the wound. However, if a dried crust forms, it is a barrier to the epidermal migration. Rather than being able to migrate straight and level across the gap between the wound edges, the epidermal cells must find a plane of

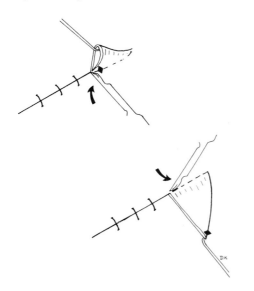

FIGURE 7-9. ■ Tenting up corner of wound with skin hook to define extent of dog ear.

migration beneath the dried crust. This leads to a shallow linear depression in the healed incision.

To prevent wound crusting and the resultant linear trough in the healed wound, an occlusive dressing is used. For such a dressing, there are a variety of commercially available products such as Bio-Occlusive or Tegaderm. However, another option is to use Dermicel tape. This is a hypoallergenic tape; its adhesive has some bacteriostatic properties. Benzoin or Mastisol is first applied to the skin. Dermicel tape is then applied directly down and over the wound. No ointment is used.

A moist environment develops under the dressing that inhibits formation of a crust and accelerates epidermal regeneration. Because of the abundant blood supply of the face, infection has not been a problem. The tape is left in place for 3 to 4 days.

Suture Removal

There are no hard and fast rules for suture removal. If there is doubt about whether sutures should be removed, remove every other or every third one and observe for another day or so. Some guidelines for the time of suture removal are as follows:

- Face: 4 to 6 days
- Neck: 6 to 10 days
- Back: 10 to 14 days
- Abdomen: 7 to 10 days
- Extremities: 10 to 18 days

It is prudent to examine wounds 4 to 5 days after surgery because this is when a wound infection is most likely to occur.

To not disrupt the wound during suture removal, the sutures may be cut with a fine scissors such as the Gradle or a No. 11 blade. For correct suture removal, the suture is pulled toward the incision line; pulling the incision away from the incision line might pull the wound apart.

The time at which sutures are removed from the face is the time when the wound is the weakest; fibroplasia is just beginning and only the epidermal bridging is holding the wound. The incision line may be reinforced with Steri-strips after suture removal.

Wound Dynamics

Wound Healing

Wound healing is divided into four phases:

- inflammatory,
- fibroblastic,
- proliferative, and
- remodeling.

However these phases overlap and blend into each other. During the beginning inflammatory phase, there is initial vasoconstriction with platelet aggregation. After 5 to 10 minutes of vasoconstriction, there is active venule dilatation and increased vascular permeability, lasting about 72 hours. Within a few hours of these vascular responses, a cellular response occurs. Polymorphonuclear leukocytes migrate into the area. There is a diapedesis of monocytes that transform into tissue macrophages. The macrophage is the dominant cell for the first 3 to 4 days. It initiates the fibroblastic phase.

While the inflammatory phase is still proceeding, the proliferative phase commences. Epidermal cells undergo changes and begin migrating into the wound. By the third day, migration of epidermal cells across an apposed incision is completed. Fibroblasts within the dermis begin to proliferate at 25 to 36 hours after the tissue injury. By the fourth day, the fibroblastic phase is heralded by the synthesis of collagen and proteoglycans by the proliferating fibroblasts. Collagen fibers are laid down in a random pattern without orientation.

Overlapping with and toward the latter part of fibroblastic phase, the remodeling phase begins. This is a phase of differentiation, resorption, and maturation. Fibroblasts disappear from the wound, and collagen fibers are modeled into organized bundles and patterns.

Wound Contraction

In an open wound healing by second intention, there is an active drawing of the full thickness of the surrounding skin toward the center of the wound. Wound contraction begins during the proliferative phase of wound healing. There is a differentiation of fibroblasts or myofibroblasts, which are responsible for this dynamic process. Wound contraction usually proceeds until the wound is closed or until surrounding forces on the skin are greater than the contractile forces of the myofibroblasts.

Contracture

All scars undergo contracture with a resultant shortening along their axes. This process of contracture is due to collagen cross-linking, which occurs during the remodeling phase. Contracture is distinct and different from wound contraction.

Wound Strength

By 2 weeks, the wound has gained 7% of its final strength; by 3 weeks, 20%; by 4 weeks, 50%. At full maturation, the healed wound regains only 80% of the strength of the original intact skin.

Documentation and Assessment

Although success or failure in cutaneous surgery may be readily apparent, it is important to document results with objective photography. Only by consistent, standardized photographs may one judge progress and analyze techniques and methods. Pre- and postoperative photographs are essential, as are intraoperative photographs. Uniform photographs are a method of self-assessment and serve as a stimulus and a direction for improvement.

SAUER'S NOTES

1. One of the more common complaints after skin surgery, especially a more extensive procedure, is numbness or altered sensation in the area. This is not a complication, but an expected effect of cutting through the skin. It is best to warn patients of this possibility before the surgery and that this change in sensation may last for 6 to 12 months and in some cases may be permanent.

2. In areas of high sebaceous gland concentration and activity such as the T area of the face and in patients with acne and rosacea, incisions tend to spread and widen no matter how meticulous and precise the surgery. This is a phenomenon of wound healing. The patient should be preadvised that this is a potential problem. "What the patient is told before surgery is informed consent; what is told after surgery may be taken as an excuse."

3. Beware of the temporal branch of the facial nerve. As it exits from the parotid gland at the superior border it runs a superficial course over the zygomatic arch and into the temporal area. Transection of this branch causes paralysis of the frontalis muscle on that side and drooping of the eyebrow. With any excision in the temporal area this is a possibility. Forewarn the patient. A drooping eyebrow can be corrected with a browpexy.

4. Beware of the spinal accessory nerve in the posterior triangle of the neck. The spinal accessory nerve pierces through the posterior border of the sternocleidomastoid muscle a little above its midportion and enters the posterior triangle of the neck. The spinal accessory nerve then travels superficially just below the subcutaneous fat in the investing fascia covering the posterior triangle. There is also a chain of lymph nodes intimately associated with the spinal accessory nerve along its course in the posterior triangle. This nerve has been transected by those aware of its superficial location as well as by those unaware. "Good judgment is based on experience, which is often based on bad judgment."

5. No matter how careful and diligent the surgeon, the response of biologic systems is not always predictable and the outcome not always anticipated or desired. "If one wants to cut, one must be prepared to cry and to pray."

Suggested Reading

McGregor IA, McGregor AD. Fundamental techniques of plastic surgery. Edinburgh, Churchill Livingstone, 1999.

Papel I. Facial plastic and reconstructive surgery, ed 2. New York, Thieme, 2002.

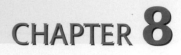

Cosmetics for the Physician

Marianne N. O'Donoghue, MD

Physicians, especially dermatologists, are often confronted by patients with cosmetic concerns. We need to explain the preferred methods of cleansing and moisturizing, safe hair care products, nail products, and skin-enhancing practices. It is important to know how cosmetics function, which products cause adverse reactions, and how we can recommend them for the better care of our patients.

The U.S. Food and Drug Administration defines cosmetics as "(1) articles intended to be rubbed, poured, sprinkled, or sprayed on, introduced into, or otherwise applied to the human body or any part thereof for cleansing, beautifying, promoting attractiveness, or altering the appearance, and (2) articles intended for use as a component of any such article: except that such term shall not include soap." Cosmetic manufacturers are not regulated as strictly as are drug manufacturers, but there is a voluntary registration for cosmetics. Cosmetic Ingredient Review is an independent panel of expert scientists and physicians established to examine all published and voluntarily submitted industry data and to summarize them in a safety monograph for each individual cosmetic ingredient or class of cosmetic ingredient.

In the United States, the regulation for labeling cosmetics is that the manufacturer should label all ingredients in descending order of predominance for all ingredients that constitute more than 1% of the product. Ingredients that compose less than 1% of the product may be listed in any order. The labels need only be on the outside wrapping.

Products intended for retail sale need a statement of identity, net quantity of content, name and place of business and the manufacturer or distributor, declaration of ingredient statement, any necessary warning statement, and directions for use. If not intended for retail sale (e.g., cosmetics in a beauty salon) those specifications need not be met.

This means that the physician should be able to trace the origin of any product to which a patient has an adverse reaction. The research and development departments of most cosmetic companies are helpful and knowledgeable, especially if the inquiring physician is not argumentative. Industry has worked very hard to be helpful to dermatologists.

Classification of Cosmetics

Cosmetics can be classified into toiletries, skin care products, fragrance products, and makeup or color products.

Toiletries

These include soaps, shampoos, hair rinses and conditioners, hair dressings, sprays and setting lotions, hair color preparations, waving preparations, straightening (relaxing) agents, deodorants, antiperspirants, and sun protective agents.

Cleansers

The purpose of cleansing is to

- remove sebum that attracts dirt,
- desquamate the skin,
- remove airborne pollutants,
- remove pathogenic organisms, and
- remove any existing makeup.

The classic cleanser, and the one that has been present for decades, is soap. This consists of a substance made up of fatty acid in oil or fat and an alkaline substance. Clear or transparent soap permits better control of the alkaline residue and rinses off more easily. Hard-milled soaps have been considered elegant for many years. Synthetic detergents (syndets) are shaped like soap in bars but consist of anionic surfactants, such as sodium lauryl sulfate, that can be adjusted for pH. This makes the syndet easier to rinse off in hard water, and the product can be adjusted to be less irritating to the skin. Special soaps can incorporate medicaments, granules, emollients, or fragrance. Soaps and synthetic detergents have been tested as to irritancy, transepidermal water loss, pH, and many other qualities. Each product has advantages and disadvantages.

Shower gels have become as popular in the United States as they are in Europe. They may have potassium lauryl sulfate as their anionic surfactant or many other ingredients. Many contain the ingredient cocamidopropyl betaine that has become a very common sensitizer. These shower gels appear to rinse off well, but may be a little more irritating in some individuals. Perfumed liquid gels using peppermint and pineapple scents have caused many cases of allergic contact and irritant dermatitis in recent years.

Cleansing cloths impregnated with a body wash–type cleanser are the newest cleansing technology. The fibered facial cloths have a textured side, which induces exfoliation, and a smooth side for rinsing that leaves behind petrolatum. This allows cleansing, exfoliation, and moisturization to occur in one product.

Shampoos

Shampoos have three major components: water, detergent, and a fatty material. Like body cleansers, the soap shampoos contain alkali plus oil and fat. Because these can leave a precipitate on the hair shaft with hard water, soap shampoos are rarely used anymore.

Most shampoos are soapless and are made of sulfonated oil. They consist of

- principal surfactants for detergent and foaming power,
- secondary surfactants to improve and condition the hair, and
- additives to complete the formulation and special effects.

Because most of the damage to the hair shaft is from chemicals that have a high pH, such as color and permanent or straightening agents, many shampoos are formulated today with an acidic or neutral pH. Because shampoo contains a large component of water, preservatives (which are considered subsequently) must be added. Formaldehyde is the most common preservative in shampoo. Because shampoo is only left on the hair for a short period, contact dermatitis does not usually occur. A more likely scenario is contact dermatitis on the hands of hairdressers. Some of the other additives beside preservatives, such as color, fragrance, and newer essential oils, occasionally can cause allergic reactions.

The major therapeutic agents added to shampoos are tar, salicylic acid, zinc pyrithione, sulfur, and, by prescription, ketoconazole, cyclopirox, cycloallamine, clobetasol and fluocinonide. It is important for physicians to know that these ingredients do not necessarily harm the hair or strip the color. The formulation of these therapeutic shampoos can contain as many conditioners and beautifying ingredients as nontherapeutic shampoos. They can even be recommended for color-treated, permed, or hair in people of color. The formulation must simply be selected for the type of hair (e.g., dry, oily, fine, or coarse).

Conditioners

Because of the trauma to the hair shaft from sun, wind, chemical treatments, and water, conditioners are often a necessary hair-grooming product for both men and women. The original rinses to remove the soap shampoo film were lemon and vinegar. These substances are still helpful when a person is "roughing it" in the wild or simply not supplied with real conditioners. The other rinses coat the hair shaft so it does not become tangled with the hair shaft next to it. These products contain wax and paraffin, and they allow the hair to shine without static cling. Balsam is a product in that category.

The major conditioners for traumatized hair are cationic surfactant conditioners. Quaternary ammonium compounds, especially stearalkonium ammonium chloride, have been used for many years to make hair manageable. It is possible to attach a polymer (such as polyvinylpyrrolidone) or other film formers to the quaternary ammonium compounds. These not only condition the hair, they add extra volume or body. There are even conditioners that contain sunscreens to protect the hair color. Occasionally, too frequent use of any of these conditioners can cause a buildup on the hair shaft so that the hair becomes too soft. This can be counteracted with an anionic shampoo to strip off the buildup, so that the hair is fresh and more easily managed.

Protein-based conditioners consist of amino acids and small polypeptide fragments of hydrolyzed protein. These can be incorporated into the cortex of the hair shaft when the hair has just been processed with color or permanent waving, or under a heat cap. This is advisable for hair that has been damaged through processing, wind, swimming, or sun. There have been reports of contact urticaria to the protein components of hair conditioners, such as quaternary derivative of hydrolyzed bovine collagen protein.

Styling aids consist of lotions, gels, mousses, or hair spray. Most of these products contain water, copolymers, polyvinylpyrrolidone, quaternary salts, and fragrance. They waterproof the hair so that perspiration or mild rain does not upset the style.

Permanent Waves and Relaxers

The three natural wave patterns of hair are straight, wavy, and kinky. To allow the hair to be curled differently, straightened, or become slightly wavy, a chemical reaction must take place in which the disulfide bond is broken with heat, high pH, or thioglycolates. For straightening, the disulfide bond is broken with sodium hydroxide, guanidine hydroxide, lithium hydroxide, heat, or thioglycolates. The hair is placed over rods or curlers, treated with the appropriate chemical until the shape of the hair shaft is changed, then neutralized with hydrogen peroxide with sodium perforate or potassium bromate. Some of the disulfide bonds are never repaired, so this process can be very hard on the hair shaft.

The mildest form of hair curling is the acid permanent—glycerol monothioglycolate. This is appropriate for fine or for color-treated hair. There are more cases of allergic contact dermatitis due to this chemical than to the other curling or straightening agents. This permanent wave must be administered in a professional salon.

The midstrength permanent wave is ammonium thioglycolate. This can be used on healthy hair for curling or on kinky hair for straightening. This may be performed at home because of its safety.

The strongest chemicals for these procedures are for resistant kinky hair and include lye (with the higher pH), sodium, lithium, or calcium hydroxide. Professionals must apply these products. If the chemicals are left on too long, the hair shaft may break. They can also burn the skin.

Hair Coloring

The five major types of hair coloring are temporary, gradual, natural, semipermanent, and permanent color. The *temporary colors* are textile dyes. These dyes lie on the top of the cuticle and come off easily with perspiration or rain. Their advantage is to let the individual try a color and not cause any permanent change. These are sage and do not cause allergic reactions. The disadvantage is that the color can come off easily onto one's face or clothes.

The *gradual coloring* consists of metallic salts. The hair can go from gray to brown or black by the action of lead acetate and sulfur. These salts precipitate on the outside of the hair shaft and allow a gradual change in color. Unfortunately, the hair looks very lusterless and can have a characteristic sulfur odor. The metal precipitate also precludes any other hair processing, such as permanent or other coloring procedures. The hair must grow out or have a stripping process before other cosmetic procedures may take place.

Natural coloring with henna from *Lawsonia inermis* is rarely used anymore. This is a vegetable dye that presents no concern for carcinogenicity. It imparts red highlights to hair. This substance can precipitate asthma and allergies. Henna also stains gray hair an unpleasant orange color.

Semipermanent dyes are a nice first step for a person going from gray to a darker color. The active ingredients are low-molecular-weight dyes specifically synthesized for hair coloring. Because the molecules are small, they can penetrate the cuticle and go into the cortex. These dyes leave the hair shiny and attractive. Because those same molecules can slip out of the cuticle just as easily, the color only lasts for four to six shampoos. These dyes have low allergenicity, are easy to apply, and cause only minimal hair shaft damage. Because there is no peroxide used, the colors can only go darker, not lighter.

By far the most common products for hair color in men and women today are the *permanent hair color dyes*. In permanent, or oxidative, hair coloring, the formation of colorless molecules from their precursors occurs inside the cortex as a result of oxidation by hydrogen peroxide. The reaction is p-phenylenediamine + $H_2O_2 \rightarrow$ amines: amines + couplers $\rightarrow$ indo dyes. The indo dye molecules are so large that they cannot slip out of the cortex of the hair shaft. This color lasts for 4 to 6 weeks, until the new growth of scalp hair at the base becomes visible. The correct procedure then is simply to color the 1 or l.5 cm of new growth.

Frosting or highlighting of the hair consists of taking strands of the hair and selectively bleaching them with the same procedure using 30 or 40 volumes percent for hydrogen peroxide (instead of 20 volumes percent, as in normal color).

For a real brunette to become a platinum blond, two processes must be used: first, a removal of all the color with peroxide and then a dying of the hair as outlined. This is the most traumatic procedure that can be performed on the hair. With all of these chemical processes, the hair can be broken off at any point on the shaft. Table 8-1 provides a summary of these color techniques.

Skin Care Products

According to the North American Contact Dermatitis Group, skin care products cause the greatest number of adverse reactions in cosmetics. These can be irritant dermatitis, allergic dermatitis, acne cosmetica, or folliculitis. To understand these products more thoroughly, it is important to study the types of ingredients compounded for these products. These consist of emollients, humectants, surfactants, preservatives, and fragrance.

Emollients

Emollients are film-forming materials that add substance to cosmetic preparations and function on the skin to retard water loss. The five categories of emollients are

- hydrocarbons,
- waxes,
- natural lipid polyesters,

Table 8-1. ■ Coloring Products and Their Key Characteristics*

Type of Coloring Product	Recognition	Skill Involved	Type of Dye	Color Change Range	Site of Action	Lasting Quality	Overall Performance	Degree of Abuse of Hair Structure	Potential for Dermatologic Complaints
Temporary color rinses	Multiple-use package	Minimal Apply and dry	High-molecular-weight acid dyes as used in textiles, and certified food colors in a hydro-alcoholic suspension	Covers gray	Surface of shaft	Poor Removed by shampooing	Poor	Negligible	Negligible
Semi-permanent	Single- or multiple-use package; more viscous than no. 1 to prevent dripping off hair	Moderate Applied to freshly shampooed hair and left in place for 15–40 minutes; skin patch test required	Low-molecular-weight dyes nitrophenylene-diamines, nitroamino-phenols, anthroquinones in shampoo vehicle or a solvent system	Covers gray; one to three shades on dark side of normal hair color	Penetrates to cortex	Gradually lost through three to five shampoos	Fair	Negligible	Negligible
Permanent oxidation type Single process	Two-unit system for mixing just before use	Moderate; skin patch test required	Several classes of dyes including PPD† intermediates in an alkaline peroxide "shampoo"	Covers gray; two or three shades on each side of normal	Cortex	Permanent; new growth touch-up every 4–8 weeks	Excellent	Moderate	Modest
Double process	Same as above	Professional attention necessary	As above, but hair must be previously decolorized (stripped)	Unlimited	Cortex	As above	Excellent	Significant	Moderate; hair breakage; local and systemic peroxide reactions
Progressive	Multiple-use package	None	Metallic salts particularly lead, in solution, cream, or pomade form	Discolors hair only	Surface and some beneath cuticle	As long as product is used regularly	Poor	Minimal	Negligible; a public health problem; incompatible with other chemical hair services
Vegetable Henna			For all practical purposes, this does not exist and is not available. Although true henna is a vegetable dye, its color properties and lasting abilities make it unacceptable. Products are being marketed currently with this name but are actually henna coloring in the second and third categories above.						

*The late Dr. Earl Brauer compiled this chart for previous editions of this book.
†p-Phenylenediamine.

- lightweight esters and ethers, and
- silicone.

The hydrocarbons that are most familiar are mineral oil and petrolatum. Because these products contain no water, there is no need to add preservatives to them. It has been shown by tagging C^+ atoms that petrolatum actually penetrates into the intercellular substance of the epithelium. These hydrocarbons are heavy and may not be as aesthetically pleasing as other moisturizers. In the temperate zones in the winter, however, they are ideal for hands, feet, and other very dry areas on the body. They probably are too occlusive for facial skin. Cosmetic-grade petrolatum has been a larger ingredient of facial cosmetics in the last few years. This grade is noncomedogenic.

Waxes consist of beeswax, synthetic beeswax, cholesterol, and lanolin. These substances usually cause no adverse reaction themselves, but esters of lanolin can occasionally be comedogenic (i.e., cause comedonal acne).

The *natural lipid polyesters* retard water loss by integrating with the proteins of the stratum corneum. Short-chain acids such as coconut oil, capric or caprylic triglycerides, esters of lanolin, and synthesized unsaturated fatty acid esters such as sorbitol oleate or lanolin linoleate can be comedogenic because of their interaction with the stratum corneum. Long-chain polyesters are less likely to be comedogenic because of their molecular size.

Lightweight esters and ethers, such as isopropyl myristate and isopropyl state, also can be comedogenic. They are acceptable if they comprise less than 2% of the formulation. Some of these products act as preservatives at lower concentrations.

By far the most helpful emollient today is *silicone.* This inert product has been pulverized into tiny particles and then added to many products for "slip". It has replaced many of the acnegenic ingredients in facial cosmetics and has performed excellently. Silicone is lubricating, protective, and water repellant. It can be soothing in patients with hypersensitive skin, such as patients with acne rosacea. There is no absorption of silicone topically, so concerns of safety with this product are absent. It has no adverse reaction regarding allergenicity or comedogenicity.

Humectants

Humectants are used to preserve moisture content of materials and attract and absorb water from their environment. Most of these products are cosmetically more pleasing to use. They are especially valuable in climates in which there is more humidity. Examples of humectants are glycerin, sodium pyroglutamic acid, sorbitol, urea, lactic acid, and propylene glycol.

Urea and lactic acid are very helpful ingredients for conditions of hyperkeratosis, such as ichthyosis, keratosis pilaris, Darier's disease, and severe dry skin. They can occasionally cause irritation or stinging but are not sensitizing. Propylene glycol is one of the favorite solvents for topical steroids. It is present in at least two thirds of the topical steroid cream products and in many of the ointments. It can be an irritant and occasionally cause allergic contact dermatitis.

Surfactants

Surfactants are surface-active ingredients that make it easier to mix the oil and water phases in an emulsion and effect a smoother contact between two surfaces. These substances can cause the skin to be more penetrable by lowering the barrier properties of the skin and allowing itself or other ingredients to penetrate the surface and cause irritation or sensitization. The four major types of surfactants are

- anionic,
- nonionic,
- cationic, and
- amphoteric.

The *anionic surfactants* are the principle ingredients in shampoos and synthetic detergent soaps. Sodium lauryl sulfate is an excellent cleanser, and it is the major workhorse for liquid facial cleansers as well as shampoos. Other anionics are alpha olefin sulfonates, NA/K stearate, triethanolamine (TEA-lauryl) sulfate, and sulfosuccinates.

The *nonionic surfactants* are gentler than the anionics. They allow for the removal of minerals from hard water and increase the viscosity and solubility of shampoos. They behave as emulsifiers. These include sorbitan fatty acids, polysorbates, polyethylene glycol lipids, and lauramine oxide.

The *cationic surfactants* function largely as conditioners for hair, thickeners for shampoo, and hair grooming aids. These include stearalkonium chloride, quaternary ammonium salts, quaternary fatty acids, and amino acids.

The *amphoteric surfactants* contain a balance of positive and negative charges. These are not as aggressive products as the anionic surfactants and are the chief ingredients in baby shampoo. Examples of these surfactants are *N*-alkyl-amino acids, betaines, and alkyl imidazoline compounds. These surfactants became more popular in the late 1990s. Cocamidopropyl betaine has been used in shampoos and shower gels more frequently. The use of cocamidopropyl betaine is widespread in the United States. Allergic contact dermatitis to these products has been reported many times in the past few years.

Preservatives

Preservatives are second only to fragrance in causing contact dermatitis. They are absolutely necessary, however, to keep the products fresh and safe. The more water that there is in a product, the more important is the content of preservatives.

Preservatives are classified into three categories: antimicrobials, ultraviolet (UV) light absorbers, and antioxidants. The allergenicity of preservatives is variable. The variables include:

- inherent sensitizing potential,
- concentration in the final product,
- whether it is a wash-off versus leave-on product,
- duration of the skin contact,
- state of the epidermal surface when applied, and
- body region.

Of all these variables, the first two are the most important. Preservatives are mixed and matched depending on whether there is a concern of gram-positive or gram-negative organisms, *Candida* sp., *Pityrosporum ovale*, or fungus.

The following is a review of five of the most commonly used groups of preservatives, their efficacy, and their disadvantages.

Formaldehyde and Formaldehyde Releasers. Free formaldehyde is present, especially in shampoos, because of its efficacy against *Pseudomonas aeruginosa*. Because it is left on for such a short time, patients usually have no reaction to it. However, hairdressers who shampoo their clients all day are likely to experience an allergic contact or an irritant dermatitis from it. Formaldehyde treatment of cornstarch in surgeons' gloves has been implicated as a potential source of sensitization. Formaldehyde-allergic people must avoid permanent press or wrinkle-resistant garments. They should wash all new clothing items before wearing and wear protective undergarments when able.

Of the formaldehyde releasers, *quaternium 15* is number one and *imidazolidinyl urea* is number two in causing contact dermatitis. Other formaldehyde releasers include BNPD (Bronopol), diazolidinyl urea (Germal II), and DMDM hydantoin (Glydant). All of these products are very effective against *Pseudomonas* sp.

Parabens. Parabens are the least allergenic and most popular of all the preservatives. They are very effective against fungi and gram-positive bacteria. They are relatively water insoluble, so are not effective against *Pseudomonas* sp. Combining two parabens in the same formulation enhances efficacy. Cross-reaction between individual parabens is the rule. As with the formaldehyde releasers,

parabens are more likely to react with dermatitic skin, but sensitization is not common with these preservatives.

Antioxidants. Antioxidants are less frequently used. These include butylated hydroxyanisole (BHA), butylated hydroxytoluene (BHT), Triclosan, and sorbic acid. BHA and BHT are important for the prevention of spoilage. These are present in lipstick and sunscreens. Their widest use is in foods. Triclosan is a disinfectant and preservative in deodorants, shampoo, and soap. Sorbic acid is used often in creams and lotions. It is fungistatic but has poor bacterial inhibition.

Kathon CG (Methylchloroisothiazoline and Methylisothiazolinone). This organic preservative was considered the most complete and safest preservative until the 1990s. It is an odorless and colorless biocide that exhibits microbiocidal activity against a wide spectrum of fungi and gram-positive and -negative bacteria.

More than 80 publications in the 1990s have reported allergic contact dermatitis to cleansing cream, hair tonics, hair balsam, wash softeners, cosmetics, and moist toilet paper. When these reports came in, a more serious study of Kathon CG took place. According to the North American Contact Dermatitis Group, the incidence of allergy is 1.9%. As long as the concentration is below 15 parts per million (ppm) in rinse-off products and less than 7.5 ppm in leave-on products, this substance is acceptable.

Fragrance and Fragrance Products

Fragrance as an ingredient in skin care products is the greatest allergen. In one study, it accounted for 149 of 536 reactions. Together, fragrance and preservatives accounted for half of all the reactions to cosmetics.

Fragrance products include perfume, cologne, toilet water, bath-water additives, bath powder, and aftershave lotions.

The most common reaction to fragrance is allergic contact dermatitis, followed by photodermatitis, contact urticaria, irritation, and depigmentation. The common fragrance allergens are:

- cinnamic alcohol,
- cinnamic aldehyde,
- hydroxycitronnellal,
- isoeugenol, and
- oak moss absolute.

The most common photoallergen is musk ambrette. This substance is not used as often currently.

Balsam of Peru as a patch test is a good screening agent for fragrance. In the past, oil of bergamot, found in Shalimar perfume, was the most common photoallergen. Now, those perfumes that contain oil of bergamot contain the bergapten-free variety, so there are fewer photodermatitis reactions.

Makeup (Color) Products

The use of color cosmetics is likened to an artist painting a picture on a canvas. Foundation is used to give a simple flawless complexion on which other color cosmetics can be applied.

Spot coverage can be achieved with several products before foundation is applied. For patients with defects after surgery, telangiectasias, or lentigines, an erase stick or a heavier concealer product is applied before foundation. For patients with rosacea, some products with a green-tinted sulfur can be used. Acne patients can use tinted spot sticks containing sulfur, salicylic acid, or benzoyl peroxide. For patients with scar tissue, laser resurfacing, face peeling, or a green or lavender tint prefoundation may be used before the regular foundation is applied.

The types of foundation vary with coverage and cream or moisture content. The concealing or covering quality varies with the amount of titanium dioxide and not the density of the product. Foundation can be transparent, imparting only color, translucent, offering more cover, or opaque, offering total coverage. This increasing amount of coverage does not affect the comedogenicity of the product.

Dermatologists are interested in the amount of cream or moisturizer in foundation. For teenagers, a shake lotion-type foundation is less likely to contribute to acne. For 20- to 50-year-old women, a heavier makeup that is labeled noncomedogenic or oil free may be appropriate. For most women 50 years old or older, any kind of moisturizing foundation is acceptable as long as they are not prone to adult acne or rosacea.

The ingredients that are more likely to be comedogenic (this term is totally relative) are:

- isopropyl myristate,
- isopropyl ester,
- oleic acid,
- stearic acid,
- petrolatum (not cosmetic grade), and
- lanolin (especially acetylated lanolin alcohols and lanolin fatty acids).

The products that have been substituted for the above ingredients, and that are less likely to be comedogenic, are low-dose mineral oil, octyl palmitate, isostearyl neopentanoate, cottonseed oil, corn oil, safflower oil, propylene glycol, spermaceti, beeswax, and sodium lauryl sulfate.

The final product, however, must be tested to determine if the compound is truly noncomedogenic or not. This is best tested on the face or back of patients who are acne prone. A good screening is with the rabbit ear, but this is not always allowed.

With the clever use of highlighting with foundation or concealer, asymmetry, scleroderma, heavy cheeks, or an unclear jaw line can be concealed. It is not necessarily a physician's place to demonstrate this to the patient, but the physician should know where to send a patient who needs help to normalize his or her appearance. Even medically tattooing burned or scarred skin can be of assistance.

Types of Color Cosmetics

Color cosmetics include foundation, eye makeup (shadow, liner, mascara), lipstick, rouge, blush, and nail enamel.

Blush adds color and the look of good health to the patient's appearance. Cream blush can be comedogenic and hard to apply. Older patients who have dry skin may best use it. Powder blush seems to be the best choice. It should be applied in the same areas that children flush in when exercising. Usually, these products do not cause adverse reactions.

Lipsticks are made of waxes that are usually nonallergenic and noncomedogenic. When eosin dyes were used for long-lasting lipsticks, there were cases of photodermatitis. They are used less frequently now. Only sunscreen may be an ingredient that causes allergic reactions.

For women who have vertical lines above and below the vermilion border, the use of a lead lipstick pencil or liner can be helpful. This stops the waxy lipstick from "bleeding" into the vertical furrows when the patient eats or drinks. Lip liner is also recommended for women with asymmetry of their lips owing to removal of a tumor, other lip surgery, or too thin lips. The desired outline of the lips can be drawn with the pencil or line, and then the color can be filled in.

Eye makeup—shadow, liner, mascara—can be used to enlarge, brighten, or accentuate the eyes. Because of the need to prevent infection, most eye makeup contains preservatives. These preservatives are listed on the outside of the package and patients can check to see if they have had an adverse reaction to them. Generally, the preservatives are EDTA, BAL, thimerosal, parabens, quaternium 15, or phenylmercuric acetate/nitrate. Usually, each cosmetic company formulates its products with its specific preservatives. Therefore, a patient who cannot use one company's eye products may be able to use another company's products. Most American eye cosmetics are formulated without fragrance and with the simplest hypoallergic formula.

Eye shadow can function to conceal flaws or enlarge the eye. Usually, if the patient has an allergic reaction to cream eye shadow, a powder eye shadow is a good substitute. *Eyeliner* may help to change the shape of the eye as well as accentuate it. These products usually are waxes and therefore produce no adverse reaction. Pencil eyeliner is preferred to liquid eyeliner for a more natural appearance.

Mascara can be water based or waterproof. The water-based products are healthier for the eyelashes because they can be removed easily with soap and water. Products with lengtheners, however, may add lacquer and may require special solvents to remove the old mascara. Waterproof mascara may have a lower concentration of preservatives and may therefore be less allergenic for some patients. It is necessary to use an eye makeup remover to take mascara off. The use of the special remover may be more traumatic to the eyelashes. Because of this, patients with fragile lashes (e.g., patients with alopecia areata) should wear water-washable mascara.

Eyelash curlers can be used to give the illusion of longer lashes and conceal blepharochalasia. The patient who is allergic to nickel or rubber should not use this instrument. If an eyelash curler is to be used, it must be used before mascara is applied.

Nail enamels, including base coats and top coats, have similar composition:

- *Film former:* nitrocellulose
- *Resin:* toluene sulfonamide/formaldehyde resin, alkyl resins, acrylates, vinyls, or polyesters
- *Plasticizers:* camphor, dibutyl phthalate, dioctyl phthalate, tricresyl phosphate
- *Solvents:* alcohol, toluene, ethyl acetate, and butyl acetate
- *Colorants:* (optional)
- *Pearlizers:* guanine and bismuth oxychloride (optional)

The major ingredient that causes allergic contact dermatitis is toluene sulfonamide. Butyl and ethyl methacrylate, which are in the glue used for sculptured nails, press-on nails, and nail mending, can also cause contact dermatitis. Cuticle remover (sodium or potassium hydroxide) is left on the cuticle to dissolve dead skin. If left on too long, this product becomes an irritant. The entire nail can be separated from the nail bed by too vigorous use of cuticle remover.

Cosmeceuticals

Cosmeceutical has been coined to describe cosmetic-type products that are promoted with aggressive claims to have a favorable impact on the condition of the skin. These products include retinoids, antioxidants (vitamins), α-hydroxy acids, β-hydroxy acids, antiperspirants, sunscreens, and self-tanners.

Retinoids

In 1984, L.H. Kligman demonstrated that connective tissue could be repaired in the rhino mouse with tretinoin. Subsequently, this same effect was established in humans with a multicenter, double-blind study over a 48-week period. This ushered in a new method of skin care for photoaging, cancer, and cosmetic reasons. The gold standard for the reversal of photoaging is tretinoin, but because of its irritant potential, many other products have been studied.

Older Retinoids, First Generation

Since 1984, many preparations of tretinoin have been made. The first products with concentrations of 0.1% were irritating to the skin of many patients. Since that time formulations of 0.02% and 0.01% have been incorporated into creams and gels. These products have been demonstrated in biopsies, photographs, and clinical observations to rejuvenate the skin. The cosmetic chemists have taken the formulations even further by incorporating the tretinoin into microsponges and special polymers and by adding moisturizers. A 4-week treatment with tretinoin in a solution of 50% ethanol and 50% propylene glycol 400 was studied by Kligman and Draelos for rapid retinization of photoaged facial skin. Almost all subjects improved on all measures of clinical grading (fine lines, mottled pigmentation, surface texture/roughness) by 4 weeks. The newer tools for assessing skin changes—digital cameras, consistent lighting, and computers—have allowed for greater accuracy in observations.

Retinoids, Third Generation

Adapaline 0.1% cream and gel is less irritating than tretinoin. This product has been used for photoaging but is used more for acne therapy. Tazarotene cream 0.1% has been compared to tretinoin emollient cream 0.05% for efficacy. The results were similar, but the tazarotene cream demonstrated quicker efficacy at weeks 12 and 20. The main side effect of this retinoid is irritation. It is a category X drug and should not be used during pregnancy.

First-Generation Cosmeceuticals

For patients who cannot tolerate retinoids, new products are discovered daily. The first sets of these products consist of vitamins, other natural occurring antioxidants, plant antioxidants, and α-hydroxy and β-hydroxy acids.

Antioxidants

Antioxidants are products that quench or offset free radicals. These free radicals occur because of sunlight, pollution, stress, heavy metals, drugs, and normal metabolism. Free radicals have a role in skin carcinogenesis, inflammation, and aging. The mechanism by which they disturb homeostasis is the combination of oxygen with other molecules, leaving an odd number of electrons. Oxygen with an unpaired electron is reactive, because it takes electrons from vital components, leaving them damaged.

DNA, cytoskeletal elements, and cellular membranes may all be adversely affected. Antioxidants couple with unpaired electrons to disarm or offset the free radicals. Naturally occurring antioxidants include:

- vitamin A,
- vitamin B_3 (niacinamide),
- vitamin B_5 (Panthenol),
- vitamin C,
- vitamin E,
- α-lipoic acid,
- β-carotene,
- catalase,
- glutathione,
- superoxide dismutase,
- ubiquinone (coenzyme Q10),
- green tea polyphenols,
- silymarin,
- soy isoflavones, and
- furfuryladenine.

These ingredients have been incorporated into many products over the past 10 years. Their success at a cellular level has been assessed with biopsies, photographs, and sun testing. The model for testing most of the antioxidants is the use of these products before, during, and after sun exposure. The results were a lack of erythema, sunburn cell production, or other signs of UV damage. Scientists have also tested the ability of the skin to keep its immunity. Sun can cause immunosuppression, which can stop cancer surveillance. These antioxidants can prevent the immunosuppression from occurring.

All of these antioxidants have been put into formulations to treat fine and coarse wrinkling, dyspigmentation, and erythema. The gold standard of improving skin quality is still tretinoin in whatever formulation it occurs. Some patients cannot tolerate the irritation from tretinoin; for those individuals, antioxidant cosmetics are appropriate.

α-Hydroxy Acids

Dermatologists have used lactic acid for many years. Research by Van Scott has ushered into widespread use the rest of the α-hydroxy acids. These natural fruit acids exert their influence by diminishing corneocyte cohesion. The most commonly used ingredients are:

- *glycolic acid:* sugar cane
- *lactic acid:* sour milk
- *malic acid:* apples
- *citric acid:* citrus fruits
- *tartatic acid:* grapes

Leyden outlines the functions of the α-hydroxy acids clearly:

1. They bind water in the skin; therefore, the stratum corneum becomes more flexible.
2. They normalize desquamation of corneocytes from the stratum corneum. This may occur by interaction with stratum corneum lipids.
3. They release cytokines locally.
4. They cause a thickening of the epidermis.
5. They increase production of hyaluronic acid within the dermis. This may be due to the increased production of transforming growth factor-β.
6. In both ichthyosis and thickening stratum corneum of dry skin, the α-hydroxy acids make the skin thin down toward normal.

The α-hydroxy acids have been incorporated into cosmetic formulation for shampoos, soap, face creams, and body creams. The difficulty in formulating these products is the need to be buffered. A 5% concentration in one product may not be as effective as a 5% concentration in another. Glycolic acid peels have also been unpredictable because of this lack of standardization. These products are being improved daily.

β-Hydroxy Acids

In the search for a less irritating and stinging compound for creams and peels, β-hydroxy acids have become very popular. There is only one ingredient in this category, salicylic acid. Dermatologists have known this keratolytic for years chiefly as an exfoliant for acne at concentration of 2% to 3%, and a therapy for warts at concentrations of 10% to 15% in creams and 40% in pastes. Salicylic acid appears to have an anti-inflammatory component and may have less sting and irritancy than glycolic acid.

β-Hydroxy acid face peels have also become popular for patients who cannot tolerate glycolic or trichloracetic acid peels.

Second-Generation Cosmeceuticals

These products have been developed from wound healing and skin repair studies. They are usually dermally active compounds. They increase fibroblast activity, increase protein and collagen syntheses, produce antioxidant enzymes, and are less irritating than retinoids. There are three categories of these cosmeceuticals:

- copper peptides,
- human growth factors, and
- pentapeptides.

Copper Peptides

These products have been shown to enhance wound healing, especially in patients undergoing Mohs and laser procedures and therapy for diabetic ulcers. They promote vascular formation, promote collagen and elastin, and are a catalyst for antioxidants.

In a poster exhibit at the American Academy of Dermatology meeting in February 2002, a study of 67 patients showed that most patients improved in fine lines and wrinkles, surface roughness, and increased skin density. At this point, copper peptide products are only available in private doctors' offices.

Human Growth Factors

These products are safe; there is no inflammatory reaction. They cause increased protein production. They are usually obtained from placental extracts or are growth factors bioengineered from human foreskin. The before and after photographs of patients using these products are very impressive. The downsides of human growth factors are that they are very expensive and they have a very unpleasant odor.

Pentapeptides

It was discovered in vitro in 1993 that a subfragment of type I collagen could stimulate type I, type III, and fibronectin. Ex vivo studies in full-thickness human skin biopsies demonstrated stimulation of collagen I. These products consisted of five amino acids that, when combined with palmitic acid, could penetrate the skin (palmitoyl-pentapeptide 3 Pal-KTTKS). When this product was compared with retinol, it decreased wrinkles in depth and volume. In vitro studies demonstrate stimulation of collagen IV and glucosaminoglucanes, including hyaluronic acid. The advantages of these products are that they stimulate matrix formation and are not irritating. These products are available over the counter and appear to be successful for both wound healing and rejuvenation.

Antiperspirants and Deodorants

Antiperspirants are considered a drug (cosmeceutical) because of their physical interaction with the sweat duct. These products, which contain aluminum salts, act by causing a precipitation in the duct itself to block the secretion of sweat. They must have a specific amount of aluminum salts and in laboratory tests must reduce sweat by at least 20% in half the people tested.

Deodorants contain bacteria-killing agents such as Triclosan, bacteria-retarding ingredients, and fragrance. They are a cosmetic because they do not change the function of the skin, just mask body odor. For efficacy, roll-on antiperspirant products are best, then the sticks, and then the spray products.

Sunscreens

Sunscreens are the most important of the cosmetics that men and women can use. Because these prevent skin cancer, they are considered a drug or cosmeceutical. These products are usually calibrated according to the sun-protective factor (SPF). The SPF value for ultraviolet B (UVB) rays is the ratio of the UVB dose required to produce the minimal erythema reaction through the applied sunscreen product (2 mg/cm^2) compared with the UVB dose required to produce the same degree of minimal erythema reaction without sunscreen. Sunscreens consist of physical sunblocks, chemical UVB sunblocks, and chemical ultraviolet A (UVA) sunblocks.

Zinc oxide has been used by lifeguards and children for many years on noses, ear tips, upper cheeks, and shoulders. The advantage of this substance is that it is inert and therefore not allergenic. The disadvantage is that it is messy. With the newer ability to pulverize this chemical, very elegant and superior products have been synthesized. The spectrum of microfine zinc oxide extends from 290 to 400 nm. This is the most complete sunscreen available.

Titanium dioxide has also been added to products for hypoallergenic coverage as well as a complete block. Without being in the microfine type, patients may look like they have a purple cast to their skin. With the advent of microfine titanium dioxide, the coverage extends from 290 to 350 nm.

Both of these physical sunblocks have good coverage and no allergic or photoallergic reactions; they are waterproof, chemical free, and provide superior coverage for UVA and good coverage for UVB. The disadvantages are that they can give a masklike or opaque appearance to the skin and may give the skin a violet color.

Chemical Absorbers UVB

p-Aminobenzoic acid (PABA) and PABA esters (padimate O, padimate A, glycerol PABA) were the major sunblocks in the United States until the mid-1980s. Their advantages were that they protect against the 290- to 320-nm wavelength, they are easy to work with cosmetically, the esters are nonstaining, and they bind to the horny layer of the skin. If a patient applied these substances 3 days in a row, he or she might still have protection on the fourth day. The disadvantages were the lack of protection for UVA, cross-sensitivity with benzoin and *p*-phenylenediamine, and that PABA itself may stain. Today, only padimate O is readily available. This is used primarily in hair products.

Cinnamates (octyl methoxycinnamate and cinoxate) have largely replaced PABA in many products. These are incorporated into many face makeups in which an SPF of 6 to 12 may be desired. These are easy to work with and rarely sensitizing. These are the most common ingredients in cosmetic products for sun protection.

Salicylates (homomenthyl, octyl, triethanolamine) have only an SPF of 3.5 but are excellent additions to formulations to increase the SPF protections. Rarely they may cause photodermatitis.

Octocrylene and *phenybenzimidazole sulfonic acid* are two other excellent UVB chemical sunscreens. They can even stabilize avobenzone (Parsol 1789), and so are helpful in combination sunscreens.

Chemical Absorbers of UVA

Benzophenones. Benzophenones were the chief UVA blockers until recently. Oxybenzone and dioxybenzone have a broad absorption spectrum of 200 to 250 nm. These ingredients are incorporated into compounds easily and are less allergenic than the PABA derivatives. There are many reports of photocontact dermatitis from oxybenzone and occasional reports of contact dermatitis and contact urticaria from dioxybenzone. The most common occurrence of the photocontact dermatitis from these products occurs with intense and very warm sun exposure such as is found near the equator. Many patients can use these products in temperate zones but react while on vacation in more tropical zones. Physical sunblocks should then be substituted.

Parsol 1789 (Avobenzone). Parsol 1789 has been available since about 1989 in the United States. It has a spectrum of 310 to 400 nm, with a peak at 358 nm. Because of this spectrum, it is the sunblock of choice for all people with special UVA needs. Of course, it must be combined with a UVB block for total protection. Cinnamates did not combine well with this ingredient. Now, octocrylene is the ingredient that stabilizes parsol and allows the attainment of a complete chemical sunblock. The physical sunblocks—microfine zinc oxide and titanium dioxide—are used very commonly in patients with UVA sensitivity.

Vitamins C and E can synergize with the chemical sunblocks. They may be included in many sunblocks in the future.

Mexoryl. This ingredient is available in Europe and Canada. This product, which is patented by L'Oreal, may be the best UVA screen available today. In combination with octocrylene, avobenzone, and titanium dioxide, it appears to be a very effective sunblock. We are awaiting its approval in the United States.

Tanning Product Categories

Self-tanning lotions consist primarily of dihydroxyacetone (DHA). These have a protein-staining effect from the DHA in the stratum corneum of the skin. These products used to be orange and streaky but have been perfected to an even-colored tone by the addition of silicone to the vehicle. They have been formulated into sprays available at salons to cover the entire body. Although these are nontoxic, they may accentuate freckles and seborrheic keratosis and therefore be unattractive. When using these products, patients should sand themselves with a loofa or cleansing granules before the application to make the color even.

Bronzing gels consist of henna, walnut, juglone, and lawsone. These are water-soluble dyes to stain the skin. They can be messy to clothes, have the stickiness of a gel, but usually look good on the face. They are also noncomedogenic.

Tanning promoters, such as 5-methoxypsoralen, have been well documented to be highly phototoxic and carcinogenic. 5-Methoxypsoralen is not available over the counter in the United States. Tanning pills consist of canthaxanthin and are toxic to both skin and eyes. These are not available over the counter in the United States.

How to Test for Cosmetic Allergy

The items on the standard tray and the TRUE test that apply to cosmetics include imidazolidinyl urea, wool (lanolin) alcohols, *p*-phenylenediamine, thimerosal, formaldehyde, colophony, quaternium 15, balsam of Peru, and Cinnamic aldehyde. The cosmetics that can be tested without dilution are antiperspirants, blushes, eyeliners, eye shadow, foundations, lipstick, moisturizers, perfumes, and sunscreens. The cosmetics that are volatile and need to be allowed to dry on the patch or chamber before 48-hour occlusion are liquid eyeliner, mascara, and nail enamel.

The cosmetics that need to be diluted for testing are soaps, shampoos, shaving preparations, hair dyes, and permanent solution. These may need open patch testing or usage testing.

SAUER'S NOTES

Cosmetics are an important part of dermatology. The physician should know how they are used, what their components are, and how best to explain them to the patient.

Suggested Reading

Adams RM, Maibach HI. A five-year study of cosmetic reactions. J Am Acad Dermatol 1985;12:1062.

Draelos ZD. Alpha-hydroxy acids and other topical agents. Dermatol Ther 2000;13:154–158.

Emerit I, Packer L, Auclair C. Antioxidants in therapy and preventative medicine. New York, Plenum Press, 1990, p. 594.

Jackson EM. Tanning without sun: Accelerators, promoters, pills, bronzing gels, and self-tanning lotions. Am J Contact Dermatitis 1994;5:38.

Kligman AM, Dogadkina D, Lavker RM. Effects of topical tretinoin on non-sun-exposed protected skin of the elderly. J Am Acad Dermatol 1993;29:25.

Leyden J. Alpha-hydroxy acids. Dialog Dermatol 1994; 34:3.

Maibach HI, Engasser PG. Dermatitis due to cosmetics. In: Fischer AA, ed. Contact dermatitis, ed 3. Philadelphia, Lea & Febiger, 2986:383.1986.

O'Donoghue, MN. Hair Care Products. In Olsen EA. Disorders of hair growth, diagnosis and treatment, ed 3. McGraw-Hill, New York, Chicago, 481–496, 2003.

Olsen EA, Katz HI, Levin N, et al. Tretinoin emollient cream for photodamaged skin: Results of 48-week, multicenter, double-blind studies. J Am Acad Dermatol 1997;37:217.

Pathak MA. Sunscreens and their use in the preventative treatment of sunlight-induced skin damage. J Dermatol Surg Oncol 1987;13:739.

Pinnell, SR. Cutaneous photodamage, oxidative stress, and topical antioxidant protection. J Am Acad Dermatol 2003;48:1–19.

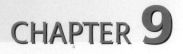

Dermatologic Allergy

John C. Hall

Contact dermatitis, industrial dermatoses, atopic eczema, and drug eruptions are included in this chapter because of their obvious allergenic factors. (However, some cases of contact dermatitis and industrial dermatitis are caused by irritants.) Nummular eczema is also included because it resembles some forms of atopic eczema and may even be a variant of atopic eczema.

Contact Dermatitis

Contact dermatitis (Figures 9-1, 9-2, 9-3, and 9-4), or dermatitis venenata, is a very common inflammation of the skin caused by the exposure of the skin either to primary irritant substances, such as soaps, or to allergenic substances, such as poison ivy resin. Industrial dermatoses are considered at the end of this section.

Presentation

Primary Lesions

Any of the stages, from mild redness, edema, or vesicles to large bullae with a marked amount of oozing, are seen. This is usually limited to the site where the contactant touched the skin, but can flare beyond the site when the inflammation is severe. With poison ivy, oak, and sumac, a black stain on skin or clothing is rarely seen.

Secondary Lesions

Crusting from secondary bacterial infection, excoriations, and lichenification occurs. A generalized eruption can occur in a symmetrical distribution in a widespread distribution when the local site is severely affected. This is called an Id or autoeczemtous eruption. It commonly causes vesicles on the palms, soles, and sides of the fingers and toes. It is very pruritic.

Distribution and Causes

Any agent can affect any area of the body. However, certain agents commonly affect certain skin areas.

- *Face and Neck* (Figure 9-5): Cosmetics, soaps, insect sprays, ragweed, perfumes or hair sprays (sides of neck), fingernail polish (eyelids), hat bands (forehead), mouthwashes, toothpaste, or lipstick (perioral), nickel metal (under earrings), necklaces and collars (neck), industrial oil (facial chloracne).
- *Hands and Forearms:* Soaps, hand lotions, wrist bands, industrial chemicals, poison ivy, and a multitude of other agents. Irritation from soap often begins under rings as does allergic reactions from nickel (common) or gold (rare). Latex from gloves can cause a contact dermatitis and contact urticaria. It can be associated with life-threatening anaphylaxis and is becoming an increasing danger because of increased use of latex gloves and latex contraceptives.
- *Axillae:* Deodorants, dress shields, detergents, bleaching agents, fabric softener, antistatic agents, and dry cleaning solutions.
- *Trunk:* Clothing (new, not previously cleaned), rubber or metal attached to, or in, clothing (central abdomen under metal clasp), and transdermal drug patches.
- *Anogenital region:* Douches, dusting powder, contraceptives, colored toilet paper, topical hemorrhoid preparations, poison ivy, or topicals for treatment of pruritus ani, candida, and fungal infections.
- *Feet:* Shoes, foot powders, topical agents for "athlete's foot" infection.
- *Generalized eruption:* Volatile airborne chemicals (paint, spray, ragweed), medicaments locally applied to large areas, bath powder, or clothing.

Course

Duration can be very short (days) to very chronic (weeks, months, and even years). As a general rule, successive recurrences become more chronic (e.g., seasonal

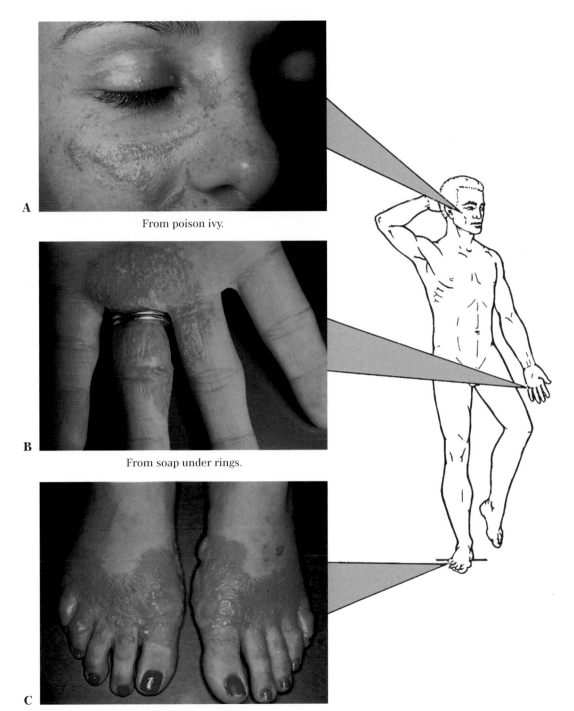

A   From poison ivy.

B   From soap under rings.

C   From shoe material.

FIGURE 9-1 ■ Contact dermatitis. (**A**) From poison ivy. (**B**) From soap under rings. (**C**) From shoe material. *(Courtesy of Burroughs Wellcome Co.)*

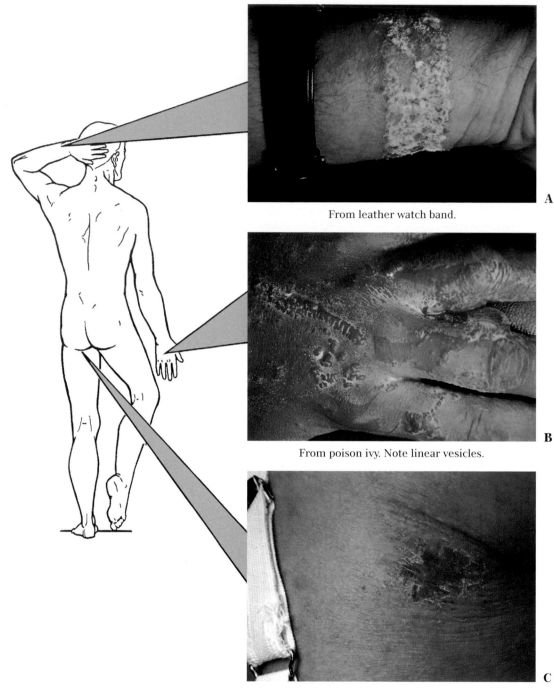

From leather watch band.

A

From poison ivy. Note linear vesicles.

B

From nickel metal in garter strap.

C

FIGURE 9-2 ■ Contact dermatitis. (**A**) From leather watch band. (**B**) From poison ivy. Note linear vesicles. (**C**) From nickel metal in garter strap. *(Courtesy of Burroughs Wellcome Co.)*

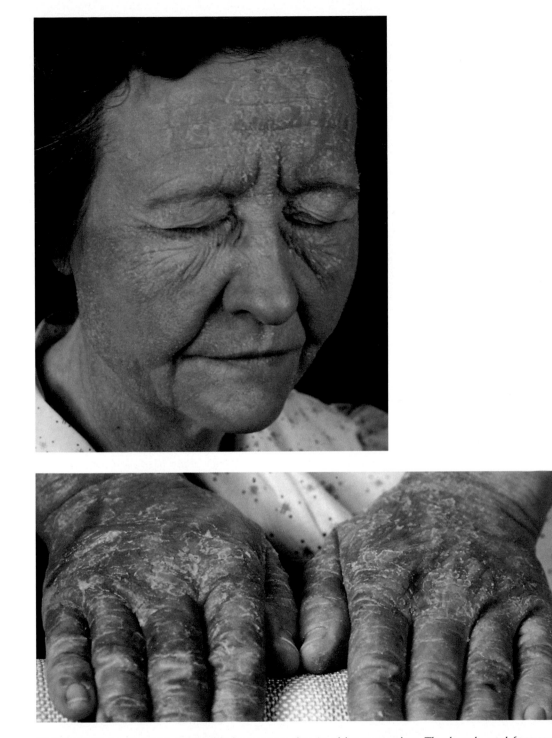

FIGURE 9-3 ■ Contact dermatitis in a nurse due to chlorpromazine. The hands and face were involved most severely. This eruption was aggravated following exposure to sunlight. *(Courtesy of K.U.M.C.; Burroughs Wellcome Co.)*

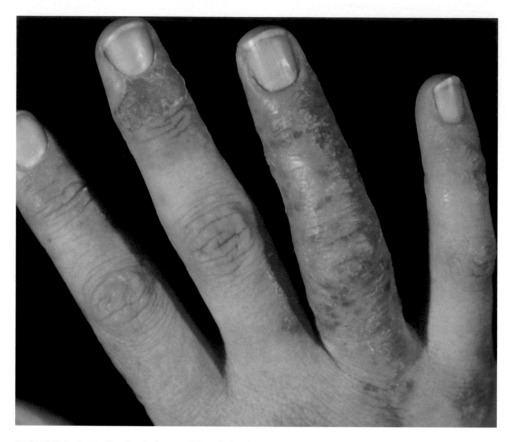

FIGURE 9-4 ■ Contact dermatitis of the hand. This common dermatitis is usually due to continued exposure to soap and water. *(Courtesy of K.U.M.C.; Burroughs Wellcome Co.)*

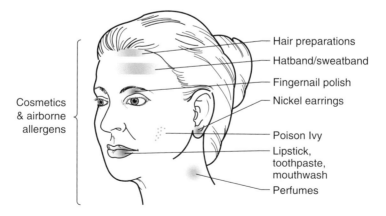

FIGURE 9-5 ■ Contact dermatitis of the face.

ragweed dermatitis can become a year-round dermatitis). An established hypersensitivity reaction is seldom lost. Also, certain people are more susceptible to allergic and irritant contact dermatitis than others. This is particularly true in patients who already have inflamed skin such as irritants in patients with eczema. A very careful seasonal history of the onset, in chronic cases, may lead to discovery of an unsuspected causative agent, such as ragweed.

Familial incidence of contact dermatitis is not evident. The eczematous reaction (e.g., the blister fluid of poison ivy) contains no allergen that can cause the dermatitis in another person or in other areas on the same person. However, if the poison ivy oil or other allergen remains on the clothes of the affected person, contact of the allergen with a susceptible person could cause a dermatitis. The hair or fur of animals, and utensils used in hunting or gardening can also transfer to allergenic resine of poison ivy.

Laboratory Findings

Patch tests (see Chap. 2) are of value in eliciting the cause in a problem case. Careful interpretation is required.

Differential Diagnosis

A contact reaction must be considered and ruled in or out in any case of eczematous or oozing dermatitis on any body area.

Treatment

Two of the most common contact dermatoses seen in the physician's office are poison ivy (or poison oak or sumac) dermatitis and hand dermatitis. The treatments for these two conditions are discussed separately.

Treatment of Contact Dermatitis Owing to Poison Ivy

Case Example. A patient comes to the office with a linear, vesicular dermatitis of the feet, hands, and face. He states that he spent the weekend fishing and that the rash broke out the next day. The itching is rather severe but not enough to keep him awake at night. He had "poison ivy" 5 years ago.

First Visit.

1. There are several mistaken notions about poison ivy dermatitis. Assure the patient that he cannot give the dermatitis to his family or spread it on himself from the blister fluid.

2. Suggest that the clothes worn while fishing be washed in warm soapy water to remove the allergenic resin.

3. Prescribe Burow's solution wet packs.

   Sig: Add one packet of powder (Domeboro) to 1 quart of cool water. Apply sheeting or toweling, wet with the solution, to the blistered areas for 20 minutes twice a day. The wet packs need not be removed during the 20-minute period. (For a more widespread case of poison ivy dermatitis, take cool baths with half box of Aveeno [colloidal oatmeal] or soluble starch to the tub, which gives considerable relief from the itching.)

4. 1% Hydrocortisone lotion q.s. 60.0 (1% Hytone [available OTC] lotion, 1% HC Pramosone lotion (contains the antipruritic antihistamine pramoxine, etc.)

   Sig: Apply t.i.d. and prn itching to the affected areas.

5. Chlorpheniramine maleate tablets, 4 mg #60

   Sig: 1 tablet t.i.d. (for relief of itching).

   Comment: Warn patient about side effect of drowsiness. This drug is available over the counter and is less expensive than if a prescription is written.

6. Use cortisone-type injection. Short- but rapid-acting corticosteroids are moderately beneficial, such as betamethasone (Celestone Phosphate) (3 mg/mL in a dose of 1 to 2 mL subcutaneously), or dexamethasone (Decadron LA) (8 mg/mL) in a dose of 1 to 1.5 mL intramuscularly. Triamcinolone (Kenalog 20) to 40 mg IM can also be given.

Subsequent Visits.

1. Continue the wet packs only as long as there are blisters and oozing. Extended use is too drying for the skin.

2. After 3 or 4 days of use, the lotion may be too drying. Substitute fluorinated corticosteroid emollient cream q.s. 60.0

   Sig: Apply small amount locally t.i.d., or more often if itching is present.

SAUER'S NOTES

1. In obtaining a history, question the patient carefully about home, over-the-counter, other physicians', and well-meaning friends' remedies. Contact dermatitis on top of a contact dermatitis is quite common.

2. When you are unable to find the cause of a generalized contact dermatitis, determine the site of the *initial* eruption and think of the agents that touch the area.

SAUER'S NOTES

1. Most failures in the therapy for severe poison ivy or oak dermatitis result from the failure to continue the oral corticosteroid for 10–14 days or longer.
2. Medrol Dosepak therapy does not provide enough days of treatment for most cases of poison ivy dermatitis.
3. Explain to the patient that it is common for new lesions, even blisters, to continue to pop out during the entire duration of the eruption.

Severe Cases of Poison Ivy Dermatitis.

1. An oral corticosteroid is indicated in severe cases of poison ivy dermatitis: prednisone, 10 mg #30

   Sig: 5 tablets each morning for 2 days, 4 tablets each morning for 2 days, 3 tablets each morning for 2 days, 2 tablets each morning for 2 days, and 1 tablet each morning for 2 days. Take with food in the morning.

The use of poison ivy vaccine orally or intramuscularly is contraindicated during an acute episode. Desensitization may occur after a long course of oral ingestion of graduated doses of the allergen, but pruritus ani, generalized pruritus, and urticaria probably make the treatment worse than the disease. Desensitization does not occur after a short course of IM injections of the vaccine, and this form of prophylactic therapy is worthless. Barrier creams may decrease dermatitis if applied before exposure; examples include Hydropel and Ivy Block.

A window of up to 2 hours may exist where washing the skin with a surfactant (e.g., Dial soap) and oil-removing compound (soap or Goop) or a chemical inactivator (Tecnu) may ameliorate or prevent the contact dermatitis.

Treatment of Contact Dermatitis of the Hand Owing to Soap

Case Example. A young housewife states that she has had a breakout on her hands for 5 weeks. The dermatitis developed about 4 weeks after the birth of her last child. She states that she had a similar eruption after her previous two pregnancies. She has used a lot of local medication of her own, and the rash is getting worse instead of better. The patient and her immediate family never had any asthma, hay fever, or eczema.

Examination of the patient's hands reveals small vesicles on the sides of all of her fingers, with a 5-cm area of oozing and crusting around her left ring finger.

SAUER'S NOTES

1. "Housewives' eczema" cannot usually be cured with a corticosteroid salve alone without observing the other protective measures.
2. After the dermatitis is clear, it is very important to advise the patient to treat the area for at least another week to prevent a recurrence. I call this "therapy plus."

First Visit.

1. Assure the patient that the hand eczema is not contagious to her family.
2. Inform the patient that soap irritates the dermatitis and that it must be avoided as much as possible. A homemaker will find this avoidance very difficult. One of the best remedies is to wear protective gloves when extended soap-and-water contact is unavoidable. Rubber gloves alone produce a considerable amount of irritating perspiration, but this is absorbed when thin white cotton gloves are worn under the rubber gloves. Lined rubber gloves are not as satisfactory because the lining eventually becomes dirty and soggy and cannot be cleaned easily. Bluettes is an excellent protective glove.
3. For body cleanliness, a mild soap, such as Dove, can be used, or any of the following: Cetaphil soapless cleanser, Basis soap, and Neutrogena soaps.
4. Tell the patient that these prophylactic measures must be adhered to for several weeks after the eruption has apparently cleared or there will be a recurrence. Injured skin is sensitive and needs to be pampered for an extended time.
5. Burow's solution soaks.

   Sig: Add 1 packet of powder (Domeboro) to 1 quart of cool water. Soak hands for 15 minutes twice a day.

6. Fluorinated corticosteroid ointment (see Formulary in Chap. 5) 15.0

   Sig: Apply sparingly, locally, q.i.d.

Resistant, Chronic Cases.

1. To the corticosteroid ointment add, as indicated, sulfur (3% to 5%), coal tar solution (3% to 10%), or an antipruritic agent such as menthol (0.25%) or camphor (2%).
2. Oral corticosteroid therapy. A short course of such therapy rapidly improves or cures a chronic dermatitis.
3. Prevention of flares of contact dermatitis can be accomplished by frequent use of emollient preparations. SBR

Lipocream, Curel, Cetaphil Hand Cream and Neutrogena Norwegian Hand Cream are examples. Bag Balm or Udder Cream are odiferous, less cosmetic choices.

Occupational Dermatoses

Sixty-five percent of all the industrial diseases are dermatoses. The most common cause of these skin problems is contact irritants, of which cutting oils are the worst offenders. Lack of adequate cleansing is a big contributing factor to cutting oil dermatitis; on the other hand, harsh or abrasive cleansers can aggravate the dermatitis.

It is not possible to list the thousands of different chemicals used in the hundreds of varied industrial operations that have the potential of causing a primary irritant reaction or an allergic reaction on the skin surface. Excellent books on the subject of occupational dermatitis are listed in the bibliography at the end of this chapter.

Management of Industrial Dermatitis

Case Example. A cutting-tool laborer presents with a pruritic, red, vesicular dermatitis on his hands, forearms, and face of 2 months' duration.

1. Obtain a careful, detailed history of his type of work and any recent change, such as use of new chemicals or new cleansing agents or exposure at home with hobbies, painting, and so on. Question him concerning remission of the dermatitis on weekends or while on vacation.
2. Question the patient concerning the first aid care given at the plant. Too often this care aggravates the dermatitis. Bland protective remedies should be substituted for potential sensitizers, such as sulfonamide and neomycin salves, antihistamine creams, benzocaine ointments, nitrofuran preparations, and strong antipruritic lotions and salves.
3. Treatment of the dermatitis with wet compresses, bland lotions, or salves is the same as for any contact dermatitis (see previous discussion). Unfortunately, many of the occupational dermatoses respond slowly to therapy. This is due in part to the fact that most patients continue to work and are reexposed, repeatedly, to small amounts of the irritating chemicals, even though precautions are taken. Also, certain industrial chemicals, such as chromates, beryllium salts, and cutting oils, injure the skin in such a way as to prevent healing for months and years, and result in a chronic eczema or chronic psoriasis (Koebner phenomena) in prone individuals.
4. Transferring a patient to a new job in the same work setting where exposure is less intensive may be helpful.

Protective clothing such as gloves (being sure not to make the patient too awkward around dangerous machines) or protective creams or sprays (Pro Q topical, OTC aerosol foam) can be beneficial.

5. The legal complications with compensation boards, insurance companies, the industry, and the injured patient can be discouraging, frustrating, and time consuming. However, most patients are not malingerers, and they do expect and deserve proper care and compensation for their injuries.

A comprehensive paper by Gordan C. Sauer on the percentages of skin impairment is entitled "A Guide to the Evaluation of Permanent Impairment of the Skin" (Arch Dermatol 1968; 97:566). A similar guide published by the American Medical Association (1990) is listed in the bibliography at the conclusion of this chapter.

Atopic Eczema

Atopic eczema (Figures 9-6, 9-7, 9-8, 9-9, and 9-10; Table 9-1), or atopic dermatitis, is a rather common, markedly pruritic, chronic skin condition that occurs in two clinical forms: infantile and adult.

Clinical Lesions

- *Infantile form:* blisters, oozing, and crusting, with excoriation.
- *Adolescent and adult forms:* marked dryness, thickening (lichenification), excoriation, and even scarring.

Distribution

- *Infantile form:* on face, scalp, arms, and legs, or generalized. The diaper area is usually clear, probably because of occlusion of the area and urea exposure from urine.
- *Adolescent and adult forms:* on cubital and popliteal fossae and, less commonly, on dorsa of hands and feet, ears, or generalized. Atopic eczema of the soles of the feet is quite common in adolescents. In adults, there is a more chronic, localized disease, especially involving genitalia, posterior scalp, and ankles (often referred to as *lichen simplex chronicus* [LSC]). Pruritus is severe and paroxysmal.

Course

The course varies from a mild single episode to severe chronic, recurrent episodes resulting in the "psychoitchical"

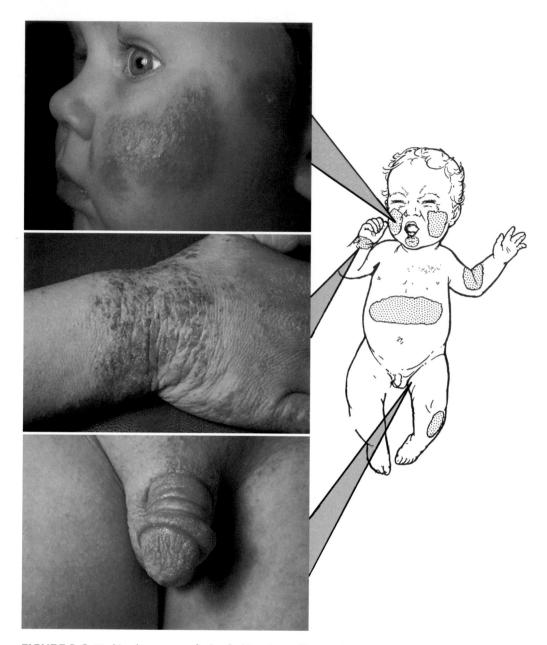

FIGURE 9-6 ■ Atopic eczema (infant). *(Courtesy of Dome Chemicals.)*

person. Eczema is referred to as "the itch that rashes." The infantile form usually becomes milder or even disappears after the age 3 or 4 years and approximately 70% of cases clear by puberty. During puberty and the late teenage years, flare-ups or new outbreaks can occur. Adult-onset eczema, once thought to be rare, is actually quite common. Young housewives or househusbands may have their first recurrence of atopic eczema since childhood because of their new job of dishwashing and child care. Thirty percent of patients with atopic dermatitis eventually develop allergic asthma or hay fever, penicillin allergy, hives, and marked reaction to insect bites are more common.

Causes

The following factors are important:

- *Heredity* is the most important single factor. The family history is usually positive for one or more of the triad of allergic diseases: asthma, hay fever, or atopic eczema. Penicillin allergy, hives, and

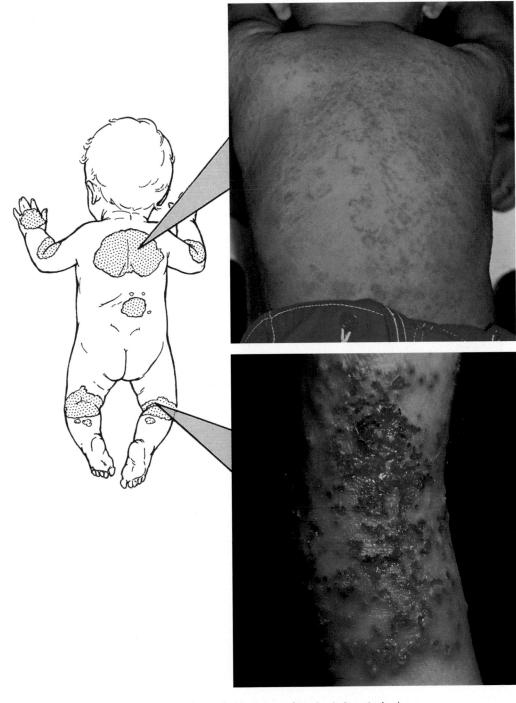

FIGURE 9-7 ■ Atopic eczema (infant). *(Courtesy of Roche Laboratories.)*

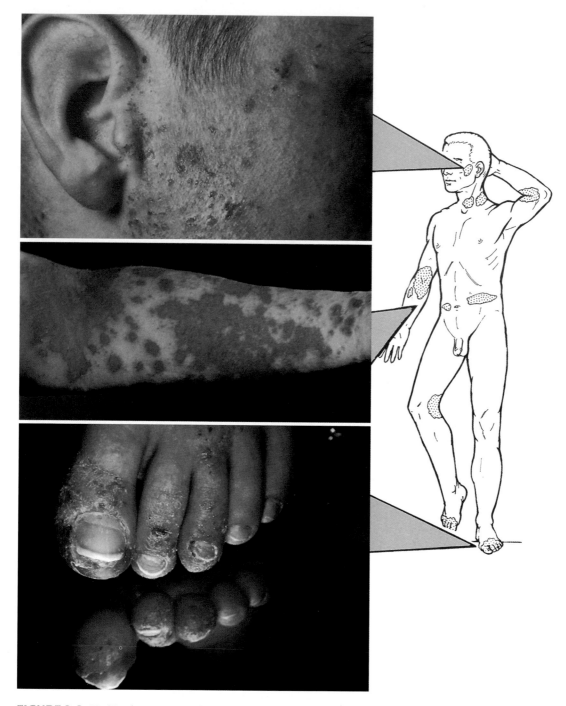

FIGURE 9-8 ■ Atopic eczema. The bottom photograph, by the use of a mirror, demonstrates the undersurface of the toes. *(Courtesy of Sandoz Pharmaceuticals.)*

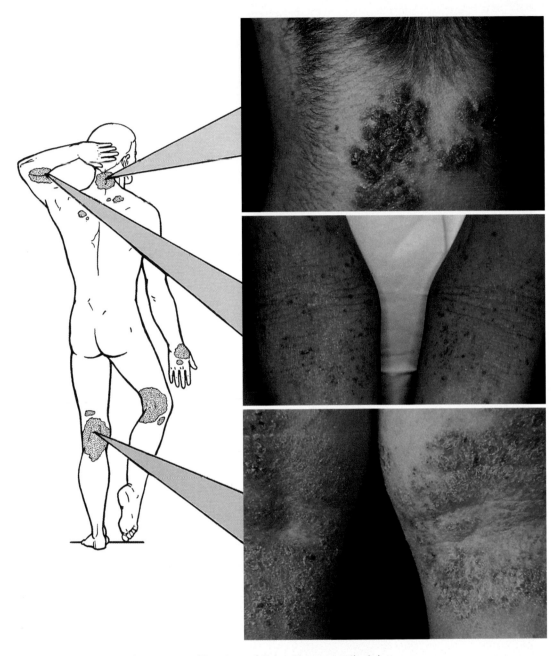

FIGURE 9-9 ■ Atopic eczema. *(Courtesy of Geigy Pharmaceuticals.)*

marked reaction to insect bites are also part of the atopic diathesis which is called Type 1 or anaphylactoid immunity. Determination of this history in cases of hand dermatitis is important because often it enables the physician, on the patient's first visit, to prognosticate a more drawn-out recovery than if the patient had a simple contact dermatitis.

■ *Dryness* of the skin is important. Most often, atopic eczema is worse in the winter owing to the decrease in home or office and outdoor humidity. For this reason, the use of soap and water should be reduced and hot water avoided. Emollients (lanolin free) can be applied after bathing.

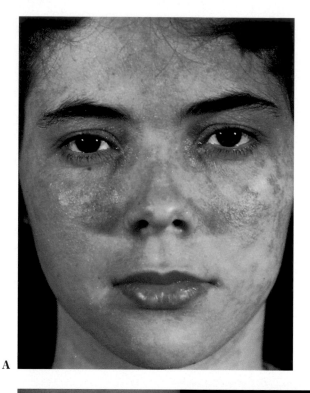

A

B

FIGURE 9-10 ■ Atopic eczema. This case of facial atopic eczema (**A**) resembled acute lupus erythematosus. The arm eruption (**B**) is on another patient and exemplifies the chronic lichenified form of atopic eczema. *(Courtesy of K.U.M.C.; Dome Chemicals.)*

TABLE 9-1 ■ Hanifin and Rajka Criteria for Diagnosis of Atopic Dermatitis

Major Criteria	Minor Criteria
Pruritus	Xerosis
Adults: flexural lichenification or linearity	Ichthyosis, palmar hyperlinearity
Children: facial or extensor involvement	Keratosis pilaris
	Type I skin test reactivity
	Elevated serum IgE
Chronic or chronically relapsing dermatitis	Early age of onset
	Tendency toward skin infections
Atopic history, personal or familial	Nipple eczema
	Cheilitis
	Recurrent conjunctivitis
	Dennie-Morgan fold (accentuated skin line on lower eyelids)
	Keratoconus
	Anterior subcapsular cataracts
	Orbital darkening
	Facial pallor/facial erythema
	Pityriasis alba
	Anterior neck folds
	Pruritus with perspiration
	Intolerance to wool and lipid solvents
	Perifollicular accentuation (especially in people of color)
	Food intolerance
	Course influenced by environmental/emotional factors
	White dermatographism/delayed blanch

Note: Three major plus four or more minor criteria should be present.

■ *Wool* and *lanolin* (wool fat) commonly irritate the skin of these patients. Wearing wool or silk clothes may be another reason for an increased incidence of atopic eczema in the winter. Cotten clothes and bed clothing are preferred.

■ *Allergy to foods* is a factor that is often overstressed, particularly with the infantile form. The mother's history of certain foods causing trouble should be a guide for eliminating foods. This can be tested by adding the incriminated foods to the diet, one new food every 48 hours, when the dermatitis is stable. Scratch tests and intracutaneous tests uncover very few dermatologic allergens.

■ *Emotional stress* and *nervousness* aggravate any existing condition such as itching, duodenal ulcers, or migraine headaches. Therefore, this "nervous" factor is important but not causative enough to label this disease *disseminated neurodermatitis.*

■ *Concomitant bacterial infection* of the skin, particularly with *Staphylococcus aureus* is common. Bacterial culture and appropriate antibiotic therapy is indicated.

Differential Diagnosis

■ *Dermatitis venenata* (contact dermatitis to plants): Positive history, usually of contactants; no family allergic history; distribution rather characteristic and often with streaking (see Chap. 9).

■ *Psoriasis:* Patches localized to extensor surfaces, mainly knees and elbows with characteristic thick silvery-white scale (see Chap. 14). Nail involvement is not uncommon.

■ *Seborrheic dermatitis in infants:* Absence of family allergy history; lesions scaling and greasy and often seen in the diaper or intertriginous areas (see Chap. 13).

General Management for Atopic Eczema

Inform the patient or family that this is usually a chronic problem; that this is an inherited condition; that skin tests usually are not helpful; and that relief can occur from the dermatitis and the itch, but there is no "cure" except time.

Treatment of Infantile Form

Case Example. A child, aged 6 months, presents with mild oozing, red, excoriated dermatitis on face, arms, and legs.

First Visit.

1. Follow regular diet except for the avoidance of any foods that the parent believes aggravated the eruption.
2. Avoid exposure of infant to excessive bathing with soaps and to contact with wool and products containing lanolin. Use mild soap sparingly. Cool to luke warm bath water.
3. Coal tar solution (liquor carbonis detergens [LCD]) or Cutar (topical, OTC) bath oil 120.0

Sig: Add ¹/₂ tbsp to the lukewarm bath water. Be sure to lubricate skin after each bath.

4. Hydrocortisone ointment, 1% 30.0

Sig: Apply sparingly b.i.d. to affected areas.

Comment: 1% Hytone ointment is in a petrolatum base without lanolin. Other proprietary corticosteroid preparations are listed in the Formulary in Chapter 5.

5. **Diphenhydramine** (Benadryl) elixir 90.0

Sig: 1 tsp b.i.d.

Comment: Warn parent that this drug may paradoxically stimulate the child.

6. If infection is present, treat with appropriate systemic antibiotic, such as erythromycin, cephalexin, or cloxacillin.

7. Pimecrolimus (Elidel) cream and tacrolimus (Protopic) ointment in .03% and 0.1% are the most significant recent advance in topical therapy for eczema. They can be used as monotherapy or as a corticosteroid-sparing drug in conjunction with topical corticosteroids. They do not cause cutaneous atrophy and striae, which are not insignificant problems with topical corticosteroids.

Subsequent Visits. Add coal tar solution such as LCD (3% to 10%) to the above ointment.

Severe or Resistant Cases.

1. Restrict diet to milk only; after 3 days, add one different food every 24 hours. An offending food causes a flare-up of the eczema in several hours.

2. Hydrocortisone liquid: Cortef (oral) 90.0

Sig: 1 tsp (10 mg) q.i.d. for 3 days, then 1 tsp t.i.d. for 1 week.

Comment: Decrease the dose or discontinue as improvement warrants. Base the dosage on the weight of the child.

3. Hospitalization with change of environment may be necessary for a severe case. This may be necessary in a case of parental negligence.

Treatment of Adult Form

Case Example. A young adult presents with dry, scaly, lichenified patches in cubital and popliteal fossae.

First Visit.

1. Counsel the patient to avoid stress, excess soap for bathing, lanolin preparations locally, and contact with wool.

> **SAUER'S NOTES**
>
> Do not initiate local corticosteroid therapy with the strongest "big guns." Save these stronger corticosteroids for later use, if necessary.

2. Coal tar solution (LCD) 5%

Fluorinated corticosteroid ointment or emollient cream (see Chap. 5) q.s. 30.0

3. Hydroxyzine, 25 mg #90

Sig: 1 tablet t.i.d.

Comment: Available generically. Warn patient about side effect of drowsiness.

4. Elidel and Protopic are topical corticosteroid-sparing drugs.

Subsequent Visits.

1. Gradually increase the concentration of the coal tar solution in the previously mentioned salve up to 10%.

2. Increase the potency of the corticosteroid ointment or emollient cream.

3. For patients with infected crusted lesions (many patients have an element of infection), an antibiotic such as erythromycin, 250 mg, may be prescribed b.i.d. or t.i.d. for several weeks.

4. Systemic corticosteroid therapy may be indicated for severe and resistant cases.

5. Topical doxepin hydrochloride (Zonalon) cream

Sig: Thin coat q.i.d. on pruritic areas.

Comment: Can cause drowsiness with overuse on large surface areas and may sting or burn when therapy is first initiated.

6. Leukotriene inhibitors have shown to be of benefit recently by some authors. An example is zafirlukast (Accolate).

Sig: 20 mg/tab; 1 tab by mouth b.i.d.

> **SAUER'S NOTES**
>
> 1. With every visit, reemphasize the fact of the chronicity of atopic eczema and the ups and downs that occur, particularly with seasons and stress.
> 2. Emollient (lanolin free) lotions are helpful in aborting recurrences.

7. Recombinant human interferon-γ has shown some benefit in some studies; 50 μg/m² is given subcutaneously daily. This is primarily experimental.
8. Rarely, immunosuppressive therapy such as methotrexate may have to be employed in recalcitrant, life-altering disease.
9. Various forms of ultraviolet (UV) light therapy can be helpful including psoralens and UVA (PUVA), narrowband UVB (TL-01), UVB, and UVA. Increased risk of skin cancer and photoaging are to be considered.
10. Topical tacrolimus is safe, beneficial, and can be important as a steroid-sparing agent.

Nummular Eczema

Nummular eczema (Figure 9-11) is a moderately common, distinctive eczematous eruption characterized by coin-shaped (nummular), papulovesicular patches, mainly on the arms and the legs of young adults and elderly patients.

Presentation

Primary Lesions

Coin-shaped patches of vesicles and papules are usually seen on the extremities and occasionally on the trunk.

Secondary Lesions

Lichenification and bacterial infection occur.

Course

This is very chronic, particularly in older people. Recurrences are common, especially in fall and winter.

Subjective Complaints

Itching is usually quite severe.

Causes

Nothing is definite, but these factors are important:

- History is usually positive for asthma, hay fever, or atopic eczema, particularly in the young adult.
- Bacterial infection of the lesions may occur.
- The low indoor humidity of winter causes dry skin, which intensifies the itching, particularly in elderly patients.

Differential Diagnosis

- *Atopic eczema:* Mainly in cubital and popliteal fossae, not coin-sized lesions (see preceding section).
- *Psoriasis:* Not vesicular; see scalp and fingernail lesions (see Chap. 14).
- *Contact dermatitis:* Will not see coin-sized lesions on both arms and legs (see beginning of this chapter).
- *"Id" reaction,* from stasis dermatitis of legs or a localized contact dermatitis: Impossible to differentiate this clinically from nummular eczema, but patient will have history of previous primary dermatitis that suddenly became aggravated.

Treatment

Case Example. An elderly man presents in the winter with five to eight distinct, coin-shaped, excoriated, vesicular, crusted lesions on the arms and the legs.

First Visit.

1. Instruct the patient to avoid excess use of soaps.
2. Use superfatted soaps such as Dove or Cetaphil and lubricate the skin immediately after every bath or shower. Use water as cool as is tolerable to bathe.
3. Corticosteroid ointment 60.0

   Sig: Apply t.i.d. locally.
   Comment: The use of an ointment base is particularly important in the therapy for nummular eczema. I find adding a mild tar such as MG 217 in a 19% concentration helpful.
4. Diphenhydramine, 50 mg #15

   Sig: 1 capsule h.s. for antipruritic and sedative effect.
   Comment: Available generically and over the counter
5. Consider Elidel and Protopic as topical nonsteriod alternatives.

Resistant Cases.

1. Add coal tar solution, 3% to 10%, to the previously mentioned salve.
2. Oral antibiotic therapy may be beneficial. Prescribe erythromycin, 250 mg, t.i.d. for several weeks.
3. A short course of oral corticosteroid therapy is effective, but relapses are common.

   Rarely methotrexate can be employed. Watch for liver and hematogic toxicity.

Drug Eruptions

It can be stated almost without exception that any drug systemically administered is capable of causing a skin eruption (Figures 9-12, 9-13 and 9-14).

To jog the memory of patients I often ask, "Do you take any medicine for any condition? What about medicated toothpaste, laxatives, vitamins, aspirin, and tonics? Have you received any shots in the past month?" As stated

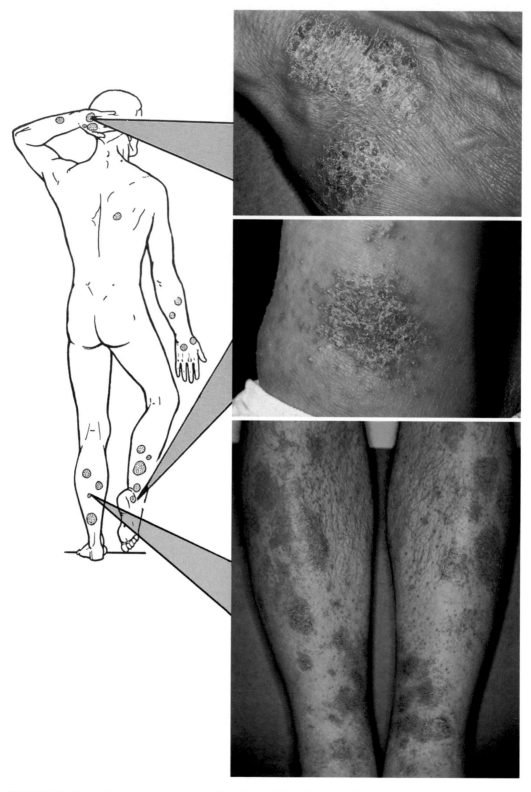

FIGURE 9-11 ■ Nummular eczema. *(Courtesy of Schering Corp.)*

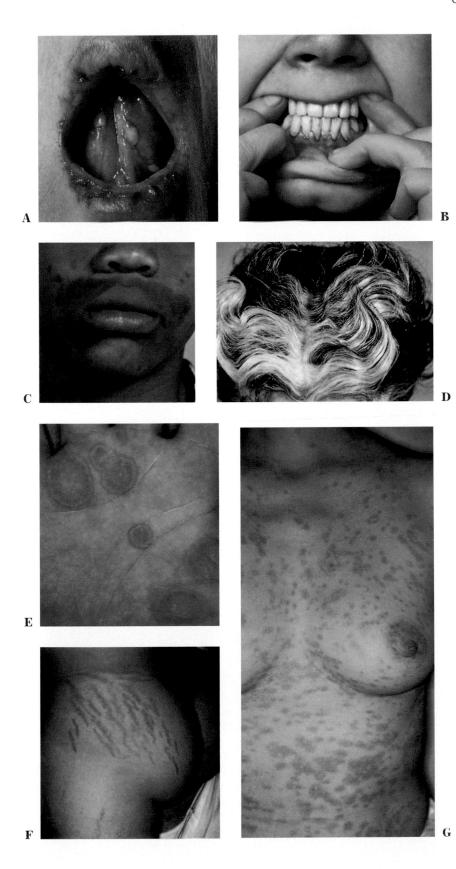

FIGURE 9-12 ■ Drug eruptions. (**A**) Erosions of tongue and lips from sulfonamides. (**B**) Bismuth line of gums. (**C**) Phenolphthalein fixed eruption of lips of an African-American boy. (**D**) Whitening of scalp hair from chloroquine therapy for lupus erythematosus. (**E**) Erythema multiforme-like eruption of palm from oral antibiotic therapy. (**F**) Striae of buttocks of 30-year-old man following 9 months of corticosteroid therapy. (**G**) Papulosquamous eruption of chest from phenolphthalein. *(Courtesy of E.R. Squibb.)*

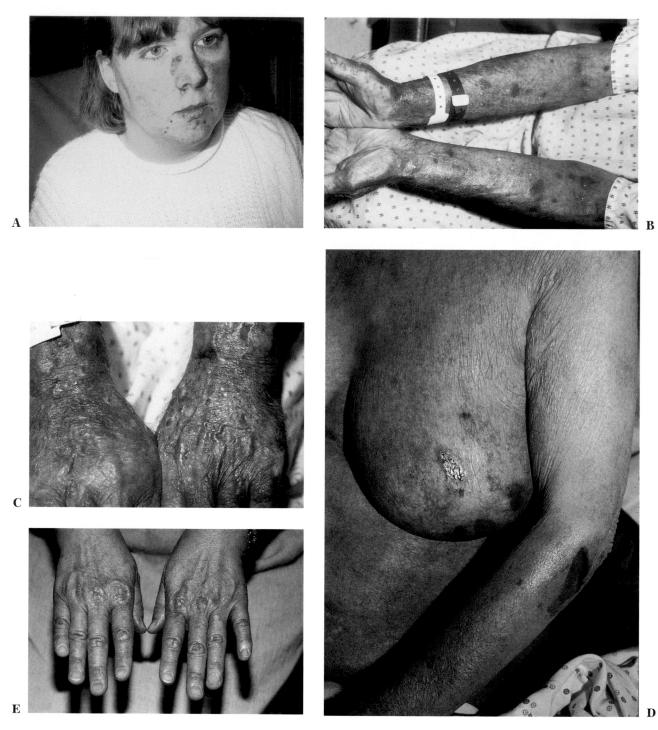

FIGURE 9-13 ■ Side effects of topical corticosteroid abuse. (**A**) Steroid rosacea. (**B**) Atrophy, telangiectasias, milia. (**C**) Purpura, atrophy. (**D**) Fragility with tearing and cigarette paper wrinkling atrophy. (**E**) Hydroxyurea dermopathy mimicking dermatomyositis.

TABLE 9-2 ■ Drugs and the Dermatoses They Cause

Drug	Dermatosis/Comments
Accutane	See *Isotretinoin*
Acetaminophen (Tylenol)	Infrequent cause of drug eruption; urticaria and erythematous eruptions are noted. Also fixed drug eruption.
Adrenocorticotropic hormones (ACTH, prednisone, IM triamcinolone)	Cushing's syndrome, hyperpigmentation, acneiform eruptions, rosacea, striae, perioral dermatitis, seborrheic dermatitis-like eruptions, and hirsutism
Allopurinol (Zyloprim)	Erythema, maculopapular rash, and severe bullae
Amantadine	Livedo reticularis
Aminosalicylic acid	Scarlatiniform or morbilliform rash, fixed drug eruption, and nummular eczema-like rash
Amiodarone	Photosensitivity reaction and blue-gray discoloration of skin
Amphetamine (Benzedrine)	Coldness of extremities; redness of neck and shoulders; increased itching in LSC
Ampicillin	See *antibiotics;* flare of morbilliform eruption in over half of patients with infectious mononucleosis
ACE inhibitors	Maculopapular eruption with eosinophilia, pemphigus, a bullous pemphigoid-like eruption, angioedema, rosacea, urticaria, and possibly flare of psoriasis
Antabuse	Redness of face and acne
Antibiotics	Various agents have different reactions, but in general: *candida overgrowth* in oral, genital, and anal orifices results in pruritus ani, pruritus vulvae, and generalized pruritus; candida skin lesions may spread out from these foci. Urticaria, morbilliform and erythema multiforme-like eruptions, particularly from penicillin.
	Ampicillin: generalized maculopapular rash, very common in patients with infectious mononucleosis
	Sulfa derivatives: particular problem in HIV+ patients. See *streptomycin* and later section on photosensitivity reactions.
Anticoagulants	*Coumadin and heparin:* severe hemorrhagic skin infarction and necrosis
Antihistamines (in Coricidin, NyQuil, and many other preparations)	Urticaria, eczematous dermatitis, and pityriasis rosea-like rash
Antineoplastic agents	Skin and mucocutaneous reactions, including alopecia, stomatitis, radiation recall reaction, and erythema
Antitoxin	*Immediate reaction:* pruritus, urticaria, and sweating
	Delayed serum sickness reaction: urticaria, redness, purpura
Apresoline	See *Hydralazine*
Aspirin and salicylates (a multitude of cold and anti-pain remedies; e.g., Pepto-Bismol)	Urticaria, purpura, bullous lesions
Atabrine hydrochloride	Universal yellow pigmentation; blue macules on face and mucosa; lichen planus–like eruption
Atropine	Scarlet fever–like rash
Barbiturates	Urticarial, erythematous, bullous, or purpuric eruptions; fixed drug eruptions

(continued)

TABLE 9-2 ■ (*Continued*)

Drug	Dermatosis/Comments
β-Blockers	Alopecia; psoriasis flare
Bleomycin sulfate injection	*Antitumor antibiotic:* gangrene, erythema, sclerosis, nail changes, characteristic striate lesions
Captopril	Pemphigus-like eruption; see *ACE inhibitors*
Cetusimab (monoclonal antibody that binds epidermal growth factor receptor)	Follicular eruption ($1/3$ of patients); acneiform eruptions, seborrheic eruptions, nail bed changes
Chemotherapy agents	See *Antineoplastic agents;* also see specific drug
Chloral hydrate	Urticarial, papular, erythematous, and purpuric eruptions
Chloroquine (Aralen)	Erythematous or lichenoid eruptions with pruritus and urticaria; ocular retinal damage from long-term use of chloroquine and other antimalarials can be irreversible
Chlorothiazide diuretics	Petechial and purpuric eruptions, especially of legs; *see* section on photosensitivity reactions
Chlorpromazine (Thorazine)	Maculopapular rash, increased sun sensitivity, purpura with agranulocytosis, and icterus from hepatitis
	Long-term therapy: slate-gray to violet discoloration of the skin
Cimetidine	Dry, scaly skin
Codeine and morphine	Erythematous, urticarial, or vesicular eruption
Collagen (bovine) injected	Skin edema, erythema, induration, and urticaria at implantation sites
Contraceptive drugs	Chloasma-like eruption, erythema nodosum, hives; some cases of acne are aggravated
Cortisone and derivatives	Allergy (rare); *see* ACTH
Coumadin	See *Anticoagulants*
Cyclosporine	Hypertrichosis, sebaceous hyperplasia, acne, folliculitis, epidermal cysts, Kaposi's sarcoma, skin precancers and cancers, gingival hyperplasia, follicular keratosis, palmoplantar paresthesias, and dysesthesias associated with temperature change
Dapsone	Red, maculopapular, vesicular eruption with agranulocytosis occurs, occasionally resembling erythema nodosum
Dextran (used in peritoneal dialysis)	Urticarial reactions
Diethylpropion hydrochloride (Tenuate, Tepanil oral)	Measles-like eruption
Dilantin	See *Phenytoin*
Docetaxel	*Cutaneous reactions:* up to 70% incidence beginning usually 2–4 days after treatment with 80% pain or itching; purple-red macules or plaques, often acral, that may peel in 3–4 weeks; if worse with repeated doses, this drug may have to be stopped; local hypothermia may be ameliorative; extravasation necrosis, nail loss, supravenous discoloration, subungual abscess, skin sclerosis
Doxorubicin (Doxil; polyethylene glycol-coated liposomal doxorubicin hydrochloride)	*Acral erythrodysthesia with desquamation:* in a few weeks; may worsen each episode and may limit dosage
	Diffuse: (10%) mild scaly erythema with follicular accentuation; does not necessarily recur
	Intertrigo eruption: due to friction from clothing; loose-fitting clothes may help

TABLE 9-2 ■ (*Continued*)

Drug	Dermatosis/Comments
	Melanotic macules: on trunk or extremities; stomatitis radiation and sunburn recall
	To ameliorate reactions: 99% DMSO four times a day, oral antioxidants (vitamins E, C, A, and selenium) and oral misoprostol (prostaglandin E, analog)
Estrogenic substances	Edema of legs with cutaneous redness progressing to exfoliative dermatitis
Feldene	See *Piroxicam*
Flagyl	See *Metronidazole*
Furosemide	Bullous hemorrhagic eruption
Gold	Eczematous dermatitis of hands, arms, and legs or a pityriasis rosea-like eruption; also, seborrheic-like eruption, urticaria, and purpura
Heparin	See *Anticoagulants*
Hydralazine (Apresoline)	SLE-like reaction
Hydroxyurea	Dermopathy mimicking cutaneous findings of dermatomyositis; atrophic, erythematous dermatitis over the back of the hands that may be photoinduced; leg ulcers; hyperpigmentation, especially nails (longitudinal bands) and palms
Ibuprofen (Motrin, Naprin, Advil)	Bullous eruptions, including erythema multiforme, Stevens–Johnson syndrome, toxic epidermal necrolysis, urticaria, photosensitivity, fixed drug reactions, morbilliform reactions
Icodextran (used in peritoneal dialysis)	Psoriasiform dermatosis, acute generalized exanthematous pustulosis
Imipramine	Slate-gray discoloration of skin
Insulin	Urticaria with serum sickness symptoms; fat atrophy at injection site
Iodides	See *Bromides;* papular, pustular, ulcerative, or granulomatous lesions mainly on acne areas or legs; administration of chloride hastens recovery
Isoniazid	Erythematous and maculopapular, generalized, purpuric, bullous, and nummular eczema-like; acne aggravation
Isotretinoin	Dry red skin and lips (common); alopecia (rare)
Lasix	See *Furosemide*
Lamotrigine	At least 10% with cutaneous drug reactions; may be similar to phenytoin cutaneous drug reactions
Lithium	Acne-like lesions on the body; psoriasis exacerbation
Meclizine HCl (Antivert)	Urticaria
Meprobamate	Small purpuric lesions, erythema multiforme-like eruption
Metronidazole (Flagyl)	Urticaria, pruritus
Minocycline	Skin (muddy skin syndrome), teeth, and scar discoloration
	Rare: hypersensitivity, sickness-like reaction, drug-induced lupus erythematosus, SLE-like syndrome, autoimmune hepatitis, *p*-ANCA–positive cutaneous polyarteritis nodosa
	Rare syndrome: hepatitis, exfoliative dermatitis, fever, lymphadenopathy, eosinophilia, lymphocytosis

(*continued*)

TABLE 9-2 ■ (Continued)

Drug	Dermatosis/Comments
Morphine	See *Codeine;* lichen planus-like eruption; fixed drug eruption, photosensitivity
Nevirapine	Unusually high incidence of potentially life-threatening Stevens–Johnson syndrome
NSAIDs (e.g., ibuprofen [Motrin], naproxen [Naprosyn], indomethacin [Indocin], piroxicam [Feldene], diclofenac [Voltaren], celecoxib (Celebrex), meloxicam [Mobic])	Urticaria, erythema multiforme-like eruption, toxic epidermal necrolysis
Penicillin	See *Antibiotics*
Penicillamine	Lupus-like rash, lichen planus-like rash, pemphigus foliaceous
Phenolphthalein (found in 4-way Cold Tablets, Ex-Lax, bile salts, and pink icing on cakes)	*Fixed drug eruption:* hyperpigmented or purplish, flat or slightly elevated, discrete, single or multiple patches
Phenothiazine group	See section on photosensitivity reactions
Phenytoin (Dilantin)	Hypertrophy of gums, erythema multiforme-like eruption; pseudolymphoma syndrome, morbilliform reaction
	Fetal hydantoin syndrome: organ defects plus nail hypoplasia
	Note: one of the most common causes of toxic epidermal necrolysis or Stevens–Johnson syndrome along with other antiseizure medications
	SLE-like reaction
Procainamide	*Rare:* drug eruption; See *β-Blockers*
Propranolol (Inderal)	See section on photosensitivity reactions
Psoralens	Edema, purpura, scarlatiniform eruption; may progress to exfoliative dermatitis
Quinidine	Diffuse eruption (any kind)
Quinine	Urticaria, photosensitivity reactions, petechial eruptions
Rauwolfia alkaloids (reserpine)	Pruritus, urticaria, acne, bullous pemphigoid, mucositis, exfoliative erythroderma, red urine, reddened soft contact lenses
Rifampin	See *Aspirin*
Salicylates	Urticaria; erythematous, morbilliform, and purpuric eruptions
Streptomycin	Urticaria, scarlatiniform eruption, erythema nodosum, eczematous flare of exudative dermatitis, erythema multiforme-like bullous eruption, fixed eruption; see later section on photosensitivity reactions, morbilliform reaction
Sulfonamides	
	AIDS patients: develop allergic drug eruptions quite often; one of the most common causes of toxic epidermal necrolysis and Stevens–Johnson syndrome
	See *Sulfonamides* and section on photosensitivity reactions
Sulfonylureas	Cutaneous reaction (80%), especially morbilliform, UV light recall (skin eruptions at site of previous UV exposure), urticaria, "suramin keratoses"
Suramin	
	Scleroderma-like skin changes, fixed drug, onycholsysis, acral erythema, erythema multiforme, pustular eruptions
Taxanes (paclitaxel, docetaxel)	
Testosterone and related drugs	Acne-like lesions, alopecia in scalp, hirsutism

TABLE 9-2 ■ (Continued)

Drug	Dermatosis/Comments
Tetracycline	Fixed drug eruption, photosensitivity, serum sickness-like reaction
	<8 years: teeth staining; see Antibiotics
Thalidomide	Erythroderma, pustulosis, toxic epidermal necrolysis
Thiazides	See section on photosensitivity reactions
Trimethoprim (Trimpex)	Rarely incriminated in drug eruptions
Vitamin A	Long-term, high-dose therapy: scaly, rough, itchy skin with coarse, dry, scant hair growth, systemic changes including liver toxicity
Vitamin D	Skin lesions rare, but headache, nausea, diarrhea, increased urination, and sore gums and joints
Vitamin B group	Urticaria, pruritic redness, and even anaphylactic reactions occur after IM or IV administration
	Nicotinic acid: red flush (common—warn patient to eliminate unnecessary alarm), pruritus (common), hives (rare, within 15– to 30 minutes after oral ingestion of 50–100 mg)
Warfarin sodium	See Anticoagulants

Abbreviations: ACE, angiotensin-converting enzyme; ACTH, adrenocorticotropic hormone; LSC, lichen simplex chronicus; NSAID, non-steroidal anti-inflammatory drug; SLE, systemic lupus erythematosus; UV, ultraviolet.

in Chapter 4, this questioning also gives the physician some general information regarding other ills of the patient that might influence the skin problem. (An eruption due to allergy or primary irritation from locally applied drugs is a contact dermatitis.)

Any of the larger dermatologic texts has extensive lists of common and uncommon drugs, with their common and uncommon skin reactions. These books must be con-sulted for the rare reactions, but the following paragraphs cover 95% of these idiosyncrasies.

Photosensitivity reactions from drugs are covered in Chapter 30. Hepatic drug metabolism pathway involving cytochrome P-450 enzymes defines the most significant and largest group of drug–drug interactions. Adverse drug interactions must always be considered.

Drugs and Associated Dermatoses

Drug eruptions are usually not characteristic for any certain drug or group of drugs, but experience has shown that certain clinical pictures commonly follow absorption of certain drugs. Common drugs causing skin eruptions are given in Table 9-2, and common skin eruptions caused by drugs are given in Table 9-3.

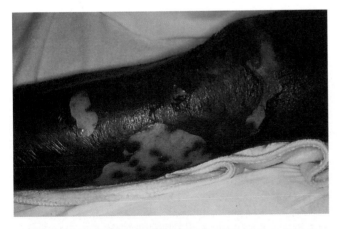

FIGURE 9-14 ■ Positive Nikelsky's sign of the right leg: sheets of skin peeling off with very light pressure. This was due to secondary therapy with a sulfur-related drug.

SAUER'S NOTES

Any patient with a generalized skin eruption should be *carefully* questioned concerning the use of oral or parenteral medicinal drugs. For a minor non life-threatening drug eruption, it may not be necessary or advisable to stop a life-saving drug. The rash may resolve on its own or be controlled with conservative therapy.

TABLE 9-3 ■ Dermatoses and the Drugs That Cause Them

Dermatosis	Drug(s)	Comments
Acne-like or pustular lesions	Bromides, iodides, lithium, testosterone, corticosteroids	
Acral erythema	Redness, pain, and swelling of the hands and feet associated with various chemotherapeutic agents including cyclophosphamide, cytosine arabinoside, docetaxel, doxorubicin, fluorouracil, hydroxyurea, mercaptopurine, methotrexate, and mitotane.	Most commonly cytarabine, doxorubicin and fluorouracil.
Actinic keratosis inflammation	First described with fluorouracil; also doxorubicin, cisplatin, fludarabine, dactinomycin, dacarbazine-vincristine sulfate.	Chemotherapy can be continued or briefly interrupted with use of topical corticosteroids.
Alopecia	Amethopterin (methotrexate) and other antineoplastic agents; colchicine, clofibrate, testosterone and other androgens; tricyclic antidepressants; β-blockers; heparin; progesterone derivatives; Coumarin derivatives; sotretinoin	
Angioedema	Aspirin, NSAIDs, ACE inhibitors	
Baboon syndrome	Mercury (most often); also ampicillin, amoxicillin, nickel, erythromycin, heparin and food additives	Systemic contact dermatitis owing to ingestion, inhalation, or percutaneous absorption; symmetric diffuse acute light red exanthema on buttocks, anogenital area, major flexural areas of extremities and peeks at day 2–5 of exposure to the involved drug; resolves within 1 week
DIDMOHS (drug-induced delayed [3–6 weeks] multiorgan hypersensitivity syndrome of Sontheimer and Houpt; also called DRESS [drug rash with eosinophil and systemic symptoms of Bocquet and Roujeau].)	Dapsone, carbamazepine, phenobarbital, minocycline, trimethoprim, sulfamethoxazole, procarbazine, allopurinol, terbinafine	Exanthematous or papulopustular febrile eruption with hepatitis (also possible lung, renal thyroid involvement), lymphadenopathy, and eosinophilia
Eczematous eruption	Quinine, antihistamines, gold, mercury, sulfonamides, penicillin, organic arsenic	
Erythema multiforme-like eruption	Penicillin and other antibiotics, sulfonamides, phenolphthalein, barbiturates, phenytoin, meprobamate	
Erythema nodosum-like eruption	Sulfonamides, iodides, salicylates, oral contraceptives, dapsone	
Exfoliative dermatitis	Particularly owing to arsenic, penicillin, sulfonamides, allopurinol, barbiturates	In the course of any severe generalized drug eruption
Fixed drug eruption	Phenolphthalein, acetaminophen, barbiturates, organic arsenic, gold, salicylates, sulfonamides, tetracycline, many others	*Fixed drug eruption:* hyperpigmented or purplish, flat or slightly elevated, discrete, single or multiple patches. Occurs at same sites on drug challenge

TABLE 9-3 ■ (*Continued*)

Dermatosis	Drug(s)	Comments
Hyperpigmentation	Contraceptives, atabrine, chloroquine, minocycline, chlorpromazine, amiodarone, bismuth and gold, silver salts, ACTH, estrogen, adriamycin, AZT, methotrexate	
Hypertrichosis	Oral minoxidil, phenytoin, cyclosporine	
	Less severe: oral contraceptives, systemic corticosteroids, psoralens, streptomycin sulfate	
Keratoses and epitheliomas	Arsenic, mercury, PUVA therapy, immunosuppressive agents	
Lichen planus-like eruption	Atabrine, arsenic, naproxen, gold, others	
Lupus erythematosus	Minocycline, hydralazine, procainamide, isoniazid, chlorpromazine, diltiazem, quinidine	
Linear IgA bullous dermatosis	Vancomycin (most common), furosemide, captopril, lithium, amiodarone, diclofenac, cefamandole, somatostatin, rifampin, topical iodine, phenytoin, trimethoprim-sulfamethoxazole, penicillin G, IL-2, interferon-γ	
Lipoatrophies from injections	Corticosteroids (e.g., triamcinolone), insulin, vasopressin, human growth hormone, iron dextron, diphtheria pertussis-tetanus immunization serum, antihistamines, TALWIN injection	
Lipodystrophy	*Partial:* proteinase inhibitors used to treat AIDS: indinavir or ritonavir plus saquinavir causes decreased subcutaneous fat on the face (cadaveric or cachetic facies) and extremities (pseudomuscular appearance) with increased prominence of the superficial veins; central adiposity with increased abdominal girth (pseudo-obesity), enlargement of breasts, increased dorsal-cervical fad pads (buffalo hump or pseudo-Cushing's syndrome)	Increased triglyceride and LDL cholesterol and low HDL cholesterol also occurs.
Measles-like eruption	Barbiturates, arsenic, sulfonamides, quinine, many others	
Mucous membrane lesions	*Pigmentation:* bismuth	
	Hypertrophy: phenytoin	
	Erosive lesions: sulfonamides, antineoplastic agents, many other drugs	
Nail changes	*Onycholysis* (distal detachment): tetracycline, apparently owing to a phototoxic reaction	
Neutrophilic eccrine hidradenitis	Bleomycin, chlorambucil, cyclophosphamide, cytarabine, doxorubicin, lomustine, mitoxantrone	

(*continued*)

TABLE 9-3 ■ (Continued)

Dermatosis	Drug(s)	Comments
Nicolau syndrome (embolia cutis medicamentosa)	Diclofenac, ibuprofen, iodine, benzathine penicillin, vitamin K, DTP immunizations, antihistamines, interferon-α, corticosteroids	At IM injection site; see dictionary index
Nummular eczema-like eruption	Combination of isoniazid and *p*-amino-salicylic acid	
Necrosis of the skin	*Localized:* coumarin and heparin derivatives; recombinant γ-interferon	
	Distant: coumarin and heparin derivatives	
Ochronosis, exogenous	Topical phenol, quinine injections, topical resorcinol	
	With prolonged use: topical hydroquinone, mainly in dark-skinned patients at the site of application only	
Pemphigoid-like lesions	Furosemide, penicllin, sulfasalazine, ibuprofen	
Pemphigus-like lesions	Rifampin, penicillamine, captopril, pyrazolone derivatives	
Photosensitivity reaction	*Sulfonamides:* sulfonylurea	Several of the newer drugs and some of the older ones cause a dermatitis on exposure to sunlight. These skin reactions can be urticarial, erythematous, vesicular, or plaquelike. The mechanism can be either phototoxic or photoallergic, but this distinction can be difficult to ascertain. This list of *photosensitizing drugs* is rather complete, but also consult Chapter 35.
	Hypoglycemics: tolbutamide (Rinase), chlorpropamide (Diabinese)	
	Antibiotics: demethylchlortetracycline (Declomycin), doxycycline (Doryx, Monodox, Vibramycin), griseofulvin (Fulvicin, Grifulvin, Gris-PEG), maxaquin (Lomefloxacin), nalidixic acid (neg-gram), tetracycline	
	Benzofurans: amiodarone	
	Chlorothiazide diuretics: chlorothiazide (Diuril); hydrochlorothiazide; methyclothiazide	
	Phenothiazines: chlorpromazine (Thorazine); prochlorperazine (Compazine); promethazine (Phenergan)	
	Psoralens: methoxsolen (Oxsoralen); tri-oxsalen (Trisoralen)	
	Oxicams: piroxicam (Feldene)	
Pityriasis rosea-like eruption	Bismuth, gold, barbiturates, antihistamines	
Porphyria cutanea tarda exacerbation	Estrogen, iron, ethanol ingestion, hexachlorobenzene, chlorinated phenols, polychlorinated biphenyls; possibly privastatin	
Pseudolymphoma	Antidepressants, diphenylhydantoin, α-agonists, ACE inhibitors, anticonvulsants, antihistamines, benzodiazepine, β-blockers, calcium-channel blockers, lipid-lowering agents, lithium, NSAIDs, phenothiazines, procainamide, estrogen, progesterone	

TABLE 9-3 ■ (Continued)

Dermatosis	Drug(s)	Comments
Pseudoporphyria cutanea tarda (PCT)	NSAIDs (naproxen, nabumetone, oxaprozin, ketoprofen, mefenamic acid, diflunisal), nalidixic acid, tetracycline, chlorothalidone, furosemide, hydrochlorothiazide/tramterene, isotretinoin, etretinate, cyclosporine, 5-fluorouracil, pyridoxine, amiodarone, flutamide, dapsone, aspirin	Skin findings but no biochemical abnormalities. May persist for months after offending drug stopped, mimics skin finding and skin biopsy of PCT
Psoriasis exacerbation	Lithium, β-blockers, ACE inhibitors, antimalarials, NSAIDs, terbinafine	
Purpuric eruptions	Barbiturates, salicylates, meprobamate, organic arsenic, sulfonamides, chlorothiazide diuretics, corticosteroids (long-term use)	
Pustulosis, acute generalized erythematous (aged or toxic pustulosis)	Antibiotics (mainly β-lactam); many others	
Scarlet fever-like eruption or "toxic erythema"	Arsenic, barbiturates, codeine, morphine, mercury, quinidine, salicylates, sulfonamides, others	
Seborrheic dermatitis-like eruption	Gold, ACTH	
Stevens–Johnson syndrome	Lamotrigine, valproic acid, penicillin, barbiturates, diphenylhydantoin, sulfonamides, rifampin, NSAIDs, salicylates	
Subacute cutaneous lupus erythematosus	Hydrochlorothiazide, ACE inhibitors, calcium channel blockers, interferons, statins	
Urticaria	Penicillin, salicylates, serums, sulfonamides, barbiturates, opium group, contraceptive drugs, Rauwolfia alkaloids, ACE inhibitors	
Vesicular or bullous eruptions	Sulfonamides, penicillin, mephenytoin	
Whitening of hair	Chloroquine, hydroxychloroquine	In blonde- or red-haired people

Abbreviations: ACE, angiotensin-converting enzyme; ACTH, adrenocorticotropic hormone; HDL, high-density lipoprotein; LDL, low-density lipoprotein; NSAID, nonsteroidal anti-inflammatory drugs; PUVA, psoralens and ultraviolet light.

Course

The course of drug eruptions depends on many factors, including the type of drug, severity of the cutaneous reaction, systemic involvement, general health of the patient, and efficacy of corrective therapy. Most cases with bullae, purpura, or exfoliative dermatitis have a serious prognosis and a protracted course.

Treatment

1. Eliminate the drug. This simple procedure is often delayed, with resulting serious consequences, because a careful history is not taken. If the eruption is mild and the drug necessary, discontinuation of the drug may not be mandatory.

SAUER'S NOTES

1. When confronted with any diffuse or puzzling eruption, routinely question the patient regarding *any* medication taken by *any* route.
2. Ask: "Are you taking any vitamins, laxatives, nerve pills, and so forth?" This jogs the patient's memory.
3. Remember, any chemical ingested can cause an eruption, such as toothpaste, mouthwash, breath freshener, and chewing gum.
4. Antiseizure medications, antibiotics, sulfa and sulfa-related drugs, nonsteroidal anti-inflammatory drugs and allopurinol cause of the majority of cutaneous drug eruptions.

2. Further therapy depends on the seriousness of the eruption. Most barbiturate, measles-like eruptions subside with no therapy. An itching drug eruption should be treated to relieve the itch. Cases of exfoliative dermatitis or severe erythema multiforme-like lesions require corticosteroid and other supportive therapy.

3. Toxic epidermal necrolysis and Stevens–Johnson's syndrome is treated with high-dose intravenous immunoglobulin G and intensive supportive hospital care. Discontinuation of the offending drug in a timely manner can be life-saving and vision-saving.

Suggested Readings

American Medical Association. Guides to the evaluation of permanent impairment, ed 3. Chicago, AMA, 1990.

DiCarlo JB, McCall CO. Pharmacologic alternatives for severe atopic dermatitis. Int J Dermatol 2001;40: 82–88.

Eichenfield LF, Hanifin JM, et al. Consensus conference on pediatric atopic dermatitis. J Am Acad Dermatol 2003;49:1088–1095.

Kanerva L, Elsner P, et al. Condensed handbook of occupational dermatology. New York, Springer, 2003.

Litt's Drug Eruption Reference Manual Including Drug Interactions, ed 10. Philadelphia, Taylor & Francis, 2004.

Physicians' desk reference to pharmaceutical specialties and biologicals. Oradell, NJ, Medical Economics, 2005.

Rietschel R, Fowler JF. Fisher's contact dermatitis, ed 5. 2000. Philadelphia, Lippincott, Williams & Wilkins.

Roujeau JC, Stern RS. Severe adverse cutaneous reactions to drugs. N Engl J Med 1994;331:1272.

Warshaw EM. Latex allergy. J Am Acad Dermatol 1998;39:1.

Williams HC. Atopic dermatitis: The epidemiology, causes, and prevention of atopic eczema. Cambridge, UK, Cambridge University Press, 2000.

CHAPTER 10

Dermatologic Immunology

Jon A. Dyer, MD

As an organism's major interface with the environment the cutaneous organ functions in multiple roles to maintain homeostasis. The immune system is active in the skin, patrolling for pathogens and participating in normal cutaneous physiology. The importance of the immune function of the skin is highlighted by the fact that many of the most important therapies utilized in dermatology involve modulation or suppression of the immune system.

Normal Cutaneous Immunity

The immune system is composed of two functional "arms," both of which are important in normal and abnormal states of the skin. First is the more recently investigated innate immune response, and second, the better characterized adaptive immune response. The synergy between the innate and acquired immune systems and their regulation of each other is currently being studied in great detail. The separation of the immune system into these two arms, while allowing for better conceptualization of various functional roles is likely artificial; in reality they function as a seamless syncytium.

Innate Immunity

Innate immunity lacks specificity and memory but is rapid in its effect. It is believed to represent a much older and more primitive method of immune response. Some form of innate immune function is thought to exist in most multicellular organisms.

The innate immune system serves as the "first responder" to infectious or traumatic cutaneous events. Whereas the adaptive immune response may take several days to reach functional levels (even longer if it is the initial exposure to an antigen), the innate immune system can begin working immediately.

Specificity in the innate immune system is mediated by pattern recognition receptors (PRRs), which recognize conserved molecular structures on pathogens (pathogen-associated molecular patterns [PAMPs]) that do not exist in higher organisms. The toll-like receptors are a major subset of PRRs for the innate immune system.

PAMPs are essential to the activity of the pathogens and exhibit a low mutation rate. A wide variety of bacterial, fungal, protozoan, and viral components are capable of stimulating the innate immune response, including

- lipopolysaccharide (LPS),
- peptidoglycan,
- lipoteichoic acid,
- lipoaraginomannan,
- lipopeptides,
- yeast wall mannans,
- bacterial DNA,
- double-stranded RNA, and
- flagellin.

The innate immune system has multiple components. Cytokines and complement play important roles. Additionally, numerous cell types participate in innate immune processes, including

- dermal mast cells,
- dendritic cells (such as Langerhan's cells),
- macrophages,
- epithelial cells,
- natural killer cells,
- neutrophils, and
- endothelial cells.

Keratinocytes are involved in innate immune responses. They produce numerous important cytokines and antimicrobial peptides.

Complement

The complement cascade functions in both the innate and adaptive arms of the immune system. It includes over 30 serum glycoproteins. There are three defined paths of complement activation:

- the classical pathway, triggered by antigen–antibody reactions;
- the alternative pathway, triggered by yeast polysaccharides and gram-negative bacterial products such as LPS; and
- the mannan-binding lectin pathway, stimulated by mannose-containing proteins present in viruses and yeasts.

All three paths converge at the central step of C3 component activation. The final outcome of this pathway is activation of a membrane attack complex composed of C5–C9, which functions as a transmembrane pore inducing osmotic cell lysis. Activation of the complement system also generates components that increase inflammatory cell chemotaxis and vascular permeability and others, which function as opsonins. Complement deposition and activation by immune complexes stimulates the adaptive immune system and lowers the threshold for B cell activation and subsequent antibody production. Complement activation is normally impaired on normal host cells by several mechanisms.

Cytokines

Cytokines are a large family of substances that play a critical role in intercellular communication. They are secreted by most cells and can function in autocrine, paracrine, or endocrine fashions. Cytokines function via binding of cell-surface receptors. Cytokines produced by white blood cells that affect other white blood cells are called *interleukins* (IL). Colony-stimulating factors induce differentiation and proliferation of progenitor cells in the bone marrow. Interferons (IFN) are so called because they were identified as substances that "interfere" with viral replication. Chemokines are cytokines with chemoattractant activities and play an important role in migration of white blood cells. Cytokines are often divided into two groups: Th1 cytokines promote cellular immunity and Th2 cytokines promote antibody production (especially IgE). CD4$^+$ T cells are divided based on their cytokine production into Th1 and Th2 types. Table 10-1 lists cytokines, their sources, and major methods of action.

Adaptive Immunity

Adaptive immune responses exhibit the qualities of specificity and immunologic memory with increased specificity of the immune response developing over time. Adaptive immune responses are orchestrated by T and B-lymphocytes, which clonally proliferate in response to a specific antigen, and antigen presenting cells (APCs) that stimulate the lymphocytic response.

Antigen Presenting Cells

Several forms of APC exist in normal human skin, including epidermal Langerhan's cells and dermal dendritic cells. Langerhan's cells are derived from the bone marrow, have a dendritic shape, and characteristic rod- or racquet-shaped granules (Birbeck granules) ultrastructurally.

APCs function by taking up antigen, digesting it into smaller pieces, migrating to skin draining lymph nodes, and then presenting these antigen-derived peptides, bound to major histocompatibility complex (MHC) molecules, to naïve T cells. Antigens derived from intracellular processing pathways, such as viral or tumor proteins are presented on MHC class I molecules. Antigens from outside the cell are typically presented on MHC class II molecules.

Langerhan's cells exist in a premature state in the skin, likely "scanning" the epidermis for antigens. Upon uptake of an antigen, Langerhan's cells undergo a change in phenotype and express molecules which play a role in priming T cells.

T Lymphocytes

T cells arise in the bone marrow and migrate very early in their development to the thymus, where a highly regulated process deletes autoreactive T cells.

T-cell selectivity is mediated through the T-cell receptor (TCR). A unique recombination process cuts, splices, and modifies the genes of the antigen-binding area of the TCR, generating an enormously diverse number of TCRs.

The TCR only recognizes antigen-derived peptides attached to APC MHC molecules. CD4$^+$ helper T cells recognize antigen bound to MHC class II molecules, and CD8$^+$ cytotoxic T cells recognize antigen bound to MHC class I.

Costimulatory signals at the time of TCR binding are critical in determining the outcome of this event. The binding of the TCR to its peptide–MHC complex is the first signal and generates the specificity of the immune response. Surface molecules and cytokines provide secondary signals necessary for clonal expansion of stimulated T cells. Without costimulation, TCR binding induces cell anergy (unreactivity).

Once stimulated by APC in the lymph node, naïve T cells undergo division and clonal expansion to become memory/effector T cells.

Effector T-Cell Functions

CD4$^+$ helper T cells typically mediate immune responses to foreign antigens. Helper T cells are divided by their cytokine

Table 10-1 ■ Cytokines: Sources and Important Methods of Action

Cytokine	Source	Method of Action
IL-1 (6)	*IL-1α*: macrophages; monocytes; dendritic cells; Langerhans' cells *IL-1β*: keratinocytes; epithelial cells	Stimulation of local immune function (costimulatory for activated T cells; chemotactic; acute phase reactant induction; synergizes with other cytokines; innate immunity)
IL-2	Th1 lymphocytes	T-cell growth factor; activates T and NK cells and promotes their growth
IL-3	T cells	Promotes growth of hematopoietic cells, including mast cells
IL-4	Th2 helper cells	Growth factor for Th2 cells; promotes IgE responses
IL-5	Th2 helper cells	Promotes B-cell and eosinophil growth
IL-6	Fibroblasts	Induces acute phase reactants
IL-7	Stromal cells	Lymphocyte growth factor
IL-8	Macrophages; T cells; keratinocytes; endothelial cells; fibroblasts; neutrophils	Neutrophil and T-cell chemotaxis; neutrophil activation
IL-10	CD4$^+$ helper cells, activated monocytes	Inhibits Th1 cell cytokine production, stops antigen presentation
IL-12	Monocytes/macrophages	γ-IFN induction and Th1 responses
IL-13	Activated T cells	B-cell stimulation
Granulocyte-colony stimulating factor	Monocytes	Promotes myeloid cell growth
Monocyte-colony stimulating factor	Monocytes	Promotes macrophage growth
Granulocyte–macrophage-colony stimulating factor	T cells	Promotes monomyelocytic cell growth in marrow; activates monocytes and neutrophils
IFN-α	Leukocytes	Activation and modulation of immune system
Interferon-β	Fibroblasts	Activation and modulation of immune system
IFN-γ	Th1 cells/NK cells	Activation and modulation of immune system
TNF-α	Macrophages; T lymphocytes; keratinocytes	Stimulates immune activation, adhesion molecule expression, IL-8 and TGF-α expression; necrosis
TNF-β	Th1 cells	Stimulates immune activation; vascular effects
TGF-β	Platelets; T cells; macrophages; B cells; mast cells	Inhibits immune system; stimulates growth of connective tissue and collagen formation
Chemokine		
CCL17	*Endothelium:* cutaneous postcapillary venules	Skin homing T-cell attraction
CCL27	Keratinocytes	CTACK; attraction of skin homing T cells

Abbreviations: CTACK, cutaneous T-cell attracting cytokine; IFN, interferon; IgG, immunoglobulin G; IL, interleukin; NK, natural killer; TGF, transforming growth factor.
Source: Data from Parkin and Cohen (2001); Dleves and Roitt (2000); and Schwartz (2003).

profile into Th1 (γ-IFN; tumor necrosis factor α [TNF-α]; and IL-2) and Th2 (IL-4, IL-5, IL-6, IL-9, IL-10, and IL-13). Th1 cells typically induce a cell-mediated inflammatory response. Th2 cells induce antibody production, promote eosinophil growth, and promote B-cell class switching in favor of immunoglobulin E (IgE) production. Thus, Th2-type responses are typically associated with allergic diseases.

Memory/effector T cells are characterized by the ability to remember the anatomic site that the lymph node in which they were activated was draining. The cutaneous lymphocyte antigen (CLA), which directs memory T cells to migrate through the skin, is expressed on 10% to 30% of all memory T cells.

Activation of T cells in the skin occurs when they bind their particular presented antigen. At this stage, antigen presentation does not require an APC and may be performed by local cells including keratinocytes, macrophages, or mast cells.

CD8$^+$ cytotoxic T cells act against tumors or viruses. CD8$^+$ T cells are directly cytotoxic to cells bearing their respective antigen. They are also separated into two classes (Tc1 and Tc2) based on their cytokine profiles.

Recently the subclass of regulatory T cells was described and includes the previously described suppressor T cell. These play a role in down regulating immune responses.

B cells

B lymphocytes produce antibodies that function as the humoral arm of the adaptive immune system. They undergo the majority of their development in the bone marrow. Early in development, the four gene segments that comprise the B-cell receptor undergo a complex process of rearrangement resulting in the generation of over 10^{10} possible antibody specificities. The protein expressed from these rearranged genes functions early in B-cell development as an antigen receptor, much like the TCR. Upon antigen recognition and binding, the antigen is internalized, processed, and reexpressed on the B-cell surface attached to MHC class II molecules. Presentation of antigen to primed T cells stimulates B-cell division and activation. Activated B cells mature into antibody-producing plasma cells.

Although immunoglobulin M (IgM) antibodies are initially produced, the final antibody type is determined by isotype switching induced by further T-cell interactions. Other modifications, including somatic hypermutation, further refine antibody affinity. Long-lived memory cells also result from final isotype switching, allowing rapid response to future challenges with the same antigen.

B cells produce five main antibody classes: immunoglobulin G (IgG), immunoglobulin A (IgA), M (IgM),

E (IgE), and immunoglobulin D (IgD). IgM predominates in the intravascular compartments; IgG in tissues and blood. IgA (either monomeric or dimeric) is the main secreted antibody functioning at mucosal surfaces. IgE antibodies can cross-link high-affinity IgE (FcεR) receptors on mast cells triggering release of preformed granules. IgG and IgM can activate complement, promoting immune responses upon binding antigen.

Skin Diseases Illustrating Immunologic Concepts

An inclusive discussion of cutaneous disorders illustrating cutaneous immunologic concepts is well beyond the scope of this chapter. Instead we include here "classic" immune-mediated skin diseases, which provide insights into basic cutaneous immunology.

Autoimmune Bullous Disease

Several immune-mediated skin diseases present with blistering. Pemphigus and pemphigoid are the two major groups of autoimmune bullous diseases.

Pemphigus describes a group of autoimmune bullous diseases characterized histopathologically by intraepidermal blistering, caused by separation of keratinocytes from each other (acantholysis). The main types are pemphigus vulgaris (PV) and pemphigus foliaceus (PF). In pemphigus, autoantibodies are the primary effectors of the disease. No secondary inflammatory mediators are required, a difference between pemphigus and pemphigoid. Direct immunofluorescence (DIF) studies are similar in both conditions and show deposition of IgG around the cell surface of keratinocytes.

Autoantibodies in PV target desmoglein 3, a component of the desmosomes that function to attach keratinocytes to each other. Desmoglein 3 is expressed in the lower epidermal cell layers and its impairment by autoantibodies leads to suprabasilar bulla formation. The antigen in PF is desmoglein 1, a desmosomal protein expressed in all epidermal cell layers. Antibody binding of desmoglein 1 in PF impairs its function, but cell–cell binding is maintained in the lower epidermis by the compensating activity of desmoglein 3. This explains the superficial blistering seen in PF.

The most common form of pemphigoid is *bullous pemphigoid* (BP), in which IgG antibodies bind proteins of the cutaneous basement membrane. Antibody binding leads to deposition and activation of complement, recruitment of inflammatory cells such as neutrophils and eosinophils, and dissolution of the basement membrane proteins. This causes separation of the epidermis from the dermis forming the classic tense bullae on noninflammatory bases seen in BP. These factors, both IgG and C3, are detectable as linear deposits on DIF examination of bullous or perilesional skin.

Psoriasis

Psoriasis is a chronic inflammatory skin disease affecting 2% to 3% of the population. It is characterized by well-demarcated, erythematous, symmetric, sometimes pruritic, patches and plaques with overlying silvery white scale.

Initially thought to result from overgrowth of keratinocytes, psoriasis is now recognized as an immune-mediated skin disease. Entry of CD4$^+$ T cells is one of the earliest detectable events in the development of psoriatic lesions. Affected skin typically shows dermal and epidermal infiltrates of T cells, macrophages, and dendritic cells. The dermal T-cell infiltrate is CD4$^+$ predominant; CD8$^+$ T cells predominate in the epidermis.

A role for the innate immune system is suggested by the tendency of psoriasis lesions to arise at sites of trauma (Koebner phenomenon). External trauma induces release of preformed cytokines from keratinocytes resulting in up-regulation of recruitment molecules on regional postcapillary venules. Resident T cells are activated and CLA$^+$ circulating T cells are recruited to the area, including those T cells that trigger psoriatic lesion development.

Psoriasis is a Th1-dominant disease (often contrasted with atopic dermatitis [AD], a Th2-dominant disease). Activated lesional psoriatic T cells produce cytokines that likely drive the phenotypic features of the disease. One such cytokine, TNF-α is increased in psoriatic skin and is the target of many new biologic agents (see below).

The role of the immune system is illustrated by the response of psoriasis to immunosuppressant medications, such as corticosteroids and cyclosporine, and its favorable response to ultraviolet light (which is immunosuppressive).

More recently, a new generation of biologic agents targeting specific events in the generation of the immune response have been created and employed in various disorders, including psoriasis. Agents targeting TNF-α, such as etanercept and infliximab, have shown efficacy in controlling psoriasis. Additionally, efalizumab, which blocks T-lymphocyte attachment to skin capillary endothelium and alefacept, which blocks costimulation between APC and T cells, also improve psoriasis.

Further investigations in the molecular participants of this "immunologic synapse" will no doubt lead to additional therapies for psoriasis as well as other immune-mediated skin diseases.

Connective Tissue Diseases

Also called *collagen vascular diseases,* this group of rheumatologic conditions often also exhibits skin lesions. These conditions are associated with antibodies against self-proteins, many of which are used in the diagnosis of the specific conditions. Table 10-2 summarizes the most common conditions, their skin findings, and laboratory findings. These conditions are typically treated using immunosuppressant or immunomodulatory medications often in collaboration with a rheumatologist.

Vasculitis

Inflammation and necrosis of the blood vessel wall can lead to wall disruption with resultant leakage of blood into surrounding tissue. This produces the classic cutaneous lesion of vasculitis, palpable purpura. Purpura are typically erythematous to dusky skin lesions that do not blanch with pressure.

The inflammation in vasculitis is thought to result from recruitment of inflammatory cells and subsequent release of inflammatory mediators in the vessel wall, often from deposition of immune complexes, which activate complement. In leukocytoclastic vasculitis, there is a neutrophilic infiltrate, whereas lymphocytic vasculitis shows an infiltrate of lymphocytes.

Various causes of complement formation and deposition can be seen. A common form of vasculitis is Henoch–Schönlein purpura, seen most often in children. The eruption is often preceded by a respiratory infection. In lesions of Henoch–Schönlein purpura, a leukocytoclastic vasculitis is seen. Immunohistochemical staining of lesional blood vessels reveals perivascular deposits of IgA and C3. These IgA deposits likely lead to complement deposition and activation with resultant vasculitis.

Vasculitis caused by mixed cryoglobulinemia may be seen in the setting of hepatitis C infection where complexes of mixed cryoglobulin deposit in vessel walls with resultant complement activation causing vascular damage.

Graft-Versus-Host Disease

Graft-versus-host disease (GVHD) is most commonly seen in the setting of bone marrow and stem cell transplantation, although it may also be seen with solid organ transplants, in the rare setting of maternofetal lymphocyte engraftment, or following transfusion of nonirradiated blood products. Increased human leukocyte antigen (HLA) mismatch between donor and recipient increases the risk of GVHD. The most common organ systems

Table 10-2 ■ **Connective Tissue Diseases: Clinical and Laboratory Findings**

Connective Tissue Disease	Clinical Findings	Laboratory Findings
SLE	*Acute*: malar "butterfly" rash; photodistributed; spares knuckles; associated systemic disease	Elevated ANA titer; positive anti-dsDNA Ab; anti-Sm Ab; anti-rRNP Ab
	Subacute: annular, red, papulosquamous lesions; chronic; no scarring; rarely associated with systemic disease; infants of affected mothers may exhibit neonatal lupus	Anti-Ro (SSA) and anti-La (SSB) antibodies present in high percentage of SCLE patients
	Chronic/discoid: chronic, papulosquamous lesions in sun exposed areas; rarely associated with systemic disease; prominent scarring	Usually (−) serologic markers
Dermatomyositis	Violaceous photodistributed poikilodermatous eruption ("heliotrope" rash) periorbital and over knuckles (Gottron's sign) progressing to papules (Gottron's papules); nailfold telangiectasia; proximal muscle weakness; calcinosis cutis; associated malignancy in 10–50% of adults	Anti-Jo1; anti-Mi-2 antibodies *Amyopathic dermatomyositis*: Anti-155kD and anti-Se antibodies; increased incidence of positive ANA
Scleroderma	Systemic form predominantly affects women; induration of skin from excess collagen; involvement of other organs; Raynaud's phenomenon; CREST syndrome is a milder variant; localized forms (morphea) without systemic involvement are more commonly seen	*ANA Anti-Scl-70*: systemic scleroderma *Anti-centromere*: CREST syndrome
Sjögren's syndrome	Primarily affects secretory glands with decreased tearing, salivation, and arthritis; palpable and nonpalpable purpura; annular erythemas; and urticarial vasculitis may be seen; dry skin	anti-Ro; anti-La; anti−α-fodrin antibodies
Juvenile idiopathic/ rheumatoid arthritis	Transient, erythematous, asymptomatic exanthem during acute febrile episodes; less commonly rheumatoid nodules and persistent plaques	Rheumatoid factor

involved are the skin, liver, and gastrointestinal tract, with resulting rash, hepatitis, and enteritis with diarrhea seen clinically.

The rash of GVHD may have a variety of presentations. Both acute and chronic forms are recognized. The acute form exhibits macular erythema, often acral with later generalization. Less commonly, the eruption may be so severe as to mimic toxic epidermal necrolysis. In its chronic form GVHD may exhibit a lichenoid or a sclerodermoid appearance.

The clinical manifestations in acute GVHD are thought to result from an attack of donor CD8⁺ T lymphocytes responding to foreign MHC molecules on the tissues of the recipient.

Allergic Contact Dermatitis

Allergic contact dermatitis (ACD) occurs when a type IV immune response develops against an allergen present on the skin. Typically these allergens are low-molecular-weight molecule (haptens), which must be coupled with a host protein to generate an immune response. The prototypic allergen is the urushiol resin present in the poison ivy plant. APCs resident in the skin process the antigen and present it to naïve T cells in the skin-draining lymph nodes. Clonal expansion of this T cell occurs, and such urushiol-specific T cells then home back to the skin, releasing cytokines and mediators leading to the inflammation that characterizes the clinical lesions. On initial exposure, this process can take 1 to 2 weeks; however, upon reexposure resident antigen-specific T cells and effector memory T cells generate a response in hours to days.

ACD skin lesions are often patterned reflecting their external application to the skin. Suppression of the immune response relieves the clinical symptoms but memory T cells persist and mediate recurrence of the eruption upon reexposure to the antigen.

Patch testing is used to detect such cutaneous allergies and involves application of controlled concentrations of purified allergens to nonlesional skin and monitoring for the development of classic ACD signs and symptoms.

Erythema Multiforme

Erythema multiforme (EM) represents a range of immune-mediated cutaneous hypersensitivity eruptions. Classic targetoid skin lesions, often on acral surfaces, with minimal mucosal involvement characterize the mildest form of EM, EM minor. Such lesions may be tender or pruritic. The most common cause of EM minor is herpes simplex virus infection. Pathophysiologically it is suspected that cytotoxic T lymphocytes attack lesional keratinocytes and induce apoptosis of affected cells, leading to the clinical lesions.

Stevens–Johnson Syndrome/Toxic Epidermal Necrolysis

Stevens–Johnson syndrome and toxic epidermal necrolysis refer to conditions with more severe cutaneous eruptions and mucosal epidermal necrosis. They may be induced by drugs (nonsteroidal anti-inflammatory medications; sulfa drugs, anticonvulsants, antibiotics) or infections (such as mycoplasma). Toxic epidermal necrolysis is often defined as involvement of more than 30% of the body surface area with epidermal denudation. Resultant defective skin barrier function and severe mucosal involvement require that such patients be managed intensively.

The cause of these severe eruptions is unknown. Lesional keratinocytes have been shown to have upregulated Fas ligand (CD95L) on their cell surface. Fas ligand, when bound by Fas (CD95), triggers apoptosis. Keratinocytes constantly express Fas on their cell surface; thus, it is thought that the upregulation of Fas ligand seen in Stevens–Johnson syndrome/toxic epidermal necrolysis allows keratinocytes to trigger apoptosis of adjacent cells, leading to widespread epidermal necrosis.

Although the role of immunosuppressive medications in the management of Stevens–Johnson syndrome and toxic epidermal necrolysis has been controversial in the past, the use of intravenous immunoglobulin (IVIG) has gained favor recently. IVIG contains antibodies to Fas, which can block Fas binding to Fas ligand, and appears to arrest the disease process. Additionally, IVIG induces expression of inhibitory receptors, which may also explain its apparent beneficial effects.

Urticaria

Urticaria (also called *hives*) is thought to represent a classic type I or immediate hypersensitivity reaction. Mast cells and mast cell–derived histamine are major initiators of urticaria. Stimuli or substances that lead to mast cell degranulation trigger lesion development.

Urticaria is described as acute (<6 weeks duration) and chronic (>6 weeks duration). Cross-linking of mast cell IgE by allergens may cause acute urticaria, but this mechanism is not thought to play an important role in chronic urticaria. Acute urticaria may be idiopathic or follow an upper respiratory infection.

An inciting cause for chronic urticaria is found in fewer than 10% of cases. In patients with chronic urticaria, autoantibodies against the high-affinity IgE receptor (FcεRI) or the Fc portion of IgE itself are present in 30% to 50% and approximately 10% of patients, respectively, suggesting an autoimmune mechanism for mast cell degranulation. Urticaria has also been associated with other autoimmune endocrine conditions such as thyroid disease, vitiligo, and rheumatoid arthritis.

Alopecia Areata

One of the most common causes of hair loss in young children, alopecia areata is thought to result from an immune attack on the hair follicles themselves. *This is substantiated* histologically by an infiltrate of T-cells at the hair bulb as well as the induction of alopecia on human skin explants on SCID mice by injection of scalp-infiltrating lymphocytes.

Normally, keratinocytes from anagen hair follicles do not express MHC antigens and are thought to represent immunologically privileged tissue. However, in alopecia areata, various HLA are expressed by the follicle cells, reflecting a possible loss of immune privilege and mechanism for cytotoxic T-cell interaction with these hair cells.

Although destruction of the hair follicle does not result, affected follicles become quiescent with lack of hair growth. Clinically this presents as well-demarcated areas, often nummular in shape, of complete alopecia, with normal follicular orifices and no other skin findings.

In rare cases, alopecia areata may be part of a spectrum of autoimmune endocrine disorders such as autoimmune hyper- or hypothyroidism, Addison's disease, inflammatory bowel disease, type I diabetes, pernicious anemia, and vitiligo.

Vitiligo

Vitiligo is characterized by the development of depigmented areas of skin that are devoid of melanocytes histologically. This is thought to result from an immune-mediated attack on melanocytes. CD8[+] T cells active against melanocytic antigens are seen in vitiligo lesions. Additionally, vitiligo also exhibits the Koebner phenomenon and thus the innate immune system may play a role. It may also be seen as part of a broader spectrum of autoimmune endocrine diseases as outlined for alopecia areata above.

Cutaneous T-Cell Lymphoma

Cutaneous T-cell lymphoma (CTCL) is characterized by the formation of well-defined, often erythematous, patches and plaques on the skin. There has been much debate on the etiology of CTCL. Some think it is a malignancy derived from skin-homing T lymphocytes. Others propose that it is a systemic disease process. Lesional T cells are clonally expanded and secrete a Th2 cytokine profile. It is proposed that homing molecules expressed by the abnormal cells determines their eventual location.

Atopic Dermatitis

AD is a common skin disease of childhood affecting 10% to 15% of children. *Atopy* refers to a hereditary predisposition to a group of diseases such as asthma, allergic rhinitis, allergic keratoconjunctivitis, urticaria, penicillin allergy, and eczema. Atopy is thought to reflect allergy or hypersensitivity to environmental allergens. In AD, T cells of a Th2 subtype are present initially, shifting to a Th1 type as lesions become chronic.

The innate immune system is thought to play a significant role in AD. A common nickname for AD is "the itch that rashes," describing not only the significant underlying pruritis in the disorder, but also the tendency for eczema to develop at sites of scratching. As discussed, exacerbation by skin trauma may indicate a role for innate immune-mediated upregulation of the immune response.

Bacteria, especially *Staphylococcus aureus,* are known to colonize AD lesions and trigger the inflammatory process. Recent studies have detected deficient production of endogenous peptide antibiotics, which function as part of the innate immune system, in response to skin infection in AD. It is suspected that Th2 cell products suppress innate immune activation, allowing bacterial overgrowth and resultant immune system activation, which lead to persistence of lesions.

Immunodeficiency-Associated Skin Diseases

There are a myriad of skin diseases associated with impaired or defective immune function. Table 10-3 summarizes some major disorders, their clinical features, and underlying defects.

Role of the Immune System in Prevention of Skin Cancer

The immune system plays a major role in the prevention and suppression of cutaneous malignancies. This is highlighted in the organ transplant patient population, where the incidence of cutaneous malignancy greatly increases with the institution of immunosuppression.

Skin cancers are the most common malignancy in transplant recipients. Squamous cell carcinoma (SCC) and basal cell carcinoma (BCC) account for over 90% of all skin cancers in transplant recipients. SCC is the most common skin cancer and although the risk for BCC appears to increase linearly with time, the risk for SCC appears to increase exponentially. These tumors in transplant recipients are more aggressive and grow more rapidly than in the immunocompetent patient.

Other cutaneous malignancies seen in transplant recipients include Kaposi's sarcoma (associated with HHV-8), melanoma (present at a lower incidence than other skin cancers in immunosuppressed patients), Merkel cell carcinoma, and lymphoma (B cell > T cell).

Imiquimod, a topical antiviral agent functioning via modulation of the innate immune system, has shown efficacy against cutaneous malignancies such as BCC and melanoma in situ. This highlights the potential of immunomodulatory therapies in the treatment of cancer.

Immunodermatologic Testing

Direct Immunofluorescence

By using secondary anti-human antibodies, DIF can detect the presence of autoantibodies bound in vivo to perilesional skin or mucous membrane from a patient. This is classically used in the identification of immunobullous

Table 10-3 ▪ Syndromes Exhibiting Immunodeficiency

Disorder	Clinical/Cutaneous Features	Defect	Inheritance
AIDS	Opportunistic infections; severe dermatitis; psoriasis; candidiasis; viral and fungal infections	HIV infection	Acquired
APECED syndrome	Addison's disease; candidiasis; hypoparathyroidism; ectodermal dystrophy	AIRE—autoimmune regulator—a DNA transcription factor	AR; AD
Ataxia telangiectasia	Progressive cerebellar ataxia; telangiectasia (eye/skin); progeric change of skin/hair; granulomatous skin lesions; sinopulmonary infections; lymphomas; increased breast cancer and lymphoma in carriers	ATM—senses DNA damage and initiates responses allowing DNA repair	AR
Chediak–Higashi syndrome	Silvery hair, abnormal skin pigment, skin/respiratory infections, photosensitivity; giant intracytoplasmic granules in leukocytes; accelerated lymphomatous phase	LYST—controls lysosomal vesicle and melanosome processing	AR
Chronic granulomatous disease	Pneumonia, hepatosplenomegaly, lymphadenopathy, cutaneous granulomas, abnormal nitroblue tetrazolium assay	Phagocyte NADPH oxidase defects (X linked); p47 phox deficiency (AR forms)	XLR (76%); AR
Chronic mucocutaneous candidiasis	Recurrent, progressive candida infections of mucosa, nails, and skin	Multiple genes	AR; AD
Common variable immunodeficiency	Late onset (~30 years of age); pyogenic upper and lower respiratory tract infections; pyoderma of skin; eczema; noncaseating granulomas of various tissues including skin; increased malignancy including lymphoma; increased autoimmune disease	Unknown	AR and AD forms
Complement deficiencies	*Early components* (C1, C2, C4): LE-like disorders, onset in childhood *Late components* (C5-9): overwhelming neisserial infections	Various	Most AR
	Hereditary angioedema	C1 INH	C1 INH: AD
Epidermodysplasia verruciformis	Infection by numerous HPV types (HPV 3, 5, 8); cutaneous malignancy; flat warts/tinea versicolor like skin lesions	EVER1; EVER2 genes; unknown function	AR
Hyper-IgE syndrome	Recurrent *Staphylococcus* and Candida infections; cold abscesses of skin; sinopulmonary infections; chronic dermatitis; characteristic facies, osteopenia, dental abnormalities	Chromosome 4; gene not identified	AD
Hyper-IgM syndrome	Sinopulmonary and GI infections; oral ulcers; recalcitrant verruca; lymphadenitis, hepatosplenomegaly	XLR (most) – CD40L defect; AR (less common) due to cytidine deaminase deficiency	XLR; AR

(continued)

Table 10-3 ■ (Continued)

Disorder	Clinical/Cutaneous Features	Defect	Inheritance
IgA deficiency	Sinopulmonary infections; autoimmune disorders, most common Ig deficiency (often asymptomatic)	Multifactorial	Heterogeneous
IPEX syndrome	Immune dysregulation; polyendocrinopathy; enteropathy (diarrhea); skin eruptions	Forkhead box P3 mutations; protein highly expressed in Tr cells	XLR
Leukocyte adhesion deficiency	Pyoderma gangrenosum–like ulcerations; gingivitis, periodontitis; poor wound healing; delayed detachment of umbilical cord; severe infections (bacterial/fungal)	Defective B2 subunit of CD18	AR
Omenn's syndrome	Seborrheic dermatitis–like eruption; eosinophilia; recurrent infections; alopecia	RAG 1 and 2 defects: impaired recombination of receptor genes with abnormal Ig diversity	AR
SCID	Recurrent infections, diarrhea, failure to thrive; in utero GVHD; increased GVHD risk from nonirradiated blood products; absence of lymphoid tissue, T-, B-, and/or NK cell deficiencies	Common γ-chain deficiency causes absent T and NK cells with normal B cells	XLR (most common); AR
Wiskott-Aldrich syndrome	Atopic dermatitis–like rash; sinopulmonary infections; thrombocytopenia leading to easy bleeding	WASP: controls assembly of actin filaments	XLR

Abbreviations: GI, gastrointestinal; GVHD, graft-versus-host disease; HPV, human papilloma virus; NK, natural killer; SCID, severe combined immunodeficiency.

diseases such as pemphigus and pemphigoid. It is considered the most reliable and sensitive test for pemphigus.

Indirect Immunofluorescence

Indirect immunofluorescence (IIF) detects the presence of circulating autoantibodies by reacting sera from patients with epithelial cell substrates. In the case of diseases showing DIF staining along the basement membrane, IIF studies on salt split skin can facilitate diagnosis of these conditions, for example, differentiating BP from epidermolysis bullosa acquisita.

Immunomapping

Immunomapping utilizes lesional skin samples from a patient and standard antibodies against normal cutaneous proteins. It can identify deficiency of or abnormal localization of these proteins. This technique has been used to subtype inherited bullous diseases of the skin such as epidermolysis bullosa.

Immunoprecipitation and Immunoblotting

These tests detect target antigens as bands of a characteristic molecular weight after electrophoretic separation. In immunoblotting the proteins are denatured, which means they are not in immunoprecipitation.

ELISA Testing

ELISA stands for enzyme-linked immunosorbent assay, and refers to a technique utilizing antigen that is prebound to ELISA plates. Patient sera are exposed to the plates and bound antibody is then detected. ELISA tests are available for both pemphigus and BP antigens. In the case of BP, serum levels of IgG and IgE to BP180 measured with ELISA testing have been shown to correlate with disease severity.

Immunology: Therapeutics

Many therapeutic agents used in dermatology work via effects on the immune system. Topical and oral corticosteroids

Table 10-4 ■ **Commonly Used Dermatologic Medications and Their Known Mechanisms of Action on the Immune System**

Drug	Immune Effect
Azathioprine	Inhibits DNA/RNA synthesis and repair via active metabolite 6-thioguanine
Biologic Agents	
Alefacept	Fusion protein of LFA-3 and Fc fragment of human IgG
Efalizumab	Antibody to CD11a, the α-subunit of LFA-1
Etanercept	TNF-α–Fc fragment of IgG fusion protein
Infliximab	Humanized monoclonal anti–TNF-α antibody
Calcipotriene	Vitamin D receptor agonist–inflammatory cytokine inhibition
Corticosteroids	Inhibition of NfκB and AP-1
Cyclosporine; tacrolimus; pimecrolimus	Calcineurin inhibition; inhibits IL-2 production and decreases NFAT-1 activity
Dapsone	Inhibition of neutrophil (? eosinophil) myeloperoxidase; endothelial integrin adhesion; impaired neutrophil chemotaxis
Hydroxychloroquine; chloroquine	Increased lysosomal pH
Imiquimod	Toll-like receptor 7 agonist
IVIG	Inhibition of Fas/FasL binding; induces FcγRIIB receptor expression
Methotrexate	Dihydrofolate reductase inhibition; AICAR transformylase inhibition
Retinoids	Modulation of toll-like receptor 2; modulation of AP-1 pathway
Thalidomide	TNF-α inhibition; suppression of IL-12 production
Ultraviolet light	Suppression of LCs; stimulation of Tr cells; increased IL-10 production

Abbreviations: IL, interleukin; IVIG, intravenous immunoglobulin; TNF, tumor necrosis factor; Tr, regulatory T cell.

are a classic example of anti-inflammatory medications widely used in Dermatology. Table 10-4 summarizes some commonly used dermatologic medications and their known mechanisms of action on the immune system.

Suggested Reading

Delves P, Roitt I. Advances in immunology: The immune system (first of two parts). N Engl J Med 2000;343:37–49.

Delves P, Roitt I. Advances in immunology: The immune system (second of two parts). N Engl J Med 2000;343: 108–117.

Duthie M, Kimber I, Norval M. The effects of ultraviolet radiation on the human immune system. Br J Dermatol 1999;140:995–1009.

Johnson M, Farmer E. Graft-versus-host reactions in dermatology. J Am Acad Dermatol 1998;38:369–392.

Korman N. Bullous pemphigoid: The latest in diagnosis, prognosis, and therapy. Arch Dermatol 1998;134: 1137–1141.

Medzhitov R, Janeway C. Advances in immunology: Innate immunity. N Engl J Med 2000;343:338–344.

Parkin J, Cohen B. An overview of the immune system. Lancet 2001;357:1777–1789.

Schwarz, T. Skin immunity. Br J Dermatol 2003;149 (Suppl 66):2–4.

von Andrian U, Mackay C. Advances in immunology: T-cell function and migration—Two sides of the same coin. N Engl J Med 2000;343:1020–1034.

INFLAMMATORY SKIN DISEASES

CHAPTER 11

Pruritic Dermatoses

John C. Hall

Pruritus, or itching, brings more patients to the physician's office than any other skin disease symptom. Itchy skin is not easily cured or even alleviated. Many hundreds of proprietary over-the-counter and prescription drugs are touted as effective anti-itch remedies, but none is 100% effective. Many are partially effective, but it is unfortunate that the most effective locally applied chemicals frequently irritate or sensitize the skin.

Pruritus is a symptom of many of the common skin diseases, such as contact dermatitis, atopic eczema, seborrheic dermatitis, hives, scabies, insect bites, some drug eruptions, and many other dermatoses. Relief of itching is of prime importance in treating these diseases.

In addition to the pruritus that occurs as a symptom of many skin diseases, there are other clinical forms of pruritus that deserve special consideration. These special types include *generalized pruritus* of the winter, senile, and essential varieties and *localized pruritus* of the lichen simplex type of the ears, anal area, lower legs in men, back of the neck in women, and genitalia. Localized pruritus of unknown etiology should alert one to the possibility of underlying peripheral nerve or central nervous system pathology.

Generalized Pruritus

Diffuse itching of the body without perceptible skin disease usually is due to winter dry skin or senile skin.

Winter Pruritus

Winter pruritus, or pruritus hiemalis, is a common form of generalized pruritus, although most patients complain of itching confined mainly to their legs. Every autumn, a certain

> ### SAUER'S NOTE
>
> When the presenting complaint is generalized itching of the skin, always stroke the skin on the forearm with your nail or a tongue depressor. After 5 minutes or so, if there is a wheal reaction at the stroking site, you have a diagnosis of dermographism. This is a common problem that is easily overlooked.

number of elderly patients, and occasionally young ones, walk into the physician's office complaining bitterly of the rather sudden onset of itching of their legs. Men often also itch around the waist. These patients have dry skin caused by the low humidity in their furnace-heated homes, or occasionally from the low humidity resulting from cooling air conditioning. Clinically, the skin shows excoriations and dry, curled, scaling plaques resembling a sun-baked, muddy beach at low tide. The dry skin associated with winter itch is to be differentiated from *ichthyosis,* a congenital, inherited dermatosis of varying severity, which is also worse in the winter.

Treatment of winter pruritus consists of the following:

1. Bathing should involve as cool water as possible and as little soap as possible. Soap can be limited to the face, axillae, groin, gentalia, hands, and feet.
2. A bland soap, such as Dove, Oilatum, Cetaphil, or Basis, is used sparingly.
3. An oil is added to the bath water, such as Lubath, Ro-Bathol, Nivea, or Alpha-Keri. (The patient should be warned to avoid slipping in the tub). The oil can be rubbed on after a shower.
4. Emollient lotions are beneficial, such as Complex 15, Curel, Eucerin, Aquaphor (quite greasy), Pen-Kera, or Moisturel (not as greasy and noncomedogenic). α-Hydroxy acid preparations include Amlactin 12% Cream and Lotion (over the counter), Lac-Hydrin 5% (over the counter), Lachydrin 12% (prescription only), and Eucerin Plus. Urea products that are beneficial include Keralotion (35%), Keracream (40%), Vanamide (40%), Carmol 40 Cream and Lotion (40%), and Eucerin Plus Lotion (also has lactic acid as an α-hydroxy acid). Lubricants should be applied immediately after bathing for the most benefit.
5. A low-potency corticosteroid ointment applied twice daily is effective. Triamcinilone ointment 0.1% is mid-potency and very inexpensive. A 1% hydrocortisone can be mixed with any of the mentioned moisturizers.
6. Oral antihistamines are sometimes effective, such as chlorpheniramine (Chlor-trimeton), 4 mg h.s. or q.i.d, or diphenhydramine (Benadryl), 50 mg h.s. There are newer nonsedating antihistamines such as Claritin 10 mg q day (over the counter), Clarinex 10 mg q day, Zyrtec 10 mg q day, and Allegra 60 or 180 mg q day. Some dermatologists do not think the nonsedating antihistamines are as effective as the sedating antihistamines. A commonly used sedating antihistamine is hydroxyzine 10 mg every 8 hours while awake. The dose can be titrated to 25 mg, 50 mg, or rarely 100 mg. The soporific effect, or drowsiness, often becomes less severe with prolonged use.

Senile Pruritus

Senile pruritus is a resistant form of generalized pruritus in the elderly patient. It can occur at any time of the year and may or may not be associated with dry skin. There is some evidence that these patients have a disorder of keratinization. This form of itch occurs most commonly on the scalp, shoulders, sacral areas, and legs. Clinically, some patients have no cutaneous signs of the itch, but others may have linear excoriations. *Scabies* should be ruled out, as well as the diseases mentioned under the next form of pruritus to be considered, essential pruritus.

Treatment is usually not very satisfactory. In addition to the agents mentioned previously in connection with winter pruritus, the injection of 30 mg of triamcinolone acetonide suspension (Kenalog-40) intramuscularly every 4 to 6 weeks for two or three injections is quite beneficial. I do not like to repeat this more often than three to four times a year to avoid systemic corticosteroid side effects. Topical antipruritic agents can be used, such as pramoxine hydrochloride (Pramosone with either 1% or 2.5% hydrocortisone is a prescription or Aveeno Anti-itch Lotion, which is available over the counter). Menthol (0.5%), phenol (0.5%), or sulfur (2% to 5%) can be added to any appropriate base (see Chapter 5).

Essential Pruritus

Essential pruritus is the rarest form of the generalized itching diseases. No person of any age is exempt, but it occurs most frequently in the elderly patient. The itching is usually quite diffuse, with occasional "bites" in certain localized areas. All itching is worse at night, and no exception is made for this form of pruritus. Before a diagnosis of essential pruritus is made, the following diseases must be ruled out by appropriate studies:

- drug reaction,
- diabetes mellitus,
- uremia,
- lymphoma (mycosis fungoides, leukemia, or lymphoma [especially Hodgkin's disease]), as a paraneoplastic syndrome from any metastatic underlying malignancy,

- primary sclerosing cholangitis which has very severe pruritis,
- liver disease (especially hepatitis B or C even without jaundice),
- bullous pemphigoid before the blisters are present,
- AIDS,
- stress or more severe psychiatric illness such as psychosis or parasitophobia,
- hyperthyroidism,
- post–brain tissue damage such as a stroke, brain cancer or trauma, and
- intestinal parasites.

Treatment is the same as for senile and winter pruritus.

Localized Pruritic Dermatoses

Lichen Simplex Chronicus

Other common terms for lichen simplex chronicus (LSC) include *localized neurodermatitis* and *lichenified dermatitis*. There are pros and cons for all the terms.

LSC (Fig. 11-1) is a common skin condition characterized by the occurrence of single or, less frequently, multiple patches of chronic, itching, thickened, scaly, dry skin in one or more of several classic locations. It is unrelated to atopic eczema according to some experts, but others feel it is an adult form of eczema.

Primary Lesions

This disease begins as a small, localized, well-demarcated, pruritic papule or patch of dermatitis that might have been an insect bite, chigger bite, contact dermatitis, or other minor irritation, which may or may not be remembered by the patient. Because of various etiologic factors, a cycle of itching, scratching, more itching, and more scratching supervenes, and chronic dermatosis develops. Emotional stress is thought to lower the itch threshold and cause exacerbation of the disease. The itching is intense and paroxysmal in nature.

Secondary Lesions

These include excoriations, lichenification, and, in severe cases, marked verrucous thickening of the skin, with pigmentary changes. In severe cases, healing is bound to be followed by some scarring.

Presentation and Characteristics

Distribution. This condition is seen most commonly at the hairline of the nape of the neck and on the wrists, the

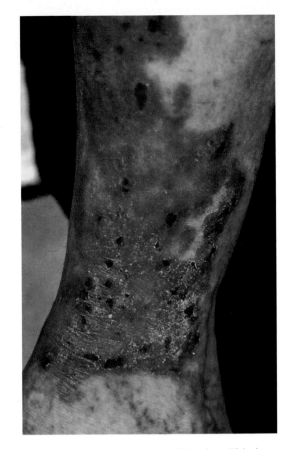

FIGURE 11-1 ■ Localized LSC of the leg. This is a common location. Note the lichenification and the excoriations owing to the marked pruritus. *(Courtesy of K.U.M.C.; Duke Labs, Inc.)*

ankles, the ears (see external otitis), anal area (see pruritus ani), and so on (Fig. 11-2).

Course. This disease is chronic and recurrent. Most cases respond quickly to potent topical corticosteroid treatment, but some can last for years and defy all forms of therapy.

Subjective Complaints. The primary symptom is intense itching, often paroxysmal, that is usually worse at night, occurs even during sleep, and may awaken the patient.

Causes. The initial cause (a bite, stasis dermatitis, contact dermatitis, seborrheic dermatitis, tinea cruris, psoriasis) may be very evanescent, but it is generally agreed that the chronicity of the lesion is due to the nervous habit of scratching. It is a rare patient who does not volunteer the information or admit, if questioned, that the itching is worse when he or she is upset, nervous, or tired. Why some people with a minor skin injury respond with the development of a

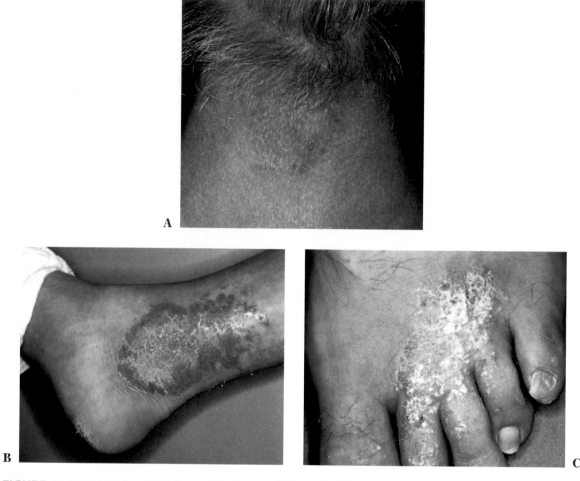

FIGURE 11-2 ■ Localized LSC in occipital area of the scalp (**A**), of the medial aspect of ankle, following lichen planus of the area (**B**), and on dorsum of the foot (**C**). *(Courtesy of Duke Labs, Inc.)*

lichenified patch of skin and others do not is possibly due to the personality of the patient or in an atopic patient due to an increase release of antihistamines with an exaggerated triple response of Lewis beginning the chronic itch–scratch cycle.

Age Group. It is very common to see localized neurodermatitis of the posterior neck in menopausal women. Other clinical types of neurodermatitis are seen at any age.

Family Incidence. This disorder may be unrelated to allergies in patient or family, thus differing from atopic eczema. Atopic people are more "itchy," however, and, as mentioned, some authors feel the two diseases are a continuum.

Related to Employment. Recurrent exposure and contact to irritating agents at work can lead to LSC.

Differential Diagnosis

- *Psoriasis:* Several patches on the body in classic areas of distribution; family history of disease; classic silvery whitish scales; sharply circumscribed patch; itching may be intense especially in the scalp and perianal areas but it is often minimal (see Chaps. 14 and 15).
- *Atopic eczema:* Allergic history in patient or family; multiple lesions; classically seen in cubital and popliteal areas and face (see Chap. 9).
- *Contact dermatitis:* Acute onset; contact history positive; usually red, vesicular, and oozing; distribution matches site of exposure of contactant; may be acute contact dermatitis overlying LSC owing to overzealous therapy (see Chap. 9).
- *Lichen planus, hypertrophic form on anterior tibial area:* Lichen planus in mouth and on other body

areas; biopsy specimen usually characteristic (see Chap. 15).

- *Seborrheic dermatitis of scalp:* Does not itch as much; is better in summer; a diffuse, scaly, greasy eruption (see Chap. 13).

Treatment

Case Example. A 45-year-old woman presents with a severely itching, scaly, red, lichenified patch on back of the neck at the hairline.

First Visit.

1. Explain the condition to the patient and tell her that the medicine is directed toward stopping the itch. If this can be done, and if she cooperates by keeping her hands off the area, the disease will disappear. Emphasize the effect of scratching by stating that if both arms were broken, the eruption would be gone when the casts were removed. However, this is not a recommended form of therapy. Do not blame the patient for this disease in your zeal to explain the importance of keeping hands off.
2. For severe bouts of intractable itching, prescribe ice-cold Burow's solution packs.

   Sig: Add 1 packet of Domeboro powder to 1 quart of ice cold water. Apply cloth wet with this solution for 15 minutes p.r.n.
3. A moderate-potency corticosteroid ointment or emollient cream 15.0

   Sig: Apply q.i.d., or more often, as itching requires.

   The moderate-potency fluorinated corticosteroid creams (Synalar, Cordran, Lidex, Diprosone, Cutivate) can be used under an occlusive dressing of plastic wrap on lesions on an extremity. The dressing can be left on overnight.

   Warning: Long-term occlusive dressing therapy with corticosteroids can cause atrophy of the skin.

Subsequent Visits.

1. Add menthol (0.25%) or coal tar solution (3% to 10%) to above ointment or cream for greater antipruritic effect.
2. Intralesional corticosteroid therapy is a very effective and safe treatment. The technique is as follows. Use a 1-inch-long No. 26 needle or 30-½ needle and a Luer-Lok–type tuberculin syringe. Inject 3 or 5 mg per cc of triamcinolone parenteral solution (Kenalog-10 or Aristocort Intralesional Suspension diluted with normal saline or xylocaine with or without epinephrine)

intradermally or subcutaneously, directly under the skin lesion. Do not inject all the solution in one area, but spread it around as you advance the needle. Usually 1 or less is injected each time. The injection can be repeated every 3 or 4 weeks as necessary to eliminate the patch of dermatitis. *Warning:* A complication of an atrophic depression at the injection site can occur. This usually can be avoided if the concentration of triamcinolone in one area is kept low, and when it occurs, it usually disappears after months.

Resistant Cases.

1. An antihistamine or antianxiety agent orally.
2. Prednisone 10 mg.

   Sig: 1 tablet q.i.d. for 3 days, then 2 tablets every morning for 7 days.
3. Dome-Paste boot or Coban wrap. Apply in office for cases of neurodermatitis localized to arms and legs. This is a physical deterrent to scratching. Leave on for 1 week at a time.
4. Psychotherapy is of questionable value.

External Otitis

External otitis is a descriptive term for a common and persistent dermatitis of the ears owing to several causes. The agent most frequently blamed for this condition is "fungus," but pathogenic fungi are rarely found in the external ear. The true causes of external otitis, in order of frequency, are as follows: seborrheic dermatitis (which is now felt to be related to *Pityosporum ovale* yeast infection), LSC, contact dermatitis, atopic eczema, psoriasis, *Pseudomonas* bacterial infection (which is usually secondary to other causes) and, last, fungal infection, which also can be primary or secondary to other factors. For further information on the specific processes, refer to each of the diseases mentioned.

Treatment

Treatment should be directed primarily toward the specific cause, such as care of the scalp for seborrheic cases or avoidance of jewelry for contact cases. When this is done, however, certain special techniques and medicines must be used in addition to clear up this troublesome area.

Case Example. An elderly woman presents with an oozing, red, crusted, swollen left external ear, with a wet canal but an intact drum. A considerable amount of seborrheic dermatitis of the scalp is confluent with the acutely inflamed ear area. The patient has had itching ear trouble off and on for 10 years, but in the past month, it has become most severe.

SAUER'S NOTES

1. Many cases of acute ear dermatitis are aggravated by an allergy to the therapeutic cream, such as Neosporin, or the ingredients in the base.
2. A corticosteroid in a petrolatum base eliminates this problem.
3. Use 1% Hytone ointment, DesOwen ointment, or Tridesilon ointment.

First Visit.

1. Always inspect the canal and the drum with an otoscope. If excessive wax and debris are present in the canal, or if the drum is involved in the process, the patient should be treated for these problems or referred to an ear specialist. An effective liquid to dry up the oozing canal is as follows:

   Hydrocortisone powder 1%
   Burow's solution, 1:10 strength q.s. 15.0
   Sig: Place 2 drops in ear t.i.d.

2. Burow's solution wet packs

   Sig: Add 1 packet of Domeboro powder to 1 quart of cool water. Apply wet cloths to external ear for 15 minutes t.i.d.

3. Corticosteroid ointment 15.0

   Sig: Apply locally to external ear t.i.d., not in canal.

Subsequent Visits. Several days later, after decreased swelling, cessation of oozing, and lessening of itching, institute the following changes in therapy:

1. Decrease the soaks to once a day.
2. Sulfur, ppt. 5%

   Corticosteroid ointment q.s. 15.0
   Sig: Apply locally t.i.d. to ear with the little finger, not down in the canal with a cotton-tipped applicator.

   For persistent cases, a short course of oral corticosteroid or antibiotic therapy often removes the "fire" so that local remedies are effective.

Pruritus Ani

Itching of the anal area is a common malady that can vary in severity from mild to marked. The patient with this very annoying symptom is apt to resort to self-treatment and therefore delay the visit to the physician. Usually, the patient has overtreated the sensitive area, and the immediate problem of the physician is to quiet the acute contact dermatitis. The original cause of the pruritus ani is often difficult to ascertain.

Pruritic diseases common in this area are seborrheic dermatitis, psoriasis, lichen sclerosis et atrophicus, candidiasis, tinea, pin worms (especially in children), and hemorrhoids in adults.

Presentation and Characteristics

Primary Lesions. These can range from slight redness confined to a very small area to an extensive contact dermatitis with redness, vesicles, and oozing of the entire buttock.

Secondary Lesions. Excoriations from the intense itching are very common, and after a prolonged time, they progress toward lichenification. A generalized papulovesicular id eruption can develop from an acute flare-up of this entity.

Course. Most cases of pruritus ani respond rapidly and completely to proper management, especially if the cause can be ascertained and eliminated. Every physician, however, will have a patient who will continue to scratch and defy all therapy.

Causes. The proper management of this socially unacceptable form of pruritus consists in searching for and eliminating the several factors that contribute to the persistence of this symptom complex. These factors can be divided into general and specific etiologic factors.

General Factors

- *Diet:* The following irritating foods should be removed from the diet: chocolate, nuts, cheese, and spicy foods. Coffee, because of its stimulating effect on any form of itching, should be limited to

---

SAUER'S NOTES

1. Do not prescribe a fluorinated corticosteroid salve for the anogenital area. It can cause telangiectasia and atrophy of the skin after long-term use.
2. One of my favorite medications for pruritus ani or genital pruritus is 1% Hytone ointment applied sparingly locally two or three times a day. The petrolatum base is well tolerated.
3. If the anogenital pruritus is resistant to therapy and especially if the involvement is unilateral, a biopsy should be performed to rule out Bowen's disease or extramammary Paget's disease.

1 cup a day. Rarely, certain other foods are noted by the patient to aggravate the pruritus.

- *Bathing:* Many patients have the misconception that the itching is caused by uncleanliness. Therefore, they resort to excessive bathing and scrubbing of the anal area. This is harmful and irritating and must be stopped.
- *Toilet care:* Harsh toilet paper contributes greatly to the continuance of this condition. Cotton or a proprietary cleansing cloth (Tucks) must be used for wiping. Mineral oil or Balneol lotion can be added to the cotton if necessary. Rarely, an allergy to the pastel tint in colored toilet tissues is a factor causing pruritus.
- *Scratching:* As with all the diseases of this group, chronic scratching leads to a vicious cycle. The chief aim of the physician is to give relief from this itching, but a gentle admonishment to the patient to keep hands off is indicated. With the physician's help, the itch–scratch cycle can be broken. The emotional and mental personality of the patient regulates the effectiveness of this suggestion.

Specific Etiologic Factors

- *Oral antibiotics:* Pruritus ani from oral antibiotic therapy is seen frequently. It may or may not be due to an overgrowth of candida organisms. The physician who automatically questions patients about recent drug ingestion will not miss this diagnosis.
- *Lichen simplex chronicus:* It is always a problem to know which comes first, the itching or the "nervousness." In most instances, the itching comes first, but there is no denying that once pruritus ani has developed, it is aggravated by emotional tensions and "nerves." However, only the rare patient has a "deep-seated" psychological problem.
- *Psoriasis:* In this area, psoriasis is common. Usually, other skin surfaces are also involved.
- *Atopic eczema:* Atopic eczema of this site in adults is rather unusual. A history of atopy in the patient or family is helpful in establishing this cause.
- *Fungal infection:* Contrary to old beliefs, this cause is quite rare. Clinically, a raised, sharp, papulovesicular border is seen that commonly is confluent with tinea of the crural area. If a scraping or a culture reveals fungi, then local or systemic antifungal therapy is indicated for cure.
- *Worm infestation:* In children, pinworms can usually be implicated. A diagnosis is made by finding eggs on morning anal smears, by applying scotch tape to the anal orifice and viewing the worms under the microscope or by seeing the small white worms when the child is sleeping. Worms are a rare cause of adult pruritus ani.
- *Hemorrhoids:* In the lay person's mind, this is undoubtedly the most common cause. Actually, it is an unimportant primary factor, but may be a contributing factor. Hemorrhoidectomy alone is rarely successful as a cure for pruritus ani.
- *Cancer:* This is a very rare cause of anal itching, but a rectal or proctoscopic examination may be indicated especially in men who have sex within the AIDS population.

Treatment

Case Example. A patient states that he has had anal itching for 4 months. It followed a 5-day course of an antibiotic for the "flu." Many local remedies have been used; the latest, a supposed remedy for athlete's foot, aggravated the condition. Examination reveals an oozing, macerated, red area around the anus.

First Visit.

1. Initial therapy should include removal of the general factors listed under *Causes* and giving instructions as to diet, bathing, toilet care, and scratching.
2. Burow's solution wet packs

   Sig: Add 1 packet of Domeboro to 1 quart of cool water. Apply wet cloths to the area b.i.d. while lying in bed for 20 minutes, or more often if necessary for severe itching. Ice cubes may be added to the solution for more antiitching effect.
3. Low-potency corticosteroid cream or ointment q.s. 15.0

   Sig: Apply to area b.i.d.
4. Diphenhydramine, 50 mg

   Sig: 1 capsule h.s. (for itching and sedation).
   Comment: Available over the counter

Subsequent Visits.

1. As tolerated, add increasing strengths of sulfur, coal tar solution, or menthol (0.25%) or phenol (0.5%) to the above cream, or Vytone cream with hydrocortisone 1% (can be given in a cheaper generic formulation).
2. Intralesional corticosteroid injection therapy is very effective. Usually, the minor discomfort of the injection is quite well tolerated because of the patient's desire to be cured. The technique is given in the section on LSC. Use only 3 mg/cc concentration

Genital Pruritus

Itching of the female vulva or the male scrotum can be treated in much the same way as pruritus ani if these special considerations are borne in mind.

Vulvar Pruritus

Etiologically, vulvar pruritus caused by Candida or Trichomonas infection; contact dermatitis from underwear, douche chemicals, contraceptive jellies and diaphragms; chronic cervicitis; neurodermatitis; menopausal or senile atrophic changes; lichen sclerosus et atrophicus; bacillary vaginosis; or leukoplakia. Pruritus vulvae is frequently seen in patients with diabetes mellitus and during pregnancy.

Treatment can be adapted from that for pruritus ani (see preceding section) with the addition of a daily douche, such as 2 tablespoons of vinegar to 1 quart of warm water.

Vulvodynia is a difficult problem to manage. The sensation of burning and pain in the vulvar area is not uncommon and requires careful etiologic evaluation. Most cases can be managed as a contact dermatitis, but there is a strong psychological element. A minimal dose of haloperidol (Haldol), 1 mg, b.i.d., amitriptyline (Elavil), 10 mg h.s. or sinequan (Doxepin), 10 mg h.s. is occasionally indicated and effective. Larger doses may be necessary. Scrotodynia is a similar variant in men.

Scrotal Pruritus

Etiologically, scrotal pruritus is due to tinea infection; contact dermatitis from soaps, powders, or clothing; or LSC (Fig. 11-3). Treatment is similar to that given for pruritus ani in the preceding section.

Notalgia Paresthetica

Notalgia paresthetica is a moderately common localized pruritic dermatosis that is usually confined to the middle

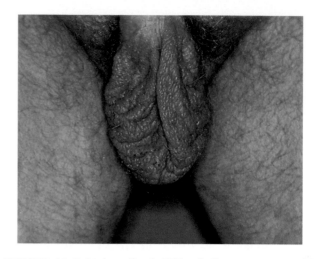

FIGURE 11-3 ■ Localized LSC of the scrotum, with marked lichenification and thickening of the skin. *(Courtesy of Duke Labs, Inc.)*

upper back or scapular area off to one side of the spine. A pigmented patch may be formed by the chronic rubbing. Spinal nerve impingement has been suggested as the etiology by some authors. Zonalon cream 4 times a day may be helpful, but when applied over large areas, it may cause drowsiness. Some evidence exists for a hereditary factor. EMLA anesthetic cream and capsaicin (Zostrix) cream may be beneficial.

Suggested Reading

Fleischer A. The clinical management of itching. New York, The Parthenon Publish Group, 2000.

Yosipovitch G, Greaves MW, et al. Itch: Basic mechanisms and therapy. New York, Marcel Dekker, 2004.

Yosipovitch G, David M. The diagnostic and therapeutic approach to idiopathic generalized pruritus. Int J Dermatol 1999;38:881–887.

CHAPTER 12

Vascular Dermatoses

John C. Hall

Urticaria, erythema multiforme and its variants, and erythema nodosum are included under the heading of vascular dermatoses because of their vascular reaction patterns. Stasis dermatitis is included because it is a dermatosis owing to venous insufficiency in the legs.

Urticaria

The commonly seen entity of urticaria (Fig. 12-1), or hives, can be acute or chronic and due to known or unknown causes. Numerous factors, both immunologic and nonimmunologic, can be involved in its pathogenesis. The urticarial wheal results from liberation of histamine from tissue mast cells and from circulating basophils.

Nonimmunologic factors that can release histamine from these cells include

- chemicals,
- various drugs (including morphine and codeine),
- ingestion of lobster, crayfish, and other foods,
- bacterial toxins, and
- physical agents.

Examples of the type caused by physical agents are the linear wheals that are produced by light stroking of the skin, known as *dermographism.* (Consult the Dictionary–Index for the triple response of Lewis reaction.)

Immunologic mechanisms are probably involved more often in acute than in chronic urticaria. The most commonly considered of these mechanisms is the type I hypersensitivity state that is triggered by polyvalent antigen bridging two specific immunoglobulin E molecules that are bound to the mast cell or basophil surface (see Chap. 10).

Lesions

Pea-sized red papules to large circinate patterns with red borders and white centers that can cover an entire side of the trunk or the thigh may be noted. Vesicles and bullae are seen in severe cases, along with hemorrhagic effusions. A severe form of urticaria is labeled *angioedema.* It can involve an entire body part, such as the lip or the hand. Edema of the glottis and bronchospasm are serious complications and are a true medical emergency.

Presentation and Characteristics

Course

Acute cases may be mild or explosive, but usually disappear with or without treatment in a few hours or days. The chronic form has remissions and exacerbations for months or years.

Causes

After careful questioning and investigation, many cases of hives, particularly of the chronic type, are concluded to result from no apparent causative agent. Other cases, mainly the acute ones, have been found to result from the following factors or agents:

- *Drugs or Chemicals:* Penicillin and derivatives are probably the most common causes of acute hives, but any other drug, whether ingested, injected, inhaled, or, rarely, applied on the skin, can cause the reaction (see Chap. 9).
- *Foods:* Foods are a common cause of acute hives. The main offenders are seafood, nuts, chocolate, strawberries, cheeses, pork, eggs, wheat, and milk. Chronic hives can be caused by traces of penicillin in milk products (see Fig. 12-1A).
- *Insect Bites and Stings:* Insect bites, stings from mosquitoes, fleas, or spiders, and contact with certain moths, leeches, and jellyfish cause hives.
- *Physical Agents:* Hives result from heat, cold, radiant energy, and physical injury. *Dermographism* is a term applied to a localized urticarial wheal produced by scratching the skin in certain people (see Fig. 12-1B).
- *Inhalants:* Nasal sprays, insect sprays, dust, feathers, pollens, and animal danders are some offenders.

125

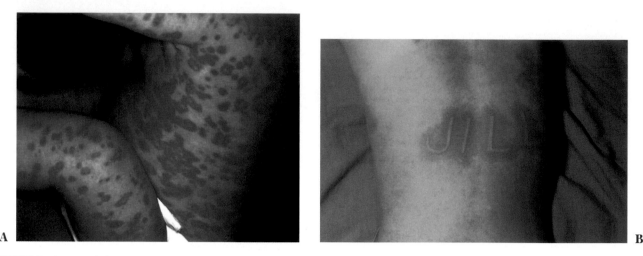

FIGURE 12-1 ■ **(A)** Acute urticaria from penicillin in 6-month-old child. **(B)** Dermographism on flexor wrist. *(Courtesy of Dermik Laboratories, Inc.)*

■ *Infections:* A focus of infection is always considered, sooner or later, in chronic cases of hives, and in unusual instances it is causative. The sinuses, teeth, tonsils, gallbladder, and genitourinary tract should be checked.

■ *Internal disease:* Urticaria has been seen with liver disease, intestinal parasites, cancer, rheumatic fever, lupus erythematosus, and others.

■ *"Nerves":* After all other causes of chronic urticaria have been ruled out, there remain a substantial number of cases that appear to be related to nervous stress, worry, or fatigue. These cases benefit most from the establishment of good rapport between the patient and the physician.

■ *Contact Urticaria Syndrome:* This uncommon response can be incited from the local contact on the skin of drugs and chemicals, foods, insects, animal dander, and plants.

■ *Cholinergic Urticaria:* Clinically, small papular welts are seen that are caused by heat (hot bath), stress, or strenuous exercise.

Differential Diagnosis

■ *Erythema multiforme:* Systemic fever, malaise, and mouth lesions are noted in children and young adults (see the next section of this chapter).

SAUER'S NOTE

Dermographism is commonly overlooked as a cause of the patient's "welts" or vague itching.

■ *Dermographism:* A common finding in young adults, especially those who present complaining of welts on their skin or vague itching of the skin with no residual lesions. To make the diagnosis, stroke the skin firmly to see if an urticarial response develops. The course can be chronic, but hydroxyzine, 10 mg b.i.d. or t.i.d., is quite helpful. (Warn the patient about the possibility of drowsiness.) Nonsedating antihistamines can also be tried.

■ *Urticarial vasculitis:* Lesions may last more than 24 hours, be painful, leave a bruise, and be associated with hypocomplementemia. Skin biopsy is confirmatory.

Treatment

Case Example. A patient presents for a case of acute hives due to penicillin injection 1 week previously for a "cold."

1. Colloidal bath

   Sig: Add 1 cup of starch or oatmeal (Aveeno) to 6 to 8 inches of lukewarm water in the tub. Bathe for 15 minutes once or twice a day.

2. Sarna Lotion, Aveeno Anti-itch Lotion or PrameGel OTC

   Sig: Apply p.r.n. locally for itching.

3. Hydroxyzine (Atarax), 10 mg #30

   Sig: Take 1 tablet t.i.d., a.c. (warn of drowsiness).

4. Diphenhydramine (Benadryl), 50 mg

   Comment: Available over the counter

5. Nonsedating antihistamines can also be used.

6. Betamethasone sodium phosphate (Celestone), 3 mg/mL

   Sig: Inject 1 to 1.5 mL subcutaneously

For a more severe case of acute hives:

1. Diphenhydramine injection

   Sig: Inject 2 mL (20 mg) subcutaneously, *or*

2. Epinephrine hydrochloride

   Sig: Inject 0.3 to 0.5 mL of 1:1000 solution subcutaneously, *or*

3. Prednisone tablets, 10 mg #30

   Sig: Take 1 tablet q.i.d. for 3 days, then 1 tablet in morning as necessary.

For treatment of patient with chronic hives of 6 months' duration when cause is undetermined after careful history and examination:

1. Hydroxyzine (Atarax), 10 to 25 mg #60

   Sig: Take 1 tablet t.i.d. depending on drowsiness and effectiveness. Continue for weeks or months.
   Clemastine (Tavist) 1.34 or 2.68 mg #30
   Sig: Take 1 tablet b.i.d., available OTC
   Cyproheptadine (Periactin) 4 mg #60
   Sig: One by mouth t.i.d.

2. Loratadine (Claritin) now OTC 10 mg #30

   Sig: Take 1 tablet once a day
   Cetirizine (Zyrtec) 5 mg or 10 mg #30
   Sig: Take 1 tablet once a day
   Fexofenadine (Allegra), 60 mg or 180 mg #30
   Sig: Take 1 tablet once a day

3. Cimetidine (Tagamet), 300 mg #60

   Sig: Take 1 tablet t.i.d. (200 mg, 400 mg or 800 mg)
   Comment: This H_2 blocker is of benefit in some cases, and can be added to H_1 blockers.

4. Suggest avoidance of seafood, nuts, chocolate, cheese and other milk products, strawberries, pork, excessively spicy foods, and excess of coffee or tea.

5. Keep a diet diary of everything ingested (including all foods, all medicines, even over-the-counter, candy, menthol cigarettes, chewing gum, chewing tobacco, mouthwash, breath fresheners) and then see what items were used 12 to 24 hours before the episode of hives occurred.

6. A mild sedative or tranquilizer such as meprobamate, 400 mg t.i.d., or chlordiazepoxide (Librium), 5 mg t.i.d., may help.

7. Doxepin (Sinequan) 10 mg #60

   Sig: 1 tablet t.i.d.
   Comment: This is a tricyclic antidepressant with potent antihistaminic properties. It can cause drowsiness, dry mouth, and other side effects of this classification of drugs.

8. Immunosuppressive drugs such as prednisone are unfortunately necessary in severe cases.

9. Zaditor (ketotifen fumarate) is a mast cell stabilizer with benefits in severe cases.

Erythema Multiforme

The term *erythema multiforme* introduces a flurry of confusion in the mind of any student of medicine. It is our purpose in this section to attempt to dispel that confusion. Erythema multiforme, as originally described by Hebra, is an uncommon, distinct disease of unknown cause characterized by red iris-shaped or bull's eye–like macules, papules, or bullae confined mainly to the extremities, the face, and the lips (Fig. 12-2). It is accompanied by mild fever, malaise, and arthralgia. It occurs usually in children and young adults in the spring and the fall, has a duration of 2 to 4 weeks, and frequently is recurrent for several years.

The only relation between Hebra's erythema multiforme and the following diseases or syndromes is the clinical appearance of the eruption:

■ *Stevens-Johnson syndrome* is a severe and rarely fatal variant of erythema multiforme. It is characterized by high fever, extensive purpura, bullae, ulcers of the mucous membranes, and, after 2 to 3 days, ulcers of the skin. Eye involvement can result in blindness. It can be related to drugs and its severest form is considered by some to be the same as toxic epidermal necrolysis (see Chap. 18).

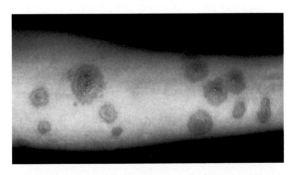

FIGURE 12-2 ■ Erythema multiforme–like eruption on arm during pregnancy. *(Courtesy of Dermik Laboratories, Inc.)*

- *Erythema multiforme bullosum* is a severe, chronic, bullous disease of adults (see Chap. 18). There is an opinion that this syndrome is completely separate from erythema multiforme. More macular, truncal lesions and more epidermal necrosis and less infiltrate may be seen in Stevens-Johnson syndrome (toxic epidermal necrolysis). Sulfonamides, anticonvulsant agents, allopurinol, chlormezanone, and nonsteroidal anti-inflammatory drugs.

- *Erythema multiforme–like drug eruption* is frequently due to phenacetin, quinine, penicillin, mercury, arsenic, phenylbutazone, barbiturates, trimethadione, phenytoin, sulfonamides, and antitoxins (see Chap. 9).

- *Erythema multiforme–like eruption* is caused rather commonly as part of a herpes simplex outbreak and also in conjunction with rheumatic fever, pneumonia, meningitis, measles, Coxsackievirus infection, pregnancy, and cancer, as well as after deep x-ray therapy, and as an allergic reaction to foods.

Differential Diagnosis

- The *erythema perstans* group or figurate erythemas of diseases includes over a dozen clinical entities with impossible-to-remember names. (See Dictionary–Index under *erythema perstans*.) All have various-sized erythematous patches, papules, or plaques with a definite red border and a less active center, forming circles, half circles, groups of circles, and linear bands. Multiple causes have been ascribed, including tick bites; allergic reactions; fungal, bacterial, viral, and spirochetal infections; and internal cancer. The duration of and the response to therapy varies with each individual case.

- *Erythema chronicum migrans* is the distinctive cutaneous eruption of the multisystem tick-borne spirochetosis Lyme disease. The deer tick, *Ixodes dammini*, is the vector for the spirochete. Early therapy with doxycycline or ampicillin may prevent late manifestations of the disease (see Chap. 22).

- *Reiter's syndrome* is a triad of conjunctivitis, urethritis, and, most important, arthritis, that occurs predominantly in men and lasts about 6 months. The skin manifestations consist of psoriasiform dermatitis that is called *balanitis circinata* on the penis and keratoderma blenorrhagica on the palms and soles.

- *Behçet's syndrome* consists of a triad of genital, oral, and ophthalmic ulcerations seen most commonly in men; it can last for years, with recurrences. Other manifestations include cutaneous pustular vasculitis, synovitis, and meningoencephalitis. It is more prevalent in eastern Mediterranean countries and Japan. Skin hypersensitivity to trauma or pathergy as observed with sterile pustular formation 24 to 48 hours after an intradermal needle prick.

- *Urticaria:* Clinically, urticaria may resemble erythema multiforme, but hives are associated with only mild systemic symptoms; it can occur in any age group; iris lesions are unusual; usually, it can be attributed to penicillin or other drug therapy; and it responds rapidly but often not completely to antihistamine therapy (see first part of this chapter). It is evanescent and dissipates or moves to a new area in less than 24 hours.

Treatment

Case Example. A 12-year-old boy presents with bull's eye–like lesions on his hands, arms, and feet; erosions of the lips and mucous membranes of the mouth; malaise; and a temperature of 101°F (38.3°C) orally. He had a similar eruption last spring.

1. Order bed rest and increased oral fluid intake.
2. Acetaminophen (Tylenol), 325 mg OTC

   Sig: Take 1 to 2 tablets q.i.d, *or*
   Prednisone, 10 mg #16
   Sig: Take 2 tablets stat and then 2 tablets every morning for 7 days.
3. For severe cases, such as the Stevens-Johnson form, hospitalization is indicated, where intravenous corticosteroid therapy (debatable), intravenous fluid replacement infusions, immune globulin, and other supportive measures can be administered.

Erythema Nodosum

Erythema nodosum is an uncommon reaction pattern seen mainly on the anterior tibial areas of the legs (Fig. 12-3). It appears as erythematous nodules in successive crops and is preceded by fever, malaise, and arthralgia.

Presentation and Characteristics

Primary Lesions

Bilateral red, tender, rather well-circumscribed nodules are seen mainly on the pretibial surface of the legs but also on the arms and the body. Later, the flat lesions may become raised, confluent, and purpuric. Only a few lesions develop at one time.

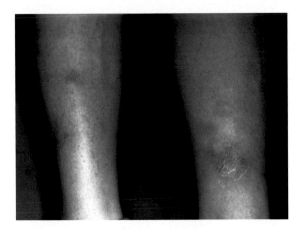

FIGURE 12-3 ■ Erythema nodosum on legs. *(Courtesy of Dermik Laboratories, Inc.)*

Secondary Lesions

The lesions never suppurate or form ulcers.

Course

The lesions last several weeks, but the duration can be affected by therapy directed to the cause, if it is known. Relapses are related to the cause. It can be idiopathic and have a chronic course.

Causes

Careful clinical and laboratory examinations are necessary to determine the cause of this toxic reaction pattern. The following tests should be performed:

- complete blood cell count,
- erythrocyte sedimentation rate,
- urinalysis,
- strep screen, serum pregnancy test, angiotensin? converting enzyme, tuberculin skin test
- serologic test for syphilis,
- chest x-ray, and
- specific skin tests, as indicated.

The causes of erythema nodosum are

- streptococcal infection (rheumatic fever, pharyngitis, scarlet fever, arthritis),
- fungal infection (coccidioidomycosis, trichophyton infection),
- pregnancy,
- sarcoidosis,
- lymphogranuloma venereum,
- syphilis,
- chancroid,

- drugs (contraceptive pills, sulfonamides, iodides, bromides), and
- tuberculosis (rare).

It is rare in children, but when it occurs group A β-hemolytic streptococcal infection (which may be occult) is the most common cause. Oral contraceptives are a common cause in adult women.

Age and Gender Incidence

The disorder occurs predominantly in adolescent girls and young women.

Laboratory Findings

Histopathologic examination reveals a nonspecific but characteristically localized inflammatory infiltrate in the subcutaneous tissue and in and around the veins.

Differential Diagnosis

- *Erythema induratum:* Chronic vasculitis of young women that occurs on the posterior calf area and often suppurates; biopsy shows a tuberculoid-type infiltrate, usually with caseation. A tuberculous causation has been suggested, again.
- *Necrobiosis lipoidica diabeticorum:* An uncommon cutaneous manifestation of diabetes mellitus, characterized by well-defined patches of reddish-yellow atrophic skin, primarily on anterior areas of legs; the lesions can ulcerate; biopsy results are characteristic, but biopsy may not be indicated because of the possibility of poor healing and the characteristic clinical presentation (see Chap. 33).
- *Periarteritis nodosa:* A rare, sometimes fatal, arteritis that most often occurs in men; 25% of patients show painful subcutaneous nodules and purpura, mainly of the lower extremities. It is a multiorgan system disease; renal failure is often a component. There is a cutaneous variety. (+) p-ANCA blood test
- *Superficial thrombophlebitis migrans (Buerger's disease):* An early venous change of Buerger's disease commonly seen in male patients, with painful nodules of the anterior tibial area; biopsy is of value. Smoking has been suggested as an important contributing factor.
- *Nodular panniculitis or Weber-Christian disease:* Occurs mainly in obese middle-aged women; tender, indurated, subcutaneous nodules and plaques are seen, usually on the thighs and the buttocks; each crop is preceded by fever and malaise; residual atrophy and hyperpigmentation occur.
- *Leukocytoclastic vasculitis:* Includes a constellation of diseases, such as allergic angiitis, allergic vasculitis,

necrotizing vasculitis, and cutaneous systemic vasculitis. Clinically, palpable purpuric lesions are seen, most commonly on the lower part of the legs. In later stages, the lesions may become nodular, bullous, infarctive, and ulcerative. Various etiologic agents have been implicated, such as infection, drugs, and foreign proteins. Treatment includes bed rest, pentoxifylline (Trental), corticosteriods, and other immunosuppressive drugs (see Chap. 10).

For completeness, the following five very rare syndromes with *inflammatory nodules of the legs* are defined in the Dictionary–Index:

1. subcutaneous fat necrosis with pancreatic disease,
2. migratory panniculitis,
3. allergic granulomatosis,
4. necrobiotic granulomatosis, and
5. embolic nodules from several sources.

Treatment

1. Treat the cause, if possible.
2. Rest, local heat, and aspirin are valuable. The eruption is self-limited if the cause can be eliminated.
3. Chronic cases can be disabling enough to warrant a short course of corticosteroid therapy. Some cases have benefited from naproxen (Naprosyn), 250 mg b.i.d. (or other nonsteroidal anti-inflammatory drugs), for 2 to 4 weeks.

Stasis (Venous) Dermatitis and Ulcers

Stasis dermatitis is a common condition owing to impaired venous circulation in the legs of older patients (Fig. 12-4). Almost all cases are associated with varicose veins, and because the tendency to develop varicosities is a familial characteristic, stasis dermatitis is also familial. The medial malleolus area of the ankle is the most common location. Stasis ulcers can develop in the impaired skin.

Differential Diagnosis before: Contact dermatitis

- Arterial or ischemic ulcers are usually more punched out and painful. Intermittent claudication and nighttime pain are relieved by exercise. Arterial duplex ultrasound or arteriography may be necessary to diagnose these ulcers. Revascularization procedures may be indicated and compression therapies can be counterproductive.

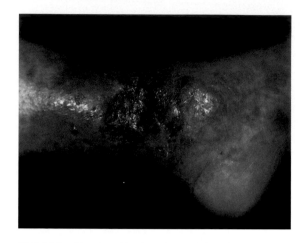

FIGURE 12-4 ■ Stasis dermatitis. *(Courtesy of Dermik Laboratories, Inc.)*

Presentation and Characteristics

Primary Lesions

Early cases of stasis dermatitis begin as a red, scaly, pruritic patch that rapidly becomes vesicular and crusted, owing to scratching and subsequent secondary infection. Bacterial infection may be responsible for the spread of the patch and the chronicity of the eruption. Edema of the affected ankle area results in a further decrease in circulation and, consequently, more infection. The lesions may be unilateral or bilateral.

Secondary Lesions

Three secondary conditions can arise from untreated stasis dermatitis:

- *Hyperpigmentation:* This is inevitable following the healing of either simple or severe stasis dermatitis of the legs. This reddish-brown increase in pigmentation is slow to disappear, and in many elderly patients it never does.
- *Stasis ulcers:* These can occur as the result of edema, trauma, deeper bacterial infection, or improper care of the primary dermatitis.
- *Infectious eczematoid dermatitis:* This can develop on the legs, the arms, and even the entire body, either slowly, or as an explosive, rapidly spreading autoeczematous or "id" eruption (see Chap. 21).

Course

The rapidity of healing of stasis dermatitis depends on the age of the patient and on other factors listed under Causes.

In elderly patients who have untreated varicose veins, stasis dermatitis can persist for years with remissions and exacerbations. If stasis dermatitis develops in a patient in the 40- to 50-year-old age group, the prognosis is particularly bad for future recurrences and possible ulcers. Once stasis ulcers develop, they can rapidly expand in size and depth. Healing of the ulcer, if possible for a given patient, depends on many factors. Ulcers less than 1 year old, less than 5 cm², and that show significant healing after 3 weeks are more likely to heal by compression and bioocclusive dressings alone. Grafting procedures may be necessary for other venous leg ulcers.

Causes

Poor venous circulation owing to the sluggish blood flow in tortuous, dilated varicose veins with incompetence of the venous valves is the primary cause. If the factors of obesity, congestive heart failure, renal failure, lack of proper rest or care of the legs, pruritus, secondary infection, low-protein diet, and old age are added to the circulation problem, the result can be a chronic, disabling disease. Table 12-1 lists tests for nonhealing ulcers.

Differential Diagnosis

- *Contact dermatitis:* History is important, especially regarding nylon hose, new socks, contact with ragweed, high-top shoes, and so on; no venous insufficiency is noted (see Chap. 9).
- *Lichen simplex chronicus:* Thickened, dry, pruritic patch; no venous insufficiency is found (see Chap. 11).
- *Atrophie blanche:* Characterized by small ulcers that heal with irregular white scars; seen mainly over the ankles and legs. Telangiectasis and hyperpigmentation surround the scars. This arterial vasculitis can respond to pentoxifylline (Trental). Another name is segmental hyalinizing vasculitis. Anticoagulants

such as aspirin, Plavix, psersantin, and coumadin may be beneficial.

Differential diagnosis for stasis ulcers includes

- pyodermic ulcers,
- arterial ulcers (such as mal perforans of diabetes),
- periarteritis nodosa,
- necrobiosis lipoidica ulcers,
- pyoderma gangrenosum,
- malignancies (especially squamous cell carcinoma),
- ulcers from hematologic problems (antiphospholipid antibodies, hemophelia, anticardiolipin antibodies, factor V Leiden defeciency),
- ulcers from autoimmune diseases especially lupus erythematosus, and
- vasculitis

Blood tests, cultures, and biopsies help to establish the type of ulcer.

Treatment of Stasis Dermatitis

Case Example. A 55-year-old laborer presents with scaly, reddish, slightly edematous, excoriated dermatitis on the medial aspect of the left ankle and leg of 6 weeks' duration.

1. Prescribe rest and elevation of the leg as much as possible by lying in bed. The foot of the bed should be elevated 4 inches by placing two bricks under the legs. Attempt to elevate the leg when sitting. Avoid prolonged standing or sitting with the legs bent. Taking time to walk on long train, car, or plane trips is a good idea.
2. Burow's solution wet packs

   Sig: Add 1 packet of powder to 1 quart of warm water. Apply cloths wet with this solution for 30 minutes, b.i.d.
3. An antibiotic and corticosteroid ointment mixture q.s. 30.0

   Sig: Apply to leg t.i.d.

For more severe cases of stasis dermatitis with oozing, cellulitis, and 3-pitting edema, the following treatment should be ordered, in addition:

1. Hospitalization or enforced bed rest at home for the purpose of (1) applying the wet packs for longer periods of time and (2) strict rest and elevation of the leg
2. A course of an oral antibiotic
3. Prednisone, 10 mg #36

   Sig: Take 2 tablets b.i.d. for 4 days, then 2 tablets in the morning for 10 days
4. Ace elastic bandage, 4 inches wide, no. 8

TABLE 12-1 ■ Clotting Tests for Patients With Nonhealing Leg Ulcers

Activated partial thromboplastin time (aPTT)
Anticardiolipin antibody
Antithrombin III
Factor II (prothrombin)
Factor V (Leiden)
Lupus anticoagulant
Prothrombin time (PTT)
Protein C and protein S
Thrombin time

After the patient is discharged from the hospital and ambulatory, give instructions for the correct application of this bandage to the leg before arising in the morning. This helps to reduce the edema that could cause a recrudescence of the dermatitis.

Treatment of Stasis Ulcer

As for any chronic difficult medical problem, there are many methods touted for successful management.

Case Example. Consider a 75-year-old obese woman on a low income who has a 4-cm ulcer on her medial right ankle area with surrounding dermatitis, edema, and pigmentation.

1. *Manage the primary problem or problems:* Attempt to remedy the obesity, make sure there is adequate nutrition, and treat systemic or other causes of the ulcer.
2. *Correct the physiologic alterations:* Control the edema with adhesive flexible bandages of adequate width (4 inches wide usually) and with correct application from foot up to knee. A Jobst-type support stocking or pump may be indicated in resistant cases.
3. *Treat contributing factors:* Control the dermatitis, itching, and infection.
4. *Promote healing:* Occlusion of the ulcer has been proved to accelerate healing. Unna boots, adhesive flexible bandage dressings, and polyurethane-type films have been used with success. Enzymatic granules have their proponents as well as collagen granules and Granulex. Accuzyme which contains papain and urea is an example of a topical debriding agent.
5. *Skin grafting may be indicated in deep, stubborn ulcers:* Artificial skin substitutes such as Apligraft may be used.

Here is the technique we would use for this case. The diagnosis is stasis or venous ulcer.

1. Advise a multiple vitamin and mineral supplement tablet once a day, including zinc and magnesium.
2. Elevate leg as much as possible lying down prone.
3. Erythromycin, 250 mg #100

   Sig: Take 2 to 3 tablets a day until ulcer is healed.
   Comment: Infection is common.
4. Prednisone, 10 mg #60

   Sig: Take 1 tablet every morning.
   Actions: Antipruritic, antiinflammatory
5. *Occlusive dressing:* This is to be applied in the office. If there is a lot of drainage and debris, the frequency of dressing should be every 3 to 4 days at first, then weekly. Use a foot-rest stand for the leg. Keep a record on the size of the ulcer.

   a. Apply Bactroban ointment to a Telfa dressing.
   b. Place gauze squares in four layers over the Telfa dressing.
   c. Apply adhesive flexible bandage wrap over the gauze, down to the foot arch and up to below the knee. More firmly wrapped distally. Do not apply too tightly at first.
   d. Wrap an adhesive flexible bandage, 4 inches wide, over the Coban.
   e. Leave the dressing on for 3 to 7 days, and then reapply.
6. Pentoxifylline (Trental) at a dosage of 1200 to 2400 mg and divided into three doses per day with food has been shown to be beneficial. Gastrointestinal upset is common.

Another variant of occlusive dressing is as follows:

1. Zeasorb powder on ulcer.
2. Midstrength cortisone cream around the ulcer.
3. Zinc oxide wrap around the entire leg with a tighter wrap distally.
4. Flexible adhesive bandage as a second wrap. Change every week, and keep dry.

No management of a venous stasis ulcer is 100% effective, but this routine with modifications is the one we use. If an ulcer is stable or decreasing in size after 4 weeks the current treatment should be continued. If it is enlarging, then alternate therapy, including surgery, should be considered.

After the ulcer has healed, which takes many weeks, advise the patient to wear an elastic bandage or support hose constantly during the day, primarily as protection against injury of the damaged and scarred skin and to decrease recurrent edema.

Purpuric Dermatoses

Purpuric lesions are caused by an extravasation of red blood cells into the skin or mucous membranes. The lesions can be distinguished from erythema and telangiectasia by the fact that purpuric lesions do not blanch under pressure applied by the finger or by a clear glass slide (diascopy) (Fig. 12-5).

- *Petechiae* are small, superficial purpuric lesions. These are most often a sign of platelet deficiency or malfunction.
- *Ecchymoses,* or bruises, are more extensive, round or irregularly shaped purpuric lesions often seen in the elderly (senile purpura), patients on chronic topical or systemic corticosteroids and patients on anticoagulants.
- *Hematomas* are large, deep, fluctuant, tumor-like hemorrhages into the skin.

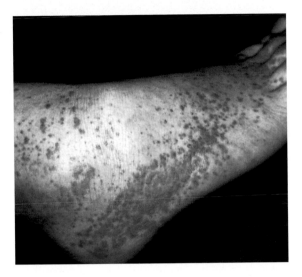

FIGURE 12-5 ■ Acute purpura, of unknown origin, in 12-year-old boy. *(Courtesy of Dermik Laboratories, Inc.)*

The purpuras can be divided into the *thrombocytopenic* forms and the *nonthrombocytopenic* forms.

- *Thrombocytopenic purpura* may be idiopathic or secondary to various chronic diseases or to a drug sensitivity. The platelet count is below normal, the bleeding time is prolonged, and the clotting time is normal, but the clot does not retract normally. This form of purpura is rare.
- *Nonthrombocytopenic purpura* is more commonly seen. *Henoch-Schönlein purpura* is a form of nonthrombocytopenic purpura most commonly seen in children that is characterized by recurrent attacks of purpura accompanied by arthritis, hematuria, IgA glomerulonephritis, and gastrointestinal disorders. Approximately 75% of the time it involves skin only.

The ecchymoses, or *senile purpura,* seen in elderly patients after minor injury are very common. Ecchymoses are also seen in patients who have been on long-term systemic corticosteroid therapy and also occur after prolonged use of the high-potency corticosteroids locally and from corticosteroid nasal inhalers. Anticoagulants make these more common.

Another common purpuric eruption is that known as *stasis purpura.* These lesions are associated with vascular insufficiency of the legs and occur as the early sign of this change, or they are seen around areas of stasis dermatitis or stasis ulcers. Frequently seen is a petechial drug eruption owing to the chlorothiazide diuretics.

Pigmented Purpuric Eruptions

A less common group of cases are those seen in middle-aged adults, classified under the name *pigmented purpuric eruptions.* They are usually asymptomatic but some cases of pigmented purpuric eruptions itch severely. The cause is unknown; most cases have a positive tourniquet test, but other bleeding tests are normal. Clinically, these patients have grouped petechial lesions that begin on the legs and extend up to the thighs, and occasionally up to the waist and onto the arms. They turn into a brown Cayenne-pepper nonpalpable discoloration that fades over weeks to months.

Some clinicians are able to separate these pigmented purpuric eruptions into

- purpura annularis telangiectodes (Majocchi's disease),
- progressive pigmentary dermatosis (Schamberg's disease), and
- pigmented purpuric lichenoid dermatitis (Gougerot and Blum disease).

Majocchi's disease commonly begins on the legs but slowly spreads, to become generalized. Telangiectatic capillaries become confluent and produce annular or serpiginous lesions. The capillaries break down, causing purpuric lesions. Schamberg's disease is a slowly progressive pigmentary condition of the lower part of the legs that fades after a period of months but may recur. The Gougerot-Blum form is accompanied by severe itching and eczematous changes; otherwise it resembles Schamberg's disease.

Treatment

For these pigmented purpuric eruptions, therapy may not be necessary. Occlusive dressing therapy with a corticosteroid cream can be beneficial. For resistant cases, prednisone, 10 mg, 1 to 2 tablets in the morning for 3 to 6 weeks, is indicated.

Telangiectases

Telangiectases are abnormal dilated small blood vessels. Telangiectases are divided into *primary forms,* in which the causes are unknown, and *secondary forms,* which are related to some known disturbance. The primary telangiectases include the simple and compound hemangiomas of infants, essential telangiectasias, and spider hemangiomas (see Chap. 32). Diseases with numerous telangiectasias include

- cirrhosis of the liver,
- Osler-Weber-Rendu disease, which also has mucous membrane involvement,
- lupus erythematosus,

- scleroderma,
- dermatomyositis,
- cutaneous polyarteritis,
- metastatic carcinoid syndrome,
- ataxia telangiectasia,
- angiokeratoma corporis diffusum,
- telangiectasia macularis eruptiva perstans, and
- rosacea.
- overlying basal cell cancers

Unilateral nevoid telangiectasia syndrome can be congenital or acquired. The acquired form appears when increased estrogen levels occur in women with puberty or pregnancy and in cirrhosis. C3, C4, and trigeminal dermatomes are the most common.

Secondary telangiectasia is very commonly seen on the fair-skinned person as a result of aging, chronic topical and systemic corticosteroid use, and chronic sun exposure. X-ray therapy and burns can also cause dilated vessels.

Treatment for the secondary telangiectasias can be accomplished quite adequately with very light electrosurgery to the vessels, which is usually tolerated without anesthesia or for many extensive lesions use of laser therapy or intense pulsed light therapy. Injectable sclerosing agents are available for therapy on the lower legs.

Vasculitis (Figs 12-6A and 12-6B)

Inflammation of the blood vessels (vasculitis) commonly affects the skin and has numerous underlying causes. It can be cutaneous only (Gougerot and Ruiter's type), but often involves other organs, most commonly joints, kidney, and gastrointestinal tract and rarely the nervous system, eye (temporal arteritis), heart, and respiratory tract.

Diagnosis is confirmed by biopsy and then appropriate tests need to be done to look for underlying causes (Table 12-2). Vasculitis classification is complex but can be helpful in trying to find an underlying cause (Table 12-3).

Presentation and Characteristics

Primary Lesions

Palpable purpura is the classic clinical appearance. Varying shades of bluish-red discoloration may be firmly indurated or difficult to feel. Lesions can be large (many centimeters) or quite small (several millimeters) with a petechial look. The dependent areas are the location where it is most commonly seen—legs on ambulatory patients, on buttocks and back in bedridden patients.

TABLE 12-2 ■ **Basic Laboratory Evaluation of Vasculitis**

Urine analysis (most crucial test because early asymptomatic renal disease can be detected and progression to renal failure prevented)

Stool screen for occult blood (stool Guaiac)

Complete blood count with platelets and coagulation screen

Hypercoagulability studies may be indicated such as anticardiolipin and antiphospholipid antibodies

Antinuclear antibody, rheumatoid factor, liver enzymes, hepatitis screen, cryoglobulins, cryofibrinogen, and complement immunoglobulins

Antineutrophil cytoplasmic antibody (ANCA) that is positive in Wegener's granulomatosis (c-ANCA) and polyarteritis nodosa (p-ANCA)

Secondary Lesions

As the vascular damage progresses, blisters, nodules, ulcers, necrosis, and gangrene may occur. Livedo reticularis (see Dictionary–Index) is a bluish-red, netlike appearing condition that can be associated with vasculitis.

TABLE 12-3 ■ **Types of Vasculitis**

I. Leukocytoclastic vasculitis (hypersensitivity angiitis or allergic vasculitis)
   A. Idiopathic
   B. Drug induced
   C. Hypocomplementemic vasculitis (often urticarial)
   D. Essential mixed cryoglobulinemia
   E. Hyperglobulinemic purpuras (Waldenström's macroglobulinemia)

II. Rheumatic vasculitis
   A. Systemic lupus erythematosus
   B. Rheumatoic vasculitis
   C. Dermatomyositis

III. Granulomatous vasculitis
   A. Allergic granulomatous vasculitis (Churg-Strauss)
   B. Wegener's granulomatosis
   C. Lymphomatoid granulomatosis

IV. Polyarteritis nodosa
   A. Classic type
   B. Cutaneous type

V. Giant cell arteritis
   A. Temporal arteritis
   B. Takayasu's disease

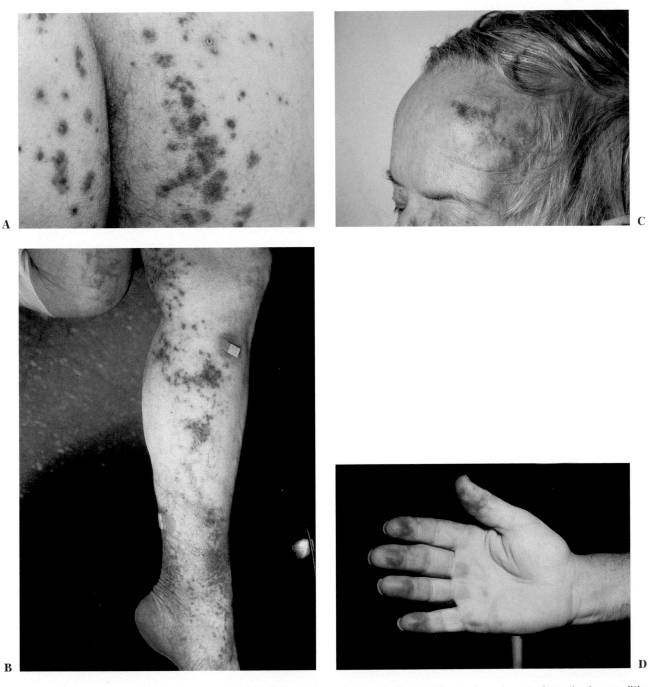

FIGURE 12-6A ■ Forms of vasculitis. (**A**) Vasculitis on buttock of a patient with renal and gastrointestinal vasculitis. Bedridden patient often erupts first on the buttock. (**B**) Vasculitis of lower extremity owing to mixed cryoglobulinemia. Patient was worse in cold weather. (**C**) Temporal arteritis. Systemic corticosteroids were used to prevent blindness. (**D**) Fingers showing vasculitis in a patient with Wegener's granulomatosis.

(continued)

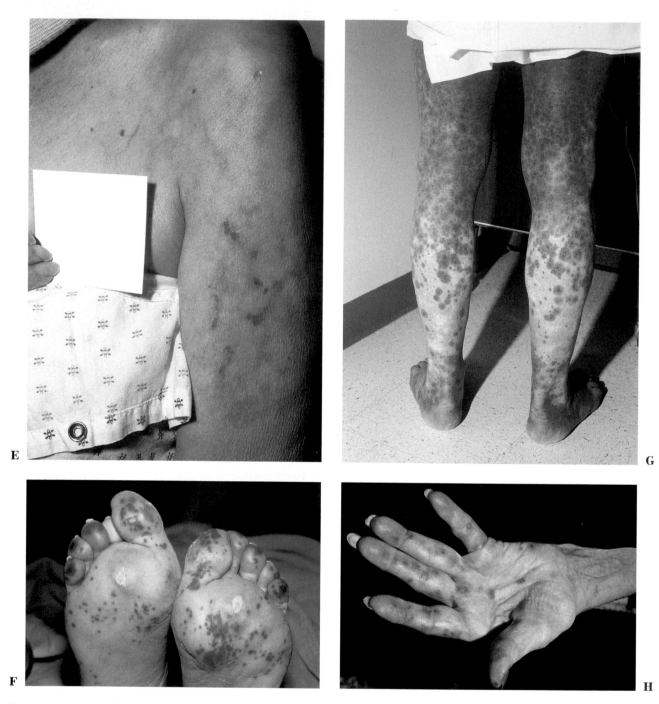

E

G

F

H

FIGURE 12-6B ■ (*Continued*) (**E**) Livedo reticularis pattern of vasculitis. This patient has systemic lupus erythematosus. (**F**) Vasculitis of the feet. Lower extremities are the location where it is most common in ambulatory patients. (**G**) Widespread, drug-induced vasculitis owing to ampicillin. (**H**) Vasculitis of the hand in a patient with rheumatoid arthritis.

Course

The disease may be very chronic and long lasting, such as in lupus erythematosus or acute and self-limited such as Henoch-Schönlein purpura (see Chaps. 12 and 33). Early diagnosis and therapy can prevent renal failure or bowel necrosis.

Causes

See Table 12-2.

Differential Diagnosis

- *Urticaria:* Evanescent, very pruritic.
- *Thrombophlebitis:* Evidence of varicosities and stasis changes and positive Doppler studies in this localized distribution of a vein almost always in the lower extremity below the knee.
- *Erythema nodosum:* May be impossible to tell without a deep skin biopsy, especially in female patients. Deep nodule and usually only in pretibial location.
- *Petechia:* Small, uniform, single-color, nonpalpable lesions associated with decreased platelets.
- *Schamberg's disease* (benign pigmented purpura, benign hemosiderosis): Cayenne pepper–colored tiny lesions. No underlying illness. Skin biopsy differentiates usually below the knees but can rarely be generalized. For several variations, see under hemosiderosis in the Dictionary–Index and discussion under petechiae in this chapter.
- *Panniculitis:* Lesions very deep and nodular. May have elevated amylase and lipase when associated with pancreatitis.
- *Cellulitis:* Lesions warm and tender. Elevated white count with fever. May have proximal, tender, red, linear lymphatic involvement. Lymph nodes may be enlarged.
- *Insect bites:* Very pruritic. History of exposure to insects, acute in onset. Can be excoriated and can be chronic.

Treatment

Systemic corticosteroids are the mainstay of early therapy. Corticosteroid-sparing drugs include colchicine, dapsone, azathioprine, methotrexate, cytoxan (drug of choice for Wegener's granulomatosis), intravenous gamma globulin, antimalarials, and plasmapheresis have all been used.

Suggested Reading

Cherry G. The Oxford European wound healing course handbook. Oxford, Oxford University Press, 2002.

Ghersetich I, Panconesi E. The purpuras. Int J Dermatol 1994;33:1.

Graves MW, Kaplan AP. Urticaria and angiodema. Marcel Dekker, 2004.

Henz BM, et al. Urticaria: Clinical diagnostic and therapeutic aspects. Springer Verlags, 1998.

Nussinovitch M, Prais D, et al. Cutaneous manifestations of Henoch-Schonlein purpura in young children. Pediatr Dermatol 1998;15:426–428.

Ollert MW, Thomas P, Korting HC, et al. Erythema induratum of Bazin. Arch Dermatol 1993;129:469.

Stein SL, Miller LC, Konnikov N. Wegener's granulomatosis: Case report and literature review. Pediatr Dermatol 1998;15:352–356.

Valencia IC, Falabella A, et al. Chronic venous insufficiency and venous leg ulceration. J Am Acad Dermatol 2001;44:401–421.

CHAPTER 13

Seborrheic Dermatitis, Acne, and Rosacea

John C. Hall

Seborrheic Dermatitis

Seborrheic dermatitis, in our opinion, is a synonym for *dandruff.* The former is the more severe manifestation of this dermatosis. Seborrheic dermatitis is exceedingly common on the scalp but less common on the other areas of predilection: ears, face, sternal area, axillae, intergluteal area, and pubic area (Figs. 13-1 & 13-2; see also Fig. 36-27). It occurs as part of the acne seborrhea complex. Dandruff is spoken of as oily or dry, but it is all basically oily. If dandruff scales are pressed between two pieces of tissue paper, an oily residue is expressed, leaving a mark on the tissue.

Certain misconceptions that have arisen concerning this common dermatosis need to be corrected. Seborrheic dermatitis cannot be cured, but remissions for varying amounts of time do occur naturally or as the result of treatment. Seborrheic dermatitis does not cause permanent hair loss or baldness unless it becomes grossly infected. Seborrheic dermatitis is not contagious. The cause is unknown, but an important etiologic factor is the yeast *Pityrosporum ovale.*

Seborrheic dermatitis in AIDS patients can be widespread and recalcitrant to therapy. It can be severe and is common in patients with Parkinson's disease.

Presentation and Characteristics

Primary Lesions

Redness and scaling appear in varying degrees. The scale is of the greasy type (see Fig. 13-1).

Secondary Lesions

Rarely seen are excoriations from severe itching and secondary bacterial infection. Lichen simplex chronicus can follow a chronic itching and scratching habit.

Course

Exacerbations and remissions are common, depending on the season, treatment, and age and general health of the patient. A true cure is impossible.

Seasonal Incidence

This condition is worse in colder weather, presumably due to lack of summer sunlight.

Age Incidence

Seborrhea occurs in infants (called *cradle cap*) but usually disappears by age of 6 months (Fig. 13-3). It may recur again at puberty.

Differential Diagnosis

Scalp Lesions

- *Psoriasis:* Sharply defined, silvery-white, dry, scaly patches; typical psoriasis lesions on elbows, knees, nails, or elsewhere (see Chap. 14)
- *Lichen simplex chronicus:* Usually a single patch on the posterior scalp area or around the ears; intense itching; excoriation; thickening of the skin (see Chap. 11)
- *Tinea capitis:* Usually occurs in a child; broken-off hairs, with or without pustular reaction; some types fluoresce under Wood's light; positive culture and KOH mount (see Chap. 25)
- *Atopic eczema:* Usually occurs in infants (where it spares diaper area) or children; diffuse dry scaliness; eczema also on face, arms, and legs; atopic personal and family history (see Chap. 9)

Face Lesions

- *Systemic lupus erythematosus:* Faint, reddish, slightly scaly, "butterfly" eruption, aggravated by sunlight, with fever, malaise, arthritis, Raynauds and positive antinuclear antibody test (see Chap. 32)
- *Chronic discoid lupus erythematosus:* Sharply defined, red, scaly, atrophic areas with large follicular openings with keratotic plugs, resistant to local therapy, often leaves scars (see Chap. 32)

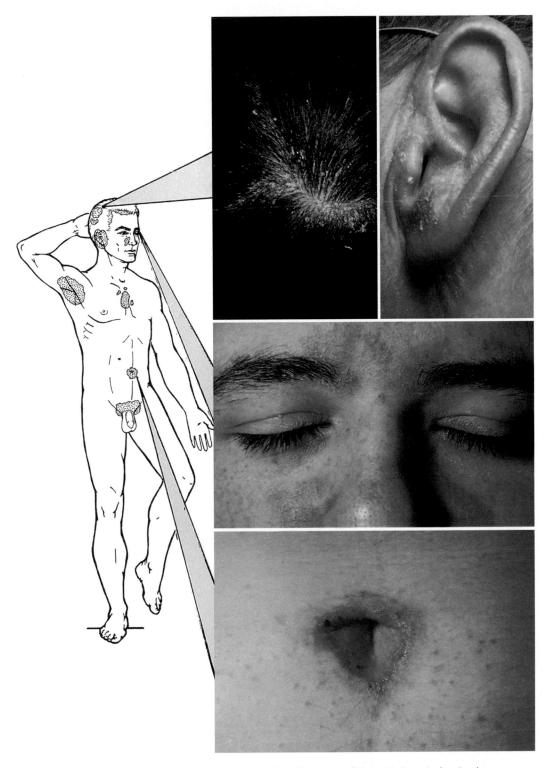

FIGURE 13-1 ■ Seborrheic dermatitis. *(Courtesy of Owen Laboratories, Inc.)*

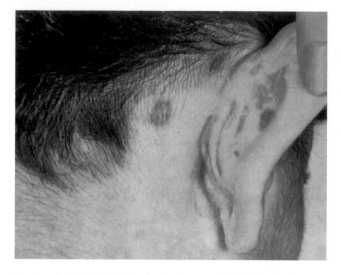

FIGURE 13-2 ■ Seborrheic dermatitis behind the ear and at the border of the scalp. (*Courtesy of Smith Kline & French Laboratories*)

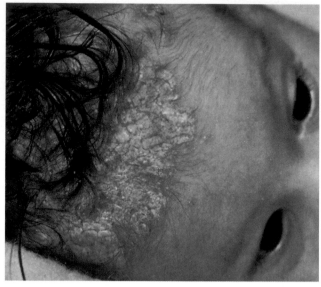

FIGURE 13-3 ■ Seborrheic dermatitis of infancy. This is one of the causes of "cradle cap." (*Courtesy of Smith Kline & French Laboratories*)

Body Lesions

- *Tinea corporis* (see Chap. 25)
- *Psoriasis* (see Chap. 14)
- *Pityriasis rosea* (see Chap. 15)
- *Tinea versicolor* (see Chap. 15)

Treatment

Case Example. A young man presents with recurrent red, scaly lesions at the border of the scalp and forehead and diffuse, mild, whitish scaling throughout the scalp.

1. Management of cases of dandruff must include explaining the disease and stating that it is not contagious, that there is no true cure, that it does not cause baldness, and that there are seasonal variations. Therapy can be very effective, but only for keeping the dandruff under control.

2. With this information in mind, tell the patient that shampooing offers the best management. There are several shampoos available, and the patient may have to experiment to find the one most suitable. The following types can be suggested:

   Selenium sulfide 2½% suspension (Selsun; Head and Shoulders Intensive Treatment, which is available over the counter; Selseb prescription shampoo, which also contains urea and zinc pyrithione) 120.0

   Sig: Shampoo as frequently as necessary to alleviate itching and scaling. Use no other soap. Refill prescription p.r.n.

   Additional shampoos:

   - Tar shampoos, such as Ionil T, Tarsum, Reme-T, Pentrax, X Seb T and T-gel. T-sal. (a salacylic acid shampoo)
   - Zinc pyrithione shampoos, such as Zincon, Head & Shoulders, and DHS Zinc
   - Ketoconazole (Nizoral) shampoo (over the counter) and as a higher percentage it is available as a prescription, Loprox Shampoo, Capex shampoo (contains fluocinolone, by prescription) or Clobex Shampoo (contains clobetasol and should be used Monday, Wednesday, and Friday by prescription).

   Sig: Shampoo as frequently as necessary to keep scaling and itching to a minimum.

3. Triamcinolone (Kenalog) spray, 63 mL

   Sig: Apply sparingly to scalp at night. Squirt the spray through a plastic tube that is supplied.

   Comment: A spray is less messy on the scalp than a corticosteroid solution, but solutions are available.

4. A low-potency corticosteroid cream 15.0

   Sig: Apply b.i.d. locally to body lesions. A good combination is 1% HC and 2% sulfur in Acid Mantle Cream. Generic Vytone cream is another safe therapy.

5. Ketoconazole 2% cream 15.0 (available over the counter)

   Sig: Apply b.i.d. on scalp or body lesions.

Comment: This is a corticosteroid-sparing agent. Ciclopirox (Loprox shampoo) and sodium sulfacetamide (Ovace) wash used as a shampoo may also be used.

6. 5% LCD, 3% salicylic acid in betamethasone solution is another example to apply twice a day to scalp

7. Fluocinolone 0.01% solution is popular because it is mixed in propylene glycol, which kills yeast.

8. Pimecrolimus (Elidel) cream and tacrolimus ointment 0.1% and 0.3% (Protopic) can be used in a thin coat b.i.d. without topical corticosteroid side effects.

9. Foam preparations such as sodium sulfacetamide foam (Ovace), betamethasone valerate (Luxiq) foam, or clobetasol (Olux) foam may be beneficial b.i.d. and after shampooing. Avoid overuse of triamcinolone and especially clobetasol.

SAUER'S NOTES

1. Do not prescribe a fluorinated corticosteroid cream for long-term use on the face or in intertriginous areas.
2. Reiterate that there is no cure for seborrheic dermatitis; long-term management is necessary.
3. Reassure the patient that seborrheic dermatitis does not cause permanent hair loss.

Acne

Acne vulgaris is a common skin condition of adolescents and young adults. It is characterized by any combination of comedones (blackheads), pustules, cysts, and scarring of varying severity (Figs. 13-4, 13-5, and 13-6).

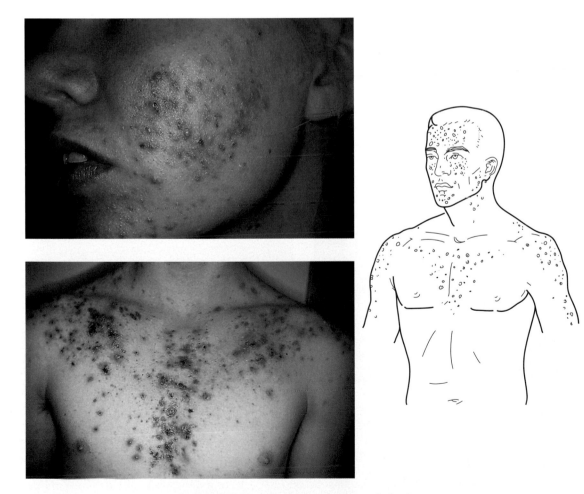

FIGURE 13-4 ■ Acne of face and chest.

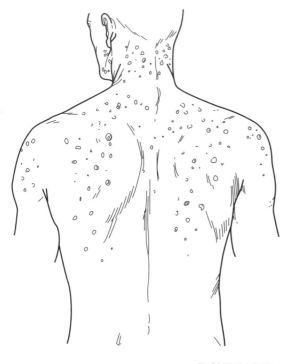

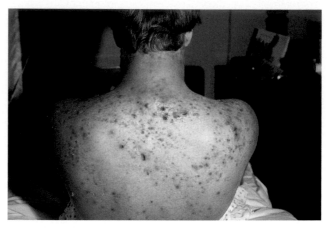

FIGURE 13-5 ■ Acne of neck and back.

Severe cystic acne is called *acne conglobata*. When accompanied by systemic symptoms such as arthralgia, leukocytosis, and fever, the term *acne fulminans* is used. *Hidradenitis suppurativa*, also termed *acne inversa*, is a debilitating disease of deep undermining cysts and fistulas in the axillary, inguinal, and perirectal areas. Treatment is difficult and includes surgery, antibiotics, and isotretinoin (Accutane).

Dissecting cellulitis of the scalp (perifolliculitis capitis abscedens et suffodiens) is an inflammatory disease of the scalp with undermining cysts and fistulas of the scalp resulting in scarring alopecia. Treatment is difficult but antibiotics, surgery, laser, x-ray, isotretinoin, azathioprine, dapsone, colchicine, methotrexate, and systemic and intralesional corticosteroids may be helpful.

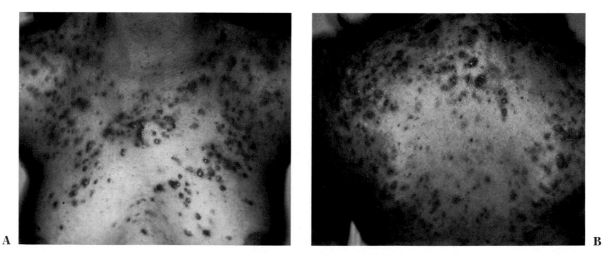

FIGURE 13-6 ■ Severe acne vulgaris of the chest (**A**) and back (**B**) of a 15-year-old girl. *(Courtesy of Hoechst-Roussel Pharmaceuticals, Inc.)*

Acne conglobata, hidradenitis suppurativa, and dissecting cellulitis of the scalp have been referred to as the *follicular occlusion triad*. Pilonidal sinus is added by some authors to make this a tetrad.

Presentation and Characteristics

Primary Lesions

Comedones, papules, pustules, and, in severe cases, cysts occur.

Secondary Lesions

Pits and scars are evident in severe cases. Excoriations of the papules are seen in some adolescents, but most often they appear as part of the acne of women in their 20s and 30s. When severe, it is called *acne excoriae des jeunes filles*. This disease may have few or no primary acne lesions. It is difficult to treat but some authors recommend selective serotonin reuptake inhibitors as anti-obsessive-compulsive therapy.

Distribution

Acne occurs on the face and neck and, less commonly, on the back, chest, and arms. More rare locations are the scalp, buttocks, and upper legs.

Course

The condition begins at ages 8 to 12 years, or later, and lasts, with new outbreaks, for months or years. It subsides in most cases by the early 20s, but occasional flare ups may occur for years. Cases tend to start earlier and be more prolonged in women. The residual scarring varies with severity of the case, individual susceptibility, and response to treatment.

Subjective Complaint

Tenderness of the large pustules and itching may be reported (rarely). Emotional upset is common as a result of the unattractive appearance.

Causes

The following factors are important:

- heredity,
- hormonal balance,
- increased heat and sweat such as with increased exercise,
- a hot, humid environment due to climate, workplace, or place of exercise,
- diet,
- use of oily cosmetics,
- sometimes exposure to oils at the workplace, and
- high glycemic diets may play a role.

In a case of severe adult acne, one should rule out an endocrine disorder. Hirsutism or abnormal menstrual periods in women are clues. Androgen abuse in male athletes can be causitive.

Season

Most cases are better during the summer due to ultraviolet light exposure.

Contagiousness

Acne is not contagious.

Differential Diagnosis

- *Drug eruption:* Note history of ingestion of lithium, corticosteroids, iodides, bromides, trimethadione, anti-estrogens used to treat estrogen receptor–positive breast cancer, testosterone (including anabolic steroids used by athletes and body builders), lithium and corticosteroids administered topically, orally, and intramuscularly (see Chap. 9).
- *Contact dermatitis from industrial oils* (see Chap. 9)
- *Perioral dermatitis* (Fig. 13-7): Red papules, small pustules, and some scaling on chin, upper lip, and nasolabial fold found almost exclusively in women. There is a perioral halo of clear skin. The cause is unknown. Corticosteroid creams locally, initially improve but eventually aggravate the eruption and usually should not be prescribed. Tetracycline, orally, as for acne, is the therapy of choice. Metronidazole gel (MetroGel) is an alternative local therapy for children under 12 years of age. Also,

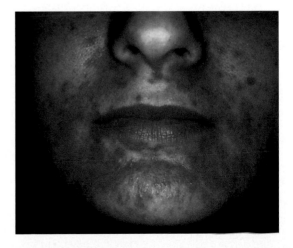

FIGURE 13-7 ■ Perioral dermatitis. *(Courtesy of Hoechst-Roussel Pharmaceuticals, Inc.)*

topical erythromycin and topical clindamycin formulations may be helpful. Some authors think this should be called *periorificial dermatitis* because it can occur around the eyes, the nares, and in the diaper area often associated with topical corticosteroid abuse. With time the eruption can become granulatous.

- *Adenoma sebaceum:* Rare; associated with epilepsy and mental deficiency. There are 2- to 4-mm papules over central face without comedones, pustules, or cysts.

Treatment

Case Example. An 11-year-old patient presents with a moderate amount of facial blackheads and pustules.

First Visit.

1. Give instructions regarding skin care (see Patient Education Sheet, "What You Should Know About Acne"). Stress to the patient and the parent that not one factor but several (heredity, hormones, diet, stress, season of the year, and greasy cosmetics) influence acne breakouts. Some of these factors cannot be altered.

2. *Bar soap:* The affected areas should be washed twice a day with a washcloth and a noncreamy soap, such as Dial, Neutrogena for Acne-Prone Skin, or Purpose.

3. Sulfur, ppt., 6%

   Resorcinol, 4%
   Colored alcoholic shake lotion (see Formulary in Chap. 5) q.s. 60.0
   Sig: Apply locally at bedtime with fingers.
   Comment: Proprietary products similar to the above lotion include Sulfacet-R, Novacet lotion, Klaron lotion, Ovace Cream, Gel and Cleanser, Plexion Cream and Cleanser, and Seba-Nil liquid and cleanser.

4. Benzoyl peroxide preparations

   Benzoyl peroxide gel (5% or 10%) as in Benzagel, Desquam-X, Benzac-W, Panoxyl, Persa-Gel,

---

WHAT YOU SHOULD KNOW ABOUT ACNE*

Acne is a disorder in which the oil glands of the skin are overactive and the duct of the oil gland is unable to drain the extra oil. It usually involves the face and frequently the chest and the back, because these areas are the richest in oil glands. When an oil gland opening becomes plugged, a blackhead is formed and irritates the skin in exactly the same way as any other foreign body, such as a sliver of wood. This irritation takes the form of red pimples or deep, painful cysts. This inflammation may destroy tissues and, when healed, may result in permanent scars.

The tendency to develop acne runs in families, especially those in which one or both parents have oily skin. Acne is aggravated by certain foods (especially highly glycemic foods, which contain large amounts of refined sugar), improper care of the skin, lack of adequate sleep, and nervous tension. In girls, acne is usually worse before a menstrual period. Even in boys, acne flares on a cyclic basis. Any or all of these factors can exaggerate the tendency of the oily skin to develop acne. Therefore, the prevention of acne depends on correcting not one but several of these factors.

Because acne is so common, is not contagious, and does not cause loss of time from school or work, many people tend to ignore it or regard it as a necessary part of growing up. We disagree with this.

REASONS FOR TREATING ACNE

There are at least two very important reasons for seeking medical care for acne. The first is to prevent the scarring mentioned. Once scarring has occurred, it is permanent. Then a patient must go through the rest of life being embarrassed and annoyed by the scars, even though active pimples are no longer present. This scarring may vary from tiny little pits, which are frequently mistaken for enlarged pores, to deep, large, disfiguring pockmarks.

The second reason for starting active treatment for acne, even without scarring, is that the condition may become the source of much psychological disturbance to a patient. Even though the acne may appear to others to be mild and inconspicuous, it may seem very noticeable to the patient and lead to embarrassment, worry, and nervousness.

TREATMENT MEASURES TO BE CARRIED OUT BY THE PATIENT

Cleaning Measures

Your face is to be washed twice a day with soap. Do not scrub too roughly. The physician may suggest a particular soap for use. Do not use any face cream, cold cream, cleansing cream, nourishing cream, or any other kind of grease on the

(continued)

WHAT YOU SHOULD KNOW ABOUT ACNE*   *(Continued)*

face. This includes the avoidance of so-called pancake-type makeup, which may contain oil, grease, or wax. Acne is related to excessive oiliness. You may think your face is dry because of the flakes on it, but these are actually flakes of dried oil or the greasy scaling of seborrhea. Later, when the treatment begins to take effect, your skin will actually become dry, even to the point where it is chapped and tender, especially around the mouth and the sides of the chin. When this point is reached, you will be advised as to suitable corrective measures for this temporary dryness. If the skin becomes red and uncomfortable between office visits, the applied remedy may be discontinued for one or two nights.

Girls may use face powder, dry rouge or blush (not cream rouge), and lipstick, but no face creams. Boys with acne should shave as regularly as necessary and should not use oils, greases, pomades, or hair tonics, except those that may be recommended by the physician. Hair should be dressed only with water.

Many cases of acne are associated with oily hair and dandruff and, for these cases, suitable local scalp applications and shampoos will be prescribed by the physician.

Plenty of rest is important. You should have at least 8 hours of sleep each night. Exercise is usually accompanied by increased activity of the oil glands and an acne flare. Wiping the skin off with a cool damp cloth and showering as soon as possible may be helpful. Moderate sun tanning is beneficial for acne, but a sunburn does more harm than good and all sun exposure adds to the cumulative risk of skin cancer. When you get out in the sun, do not use oily or greasy suntan preparations.

Diet

Recent studies have indicated that high glycemic-load carbohydrates may worsen acne. This is controversial, but I think for completeness and for the patient who wants to try diet therapy, it is important to list the diet. It is advisable to avoid or limit the following foods.

Chocolate

This includes chocolate candy, chocolate ice cream, chocolate cake, chocolate-covered nuts, chocolate sodas, cocoa, and cola drinks.

Nuts

Especially avoid peanuts, peanut butter, Brazil nuts, and coconuts. Almonds, walnuts, and pecans can be eaten in moderation.

Milk Products

Avoid whole milk (homogenized) and 2% butterfat milk. You can drink up to two glasses of skim milk a day. Avoid sour cream, whipped cream, butter, margarine (allowed in moderation), rich creamy cheeses, ice cream, and sharp cheeses. Cottage and cheddar cheese are permitted. Sherbet can be eaten.

Fatty Meats

Avoid meats such as lamb, pork, hamburgers, and tender steaks. Fish, chicken, and turkey can be eaten unless fried in coconut oil or animal fat. Mazola oil or other corn oils should be used in cooking. French fried potatoes should be avoided.

Spicy Foods

Reduce as much as possible the use of spicy sauces, Worcestershire sauce, chili, catsup, spicy smoked meats, delicatessen products, and pizzas.

Following this diet does not mean that you should starve yourself. Eat plenty of lean meats, fresh and cooked vegetables, fruits (and their juices), and all breads. Drink plenty of water (4 to 6 glasses) daily. Foods that are highly glycemic may be the most important to avoid.

MEDICAL TREATMENT OF ACNE

In addition to the prescribed treatment you apply yourself, there are several aspects of the treatment of acne that must be carried out by the physician or the nurse.

One important method of treatment is the proper removal of blackheads. This is often part of the physician's job. Pimples that have pus in them and are ready to open should be opened by the physician or the nurse. This is done with surgical instruments that are designed for the purpose and do not damage tissue or cause scars. Picking of pimples by the patient can cause scarring and should be avoided. When the blackheads are removed and the pustules opened in the physician's office, the skin heals faster and scarring is minimized.

(continued)

WHAT YOU SHOULD KNOW ABOUT ACNE* (Continued)

Tetracycline or other antibiotics are frequently prescribed for the acne patient who is developing scars or pits. This antibiotic therapy may be continued by the physician for many months or even years. Occasionally, one develops an upset stomach, diarrhea, or a genital itch from an overgrowth of yeast organisms. Oral fluconazole (Diflucan) has made control of vaginal yeast infection much easier. If these problems develop, stop the medication and call the physician.

Here are other important comments about oral tetracycline therapy:

1. Tetracycline may make the skin more sensitive to sunlight. Therefore, if you go skiing or to a sunny climate it may be necessary to lower the dosage or stop the tetracycline 4 days before the trip. This sun sensitivity is more common with doxycycline and less common with minocycline.
2. If a woman is on birth control pills and also on tetracycline, there is the remote possibility that the birth control pills may be less effective. Additional birth control measures are indicated at possible times of conception.
3. Do not take tetracycline or a similar antibiotic if you become pregnant because, after the fifth month of pregnancy, it can permanently discolor the teeth of the child.
4. The effectiveness of the tetracycline medication is decreased if iron or milk products are ingested at the same time as the tetracycline capsules. The best rule is for you to take tetracycline 30 minutes before meals or 2 hours after a meal.
5. Serious side effects from long-term therapy are almost nonexistent, but if there is any question concerning an illness and the taking of the antibiotic, call your physician. Do not continue taking an antibiotic unless you are under the continued care of your physician. Stop the antibiotic for acne while taking an antibiotic for another condition.

Other internal medications may be prescribed by the physician for acne, such as vitamin A. For very severe cases of cystic scarring acne, isotretinoin can be prescribed, with suitable precautions. Women of childbearing age should be aware of the fact that isotretinoin can cause birth defects if the woman is or becomes pregnant during therapy.

Ultraviolet light treatments are also beneficial for some cases, but the danger of photodamage must be considered. Newer, long-wave ultraviolet light called IPL therapy appears to be safe and beneficial.

Do not take any other medicines internally while under acne therapy without informing your physician.

FOLLOW-UP CARE FOR YOUR COMPLEXION PROBLEMS

When active therapy for your complexion problem by the physician is terminated, this does not mean that you also stop the home care. The routine that was outlined for you on the first visit to the physician should be adhered to so that your complexion can continue to remain as clear as possible.

First, it is important that you continue using the soap that was prescribed for you. Second, it is important that you continue to observe the diet. As the months go by and your skin matures, however, you will find that it is less important to watch your diet strictly. Third, any local preparation that was prescribed should be continued for several months, or even years, if you continue to have complexion problems. These have been prescribed especially for you and probably are stronger than any other product that can be bought over the counter. Fourth, there are certain times when your complexion can flare up again. This especially happens in the fall. If this happens, it is imperative that you begin active medical therapy with your physician as soon as possible to prevent any scarring of the skin.

If you follow these measures, you should continue to have a good complexion so that after you have passed through this stage of complexion problems you will not have any scars on your face. It is only rarely that we have complexion-problem cases so difficult that nothing can be done to prevent or minimize the scarring tendency.

CONCLUSION

Do not become discouraged! Treatment is effective in at least 95% of all cases. It may be 4 to 6 weeks before noticeable improvement appears. There may be occasional mild flare ups, but eventually your skin will improve and you and your friends will notice the difference.

It is very important for you and your parents to realize that your physician cannot shorten the length of time it takes for your oil glands to work normally. This maturing process of your skin can take several years, even into the 20s, 30s, or, for a few persons, (especially women) longer.

*This information is from an instruction sheet that I give to my acne patients. I am well aware of differences of opinion regarding the role of diet in acne, but I am presenting my belief.

Brevoxyl, Zoderm (also contains urea to decrease dryness), and others. Some of these are also available as emollient gels.

Sig: Apply locally once a day.

Comment: Some dryness of skin is to be expected. Fabric can be bleached by the benzoyl peroxide.

5. Tretinoin (Retin A) gel (0.01% or 0.025%) or cream (0.025%, 0.05% or 0.1%) is available generically, tretinoin (Retin A Micro 0.04% and 0.1%), tretinoin (Avita).

   Sig: Apply locally once a day at night. Patient toleration varies considerably.

   Comment: Especially valuable for comedo acne

6. Local antibiotic solutions, pledgets, and gels

   Clindamycin 1% (also as a gel called Clindagel) or erythromycin 2% lotion q.s. 30.0

   Sig: Apply locally once or twice a day.

7. Adapalene (Differin) 0.1% q.s. 15 g

   Sig: Thin coat each night

   Comment: May be less irritating and more effective than Retin A.

8. Remove the blackheads with a comedone extractor (Fig. 13-8) in the office.

9. Sulfur preparations with low incidence of odor or drying such as Klaron, Novacet, Ovace (cream, gel, foam or cleanser), Plexion TS (also comes as a cleanser), thin coat b.i.d.

10. Benzoyl peroxide plus antibiotic; lasts longer if kept refrigerated. Can bleach fabric. Benzamycin (benzoyl

peroxide plus erythromycin), Benzaclin (benzoyl peroxide plus clindamycin), thin coat b.i.d. Duac (benzoyl peroxide plus clindamycin) thin coat b.i.d. It does not need to be refrigerated.

11. Akne-mycin ointment and Cleocin T lotion may be good options in patients with dry sensitivity skin.

Treatment for a Case of Scarring Acne

1. Tetracycline, or similar antibiotic, 250 or 500 mg #100

   Sig: Take 1 capsule q.i.d. for 3 days, then 1 capsule b.i.d. This dose can be continued for weeks, months, or years, or the dose can be lowered to 1 capsule a day for maintenance, depending, of course, on the extent of the involvement. Severe cases respond to 3 to 6 capsules a day.

   Tetracycline should be taken 30 minutes before meals or 2 hours after a meal, and not concurrently with iron or calcium for optimal absorption.

   Comment: Other effective antibiotics include erythromycin, 250 mg b.i.d. or t.i.d., minocycline, 100 mg/d, doxycycline (Monodox is doxycyline monohydrate with a decreased chance of esophageal inflammation; Doryx is a preparation that only needs to be given once a day with a decreased gastrointestinal upset and less photosensitivity) 100 mg b.i.d. and minocycline (Minocin may be better absorbed) 100 mg b.i.d. Other antibiotics include clindamycin 150 or 300 mg b.i.d. and trimethoprim 100 mg b.i.d. Azithromycin (Zithromax) pulse in a 5-day dose pack 500 mg

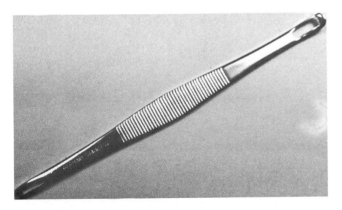

FIGURE 13-8 ■ Comedone extractor. The most frequently used instrument in my office. Firm but gentle pressure with the smaller end over a comedone forces the comedone out of the sebaceous gland opening. Gentle opening of the pimple with an 11 Bard Parker blade before using the comedone extractor may be helpful.

the first day, 250 mg for 4 days (Z-pack) can be used monthly or bimonthly

2. Other treatments

a. Vitamin A (water-soluble synthetic A), 50,000 #100

   Sig: Take 1 capsule b.i.d. for 5 months, then not for 2 months to prevent liver toxicity. Avoid if pregnancy is a possibility.

b. Abrasive cleansers are somewhat effective in removing comedones, but if too irritating may actually aggravate acne.

c. Large papules or early cysts. Intralesional corticosteroid can be injected with care. Dilute triamcinolone suspension (4 mg/mL) with equal part of saline or lidocaine (Xylocaine) with epinephrine, and inject about 0.1 mL into the lesion. Atrophy can result if too large a quantity or too high a concentration is injected.

d. Incision of fluctuant acne cysts: *never* incise these widely, but if you believe the pus must be drained, do it through a very small incision and possibly an acne stylet. A zero or ear curette can be useful.

e. Short-term prednisone systemic therapy is effective for severe cystic acne, especially for acne fulminans, an acute, disabling form of acne.

f. Isotretinoin: For severe, scarring, cystic acne this therapy has proved very beneficial. The usual dosage is 1 mg/kg per day given for 4 to 5 months. There are many minor and major side effects with this therapy (notably teratogenic effects in pregnant women), so isotretinoin should only be prescribed by those knowledgeable in its use. Depression may also be a side effect.

3. The residual scarring of severe acne (Fig. 13-9) can be lessened by surgical dermabrasion, using a rapidly rotating wire brush, diamond fraise, or laser resurfacing. These procedures are being done by many dermatologists and plastic surgeons.

4. Nicomide, 1 b.i.d. is a vitamin therapy that may be helpful.

5. Spirinolactone 25 or 50 mg b.i.d. may be beneficial in women especially if they flare during the last week of their menstrual cycle.

6. Long-wave ultraviolet light in the form of blue or red light or a combination is called intense pulsed light (IPL) therapy. It appears to be safe and can be helpful.

Rosacea

A common pustular eruption with flushing and telangiectasias of the butterfly area of the face may occur in adults especially in the 40- to 60-year-old age group (Fig. 13-10).

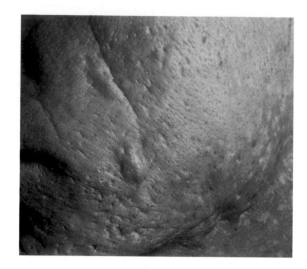

FIGURE 13-9 ■ Acne scars on the cheek.

Presentation and Characteristics

Primary Lesions

Diffuse redness, papules, pustules, and, later, dilated venules, mainly of the nose, cheeks, and forehead, are seen.

Secondary Lesions

Severe, longstanding cases eventuate in the bulbous, greasy, hypertrophic nose characteristic of rhinophyma.

Course

The pustules are recurrent and difficult to heal. Rosacea keratitis of the eye may occur.

Causes

Several factors influence the disease:

1. heredity (oily skin);
2. excess ingestion of alcoholic beverages, hot drinks, and spicy foods;
3. *Demodex* mites (may be causative);
4. increased exercise;
5. increased exposure to hot or cold environment; and
6. topical or systemic corticosteroids.

Excess sun exposure and emotional stress can aggravate some cases of rosacea.

Differential Diagnosis

■ *Systemic lupus erythematosus:* No papules or pustules; positive ANA blood test (see Chap. 32)

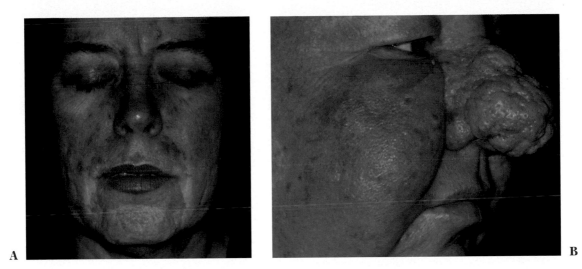

FIGURE 13-10 ■ (**A**) Rosacea of a 47-year-old woman. (**B**) Rosacea, chronic, with rhinophyma. *(Courtesy of Hoechst-Roussel Pharmaceuticals, Inc.)*

- *Boils:* Usually only one large lesion; can be recurrent but may occur sporadically; an early case of rosacea may look like small boils. Bacterial culture shows *Staphylococcus aureus* or group A β-hemolytic streptococci. Responds to anti-*Staphylococcus* antibiotics (Chap. 20).
- *Iodide or bromide drug eruption:* Clinically similar, but drug eruption usually is more widespread; history positive for drug (see Chap. 9)
- *Seborrheic dermatitis:* Pustules uncommon; red and scaly; also in scalp
- *Rosacea-like tuberculid of Lewandowsky:* Mimics small papular rosacea clinically and tuberculids histologically, rare; biopsy helpful

Treatment

Case Example. A 44-year-old man presents with redness and pustules on the butterfly area of the face.

1. Prescribe avoidance of these foods: chocolate, nuts, cheese, cola drinks, iodized salt, seafood, alcohol, spices, and very hot drinks.
2. Metronidazole gel (MetroGel, Metrocream, Metrolotion or Noritate cream)

    Sig: Apply thin coat b.i.d. Response to therapy is slow, taking 4 to 6 weeks to benefit.
3. Sulfur, ppt. 6%

    Resorcinol 4%

    Colored alcoholic shake lotion q.s. 60.0

    Sig: Apply to face h.s.

    Similar proprietary lotions are Sulfacet-R lotion Rosac Cream (contains a sunscreen), Rosula (contains urea to decrease irritation), sodium sulfacetamide topical preparations, Plexion topical preparations, Novacet lotion, Avar Green (contains green tint to hide redness).
4. Tetracycline, 250-mg capsules

    Sig: Take 1 capsule q.i.d. for 3 days, then 1 capsule b.i.d. for weeks, as necessary for benefit. Other antibiotics that can be used, as for acne, include doxycycline, minocycline, and erythromycin.
5. Therapy for *Helicobacter pylori* in the same treatment regimens as for peptic ulcer disease has been tried with some benefit in severe cases.
6. Azeleic acid (Azelex, Finacea) in thin coat b.i.d.
7. Crotamiton (Eurax) lotion in thin coat b.i.d.

Suggested Reading

Cordain L, Lindeberg S, Hurtado M, et al. Acne vulgaris: A disease of Western Civilization. Arch Dermatol 2002;138:1584–1590.

Gollnick H, Gunliffe W, Berson D, et al. Management of acne: A report from a Global Alliance to Improve Outcomes in Acne. J Am Acad Dermatol 2003;49 (1 Suppl):S1–37.

CHAPTER 14

Psoriasis

Micole Tuchman, MS, Robin Buchholz, MD, and Jeffrey M. Weinberg, MD

Psoriasis is a hereditary, papulosquamous skin disorder that affects 1.5% to 2% of the population in Western societies. In the United States, there are 3 to 5 million people with psoriasis, affecting men and women equally. Psoriasis can have multiple clinical presentations and varies widely among different individuals. It is typically a chronic and recurring disease that is best characterized by well-demarcated erythematous plaques with scaling. The plaques can be localized, which is the most common presentation, and are confined to only certain delineated areas of the body. Typically, plaques are seen most commonly on the elbows, knees, and scalp. There are other variants of psoriasis. In *palmoplantar psoriasis*, lesions are limited to the soles of the feet and palms of the hands. In contrast, *generalized pustular psoriasis* and *generalized erythrodermic psoriasis* can involve the entire body and be a life-threatening condition, even necessitating hospitalization, especially when seen in association with acute respiratory distress syndrome. Inverse psoriasis in intertriginous and tends to be on flexural areas of the skin.

Presentation and Characteristics

Primary Lesions

Plaque Psoriasis

These lesions are well-demarcated, salmon-colored papules and plaques with thick silvery scaling that typically bleeds when removed (Auspitz's sign). Lesions can vary greatly in size and shape in addition to distribution, which may be localized or generalized.

Pustular Psoriasis

The lesions are typically yellow pustules that can coalesce and evolve into dark red crusty lesions.

Secondary Lesions

Secondary lesions are less common, but can include excoriations, lichenification, (thickening) oozing, and secondary infection.

Distribution

Psoriatic patches most commonly occur on the elbows, knees, and scalp, although involvement can occur on any area of the body, including palms, soles, and even nails (Figs. 14-1 and 14-2).

Course

Psoriasis is typically a chronically recurring disease, although cases of complete resolution do occur. The onset of the disease can occur at any age, but the peaks of onset are in the 20s and 50s. HIV-positive patients can have recalcitrant psoriasis.

SAUER'S NOTES

1. Education and support are keys to the treatment of psoriasis. Give written information to the patient regarding the disease and potential treatment options. Carefully counsel the patient as to the risks and benefits of their therapies. Encourage the patient to join the National Psoriasis Foundation, which provides comprehensive patient support.
2. Encourage the patient not to pick or scratch their skin or scalp. This can aggravate their psoriasis (Koebner phenomenon).
3. With the use of topical corticosteroids, observe closely for the development of striae and skin atrophy. Avoid high-potency steroids on the face and intertriginous areas.
4. When considering biologic or systemic therapy, patient selection is critical. Take a thorough medical history and review of systems.
5. Remain cognizant of the quality of life and emotional toll of psoriasis. Provide referrals for counseling when appropriate.

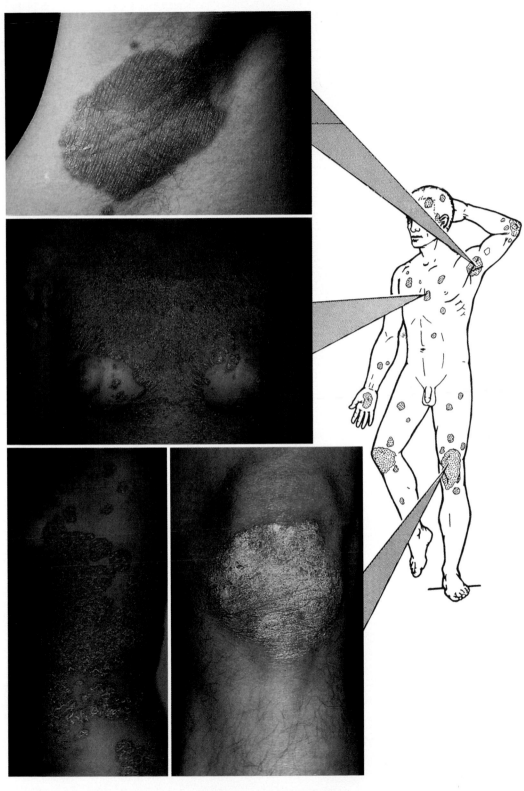

FIGURE 14-1 ■ Psoriasis.

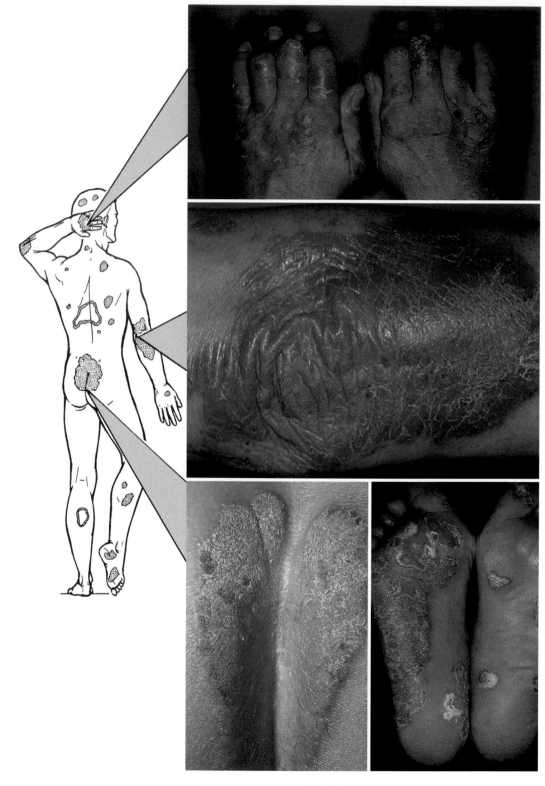

FIGURE 14-2 ■ Psoriasis.

Causes

Although the exact etiology of psoriasis is unknown, there is clearly a hereditary component. When one parent has psoriasis, a child has an 8% chance of having the disease; if both parents have psoriasis, the child's chance of developing psoriasis increases to as high as 41%. Specific HLA types have been noted to have a higher frequency of association with psoriasis, specifically HLA-B13, HLA-B17, HLA-Bw57, and most notably HLA-Cw6.

An acute form of guttate psoriasis, which characteristically develops in children and younger adults, often follows a streptococcal infection and has characteristic smaller sized, drop-shaped lesions (Fig. 14-3).

Triggering factors include physical trauma, which can elicit the lesions (Fig. 14-4), or any type of excessive rubbing or scratching, which can stimulate the proliferative process. Aggravating factors include psychological stress

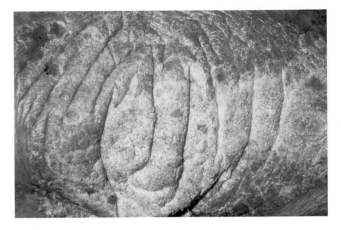

FIGURE 14-4 ■ Psoriasis on the knee with Auspitz's sign of pin-head size bleeding after scale removal.

and certain medications such as systemic glucocorticoids, oral lithium, antimalarial drugs, systemic interferon, β-blockers, and potentially angiotensin-converting enzyme inhibitors. Alcohol and smoking (especially pustular psoriasis) may also aggravate psoriasis. Rarely, ultraviolet light worsens psoriasis especially after a sunburn.

Subjective Complaints

Thirty percent of patients present with a complaint of pruritus, especially when psoriasis involves the scalp and anogenital area (Fig. 14-5). Also common are complaints of joint pain, termed *psoriatic arthritis*, found in 5% to 8% of patients with psoriasis. Interestingly, 10% of patients with psoriatic arthritis have no skin manifestations of the disease. Finally, in a rare acute onset of generalized pustular psoriasis called *von Zumbusch syndrome*, there is associated weakness, chills, and fever.

Season

Exacerbation is typically seen in the winter, most likely owing to the lack of sunlight and low humidity. Natural ultraviolet light typically cause psoriatic symptoms to improve.

Age Group

The disease can occur at any age. However, the average onset is typically bimodal, with one peak at approximately 23 years old (although in children, mean onset is 8 years old), and another at age 55.

Contagiousness

Psoriasis is not contagious.

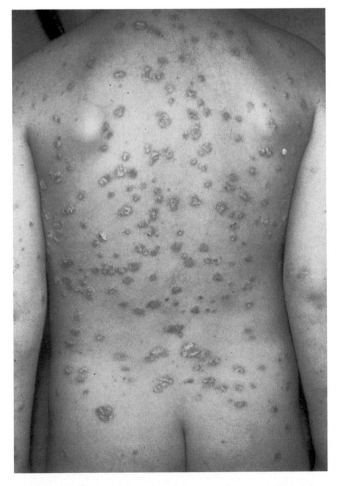

FIGURE 14-3 ■ Guttate psoriasis as a result of Group A streptococcus throat infection.

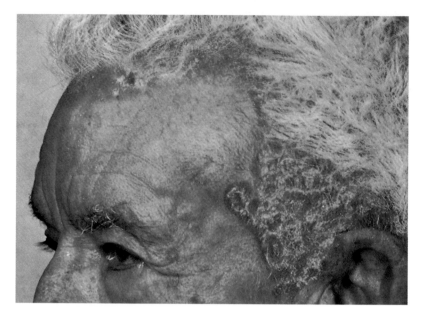

FIGURE 14-5 ■ Psoriasis of the border of the scalp. Psoriasis in this location is often difficult to distinguish from seborrheic dermatitis. *(Courtesy of Smith Kline & French Laboratories.)*

Relation to Employment

Psoriatic lesions occur more typically in areas of skin injury or repeated skin stress or pressure. This is known as the *Koebner phenomenon*. Psoriasis can be exacerbated by work place trauma and severe psoriasis (especially of the hands) can make jobs intolerable.

Laboratory Findings

The diagnosis of psoriasis is usually made on clinical grounds, and biopsy is not necessary. If biopsy is performed, histologic findings include the following:

1. acanthosis (thickening of the skin);
2. increased mitosis of keratinocytes, fibroblasts, and endothelial cells; and
3. inflammatory cells in the dermis and epidermis;

Differential Diagnosis

- *Seborrheic dermatitis:* Lesions are more yellowish and greasy than those of psoriasis. In the scalp, the scale is usually less thick than in psoriasis. Seborrheic dermatitis and psoriasis can often coexist in some patients. *Sebopsoriasis* or *seborrhiasis* are used when seborrhea and psoriasis are indistinguishable.
- *Lichen simplex chronicus:* Usually fewer patches than psoriasis, with less of a thick scale. Marked paroxysmal pruritus.

- *Tinea corporis:* Usually single lesion, with outer scale and central clearing. Potassium hydroxide preparation and fungal culture are positive for fungi.
- *Psoriasiform drug eruptions:* Check medication history.
- *Pityriasis rosea:* "Christmas tree" configuration of oval, papulosquamous lesions. Herald patch usually precedes wider eruption.
- *Atopic eczema:* Ask about family history of asthma, allergic rhinitis, eczema. Involvement typically occurs on flexural surfaces, face, and neck.
- *Secondary or tertiary syphilis:* These can appear psoriasiform. Inquire regarding history of sexually transmitted diseases and recent symptoms. Check syphilis serology if indicated.
- *Mycosis fungoides:* Biopsy in chronic cases, especially with involvement of bathing trunk area.
- *Nail dystrophy:* Psoriasis is in the differential diagnosis of nail dystrophy. Other entities to consider include onychomycosis, trauma, eczema, and lichen planus.

Treatment

Although there is no definitive cure for psoriasis there are many methods of management that can greatly improve and sometimes almost completely eradicate the skin manifestations of psoriasis, leading to a much improved quality of life. There are many new therapies available or in development for the treatment of the disease.

Case Example. A patient presents with mild to moderate localized lesions on the body, face, and scalp.

First Visit

For Body Lesions.

1. Medium- to high-potency fluorinated corticosteroid cream or ointment
   Sig: Apply b.i.d. to body lesions.
2. Calcipotriene (Dovonex) ointment
   Sig: Apply b.i.d. to body lesions. Can alternate with topical corticosteroids.
3. Tazorotene (Tazorac) gel or cream, 0.05% or 0.1%
   Sig: Apply q.h.s. to body lesions. Can be irritating and can alternate with topical corticosteroids.
4. Intralesional triamcinolone 4 to 8 mm/cc
   Sig: Subcutaneously to body lesions. This treatment can be very valuable for discrete, recalcitrant lesions.

For Facial (Less Common) and Intertriginous Lesions.

1. Low-potency corticosteroid cream or ointment
   Sig: Apply b.i.d. to facial lesions.
2. Pimecrolimus (Elidel) cream 0.1% or tacrolimus (Protopic) ointment 0.03% or 0.01%. Can be used q.o.d. alternating with topical corticosteroid.
   Sig: Apply b.i.d. to facial lesions

For Scalp Lesions.

1. Tar shampoo or Capex (fluocinolone) shampoo
   Sig: Shampoo frequently.
2. Topical corticosteroid lotion (Clobex, Diprolene), solution (Cormax, Lidex), or foam (Olux, Luxiq)
   Sig: Apply b.i.d. to scalp.
3. Derma-Smoothe FS Scalp Oil
   Sig: Apply overnight to scalp as directed.
4. Calcipotriene (Dovonex Scalp Solution) 0.0005%
   Sig: Apply b.i.d. to scalp. Can alternate q.o.d. with topical corticosteroid.
5. Tazorotene gel 0.05 or 0.1%
   Sig: Apply q.h.s. to scalp.

Subsequent Visits

1. For body lesions, the potency of the corticosteroid utilized can be increased.

2. Occlusive dressings with corticosteroid can be applied at night and left overnight.
3. Intralesional corticosteroid therapy can be given whereby individual small lesions are injected with intralesional triamcinolone as described.
4. Tazorotene gel or cream, 0.05% or 0.1% as described.
5. Ultraviolet therapy: Options include broadband or narrowband ultraviolet B, each three times per week, and oral psoralen plus ultraviolet A (PUVA), two to three times per week. PUVA has been associated with an increased risk of squamous cell carcinoma and, with long-term use, melanoma.

Case Example. A patient presents with moderate to severe generalized psoriasis.

First Visit.

1. Topical therapies listed for mild to moderate disease are utilized, possibly in combination with other therapies listed hereafter.
2. Broadband or narrowband ultraviolet B, three times per week
3. PUVA, two to three times per week.
4. Biologic therapies - TB skin test should be done before initiating therapy.
   a. Alefacept (Am evive) 15 mg IM for 12 weeks. A second and subsequent course can be initiated after 12 weeks off of the drug. T-cell counts must be monitored weekly.
   b. Efalizumab (Raptiva) 1 mg/cc SQ q. week. This drug can be given as continuous therapy after a conditioning dose of 0.7 mg/cc. Intermittent platelet counts should be checked. Worsening of psoriasis has been noted on abrupt discontinuation of the drug.
   c. Etanercept (Enbrel) 50 mg b.i.w. SQ for 3 months, followed by 25 mg b.i.w. This drug can be given as continuous therapy long term and is beneficial for psoriatic arthritis. Injection site reactions have been observed. Exercise caution in patients with multiple sclerosis, congestive heart failure, tuberculosis exposure and lupus erythematosus.
5. Methotrexate: This oral drug can be used weekly. This drug has potential side effects, including liver, hematologic, and pulmonary toxicity. Patients should be monitored closely.
6. Acitretin (Soriatane) therapy 10 to 25 mg q.d. This drug is especially useful in cases of palmoplantar, erythrodermic, and pustular psoriasis. This drug is teratogenic, and should not be used if pregnancy is possible. There are several other potential side effects, including alopecia, bone loss, and hyperlipidemia. Patients should be

monitored closely. This drug can be combined with PUVA (Re-PUVA: combination retinoid and PUVA therapy).

Subsequent Visits

1. Continue or rotate therapies as per first visit.
2. Occasionally some of these therapies can be combined. Check the package inserts and published data before combining different systemic therapies.
3. Cyclosporine (Neoral). This oral immunosuppressive therapy is highly effective for short-term, rapid treatment of severe psoriasis. It has many potential side effects, including hypertension and renal toxicity. Patients should be monitored closely.
4. Other biologic therapies: Infliximab (Remicade) can be given intravenously. Adalimumab (Humira) has been studied, but not yet approved for psoriasis. Check the package inserts and published data for the correct usage of these drugs.
5. Mycophenolate mofetil (Cellcept): This oral immunosuppressive drug has been reported to be effective in some patients with psoriasis. There is less organ toxicity with this than with methotrexate or cyclosporine. There is a small increased risk of lymphoma with chronic use of the drug.

Suggested Reading

Camisa C. Handbook of Psoriasis, ed 2. Malden, MA, Backwell Science, 2004.

Chaudhari U, Romano P, Mulcahy L, et al. Efficacy and safety of infliximab monotherapy for plaque-type psoriasis: a randomized trial. Lancet 2001;357: 1842–1847.

Cribier B, Frances C, Chosidow, O. Treatment of lichen planus. Arch Dermatol 1998;134:1521.

Fox BJ, Odum RB. Papulosquamous diseases: A review. J Am Acad Dermatol 1985;12:597.

Krueger G, Koo J, et al. The impact of psoriasis on quality of life. Arch Dermatol 2001;137:280.

Leonardi C, Powers J, Matheson R, et al. Etanercept as monotherapy in patients with psoriasis. N Engl J Med 2003;349:2014–2022.

Rapp SR, Feldman SR, et al. Psoriasis causes as much disability as other major medical diseases. J Am Acad Dermatol 1999;41:401.

Roenigk HH, Auerbach R, et al. Methotrexate in psoriasis: Consensus conference. J Am Acad Dermatol 1998; 38:3.

Sunenshine PJ, Schwartz RA, Janniger CK. Tinea versicolor. Int J Dermatol 1998;37:648.

CHAPTER 15

Other Papulosquamous Dermatoses

John C. Hall

Pityriasis Rosea

Pityriasis rosea is a moderately common papulosquamous eruption, mainly occurring on the trunk of young adults (Figs. 15-1, 15-2, and 15-3). It is mildly pruritic and occurs most often in the spring and fall.

Presentation and Characteristics

Primary Lesions

Papulosquamous, oval erythematous discrete lesions are seen. A larger "herald patch" resembling a patch of "ringworm" may precede the general rash by 2 to 10 days. A collarette of fine scaling is seen around the edge of the lesions. It begins just inside the pink plaque.

Secondary Lesions

Excoriations are rare. The effects of overtreatment or contact dermatitis are commonly seen.

Distribution

The lesions appear mainly on the chest and trunk along the lines of cleavage in the skin. Many cases have the oval lesions in a "Christmas tree branches" pattern over the back. In atypical cases, the lesions are seen in the axillae and the groin only. This is sometimes referred to as *inverse pityriasis rosea.* Facial lesions are rare in light-skinned adults, but are rather commonly seen in children and people of color.

Course

After the development of the "herald patch," new generalized lesions continue to appear for 2 to 3 weeks. The entire rash most commonly disappears within 6 to 8 weeks. Recurrences are rare. There are recurrent and long-lasting variants.

Subjective Complaints

Itching varies from none to severe, but is usually mild.

Cause

The cause is unknown. Some authors have incriminated HSV10 (herpes simplex).

Season

Spring and fall "epidemics" are common.

Age Group

Young adults and older children are most often affected.

Contagiousness

The disease is not contagious.

Differential Diagnosis

- *Tinea versicolor:* Lesions are tannish and irregularly shaped; fungi seen on scraping, fine dry adherent scale becomes apparent when the physician scratches the area with the fingernail.
- *Drug eruption:* No "herald patch"; positive drug history for gold, bismuth, or sulfa (see Chap. 9).
- *Secondary syphilis:* No itching (99% true); history or presence of genital lesions; positive blood serology (see Chap. 22).
- *Psoriasis:* Also usually on elbows, knees, and scalp; lesions have silvery-white scale.
- *Seborrheic dermatitis:* Greasy, irregular, scaly lesions on sternum, central face, external auditory canals, scalp, between buttocks and genitalia (see Chap. 13).
- *Lichen planus:* Lesions more papular and violaceous; on mucous membranes of mouth and lip.

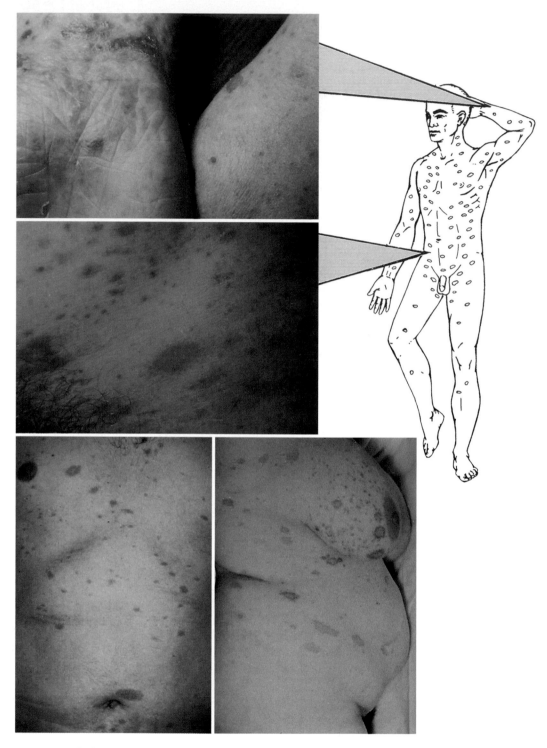

FIGURE 15-1 ■ Pityriasis rosea. *(Courtesy of Westwood Pharmaceuticals.)*

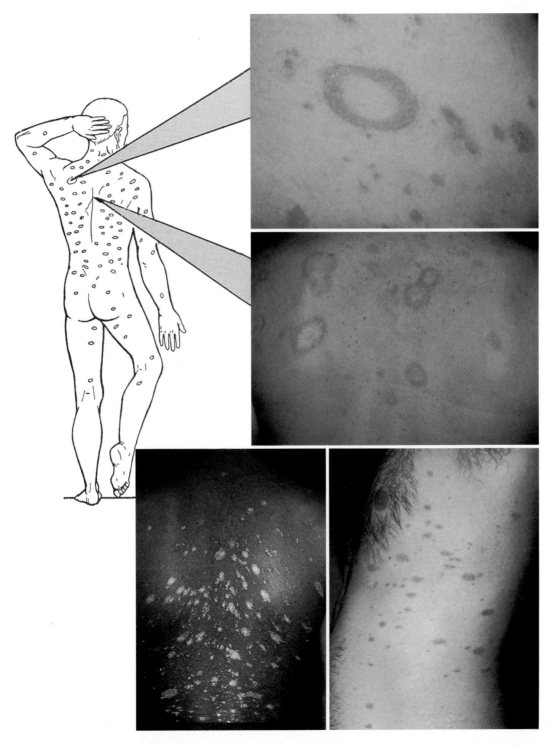

FIGURE 15-2 ■ Pityriasis rosea. Bottom left photograph is of an African-American patient. *(Courtesy of Westwood Pharmaceuticals)*

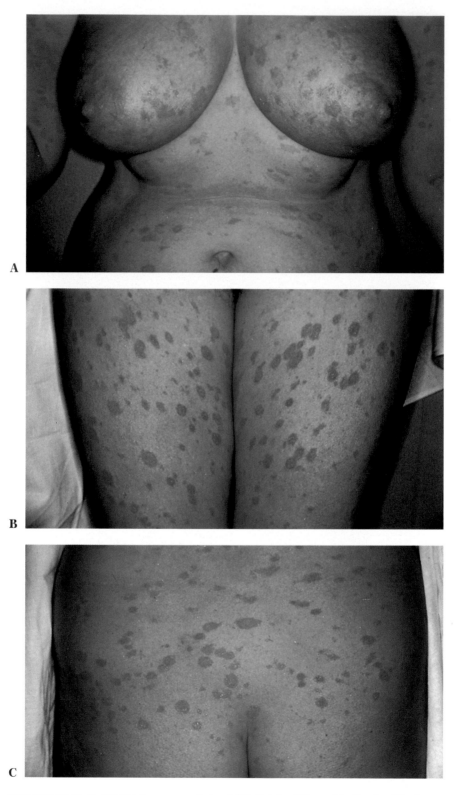

FIGURE 15-3 ■ Pityriasis rosea of chest (**A**), thighs (**B**), and buttocks (**C**) of one patient. *(Syntex Laboratories, Inc.)*

- *Parapsoriasis:* Rare; chronic form may have fine "cigarette paper" atrophy. Can develop into mycosis fungoides.

Treatment

First Visit

1. Reassure the patient that he or she does not have a "blood disease," that the eruption is not contagious, and that it would be rare to get it again.

2. Colloidal bath

   Sig: Use 1 packet of Aveeno oatmeal preparation to the tub containing 6 to 8 inches of lukewarm water. Bathe for 10 to 15 minutes every day or every other day.

   Comment: Avoid soap and hot water as much as possible to reduce any itching.

3. Nonalcoholic white shake lotion or Calamine lotion q.s. 120.0

   Sig: Apply b.i.d. locally to affected areas.

4. If there is itching, prescribe an antihistamine.

   Cyproheptadine (Periactin), 4 mg #60

   Sig: Take 1 tablet a.c. and h.s.

5. UVB therapy in increasing suberythema doses once or twice a week may be given. The severity is decreased but itching and disease duration are probably not altered.

Subsequent Visits

1. If the skin becomes too dry from the colloidal bath and the lotion, stop the lotion or alternate it with the following

   Hydrocortisone cream or ointment, 1% q.s. 60.0
   Sig: Apply b.i.d. locally to dry areas.

2. Continue the ultraviolet treatments.

Severely Pruritic Cases

1. In addition to the above, add

   Prednisone, 5 mg #40
   Sig: Take 1 tablet q.i.d. for 3 days, then 1 tablet t.i.d. for 4 days, then 2 tablets every morning for 1 to 2 weeks, as symptom of itching demands.

2. Erythromycin 250mg b. i. d × 2 weeks has been tried by some authors.

Tinea Versicolor

Tinea versicolor is a moderately common skin eruption with characteristics of tannish-colored, irregularly shaped

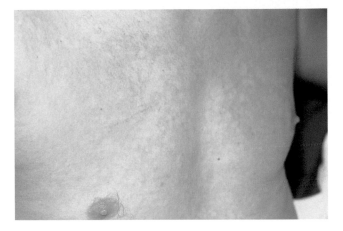

FIGURE 15-4 ■ Tinea versicolor on the chest. The dark areas of the skin are the areas infected with the fungus. *(K.U.M.C.; Sandoz Pharmaceuticals.)*

scaly patches causing no discomfort that are usually located on the upper chest and back (Fig. 15-4). It is caused by a lipophilic yeast (see Chap. 25). Dry scaling can be revealed by stroking the skin with a fingernail (coup d'ongle).

Presentation and Characteristics

Primary Lesions

Papulosquamous or maculosquamous, tan, and irregularly shaped, well demarcated lesions occur.

Secondary Lesions

Relative depigmentation results because the involved skin does not tan when exposed to sunlight. On skin not exposed to ultraviolet, the skin is slightly hyperpigmented. This cosmetic defect, obvious in the summer, often brings the patient to the office. Hence the name veriscolor (varied color).

Distribution

The upper part of the chest and the back, neck, and arms are affected. Rarely are the lesions on the face or generalized.

Course

The eruption can persist for years unnoticed. Correct treatment is readily effective, but the tinea usually recurs.

Cause

The causative agent is a lipophilic yeast, *Pityrosporum orbiculare*, which has a hyphae form called *Pityrosporum or Malassezia furfur.*

SAUER'S NOTES

1. It is important to tell the patient that depigmented spots may remain after the tinea versicolor is cured. These can be tanned by gradual exposure to sunlight or ultraviolet light.
2. A topical imidazole cream (clotrimazole, econazole, ketoconazole, miconazole) twice a day topically for 2 weeks with or without a sulfur soap can be used. Terbinafine spray (Lamisil) twice a day for 1 week.
3. Ketoconazole (Nizoral) orally in various short term regimens and itraconazole (Sporanox) 200 mg orally for 1 week have been used.

Contagiousness

The disease is not contagious and is not related to poor hygiene.

Laboratory Findings

A scraping of the scale placed on a microscopic slide, covered with a 20% solution of potassium hydroxide and a coverslip, shows the hyphae. Under the low-power lens of the microscope, very thin, short, mycelial filaments are seen. Diagnostic grape-like clusters of spores are seen best with the high-power lens. The appearance of spores and hyphae is referred to as "spaghetti and meatballs." The dimorphic organism does not grow on routine culture media.

Differential Diagnosis

- *Pityriasis rosea:* Acute onset; lesions oval with collarette of fine adherent dry scale (see earlier in this chapter)
- *Seborrheic dermatitis:* Greasy scales mainly in hairy areas (see Chap. 13)
- *Mild psoriasis:* Thicker scaly lesions on trunk and elsewhere (see earlier in this chapter)
- *Vitiligo:* Because tinea versicolor commonly manifests with depigmentation of the skin, many cases are misdiagnosed as vitiligo. This is indeed unfortunate because tinea versicolor is quite easy to treat and has a much better prognosis than vitiligo (see Chap. 31). No pigment (depigmentation) in vitiligo and decreased pigment (hypopigmentation) in tinea versicolor.
- *Secondary syphilis:* Lesions are more widely distributed and present on palms and soles (see Chap. 22)

SAUER'S NOTE

If the pityriasis rosea-like rash does not itch, obtain blood serologic test for syphilis if you have any uncertainty about the diagnosis and especially if palm and sole lesions are present with adenopathy.

Treatment

1. Selenium (Selsun or Head and Shoulders Intensive Treatment) suspension 120.0

    Sig: Bathe and dry completely. Then apply medicine as a lotion to all the involved areas, usually from neck down to pubic area. Let it dry. Bathe again in 24 hours and wash off the medicine. Repeat procedure again at weekly intervals for four treatments. This can be irritating.

2. Topical imidazole creams such as miconazole (available over the counter), ketaconazole (available over the counter), chlortimazole (available over the counter), econazole (Specatzole), and oxiconazole (Oxistat) twice a day for 2 weeks. Compounding 2% to 5% sulfur may add to the efficacy.

3. If lesions are extensive, 200 mg of ketaconazole orally twice a day for 5 days to cause a remission and the first day of each month for 6 months beginning April 1 can be used to prevent summer recurrences, which are common in warm, humid climates.

    Comment: Recurrences are rather common and can be easily retreated.

Lichen Planus

Lichen planus is an uncommon, chronic, pruritic disease characterized by violaceous flat-topped papules that are usually seen on the wrists and the legs (Figs. 15-5, 15-6, 15-7, and 15-8; see also Fig. 3-1B). Mucous membrane lesions on the cheeks or lips are milky white and net-like.

Presentation and Characteristics

Primary Lesions

Flat-topped, violaceous papules and papulosquamous lesions appear. On close examination of a papule, preferably after the lesion has been wet with an alcohol swipe, intersecting small white lines or papules (Wickham's striae) can be seen. These confirm the diagnosis. Uncommonly, the lesions may assume a ring-shaped configuration

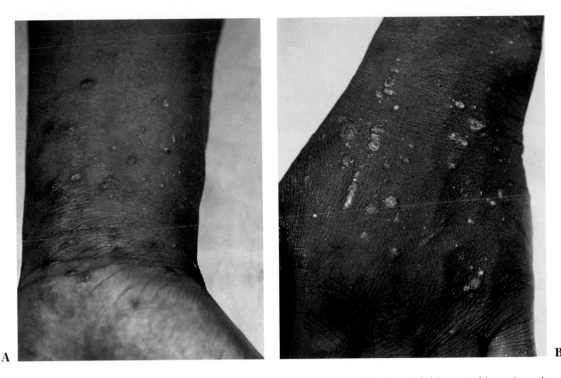

FIGURE 15-5 ■ Lichen planus on the wrist (**A**) and the dorsum of the hand (**B**) in an African-American patient. Note the violaceous color of the papules and the linear Koebner phenomenon on the dorsum of the hand. *(Courtesy of E.R. Squibb.)*

(especially on the penis) or may be hypertrophic (especially pretibial), atrophic, or bullous. On the mucous membranes, the lesions appear as a whitish, lacy network. When mucous membrane involvement is severe, ulcerations may occur and there is an increased occurrence of squamous cell cancer.

Secondary Lesions

Excoriations and, on the legs, thick, scaly, lichenified patches have been noted. Lesions are often rubbed rather than scratched because scratching is painful.

Distribution

Most commonly the lesions appear on the flexural aspects of the wrists and the ankles, the penis, and the oral mucous membranes, but they can be anywhere on the body or become generalized.

Course

Outbreak is rather sudden, with the chronic course averaging 9 months' duration. Some cases last several years. There is no effect on the general health except for itching. Recurrences are moderately common.

Cause

The cause is unknown. The disorder is rather frequently associated with nervous or emotional upsets. It may represent an autoimmune process, and some cases have a distinct pattern on direct immunofluorescence. Hepatitis C or hepatitis B is present in some cases (possibly up to 20%). This is more common when associated with HIV.

Subjective Complaints

Itching varies from mild to severe (severe is more common).

Contagiousness

Lichen planus is not contagious.

Relation to Employment

As in psoriasis, the lichen planus lesions can develop in scratches or skin injuries (Koebner phenomenon).

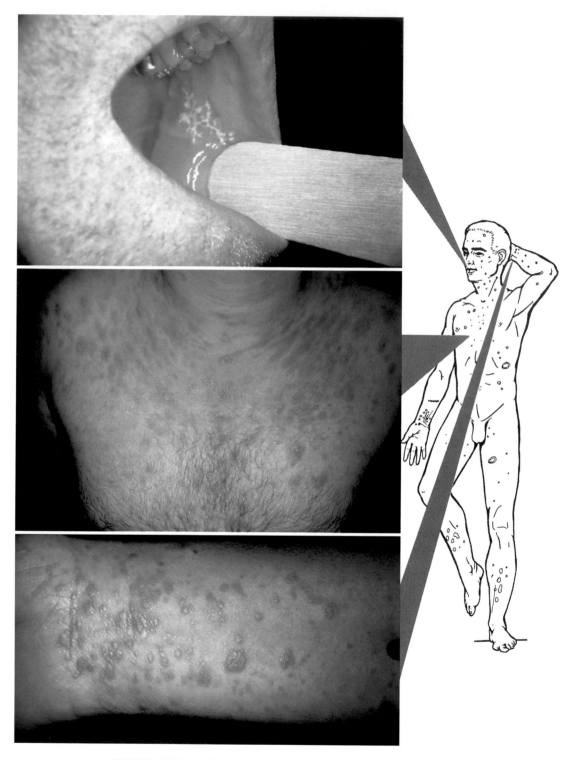

FIGURE 15-6 ■ Lichen planus. *(Courtesy of Johnson & Johnson.)*

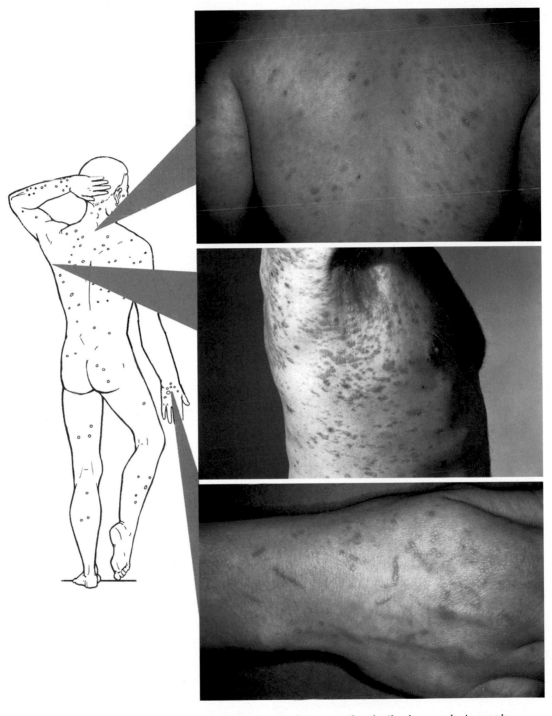

FIGURE 15-7 ■ Lichen planus. Note the Koebner reaction in the lower photograph.

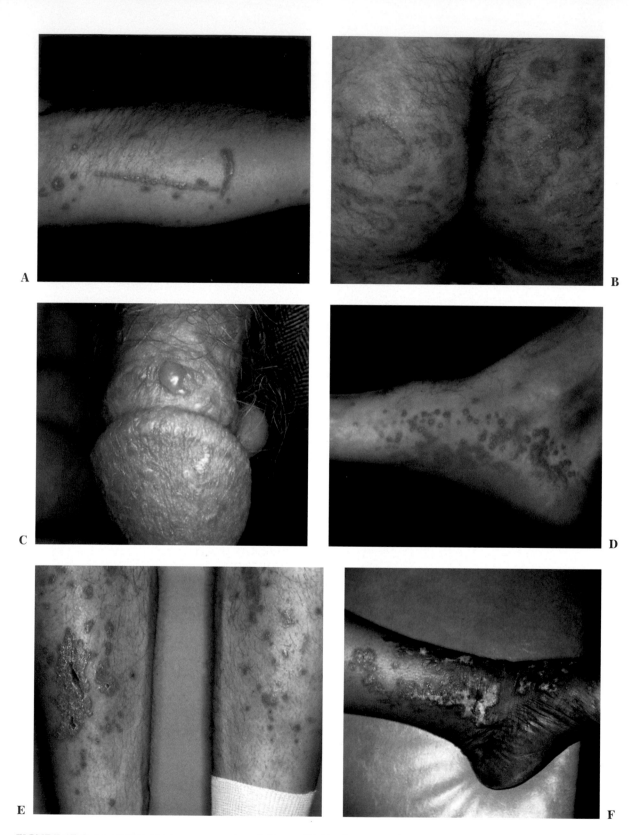

FIGURE 15-8 ■ Lichen planus, unusual variations. (**A**) Koebner reaction in scratched areas on arm. (**B**) Atrophic scarring lesions on buttocks. (**C**) Bullous and vesicular lesions on penis. (**D**) Lichen planus on sole of foot. (**E**) Hypertrophic lesions on anterior tibial area of legs. (**F**) Hypertrophic lesions on leg of an African-American woman. *(Courtesy of Neutrogena Corp.)*

Laboratory Findings

Microscopic section is quite characteristic.

Differential Diagnosis

- *Secondary syphilis:* No itching; blood serology positive (see Chap. 22)
- *Drug eruption:* History of taking atabrine, arsenic, or gold (see Chap. 9)
- *Psoriasis:* Lesions more scaly, whitish on knees and elbows (see Chap. 14)
- *Pityriasis rosea:* "Herald patch" mainly on trunk (see earlier in this chapter)

Lichen planus on leg may resemble neurodermatitis (usually one patch only; intensely pruritic; no mucous membrane lesions; see Chap. 11) or keloids (secondary to injury with no Wickham's striae)

Treatment

Case Example. A patient presents with generalized papular eruption and moderate itching.

First Visit.

1. Assure the patient that the disease is not contagious, is not a blood disease, and is chronic but not serious. Explain that a hepatitis screen is necessary since up to 20% of patients may have hepatitis B or hepatitis C.
2. Avoid excess bathing with soap.
3. Low-potency corticosteroid cream 60.0

   Sig: Apply locally b.i.d.
4. Over-the-counter antihistamine such as chlorpheniramine, 4 mg #60

   Sig: Take 1 tablet b.i.d. for itching.

   Comment: Warn the patient of drowsiness at onset of therapy

Subsequent Visits.

1. Occlusive dressing with corticosteroid therapy. This is quite effective for localized cases. I have also found that if occlusive dressings are applied only to the lichen planus on the legs, the rest of the body lesions improve.
2. Meprobamate, 400 mg #100

   Sig: Take 1 tablet t.i.d., *or*
   Chlordiazepoxide (Librium), 5 mg
   Sig: Take 1 tab t.i.d.
3. It is important in some resistant cases to rule out a focus of infection in teeth, tonsils, gallbladder, genitourinary system, and so on.
4. Corticosteroids orally or by injection are of definite value for temporarily relieving the acute cases that have severe itching or a generalized eruption.
5. Intralesional corticosteroids especially for localize hypertrophic disease.
6. Griseofulvin on rare occasions can decrease disease severity.
7. Treating hepatitis when present can benefit the disease (specifically hepatitis C).
8. Hydroxychloroquine sulfate (Plaquenil) orally can sometimes be helpful. See an ophthalmologist every 6 months to check for retinal toxicity.

Suggested Reading

Boyd AS, Neldner KH. Lichen planus. J Am Acad Dermatol 1991;25:593.

Cribier B, Frances C, Chosidow O. Treatment of lichen planus. Arch Deramtol 1998,134:1521.

Fox BJ, Odum RB. Papulosquamous diseases: A review. J Am Acad Dermatol 1985;12:597.

Sunenshine PJ, Schwartz RA, Janniger CK. Tinea versicolor. Int J Dermatol 1998;37:648.

CHAPTER 16

Granulomatous Dermatoses

John C. Hall

When considered singularly, granulomatous diseases are uncommon, but when all of them are considered together, they form a group that is interesting, varied, and ubiquitous.

A *granuloma* is a focal chronic inflammatory response to tissue injury manifested by a histologic picture of an accumulation and proliferation of leukocytes, principally of the mononuclear type and its family of derivatives, the mononuclear phagocyte system. The immunologic components in granulomatous inflammation originate from cell-mediated or delayed hypersensitivity mechanisms controlled by thymus-dependent lymphocytes (T lymphocytes). Five groups of granulomatous inflammations have been promulgated:

- Group 1 is the *epithelioid granulomas*, which include sarcoidosis, tuberculosis in certain forms, tuberculoid leprosy, tertiary syphilis, zirconium granuloma, beryllium granuloma, mercurial granuloma, and lichen nitidus.
- Group 2, *histiocytic granulomas*, include lepromatous leprosy, histoplasmosis, and leishmaniasis.
- Group 3 is the group of *foreign-body granulomas*, including endogenous products (*e.g.*, hair, fat, keratin), minerals (*e.g.*, tattoos, silica, talc), plant and animal products (*e.g.*, cactus, suture, oil, insect parts), and synthetic agents such as synthetic hair.
- Group 4 is the *necrobiotic/palisading granulomas*, such as granuloma annulare, necrobiosis lipoidica, rheumatoid nodule, rheumatic fever nodule, cat-scratch disease, and lymphogranuloma venereum.
- Group 5 is the *mixed inflammatory granulomas*, including many deep fungus infections such as blastomycosis and sporotrichosis, mycobacterial infections, granuloma inguinale, and chronic granulomatous disease.

Most of these diseases are discussed with their appropriate etiologic classifications in the Dictionary–Index. Two of these granulomatous inflammations are discussed in this chapter: *sarcoidosis*, which is an epithelioid granuloma in Group 1, and *granuloma annulare*, which is in Group 4 of necrobiotic/palisading granulomas.

Sarcoidosis

Sarcoidosis is an uncommon systemic granulomatous disease of unknown cause that affects skin, lungs, lymph nodes, liver, spleen, parotid glands, and eyes. Less commonly involved organs indicative of more severe disease are the central nervous system, heart, bones, and upper respiratory tract. Any one of these organs or all of them may be involved with sarcoid granulomas. Lymphadenopathy is the single most common finding. People of color are affected more often than white patients (14:1). Only the skin manifestations of sarcoidosis are discussed here (Fig. 16-1; see also Fig. 33-16).

Presentation and Characteristics

Primary Lesions

Cutaneous sarcoidosis is a great mimic of other skin diseases. Superficial lesions consist of reddish papules, nodules, and plaques, which may be multiple or solitary and of varying size and configuration. Annular forms of skin sarcoidosis are common. These superficial lesions usually involve the face, shoulders, and arms. Infiltration of sarcoidal lesions frequently occurs at scar sites. Subcutaneous nodular forms and telangiectatic, ulcerative, erythrodermic, and ichthyosiform types are rare. Sarcoidosis is often associated with chronic systemic disease.

Secondary Lesions

Central healing can result in atrophy and scarring.

Course

Most cases of sarcoidosis run a chronic but benign course with remissions and exacerbations. Spontaneous "cure" is not unusual. Erythema nodosum is characteristic of acute

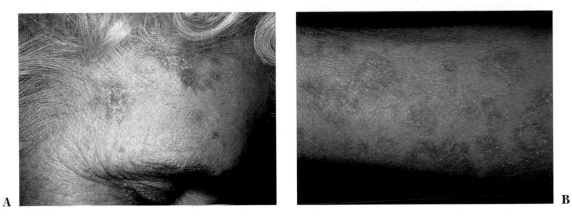

FIGURE 16-1 ■ **(A)** Sarcoid of the forehead. **(B)** Sarcoid on the forearm. *(Courtesy of Hoechst-Roussel Phar-maceuticals Inc.)*

benign sarcoidosis (see Chap. 12). Lupus pernio (indurated violaceous lesions on ears, nose, lips, cheeks, and forehead) and plaques are characteristic of chronic, severe, systemic disease. It is seen most often in African American women and girls.

Causes

The cause of sarcoidosis is unknown.

Laboratory Findings

The histopathologic appearance of sarcoidosis is quite characteristic and consists of epithelioid cells surrounded by Langerhans' giant cells, CD4 lymphocytes, some CD8 lymphocytes, and mature macrophages. No acid-fast bacilli are found, and caseation necrosis is absent. The Kveim test, using sarcoidal lymph node tissue, is positive after several weeks. This is not commonly used. Tuberculin-type, *Candida,* and other skin tests are negative (anergic). The total blood serum protein is high and ranges from 7.5 to 10.0 g/dL, mainly because of an increase in the globulin fraction.

Angiotensin-converting enzyme deficiency may be noted.

Differential Diagnosis

- *Other granulomatous diseases:* These can be ruled out by biopsy and other appropriate studies.
- *Silica granulomas:* Histologically similar; a history of such injury can usually be obtained.

Treatment

Time appears to cure or cause remission of most cases of sarcoidosis, but corticosteroids and immunosuppressant drugs may be indicated for extensive cases. Hydroxychloroquine and methotrexate may be beneficial. Anecdotal use of allopurinol has been reported. Doxycycline (100 mg b.i.d.) or minocycline (100 mg b.i.d.) has shown benefit in some studies.

Granuloma Annulare

Granuloma annulare is a moderately common skin problem. The usually encountered ring-shaped, red-bordered lesion is often mistaken for ringworm by inexperienced examiners (Fig. 16-2; see also Fig. 24-10) but there is no scaling. Several clinical variations exist. The two most common are the *localized form* and *generalized form*. There is also an annular form often seen on the glans of the penis and tongue, a rare linear form, a subcutaneous deep form, a papular variety, and a perforating form mimicking a perforating folliculitis. Some authors have described a subtle rare patch type of disease.

Women and girls with granuloma annulare predominate over men and boys in a ratio of 2.5 to 1. No ages are exempt, but the localized form is usually seen in patients in the first three decades of life and the generalized form in patients in the fourth through seventh decades. A granuloma annulare–like eruption has been reported in HIV-positive and chronic Epstein-Barr–positive patients.

Presentation and Characteristics

Primary Lesions

In both the localized and generalized forms, the lesion is a red asymptomatic papule with no scaling. The papule may be solitary. Most frequently the lesion assumes a ring-shaped or arcuate configuration of papules that tends to

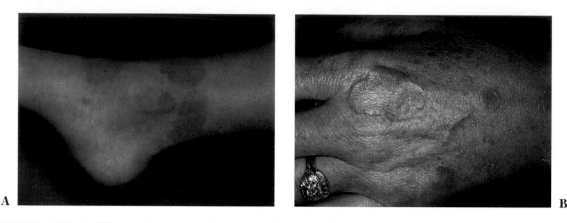

FIGURE 16-2 ■ **(A)** Granuloma annulare on ankle area. **(B)** Granuloma annulare on dorsum of hand. *(Courtesy of Hoechst-Roussel Pharmaceuticals Inc.)*

enlarge centrifugally. Rarely are the rings over 5 cm in diameter. In the localized form of granuloma annulare, the lesions appear mainly over the joints on hands, arms, and feet and on the legs. In the generalized form, there may be hundreds of the red or tan papular circinate lesions on the extremities and on the trunk. This is the most common form in HIV-positive patients. Diabetes may be increased in this form.

Secondary Lesions

On healing, the red color turns to brown before the lesions disappear.

Course

Both forms of granuloma annulare can resolve spontaneously after 1 to several years, but the generalized form is more long lasting. It does not lead to scar formation.

Causes

The cause is unknown. An immune-complex vasculitis or a cell-mediated immunity has been proposed to be a factor in the disease, as has trauma.

Laboratory Findings

The histopathologic appearance of granuloma annulare is quite characteristic. The middle and upper dermis have focal areas of altered collagenous connective tissue surrounded by an infiltrate of histiocytic cells and lymphocytes. In some cases, these cells infiltrate between the collagen bundles, giving a palisading effect. *Necrobiosis* has been used to describe these changes. Some believe that the

generalized form of granuloma annulare is associated with a higher incidence of diabetes mellitus.

Differential Diagnosis

- *Tinea corporis:* Usually itches and has a scaly red border; the fungus can be demonstrated with a potassium hydroxide scraping or Sabouraud culture (see Chap. 19).
- *Lichen planus, annular form:* Characterized by violaceous flat-topped papules with Wickham's striae; mucous membrane lesions are often seen (see Chap. 15).
- *Secondary syphilis:* Can be clinically similar but has a positive serology (see Chap. 22).
- *Other granulomatous diseases:* Can usually be distinguished by biopsy.

There is a subcutaneous form of granuloma annulare that is difficult to distinguish histologically from the rheumatoid nodule or a soft tissue tumor.

Treatment

Localized Form

Some cases respond to the application of a corticosteroid cream covered for 8 hours a day with an occlusive dressing such as Saran Wrap. Intralesional corticosteroids are effective for a case with only a few lesions. Light liquid nitrogen therapy is sometimes beneficial.

Generalized Form

Numerous remedies have been tried with anecdotal benefit. Dapsone and hydroxychloroquine have been used.

Suggested Reading

English JC, Patel PJ, Greer KE. Sarcoidosis. J Am Acad Dermatol 2001;44:725–743.

Hirsh BC, Johnson WC. Concepts of granulomatous inflammation. Int J Dermatol 1984;23:90.

Newman LS, Rose CS, Maier LA. Sarcoidosis. N Engl J Med 1997;336:17.

Smith MD, Downie JB, DiCostanzo D. Granuloma annulare. Int J Dermatol 1997;36:326.

Young RJ, Gilson RT, et al. Cutaneous sarcoidosis. Int J Dermatol 2001;40:249–253.

CHAPTER 17

Dermatologic Parasitology

John C. Hall

Dermatologic parasitology is an extensive subject and includes the dermatoses caused by three main groups of organisms: protozoa, helminthes, and arthropods.

- The *protozoal dermatoses* are exemplified by the various forms of trypanosomiasis and leishmaniasis (see Chap. 37).
- *Helminthic dermatoses* include those due to roundworms (ground itch, creeping eruption, filariasis, and other rare tropical diseases) and those due to flatworms (schistosomiasis, swimmer's itch, and others) (see Chap. 37).
- *Arthropod dermatoses* are divided into those caused by two classes of organisms: the arachnids (spiders, scorpions, ticks, and mites) and the insects (lice, bugs, flies, moths, beetles, bees, and fleas). Lyme disease is caused by a spirochete that is transmitted by a tick and is discussed in Chap. 22.

In this chapter scabies, caused by a mite, and pediculosis, caused by lice, are discussed. Flea bites, chigger bites, creeping eruption, swimmer's itch, and tropical dermatoses are discussed in Chap. 35.

Scabies

Scabies (Figs. 17-1 and 17-2; see also Fig. 37-9) is usually more prevalent in a populace ravaged by war, famine, or disease, when personal hygiene becomes relatively unimportant. However, there are unexplained cyclic epidemics of this parasitic infestation. In the 1970s and 1980s, such a cycle plagued Americans. In normal times, scabies is seen in schoolchildren, among the elderly in nursing care centers, in poorer populations under crowded conditions, and in sexually active patients with multiple sex partners.

Presentation and Characteristics

Primary Lesions

A burrow caused by the female of the mite *Sarcoptes scabiei* (see Fig. 17-2) measures approximately 2 mm in length and

---

> **SAUER'S NOTES**
>
> 1. Scabies should be ruled out in any generalized excoriated eruption.
> 2. The patient should always be asked if other members of the household itch.

can be hidden by the secondary eruption. Small vesicles may overlie the burrows. *Scabies incognito* is a form of the disease in which the burrows are not easily identified. *Norwegian*, or *keratotic, scabies* occurs in immunosuppressed patients. Hundreds of organisms create a psoriasiform dermatitis.

Secondary Lesions

Excoriations of the burrows may be the only visible pathologic process. In severe, chronic cases, bacterial infection may be extensive and may take the form of impetigo, cellulitis, or furunculosis.

Residual nodular lesions may persist as an allergic reaction for many weeks or months after the organism is eliminated. They are often recalcitrant to therapy and topical, intralesional, and even systemic corticosteroids may be necessary. Nodular scabies is not contagious.

Distribution

Most commonly, the excoriations are seen on the lower abdomen and the back, with extension to the pubic, genital, and axillary areas, the legs (ankles especially), the arms (flexor wrists especially), and the webs of the fingers.

Subjective Complaints

Itching is intense, particularly at night, when the patient is warm and in bed and the mite is more active. However, many skin diseases itch worse at night, presumably due to a lower itch threshold when relaxation occurs.

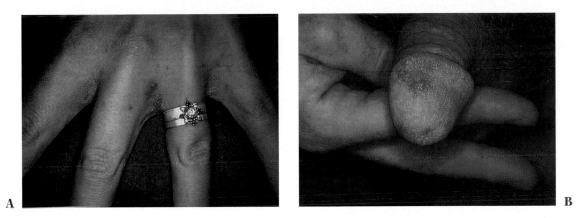

A   B

FIGURE 17-1 ■ **(A)** Scabies on the hand. **(B)** Scabies on the penis. *(Courtesy of Hoechst-Roussel Pharmaceuticals.)*

Course

The mite can persist for months and years ("7-year itch") in untreated persons.

Contagiousness

Other members of the household or intimate contacts may or may not have the disease, depending on exposure and the severity of the infestation.

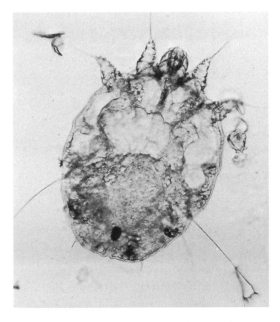

FIGURE 17-2 ■ The female of the mite *Sarcoptes scabiei*. The small, oval, black body near the anal opening is a fecal pellet. Proximal to it is a vague, much larger, oval, pale-edged mass—an egg. *(Courtesy of Dr. H. Parlette.)*

Laboratory Findings

The female scabies mite, ova, and fecal pellets may be seen in curetted burrows examined under the low-power magnification of the microscope (see Fig. 17-2). Potassium hydroxide (20% solution) can be used to clear the tissue, as with fungus smears. Another method of collection is to scrape the burrow through immersion oil and then transfer the scrapings to the microscopic slides. Skill is necessary to uncover the mite by curetting or scraping.

Differential Diagnosis

- *Pyoderma:* Rule out concurrent parasitic infestation; positive history of diabetes mellitus; only mild itching (see Chap. 21).
- *Pediculosis pubis:* Lice and eggs on and around hairs; distribution different (see following section).
- *Winter itch:* No burrows; seasonal incidence; elderly patient, usually; worse on legs and back (see Chap. 11).
- *Dermatitis herpetiformis:* Vesicles, urticaria; excoriated papules; eosinophilia; no burrows; characteristic histopathologic appearance (see Chap. 18).
- *Neurotic excoriations:* Nervous person; patient admits picking at lesions; present in areas where patient can easily reach; no burrows; characteristic stellate hypopigmented scars indicate a prolonged illness.
- *Parasitophobia* (see Chap. 20): Usually the patient brings to the office pieces of skin and debris; showing the patient the debris under a microscope helps to convince him or her of the absence of parasites. This is a difficult problem to manage. Pimozide (ORAP) can be used by a physician experienced in its use.

Treatment

Adults and Older Children

1. Inspect or question concerning itching in other members of the family or intimate contacts to rule out infestation in them. Any household members or intimate contacts must be treated at the same time as the patient to prevent "ping-pong" infestation. This is true even if itching is not present.

2. Instruct patient to bathe thoroughly and then apply a scabicide.

3. Permethrin (Elimite, Acticin) 5% cream 60.0

   or gamma benzene hexachloride (Lindane, Kwell) 120.0

   Sig: Apply to the entire body from the neck down. Repeat therapy in 1 week.

4. After 24 hours, the patient should bathe carefully and change to clean clothes and bedding.

5. Washing, dry cleaning, or ironing of clothes and bedding is sufficient to destroy the mite. Sterilization is unnecessary.

6. Itching may persist for a few days, even for 2 to 3 weeks or longer, in spite of the destruction of the mite. The itching may be worse for the first several days after treatment. For this apply b.i.d.:

   a. Crotamiton (Eurax) cream q.s. 60.0

   Comment: This cream has scabicidal power and antipruritic action combined.

   b. A topical corticosteroid ointment can be used or, if the pruritis persists, a 10- to 14-day course of systemic corticosteroids may have to be given.

7. If itching persists after 4 weeks, reexamine the patient carefully, and repeat the KOH preparation to be sure reinfestation or inadequate treatment has not occurred. Ask if all people who are potential contacts have been treated. It takes a lot of reassurance to convince these itchy patients that they are not still infested with scabies. Repeated unnecessary topical therapy may only increase the itching because these topical agents can act as irritants. Overuse of gamma benzene hexachloride can cause siezures.

8. Oral ivermectin is a therapy advocated by some authors. It is helpful in crusted scabies, which also may need keratolytic agents to remove the crusts before using topical therapy.

Newborns and Infants

1. General instructions are as for older patients.

2. Lindane lotion used in newborns and infants has caused convulsions.

3. Elimite, Actin, or Eurax cream 60.0

   Sig: Apply b.i.d. locally to affected areas only, *or*

4. Sulfur, ppt. 5%

   Water-washable cream base or Aquaphor q.s. 60.0
   Sig: Apply b.i.d. to affected areas.
   This is a good choice of therapy in pregnant and breastfeeding patients due to its extreme safety. However, it is malodorous and stains clothing.

5. In patients younger than 1 year of age, the bite may occur above the neck. There have been rare reports of disease above the neck in adults. The immunocompromised patient is a candidate for this manifestation.

Pediculosis

Lice infestation affects persons of all ages, but usually those in the lower income strata and military personnel in the field are affected most often because of lack of cleanliness and infrequent changes of clothing. It is also seen as a sexually transmitted disease. Three clinical entities are produced:

- infestation of the hair by the head louse *Pediculus humanus capitis*,
- infestation of the body by *Pediculus humanus corporis*, and
- infestation of the pubic area by the pubic louse *Pthirus pubis* (Fig. 17-3).

Pthirus pubis can also involve the hairy areas over the abdomen and chest and the eyelids. Because lice bite the skin and live on the blood, it is impossible for them to live without human contact. The readily visible oval eggs or nits are attached to hairs or to clothing fibers by the female louse. After the eggs hatch, the newly born lice mature within 30 days. The female louse can live for another 30 days and deposit a few eggs daily.

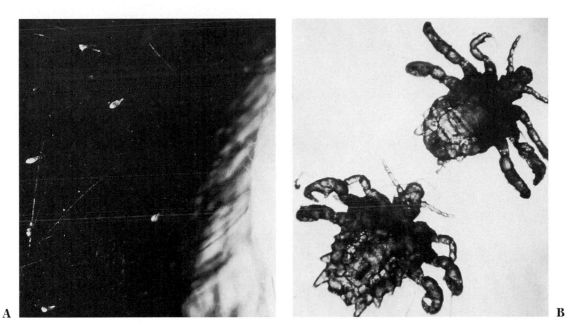

FIGURE 17-3 ■ Pediculosis. (**A**) Nits on scalp hair behind ear. *(Courtesy of Dr. L. Hyde.)* (**B**) Pubic louse, or *Pthirus pubis,* as seen with the 7.5× lens of a microscope. *(Courtesy of Dr. J. Boley.)*

Presentation and Characteristics

Primary Lesions

The site of the bite is seldom seen because of the secondary changes produced by the resulting intense itching. In the scalp and pubic forms, the nits are found on the hairs, but the lice are found only occasionally. In the body form, the nits and the lice can be found after careful searching in the seams of the clothing.

Secondary Lesions

In the scalp form, the skin is red and excoriated, with such severe secondary bacterial infection, in some cases, that the hairs become matted together in a crusty, foul-smelling "cap." Regional lymphadenopathy is common. A morbilliform rash on the body or a generalized papular "id" reaction can be seen in longstanding cases.

In the body form, linear excoriations and secondary infection, seen mainly on the shoulders, the belt line, and the buttocks, mask the primary bites.

In the pubic form, secondary excoriations are again dominant and produce some matting of the hairs. This louse can also infest body, axillary, and eyelash hairs. An unusual eruption on the abdomen, the thighs, and the arms, called *maculae cerulea* because of the bluish gray, pea-sized macules, can occur in chronic cases of pubic pediculosis.

> ### SAUER'S NOTE
>
> All cases of scalp pyoderma must be examined closely for a primary lice infestation.

Differential Diagnosis

Pediculosis Capitis

- *Bacterial infection of the scalp:* Responds rapidly to correct antibacterial therapy (see Chap. 21)
- *Seborrheic dermatitis or dandruff:* The scales of dandruff are readily detached from the hair, but oval nits are not so easily removed (see Chap. 13). Nits are easily seen when affected hairs are examined under low power on the microscope
- *Hair casts (pseudonits):* Resemble nits but usually can be pulled off more easily; no eggs are seen on microscopic examination

Pediculosis Corporis

- *Scabies:* May be small burrows; distribution of lesions different; no lice in clothes or nits on hairs (see beginning of this chapter)
- *Senile or winter itch:* History helpful; dry skin, aggravated by bathing; will not find lice in clothes or nits on hairs (see Chap. 11)

Pediculosis Pubis

- *Scabies:* No nits; burrows in pubic area and elsewhere (see beginning of this chapter)
- *Pyoderma* secondary to contact dermatitis from condoms, contraceptive jellies, new underwear, douches: History important; acute onset, no nits (see Chap. 21)
- *Seborrheic dermatitis,* when in eyebrows and eyelashes: No nits found; scaling on hairs less adherent than nits (see Chap. 13)

Treatment

Pediculosis Capitis

1. Shampoos or rinses

   a. Permethrin (Nix) creme rinse 60.0

   Sig: Use as a rinse for 10 minutes after shampooing. Only one application is necessary.

   b. Lindane (Kwell) shampoo 60.0

   Sig: Shampoo and comb hair thoroughly. Leave on the hair for 4 minutes. Repeat medicated shampoo in 3 days. Regular shampoo can be restarted in 24 hours.

   c. Pyrethrins (RID) 60.0

   Sig: Apply to scalp for 10 minutes and rinse off. Apply again in 7 days (nonprescription).

   d. Step Two (formic acid) solution (obtainable without a prescription) can be used to help remove nits from the hair.

   e. Permethrin 5% (Elimite) cream 60.0

   Leave on overnight under shower cap. May be the most effective topical treatment of all for recalcitrant cases.

   f. A single oral dose of ivermectin (Stromectol), 200 μg/kg, repeated in 10 days may be the most effective oral agent in persistent cases. Some authors are concerned about the safety of this therapy.

   g. Topical malathion (Ovide), available in a scalp preparation and quite safe.

2. For secondary scalp infection:

   a. Trim hair as much as possible and agreeable with the patient.

   b. Shampoo hair daily with a salicylic acid shampoo (T-Sal)

   c. Bactroban or polysporin ointment 15.0

   Sig: Apply to scalp b.i.d.

3. Change and clean bedding and headwear after 24 hours of treatment. Storage of headwear for 30 days destroys the lice and nits.

4. Mayonaisse (not reduced fat) left overnight for 3 nights is effective and very safe.

Pediculosis Corporis

1. Calamine lotion q.s. 120.0

   Sig: Apply locally b.i.d. for itching (the lice and nits are in the clothing).

2. Premethrin 5% (Elimite) cream overnight

3. Have the clothing laundered or dry cleaned. If this is impossible, dusting with 10% lindane powder kills the parasites. Care should be taken to prevent reinfestation. Storage of clothing in a plastic bag for 30 days kills both nits and lice.

Sulfur 5% to 10% in petrolatum overnight for 3 nights is effective and very safe. It is malodorous and stains bed clothes.

Pediculosis Pubis

Treatment is the same as for the scalp form.

When it occurs on the eylids, sulfacetamide ophthalmic ointment b.i.d for 5 days is very safe and effective.

Suggested Reading

Buntin DM, Rosen T, Lesher JL, et al. Sexually transmitted diseases: viruses and ectoparasites. J Am Acad Dermatol 1991;25:527.

Centers for Disease Control and Prevention. Scabies in health-care facilities: Iowa. Arch Dermatol 1988; 124:837.

Ko CJ, Elston DM. Pediculosis. J Am Acad Dermatol 2004; 50:1–12.

Zhu YI, Stiller MJ. Arthropods and skin diseases. Int J Dermatol 2002;41:533–549.

CHAPTER 18

Bullous Dermatoses

John C. Hall

To medical students and practitioners alike, the bullous skin diseases appear most dramatic. One of these diseases, pemphigus is undoubtedly greatly responsible for the aura that surrounds the exhibition and the discussion of an unfortunate patient with a bullous disease. Happy would be the instructor who could behold such student interest when a case of acne or hand dermatitis is being presented.

In almost all cases of bullous diseases, it is necessary to examine a fresh tissue biopsy specimen for deposits of immune reactants, immunoglobulins, and complement components, at or near the basement membrane zone. Routine histologic examination of a formalin-fixed biopsy specimen is, of course, also usually indicated (see Chap. 10).

Three bullous diseases are discussed in this chapter: pemphigus vulgaris, dermatitis herpetiformis, and erythema multiforme bullosum. However, other bullous skin diseases do occur, and in this introduction they are differentiated from these three:

- *Bullous impetigo:* Bullous impetigo is to be differentiated from the other bullous diseases by its occurrence in infants and children, rapid development of the individual bullae, presence of impetigo lesions in siblings, bacterial culture positive for *Staphylococcus aureus,* and rapid response to antibiotic therapy (see Chaps. 15 and 33). It can be a recurrent problem in HIV-positive patients in the groin area.
- *Contact dermatitis* due to poison ivy or similar plants: Bullae and vesicles are seen in linear configuration. A history of pulling weeds, cleaning out fence rows, or burning brush is usually obtained, and a past history of poison ivy or related dermatitis is common. It is important to remember that this is a form of delayed hypersensitivity and the exposure causing the eruption and the onset of symptoms can be anywhere from 1 to 2 days to 1 to 2 weeks. This delayed nature of the disease commonly leads to an erroneous diagnosis or a correct diagnosis with inability to establish when the exposure occurred and to therefore eliminate all traces of the plant oil from objects where *it* may be contacted again and result in another outbreak of the disease. The duration of disease is 10 to 21 days if untreated and is quite uncomfortable (see Chap. 9).
- *Drug eruption:* Elicit drug history (particularly of sulfonamides, nonsteroidal anti-inflammatory drugs [NSAIDs], and antiseizure medications). Fixed drug eruptions are not uncommonly bullous. Fixed drug eruptions are localized, very inflammatory, may blister, leave marked hyperpimentation and occur at the same site on drug rechallenge. The eruption usually clears on discontinuing drugs but can delay for 2 or more weeks. If the patient is not better within a few days of stopping the drug this does not mean that the drug is not the cause of the eruption. Bullae appear rapidly (see Chap. 9).
- *Epidermolysis bullosa* (see Fig. 31-3): This rare, chronic, hereditary skin disease is manifested by the formation of bullae, usually on the hands and the feet, following trauma. The full clinical and immunologic spectra of these diseases is protean in form of inheritance, severity of disease, and tendency to improve with age.
  - The simple form (epidermolysis bullosa simplex) of dominant inheritance can begin in infancy or adulthood with the formation of tense, slightly itching bullae at the sites of pressure, which heal quickly without scarring. Forced marches or jogging can initiate this disease in patients who have the heredity factor. Such cases are usually treated erroneously as athlete's foot. The disease is worse in the summer or in climates with high humidity or may be present only at this time. Often improves with age.
  - The dystrophic form of recessive inheritance begins in infancy and as time elapses the bullae

become hemorrhagic, heal slowly, and leave scars that can amputate digits; death can result from secondary infection and metastatic squamous cell carcinomas. Mucous membrane lesions are more common in the dystrophic form than in the simple form. Treatment is supportive. Gene therapy may be a future modality, but has been disappointing so far. Surgical dressings and skin substitutes (Apligraft) are an important part of care. Various surgical dressings may be helpful. Mepotil is a dressing I have found especially useful. The blisters should be immediately drained to relieve pain and keep them from enlarging. Secondary infection should be watched for carefully and treated immediately.

- A lethal, nonscarring form is of recessive inheritance also, but is usually fatal within a few months (see Chap. 35).

- *Epidermolysis bullosa acquisita:* An autoimmune response to collagen where skin lesions can appear similar to bullous pemphigoid, cicatricial pemphigoid, and recessive epidermolysis bullosa. Bulla, scarring, and esophageal disease all occur in this acquired illness. Direct immunofluorescence (DIF) is positive in a linear pattern in the epidermal basement membrane. Dapsone and systemic corticosteroids may be helpful. Trauma can induce blisters which result in scarring.

- *Familial benign chronic pemphigus* (Hailey-Hailey Disease): This is a rare, hereditary bullous eruption that is most common on the neck, groin, and in the axillae. It can be distinguished from pemphigus by its chronicity and benign nature and by its histologic picture (see Chap. 35). Some consider this disease to be a bullous variety of keratosis follicularis (Darier's disease). It is very painful and can be debilitating. It is caused by mutation of *ATP2C1* gene.

- *Porphyria:* The congenital erythropoietic type and the chronic hepatic type (porphyria cutanea tarda) commonly have bullae on the sun-exposed areas of the body (see the Dictionary–Index under *Porphyria* and Chap. 34).

- *Bullous pemphigoid:* This chronic bullous eruption most commonly occurring in elderly adults is usually not fatal. It is differentiated from pemphigus vulgaris by the histologic presence of subepidermal bullae without acantholysis and quite specific immunofluorescent autoantibodies in the basement membrane zone; from erythema multiforme by its chronicity, absence of iris lesions, and histology; and

from dermatitis herpetiformis by the absence of response to sulfapyridine or dapsone therapy (some bullous pemphigoid cases do respond to this therapy), by histology, immunofluorescent antibodies, and absence of nontropical sprue.

- *Cicatricial pemphigoid:* This disabling but nonfatal bullous eruption of the mucous membranes most commonly involves the eyes. The skin and mucous membranes may be involved usually in a localized pattern. As the result of scarring, which is characteristic of this disease and separates it from true pemphigus, eyesight is eventually lost. Over 50% of the cases have skin lesions. Histologically, the bullae are subepidermal and do not show acantholysis. There is quite a bit of immunologic similarity between this disease and bullous pemphigoid.

- *Linear IgA bullous disease:* Most of the children and adults with this disease differ from classic dermatitis herpetiformis in the morphology and distribution of their lesions, have a poorer response to dapsone, and have linear IgA antibasement membrane zone antibodies. Nontropical sprue is not a part of this illness.

- *Incontinentia pigmenti:* The first stage of this rare disease of infants manifests itself with bullous lesions, primarily on the hands and feet (see Chap. 36). This stage may appear in utero and not be seen clinically.

- *Toxic epidermal necrolysis* (TEN): This rare disease is characterized by large bullae and a quite generalized Nikolsky's sign, in which large sheets of epidermis become detached from the underlying skin with gentle pressure from a finger. The mucous membranes are frequently involved. The patient is toxic. Adults are most commonly affected. In many instances it is difficult to separate this disease clinically from severe erythema multiforme–like disease (Stevens-Johnson syndrome) and it is now thought by most dermatologists that Stevens-Johnson syndrome is a variant of TEN with more mucous membrane disease. Drugs are usually the causative factor especially in adults. Most commonly implicated are sulfonamides, anticonvulsants, and NSAIDs. There may be a genetic predisposition to this bullous drug reaction. Therapy is supportive, and an appreciable number of cases are fatal. Intravenous immunoglobulins (IVIG) may be life saving. Cyclosporine is a preferred mode of therapy by some authors. High-dose systemic corticosteroids are controversial with opinions ranging from contraindicated to life saving if given in very high doses very early in the course of the disease. Wound care is essential. Debridement should be avoided. Silver nitrate irrigation and soft gauze dressings (Sof Sorb Gauze, which may be fitted on as a garment) are used in wound care. This is usually done in an intensive care unit because electrolyte and fluid balance is crucial. A central venous line helps greatly in managing these patients. The most crucial factor in survival is stopping any potential offending drug as quickly as possible. Acute graft-versus-host disease can be an identical disease process and should be treated in a similar manner.

- *Staphylococcal scalded skin syndrome:* Clinically, this disorder is similar to TEN but has been separated from this disease because of the finding that phage group 2 *S. aureus* is the usual cause. In newborns, this formerly was known as Ritter von Ritterschein's disease. It also occurs in children and rarely adults. The prognosis is very favorable. If suspected, anti-staphylococcus drugs should be started intravenously immediately. The break in the skin is higher in the epidermis than in drug-induced TEN and this can be rapidly ascertained with a skin biopsy.

- *Impetigo herpetiformis:* One of the rarest of skin diseases, this disease is characterized by groups of pustules mainly seen in the axillae and the groin, high fever, prostration, severe malaise, and, generally, a fatal outcome. It occurs most commonly in pregnant or postpartum women. It can be distinguished from pemphigus vegetans or dermatitis herpetiformis by the fact that these diseases do not produce such general, acute, toxic manifestations. Laboratory abnormalities include elevated white blood count, elevated sedimentation rate, and low calcium, phosphate albumin, and vitamin D levels. Bacterial cultures of skin and blood are negative, high-dose (60 to 100 mg/d) prednisone and fluid and electrolyte replacement can be life saving.

In spite of high medical student and general practitioner interest in the bullous skin conditions, the diagnosis and the management of the three main bullous skin diseases, bullous pemphigoid, pemphigus vulgaris, and dermatitis herpetiformis, should be in the realm of the dermatologist. In this chapter, the salient features of these diseases are presented, with therapy briefly outlined.

Pemphigus Vulgaris

Pemphigus vulgaris is rare. These patients are miserable, odoriferous, and debilitated (Fig. 18-1; see also Fig. 3-1F and Chap. 10). Before the advent of corticosteroid therapy, the disease was fatal.

Presentation and Characteristics

Primary Lesions

The early lesions of pemphigus are small vesicles or bullae that appear on apparently normal skin. Redness of the base of the bullae is unusual. Without treatment, the bullae enlarge and spread, and new ones balloon up on different areas of the skin or the mucous membranes. Rarely, mucous

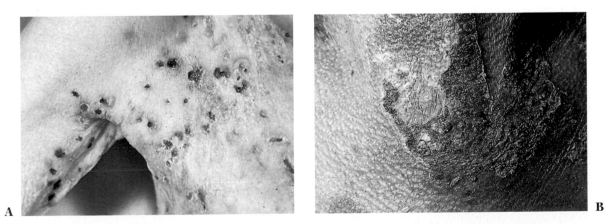

FIGURE 18-1 ■ **(A)** Pemphigus vulgaris on anterior chest and right arm areas. **(B)** Pemphigus vulgaris on neck area. *(Courtesy of Roche Laboratories.)*

membrane lesions may be the main or only manifestation of the disease. Rupturing of the bullae leaves large eroded areas. Nikolsky's sign is positive; that is, a top layer of the skin adjacent to a bulla readily separates from the underlying skin after firm but gentle pressure.

Secondary Lesions

Bacterial infection with crusting is marked and accounts, in part, for the characteristic mousy odor. Lesions that heal spontaneously or under therapy do not leave scars.

Course

When untreated, pemphigus vulgaris can be rapidly fatal or assume a slow lingering course, with debility, painful mouth and body erosions, systemic bacterial infection, and toxemia. Spontaneous temporary remissions do occur without therapy. The following clinical variations of pemphigus also exist:

- *Pemphigus vegetans* is characterized by the development of large granulomatous masses in the intertriginous areas of the axillae and the groin. Secondary bacterial infection, although often present in all cases of pemphigus, is most marked in this form. Pemphigus vegetans is to be differentiated from a granulomatous ioderma or bromoderma (see Chap. 9) and from impetigo herpetiformis (see beginning of this chapter). This type of pemphigus can often be treated more conservatively such as with potent topical corticosteroids.
- *Pemphigus foliaceus* (fogo selvagem) appears as a scaly, moist, generalized exfoliative dermatitis. The characteristic mousy odor of pemphigus is dominant in this variant, which is also remarkable for its chronicity. The response to corticosteroid therapy is less favorable in the foliaceus form than in the other types (see also Chap. 37 for a Brazilian form). Complimentary DNA cloning has shown the autoimmune target to be desmolgein 1. There is some evidence that this may be a disease born by an insect vector in tropical areas near rivers.
- *Pemphigus erythematosus* clinically resembles a mixture of pemphigus vulgaris, seborrheic dermatitis, and lupus erythematosus. The distribution of the red, greasy, crusted, and eroded lesions is on the butterfly area of the face, the sternal area, the scalp, and occasionally in the mouth. The course is more chronic than for pemphigus vulgaris, and remissions are common.
- *Pemphigus herpetiformis* appears as grouped vesicles, bullae, erythematous papules that are very pruritic. DIF of IgG in upper or entire epidermal cell surfaces and circulating IgG autoantibodies.
- *IgA pemphigus* shows flaccid, pruritic vesicles or pustules in an annular pattern with central crusting. DIF with IgA or epidermal cell surfaces in upper, lesion, or entire surface. Fifty percent of patients have circulating IgA autoantibodies.
- *Paraneoplastic pemphigus* is an often fatal, severe, rare, polymorphous eruption with erosions, bullae, or targetoid lesions and severe mucous membrane disease. DIF shows IgG on all epidermal surfaces and often linear confluent deposits at dermoepidermal junction; complement may also be on epidermal surfaces. Circulating IgG autoantibodies and 75% with circulating IgG to rat bladder epithelium. Non-Hodgkin's lymphoma is the commonest underlying malignancy.

Some dermatologists believe that pemphigus foliaceus and pemphigus erythematosus may be distinct diseases from pemphigus vulgaris and vegetans.

Causes

The cause of pemphigus vulgaris is unknown, but autoimmunity is a factor. Some cases are associated with underlying malignancy (paraneoplastic pemphigus). Paraneoplastic pemphigus has unique immunofluorescent findings and is usually rapidly fatal. Human herpesvirus 8 has been isolated from the skin lesions of some patients.

Laboratory Findings

The histopathology of early cases is characteristic and serves to differentiate most cases of pemphigus vulgaris from dermatitis herpetiformis and the other bullous diseases. Acantholysis, or separation of intercellular contact between the keratinocytes, is characteristic. The bulla is intraepidermal. Cytologic smears (Tzanck test) for diagnosis of pemphigus vulgaris reveal numerous rounded acantholytic epidermal cells with large nuclei in condensed cytoplasm. Antiepithelial autoantibodies against the intercellular substance are found by direct and indirect immunofluorescent tests. Fresh tissue biopsy specimens taken from noninvolved skin best show immunoglobulins. Indirect immunofluorescent tests are performed on serum. Complimentary DNA cloning shows the autoimmune target to be desmoglein 3.

Differential Diagnosis

See introduction to this chapter as well as the sections on dermatitis herpetiformis and erythema multiforme bullosum.

Treatment

1. If possible, a dermatologist and internist should be called in to share the responsibility of the care.
2. Hospitalization is necessary for the patient with large areas of bullae and erosions. Mild cases of pemphigus can be managed in the office.
3. Prednisone, 10 mg #100

   Sig: One or 2 tablets q.i.d. until healing occurs; then reduce the dose slowly as warranted.

   Comment: Very high doses of prednisone may be needed to produce a remission in severe cases.

4. Local therapy is prescribed to make the patient more comfortable and to decrease the odor by reducing secondary infection. This can be accomplished by the following, which must be varied for individual cases:

   a. Potassium permanganate crystals 60.0

      Sig: Place 2 teaspoonfuls of the crystals in the bathtub with approximately 10 inches of lukewarm water.

      Comment: To prevent crystals from burning the skin they should be dissolved completely in a glass of water before adding to the tub. The solution should be made fresh daily. The tub stains can be removed by applying acetic acid or "hypo" solution.

   b. Talc 120.0

      Sig: Dispense in powder can. Apply to bed sheeting and to erosions twice a day (called a "powder bed").

   c. Polysporin, Bactroban, or other antibiotic ointment q.s. 60.0

      Sig: Apply to small infected areas b.i.d.

5. Supportive therapy should be used when necessary. This includes vitamins, iron, blood transfusions, and oral antibiotics. Dapsone and gold therapy can be used with benefit in some cases as a corticosteroid-sparing agent. Methotrexate, azathioprine, cyclosporine, and other immunosuppressive therapy are also being used. IVIG may invoke long-term remission in some patients.

6. Nursing care of the highest caliber is a prerequisite for the severe case of pemphigus with generalized erosions and bullae. The nursing personnel should be told that this disease is not contagious or infectious. Surgical dressings such as Mepotil that are not adherent but quite protective may be of great benefit.

7. Mycophenolate mofetil may be an effective and safer immunosuppressive drug according to some authors.

8. Sun avoidance and sunscreen use may be beneficial especially in pemphigus vulgaris and pemphigus foliaceus.

9. Plasmapheresis has been used with some success.

10. Immunoablative cytoxan has been used in paraneoplastic pemphigus and life-threatening recalcitrant disease.

Dermatitis Herpetiformis (Duhring's Disease)

Dermatitis herpetiformis is a rare, chronic, markedly pruritic, papular, vesicular, and bullous skin disease of unknown etiology (Fig. 18-2). It is probably an autoimmune disease and activated via the alternate complement pathway. The patient describes the itching of a new blister as a burning itch that disappears when the blister top is scratched off. The severe scratching results in the formation of excoriations and papular hives, which may be the only visible pathology of the disease. Individual lesions heal, leaving an area of hyperpigmentation that is very

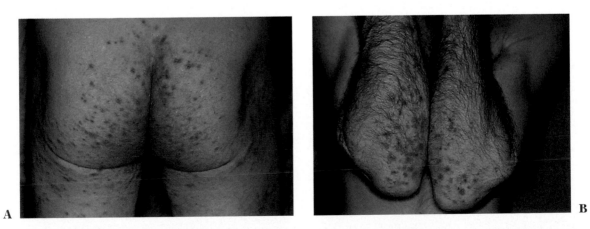

FIGURE 18-2 ■ Dermatitis herpetiform on buttocks (**A**) and on elbows (**B**) of same patient. *(Courtesy of Roche Laboratories.)*

characteristic. The typical distribution of the blisters or excoriations is on the scalp, sacral area, buttocks, scapular area, forearms, elbows, and thighs. Large spared areas especially over the trunk are sometimes seen. In some cases, the resulting bullae may be indistinguishable from pemphigus or bullous pemphigoid.

The duration of dermatitis herpetiformis varies from months to as long as 40 years, with periods of remission scattered in between. The illness is associated with nontropical sprue.

Laboratory tests should include fixed tissue and fresh tissue biopsy. The latter shows in most cases granular IgA in the dermal papillae of perilesional, along with the third component of complement (C3). The finding of endomysial antibodies in the blood is highly specific for the disease. A blood cell count usually shows an eosinophilia.

Herpes gestationis (see Fig. 33-11D–E) is a vesicular and bullous disease that occurs in relation to pregnancy. It usually develops during the second or the third trimester and commonly disappears after giving birth, only to return with subsequent pregnancies. The histologic features are believed significantly distinctive so that this disease can be separated from dermatitis herpetiformis. Immunologic findings of C3 bound to the basement membrane of the epidermis and occasional IgG deposition may be significant. Therapy with systemic corticosteroids is usually indicated.

Differential Diagnosis

- *Pemphigus vulgaris:* Large, flaccid bullae; mouth involvement more common; debilitating course; biopsy specimen characteristic; eosinophilia is uncommon (see Pemphigus)
- *Erythema multiforme bullosum:* Bullae usually arise on a red, iris-like base; burning itch is absent; residual pigmentation is minor; course is shorter and palmar–plantar lesions are common (see following section)
- *Neurotic excoriations:* If this diagnosis is being considered, it is very important to rule out dermatitis herpetiformis. In a case of neurotic excoriations one usually does not find scalp lesions, blisters, or eosinophilia. Skin lesions seen only where the patient can reach. If right handed then it is often worse on the left side of the body. The skin biopsy is helpful.
- *Scabies:* No vesicles (rarely can occur) or bullae; burrows and lesions are found in other members of the household (see Chap. 21). KOH scraping is diagnostic.

- *Subcorneal pustular dermatosis (Sneddon Wilkinson Disease):* Rare, chronic dermatosis characterized by an annular and serpiginous arrangement of pustules and vesiculopustules on the abdomen, groin, and axillae. Histopathologically, the pustule is found directly beneath the stratum corneum. Dapsone (avlosulfone) or sulfapyridine therapy is effective.

Treatment

A dermatologist should be consulted to establish the diagnosis and to outline therapy, which consists of local and oral measures to control itching and a course of one of the following quite effective drugs: sulfapyridine (0.5 g q.i.d.) or dapsone (25 mg t.i.d.). Rapid response to these medicines should make the diagnosis suspect. These initial doses should be decreased or increased depending on the patient's response. These drugs can be toxic, and the patient must be under the close surveillance of the physician. They should be avoided in the presence of a G6PD deficiency. Mild to moderate anemia is present in almost all patients on chronic dapsone therapy, but is usually well tolerated. Dapsone can cause liver damage and pancytopenia. A diet that is gluten free is curative for both the skin and the bowel disease, but it must be maintained for a lifetime and is a very difficult diet to follow. It takes a committed physician and patient to maintain a gluten-free diet.

Erythema Multiforme Bullosum

Erythema multiforme bullosum has a clinical picture and course distinct from that of erythema multiforme (Fig. 18-3; see Chap. 12). Many drugs can cause an erythema multiforme bullosum–like picture, but then this manifestation should be labeled a "drug eruption."

True erythema multiforme bullosum has no known cause. Clinically, one sees large vesicles and bullae usually overlying red, iris-like macules. The lesions most commonly appear on the arms, legs, and face, but can occur elsewhere, including, on occasion, the mouth. Erythema multiforme bullosum can last from days to months.

Slight malaise and fever may precede a new shower of bullae, but for the most part the patient's general health is unaffected. Itching may be mild or severe enough to interfere with sleep.

When the characteristic iris lesions are absent, it is difficult to differentiate this bullous eruption from early pemphigus vulgaris, dermatitis herpetiformis, and bullous pemphigoid. However, the histopathology and immunofluorescent studies are often helpful. Direct and indirect immunofloarescence studies are negative.

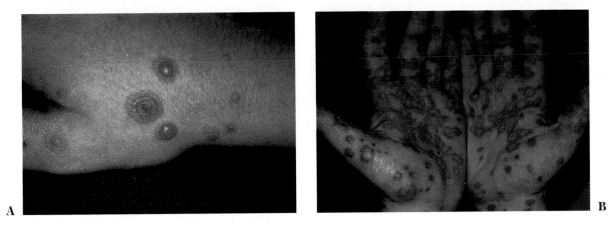

FIGURE 18-3 ■ Erythema multiforme bullosum on dorsum of hand (**A**) and on palms (**B**) 5 days later in same patient. *(Courtesy of Roche Laboratories.)*

Treatment

These patients should be referred to a dermatologist or an internist to substantiate the diagnosis and initiate therapy. Corticosteroids orally and by injection are the single most effective drugs in use today. For widespread cases requiring hospitalization, the local care is similar to that for pemphigus.

Suggested Reading

Ahmed AR, Kurgis BS, Rogers RS III. Cicatricial pemphigoid. J Am Acad Dermatol 1991;24:987.

Bastuji-Gavin S, Rzany B, Stern RS, et al. Clinical classification of cases of toxic epidermal necrolysis, Stevens-Johnson syndrome, and erythema multiforme. Arch Dermatol 1993;129:92.

Diaz LA, Sampaio SA, Rivitti EA, et al. Endemic pemphigus foliaceus (fogo selvagem). J Am Acad Dermatol 1989;20:657.

Jordon RE. Atlas of Bullous Disease. Philadelphia, WB Saunders, 2000.

Rogers RS III. Bullous pemphigoid: Therapy and management. J Geriatr Dermatol 1995;3:91.

Stanley JR. Therapy of pemphigus vulgaris. Arch Dermatol 1999;135:76–78.

Zemstov A, Neldner KH. Successful treatment of dermatitis herpetiformis with tetracycline and nicotinamide in a patient unable to tolerate dapsone. J Am Acad Dermatol 1993;28:505.

CHAPTER 19

Exfoliative Dermatitis

John C. Hall

As the term implies, *exfoliative dermatitis* is a generalized scaling eruption of the skin. The causes are many. This diagnosis should never be made without additional qualifying etiologic terms.

This is a rare skin condition, but many general physicians, residents, and interns see these cases because the patients are occasionally hospitalized. Hospitalization serves two purposes, namely to (1) perform a diagnostic workup, because the cause, in many cases, is difficult to ascertain and (2) administer intensive therapy under close supervision, especially in cases where the overall condition of the patient is poor. Exfoliative dermatitis can lead to sepsis, high-output congestive heart failure, and dehydration.

Classification of the cases of exfoliative dermatitis is facilitated by dividing them into primary and secondary forms.

Primary Exfoliative Dermatitis

These cases develop in apparently healthy persons from no ascertainable cause.

SAUER'S NOTES

1. From the history, ascertain where the exfoliative eruption began on the body. This information can aid in establishing the cause.
2. Look at the edge of an advancing exfoliative dermatitis for the characteristic lesions of the primary disease, if present.
3. As the exfoliative dermatitis becomes more widespread the characteristics of the original skin disease become less obvious or completely disappear. History, therefore, may be critical in making the correct diagnosis.
4. The underlying cause may not be apparent at the first evaluation and a nonspecific skin biopsy may be present. With time, however, the underlying cause, such as CTCL, may become evident. This is why close follow-up with repeated skin biopsy attempts is important.

Presentation and Characteristics

Skin Lesions

Clinically it may be impossible to differentiate this primary form from the one in which the cause is known or suspected. Various degrees of scaling and redness are seen, ranging from fine, generalized, granular scales with mild erythema to scaling in large plaques, with marked erythema (generalized erythroderma) and lichenification. Widespread lymphadenopathy is usually present. The nails become thick and lusterless, and the hair falls out in varying degrees.

Subjective Complaint

Itching, in most cases, is intense. The patient may be toxic.

Course

The prognosis for early cure of the disease is poor. The mortality rate is high in older patients because of generalized debility and secondary infection.

Causes

Various authors have studied the relationship of lymphomas to cases of exfoliative dermatitis. Some believe the incidence to be low, but others state that from 35% to 50% of these exfoliative cases, particularly those in patients older than the age of 40 years, are the result of lymphomas. However, years may pass before the lymphoma becomes obvious.

Laboratory Findings

There are no diagnostic changes, but the patient with a usual case has an elevated white blood cell count with eosinophilia. Biopsy of the skin is not diagnostic in the primary type, but may help to rule out a more specific diagnosis. Biopsy of an enlarged lymph node, in either the primary or the secondary form, reveals lipomelanotic reticulosis (dermatopathic lymphadenopathy) which is benign.

Treatment

Case Example. A 50-year-old man presents with a generalized, pruritic, scaly, erythematous eruption that he has had for 3 months.

First Visit.

1. A general medical workup is indicated.
2. A high-protein diet should be prescribed because these patients have an increased basal metabolic rate and catabolize protein.
3. Bathing instructions are variable. Some patients prefer a daily cool bath in a colloid solution for relief of itching (one box of soluble starch or 1 cup of Aveeno to 10 inches of water). For most cases, however, generalized bathing dries the skin and intensifies the itching.
4. Provide extra blankets for the bed. These patients lose a lot of heat through their red skin and consequently feel chilly.
5. Locally, an ointment is most desired, but some patients prefer an oily liquid. Formulas for both follow:

    a. White petrolatum 240.0

    or a generic corticosteroid ointment, such as triamcinolone 0.025% ointment 240.0
    Sig: Apply locally b.i.d.

    b. Zinc oxide 40%

    Olive oil q.s. 240.0
    Sig: Apply locally with hands or a paintbrush b.i.d.
    Comment: Antipruritic chemicals can also be added to this.

6. Oral antihistamine, for example:

    Chlorpheniramine, 8 or 12 mg #100
    Sig: 1 tablet b.i.d. for itching. Warn patient of possible drowsiness.

Subsequent Visits.

1. Systemic corticosteroids: For resistant cases, the corticosteroids have consistently provided more relief than any other single form of therapy. Any of the preparations can be used; for example:

    Prednisone, 10 mg #100
    Sig: 4 tablets every morning for 1 week, then 2 tablets every morning.
    Comment: Regulate dosage as indicated.

2. Systemic antibiotics may or may not be indicated.

Secondary Exfoliative Dermatitis

Most patients with secondary exfoliative dermatitis have had a previous skin disease that became generalized because of overtreatment or for unknown reasons. There always remain a few cases of exfoliative dermatitis in which the cause is unknown but suspected.

Presentation and Characteristics

Skin Lesions

The clinical picture of this secondary form is indistinguishable from the primary form unless some of the original dermatitis is present. As the exfoliation and erythroderma spread the characteristics of a primary skin disease, such as psoriasis, become harder to ascertain (Fig. 19-1).

Course

The prognosis in the secondary form is better than for the primary form, particularly if the original cause is definitely known and more specific therapy can be administered.

Causes

The more common causes of secondary exfoliative dermatitis are as follows.

- Contact dermatitis (see Chap. 9)
- Drug eruption (see Chap. 9)
- Psoriasis (see Chap. 14)
- Atopic eczema (see Chap. 9)
- Pyoderma or other severe localized inflammation with a secondary id reaction (see Chap. 21)
- Inflammatory fungal disease (i.e., a kerion) with id reaction (see Chap. 25)
- Seborrheic dermatitis, especially in a newborn or an AIDS patient (see Chap. 13)
- T-cell lymphoma, especially cutaneous T-cell lymphoma (CTCL) (see Chap. 26). A useful rule is that 50% of all patients older than age 50 years who have an exfoliative dermatitis have a lymphoma. The Sézary syndrome form of lymphoma is a rare cause of exfoliative dermatitis. It is considered the leukemic form of CTCL.
- Internal cancer, leukemia, and other lymphomas

Treatment

The treatment of these cases consists of a combination of the treatment for the primary form of exfoliative dermatitis plus the cautious institution of stronger therapy directed toward the original causative skin condition. This therapy should be reviewed in the section devoted to the specific disease (see above).

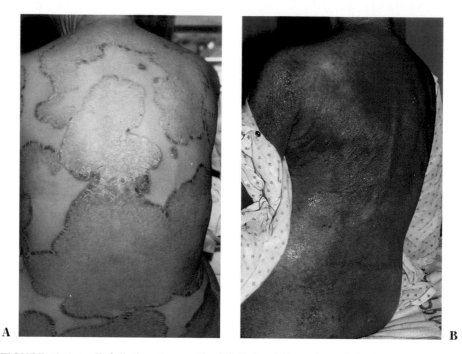

FIGURE 19-1 ■ Exfoliative dermatitis. (**A**) Only at the edge of the large plaques is there a suggestion of psoriasis as the underlying diagnosis. (**B**) Exfoliative dermatitis due to a Dilantin drug eruption.

Suggested Reading

Botella-Estrada R, Sanmartin O, Oliver V, et al. Erythroderma. Arch Dermatol 1994;130:1503.

Pal S, Haroon TS. Erythroderma: A clinico-etiologic study of 90 cases. Int J Dermatol 1998;37:104.

Wilson DC, Jester JD, King LE Jr. Erythroderma and exfoliative dermatitis [review]. Clin Dermatol 1993;11:67.

CHAPTER 20

Psychodermatology

John Koo and Ellen de Coninck

Psychodermatology and *psychocutaneous medicine* are unfamiliar terms to many physicians. These terms describe a field of medicine that focuses on the interface between psychiatry and dermatology. In a surprisingly large proportion of dermatologic disorders, understanding of the psychosocial and, sometimes, the occupational context is critical to optimal management. Examples range from common skin rashes, such as eczema or psoriasis, to flaring under emotional stress, to cases in which there is no real skin disorder, but the patient targets his or her skin to express an underlying psychopathologic condition; neurotic excoriations, trichotillomania, and delusions of parasitosis are examples. Moreover, because skin disease is visible, patients commonly experience significant negative impact on their psychological stability resulting from disfigurement caused by the skin disorder. Patients with disfiguring skin disorders, such as alopecia areata, vitiligo, and psoriasis frequently report problems with self-esteem, depression, and social anxiety.

The management of psychodermatologic disorders requires special skills. First, to understand what is going on and what the actual diagnosis is, a clinician must not only evaluate the skin manifestation based on the usual dermatologic differential diagnosis, but also evaluate the underlying psychopathology and the relevant social, familial, and occupational issues. Once the diagnosis is made, optimal management often requires a dual approach to address both the dermatologic and the psychological aspects. Even in cases where the main problem is psychopathologic and the skin manifestation are entirely self-induced, the authors cannot overemphasize the importance of maintaining supportive dermatologic care to avoid secondary complications such as infection and to ensure that the patient does not feel "abandoned" by the nonpsychiatric physician. Such demonstrated support by the nonpsychiatric physician can enhance acceptance by the patient of a psychiatric consultation or referral, should there be a need for one. At the same time, it is important for the clinician to try to understand the nature of the underlying psychopathology so the appropriate psychiatric management can be initiated. This ranges from providing appropriate psychotropic medication and encouraging the patient to attend stress-management courses to making a formal referral to a psychiatrist, depending on severity of the underlying psychopathology. Psychodermatology cases, just like those in any other field of medical practice, can range from mild to severe. In fact, when a clinician becomes aware of the mind–skin interaction and looks for psychological elements in skin patients, he or she finds that the large majority of these patients have easily treatable psychopathologies impacting on their skin disease, such as situational stress or mild depression. On the other hand, clinicians who are not fully aware of this field are often only reminded of the skin–mind interaction when they encounter the most difficult and most florid cases, such as delusions of parasitosis. It is the recommendation of the authors that clinicians become familiar with the entire range of psychodermatologic disorders so that their perception of this field is not warped by only being forced to deal with the most difficult and most frustrating cases.

Classification

Psychodermatologic disorders can be broadly classified into four categories: psychophysiologic disorders, primary psychiatric disorders, secondary psychiatric disorders, and miscellaneous cases. *Psychophysiologic disorder* refers to a situation where a real skin disorder, such as eczema or psoriasis, is worsened by emotional stress. *Primary psychiatric disorder* refers to cases such as trichotillomania where the primary problem is psychological; there is no primary skin disorder and all the manifestations are self-induced. *Secondary psychiatric disorder* refers to those cases where significant psychological problems, such as profoundly negative impact on self-esteem and body image, depression, humiliation, frustration, and social phobia, develop as a consequence of having a disfiguring skin disorder. The "miscellaneous" category refers to less well-defined situations where involvement of the central nervous system is suspected, such as cutaneous sensory syndrome. In this condition, a patient with no visible rash presents to a clinician with a purely sensory complaint, such as itching, burning, or stinging, but an extensive medical workup fails to reveal an underlying diagnosis. These patients usually respond better to psychotropic medications than to usual dermatologic therapeutics, such as topical steroids.

It is important to be able to distinguish between these broad categories for several reasons. First, the severity of the underlying psychopathologic condition tends to be different depending on the categories, with psychophysiologic disorders generally involving "milder" psychopathologies (such as situational stress) than the primary psychiatric disorders. Second, the approach to patients is frequently different among these categories. For example, with psychophysiologic cases, it is easy to talk to the patient about their situation, whereas in certain cases of primary psychiatric disorder, such as delusions of parasitosis or neurotic excoriation with underlying depression that is being denied by the patient, one must be extremely diplomatic, because these patients may not be ready to be confronted with the psychogenic aspect of their condition.

Psychophysiologic Disorders

Psychophysiologic disorders are skin disorders that are known to be frequently precipitated or exacerbated by emotional stress. However, with each of these conditions, there are "stress responders" and "non–stress responders," depending on whether a patient's skin disease is or is not frequently and predictably exacerbated by stress.

The proportion of stress responders depends on the particular dermatologic diagnosis involved. In minor, treatment-responsive cases of eczema, psoriasis, or acne, the issue of stress may not be that important. However, when a clinician is faced with a more recalcitrant case, it is important to remember to ask the patient whether psychological, social, or occupational stress might be contributing to the activity of the skin disorder. Because of the propensity of so many chronic dermatoses to be exacerbated by emotional stress, and because emotional stress can initiate a vicious cycle referred to as the *itch–scratch cycle,* recalcitrant patients with chronic dermatoses may be difficult to "turn around" without addressing stress as an exacerbating factor.

With regard to psychological issues, patients often feel embarrassed discussing it, especially if they feel hurried. Once the clinician inquires, patients are frequently glad to share whatever psychosocial or occupational stress might be exacerbating or perpetuating the dermatitis. If the situation is relatively mild, simple encouragement by an authority figure (the physician) to join a stress-management class, study relaxation techniques, or even use music or exercise as a stress reducer might suffice. If there is a specific psychosocial or occupational or issue that needs to be vented, referral to a therapist or counselor is appropriate.

If the stress or tension is of significant intensity to warrant considering the use of an anti-anxiety agent, there are three general types of agents available to meet these clinical needs. The first type, the benzodiazepines, can be used on an as-needed basis and can provide relatively quick relief from anxiety, "stress," and tension. The authors generally recommend relatively "newer" benzodiazepines, such as alprazolam (Xanax), available generically, rather than the much older ones, such as diazepam (Valium) or chlordiazepoxide (Librium), that are more often associated with possible cumulative side effects owing to their longer or unpredictable half-lives. Benzodiazepines should be reserved for short-term situations whenever possible because continued usage for more than several weeks can be associated with tolerance, dependence, and withdrawal.

On the other hand, if the "stress" proves to be a chronic predicament, a nonsedating and nonaddictive anti-anxiety agent such as buspirone (BuSpar) is safer for long-term use. Because of its slower onset of action, which may take up to 2 weeks or more, buspirone cannot be used on an as-needed basis. A common starting dose is 15 mg/d in divided doses, followed by 15 mg twice a day for 1 week, and up to 60 mg/d if required. The therapeutic range for most patients is between 15 and 30 mg/d. It is not uncommon for a benzodiazepine to be started in conjunction with buspirone and then tapered after 2 or 4 weeks after the therapeutic effect of buspirone is achieved.

Antidepressants are the third type of agents used in the treatment of anxiety. The antidepressant agent paroxetine (Paxil) and venlafaxine (Effexor) are examples of selective serotonin reuptake inhibitors (SSRIs) that are useful not only in the treatment of depression, but also in the treatment of chronic anxiety. It was found in an open-label study of paroxetine, imipramine, and a benzodiazepine that by the fourth week of treatment, paroxetine and imipramine were superior to the benzodiazepine for the relief of anxiety symptoms. Furthermore, the effectiveness of a venlafaxine extended-release preparation (Effexor XR) was demonstrated in a series of double-blind randomized, placebo-controlled trials in the treatment of patients with generalized anxiety disorder.

If the intensity and the complexity of the anxiety disorder warrants a psychiatric referral, such a referral should be discussed with the patient in a most supportive and diplomatic way so as to maximize the chance of the patient accepting the referral as an adjunct to continuing dermatologic therapy.

Primary Psychiatric Disorders

Primary psychiatric disorders are less commonly encountered than those in which stress exacerbates a common dermatosis. However, they tend to be more "florid" with striking presentation.

Delusions of Parasitosis

Delusions of parasitosis belong to a group of disorders called *monosymptomatic hypochondriacal psychosis* (MHP), where seemingly "normal" patients present with an encapsulated, somatic delusional ideation of a hypochondriacal nature. Because of the truly encapsulated nature of the delusional disorder, these cases are usually quite different from schizophrenia, which involves multiple functional defects, including auditory hallucinations, lack of social skills, and flat affect in addition to delusional ideation.

The most common form of MHP encountered by dermatologists is called *delusion of parasitosis.* In this type of MHP, patients firmly believe that their bodies are infested by some type of organism. They frequently present with elaborate ideation involving how these "organisms" mate, reproduce, move in the skin, and, sometimes, come out of the skin. Patients often present with the "matchbox" sign, in which bits of excoriated skin, debris, or unrelated insects or insect parts are brought in matchboxes or other containers as proof of infestation (Figs. 20-1 and 20-2).

Differential Diagnosis

The psychiatric differential diagnosis includes

- schizophrenia,
- psychotic depression,

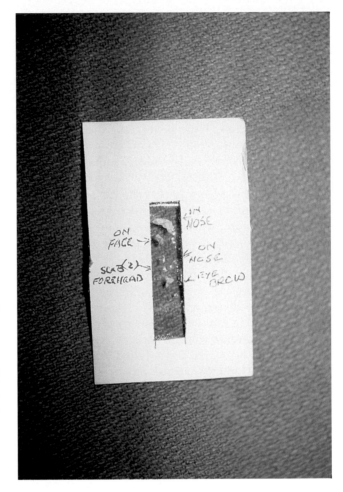

FIGURE 20-2 ■ A carefully constructed specimen board of alleged parasites from another patient with delusions of parasitosis.

- psychosis with florid mania,
- drug-induced and other forms of psychosis, and
- formication without delusions, in which the patient experiences crawling, biting, and stinging sensations without believing that they are due to organisms.

The other organic forms of psychosis include

- vitamin B_{12} deficiency,
- withdrawal from cocaine, amphetamines, or alcohol,
- multiple sclerosis,
- cerebrovascular disease, and
- syphilis.

If any of these other underlying diagnoses are made, the separate diagnosis of delusions of parasitosis is not made.

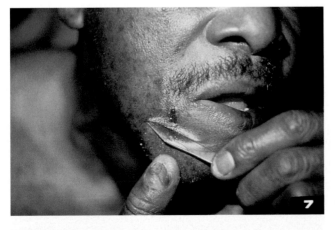

FIGURE 20-1 ■ A man with delusions of parasitosis uses his knife to dig out a "parasite" to demonstrate it to the author (J.K.).

Once again, delusions of parasitosis is a separate psychiatric entity characterized by very encapsulated ideation, where none of the other psychiatric diagnoses are involved.

Treatment

Currently, the treatment of choice for delusions of parasitosis is an antipsychotic medication called pimozide (ORAP). This antipsychotic medication with a chemical structure and potency similar to haloperidol (Haldol) has been known to be uniquely effective for this condition, especially in decreasing formication (crawling, stinging, and biting sensations). The dosage used is much lower than that used for chronic schizophrenics. Pimozide is generally started at the lowest possible dose of half a tablet (1 mg) and increased by 1 mg per week. By the time the dosage of 4 to 6 mg (two to three tablets) is reached, most patients experience a great decrease in crawling and biting sensations, as well as the sensations of "organisms" moving in their skin. At the same time, patients generally become much less agitated. In younger patients, pimozide can often be continued at the lowest effect dose for several months then gradually tapered off without necessarily inviting recurrence of the symptoms. If the condition recurs, another course of therapy with pimozide can be instituted.

The main adverse effects of pimozide are its extrapyramidal side effects (EPS), just as with many other antipsychotic agents. The most common of these, namely stiffness and restlessness, can be effectively treated with benztropine (Cogentin) 2 mg up to 4 times per day. Diphenhydramine (Benadryl) 25 mg can also be substituted for benztropine. In elderly patients, long-term maintenance with a very small dose of pimozide (1 to 2 mg/d) is sometimes required. Although the long-term side effect of tardive dyskinesia is a possibility, the risk appears to be minimal in dermatology patients where a low dose (6 mg/d or less) is generally adequate and where the medication is often used intermittently. If the patient has a cardiac rhythm disorder, is elderly, or if a dosage higher than 10 mg/d is needed, then serial electrocardiograms are required.

A new generation of antipsychotic agents, called *atypical antipsychotics* have recently been introduced into clinical practice. These atypical antipsychotics, which include risperidone (Risperdal), olanzapine (Zyprexa), and quetiapine (Seroquel), are as effective as conventional antipsychotics for the treatment of psychosis in general, are better tolerated, and cause significantly less EPS and tardive dyskinesia in placebo-controlled studies as well as in clinical practice. Given this much safer side effect profile, atypical antipsychotics may prove useful in the treatment of MHP, although studies comparing pimozide with the new atypical antipsychotics in the treatment of delusions of parasitosis have not yet been performed.

A word of caution when using atypical antipsychotics in patients with a history of seizures or with conditions such as Alzheimer's disease that potentially lower the seizure threshold: Premarketing testing found that seizures occurred in 22 (0.9%) of 2500 olanzapine-treated patients, 18 (0.8%) of 2387 quetiapine-treated patients, and 9 (0.3%) of 2607 risperidone-treated patients.

Neurotic Excoriations/Factitial Dermatitis

Neurotic excoriations is used when individuals self-inflict excoriations (scratch marks) with the fingernails. Although *neurotic excoriations* and *factitial dermatitis* are sometimes used interchangeably, *factitial dermatitis* should be used more selectively to refer to situations where the patient uses something more elaborate than the fingernails, such as lit cigarette butts, chemicals, or sharp instruments, to damage his or her own skin. Although *neurotic excoriations* contains the word *neurotic*, clinicians need to recognize that this term is essentially dermatologic and does not imply any particular psychopathology in the patient. In fact, the clinician needs to go a step further and determine what the underlying psychopathology is. The most common underlying psychopathologies encountered are major depressive episodes, anxiety, and obsessive–compulsive disorders. Rarely, patients excoriate their skin in response to a delusional ideation, in which case psychosis is the appropriate diagnosis. Patients with neurotic excoriations are usually suffering from depression or anxiety, whereas those with factitial dermatitis tend to be much "sicker" psychologically and they more frequently represent manifestations of underlying psychosis characterized by a delusional ideation (Fig. 20-3).

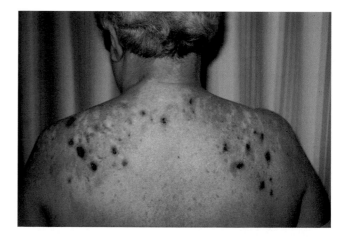

FIGURE 20-3 ■ Multiple neurotic excoriations are present only in the areas easily accessed by the patient's hands on the back of this depressed woman.

Treatment

The management of anxiety is as discussed. However, if the patient proves to have underlying depression resulting in neurotic excoriations, one antidepressant that is frequently used by dermatologists is doxepin (Sinequan). Doxepin is a tricyclic antidepressant with one of the most powerful antiitch and antihistamine effects, as well as sedative/tranquilizing effects. Because many people with depression who excoriate their skin tend to be agitated ("agitated depression"), the sedative and tranquilizing effects of doxepin frequently prove to be therapeutic in addition to its antidepressant effects. Moreover, the profound antipruritic effect is also an added benefit; even though these patients create their own skin lesions, as they keep picking on their skin and not letting them heal, the itch–scratch cycle can become an issue, which can effectively be addressed with the antipruritic effect of doxepin (Fig. 20-4).

The use of doxepin requires all of the usual precautions regarding the use of older tricyclic antidepressants, including absence of cardiac arrhythmias; doxepin can cause QT prolongation. A detailed description is beyond the scope of this chapter; however, it should be mentioned that if the patient is truly depressed, an antidepressant dosage of 100 mg/d or higher is usually required so that the patient is not undertreated. Elderly patients may respond to a lower dose.

Trichotillomania

Trichotillomania, according to the dermatologic usage of the word, refers to any patient who pulls out his or her own hair. The psychiatric definition of trichotillomania requires the presence of "impulsivity." However, using the less specific dermatologic definition, the clinician once again needs to ascertain the nature of the underlying psychopathology to select the most appropriate treatment. The most common underlying psychopathology is obsessive–compulsive behavior, whether or not it formally meets the DSM-IV criteria for obsessive–compulsive disorder. The other possible underlying psychiatric diagnosis includes depression with or without anxiety, as well as extremely rare cases of delusion, in which the patient pulls out his or her hair based on the delusional belief that something in the roots needs to be "dug out" for the hair to grow normally. This latter, rare clinical condition is called *trichophobia.*

Trichotillomania is one of the rare conditions in which a pathologic examination of the skin can be diagnostic. There is a unique change in the hair root called *trichomalacia,* which is only seen in trichotillomania. Therefore, if the patient continues to deny pulling his or her own hair, a scalp biopsy can be helpful in determining the diagnosis.

Treatment

As with other conditions, treatment is based on the nature of the underlying psychopathology. Because the most common underlying psychopathology is obsessive–compulsive tendency, medications such as fluoxetine (Prozac), paroxetine (Paxil), fluvoxamine (Luvox), sertraline (Zoloft), and clomipramine (Anafranil) in dosages appropriate for the treatment of obsessive–compulsive disorder can be helpful in pharmacologic management. It should be noted that when these medications are used in the treatment of obsessive–compulsive disorder, the dosage tends to be higher and the time to initial response is longer than when treating depression. For example, 20 mg/d

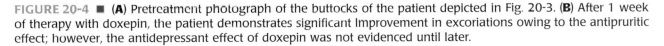

FIGURE 20-4 ■ **(A)** Pretreatment photograph of the buttocks of the patient depicted in Fig. 20-3. **(B)** After 1 week of therapy with doxepin, the patient demonstrates significant improvement in excoriations owing to the antipruritic effect; however, the antidepressant effect of doxepin was not evidenced until later.

of fluoxetine or paroxetine is often adequate for the treatment of depression. In contrast, when treating obsessive–compulsive disorder, the required dosage may be in the 40 to 80 mg/d range. The initial treatment response time in obsessive–compulsive disorder may take 4 to 8 weeks with a maximal response time of up to 20 weeks. Once a therapeutic response is achieved, therapy should be continued for 6 months to 1 year. Many clinicians have found that a complete remission is unusual. The nonpharmacologic approach includes psychotherapy, which can be useful if there is a definable issue that can be discussed. The other treatment modality includes behavioral therapy conducted by a behaviorally oriented psychologist.

Secondary Psychiatric Disorders

Although skin conditions are usually not life threatening, because they are visible, they can be life ruining. Patients frequently feel psychologically and socially devastated, because of the disfigurement (Fig. 20-5). Moreover, it is difficult for patients with skin disorders to get jobs where appearance is important. It is also well documented that patients with visible disfigurement, especially if the condition is perceived to be contagious, are generally treated worse than those with obvious physical disabilities. Even though many patients adjust to their skin disease, if the clinician notes significant distress on the part of the patient, it is important to explore this issue and evaluate whether referral to a mental health professional or dermatologic support group might be of benefit. If the

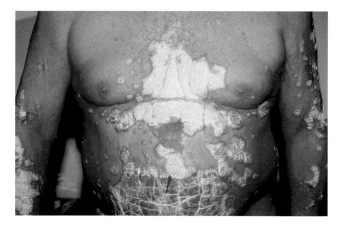

FIGURE 20-5 ■ The disfiguring effects of psoriasis are seen on the arms and torso of this patient with plaque psoriasis. This man experienced severe social, sexual, occupational, as well as psychological, impact due to his psoriasis.

depression, social phobia, or any secondary psychopathology is of significant intensity, a referral to a psychiatrist might be warranted.

Miscellaneous Cases

There are some cases that do not neatly fit into the above three categories. For example, there are patients with cutaneous sensory syndrome, who present to the clinician with nothing but a sensory complaint. There is no visible rash and an extensive workup fails to reveal any underlying medical condition that can be associated with the chief complaint. The chief complaints can vary from itching, stinging, and biting sensations to other forms of cutaneous discomfort. It is well documented that itching can occur as the manifestation of central nervous system insult, such as multiple sclerosis, brain abscess, brain tumor, or sensory stroke. However, in many of these cases, it is not possible to demonstrate a focal neurologic deficit. In general, patients with chronic sensory disorders are frustrated because they often do not respond to the usual dermatologic treatment modalities such as topical steroids, emollients, and antibiotics. However, the authors' experience is that they frequently do respond to an empirical use of psychotropic medications.

Treatment

If the primary complaint is pruritus, patients often respond to doxepin in doses that are significantly lower than those used for the treatment of depression. Often a dosage from less than 10 mg at bedtime to 50 to 75 mg during the day suffices (Fig. 20-6). If chronic pruritus can be suppressed this way and suppression is maintained with the lowest effective dose of doxepin for several months, the pruritus frequently does not return if the doxepin is gradually tapered.

If the primary sensory complaint relates to pain, including burning sensations, amitriptyline (Elavil), once again in a dosage lower than the antidepressant dosage, is frequently effective. If the patient cannot take amitriptyline because older tricyclics are associated with more side effects than new ones, then desipramine (Norpramin) can be a good substitute. If the patient cannot tolerate any tricyclic antidepressants, the last option would be the newer, nontricyclic agents such as the SSRIs. This is because the SSRIs have the last documentation regarding their efficacy as analgesics, in contrast to tricyclics, which are better documented for their analgesic therapeutic effect.

It is important to tell the patient ahead of time that improvement occurs extremely slowly whether one is treating

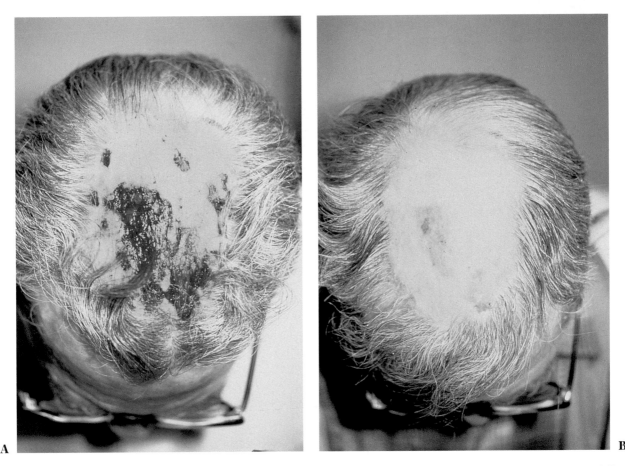

A   B

FIGURE 20-6 ■ **(A)** For decades this older man experienced severe, intermittent attacks of scalp pruritus that failed conventional dermatologic therapy and for which no primary skin lesion or systemic organic etiology was ever identified. A mental status examination by the author *(J.K.)* was entirely negative for any diagnosable psychiatric disorder. **(B)** After 2 weeks of empirical treatment with 25 to 50 mg/d of doxepin, the patient experienced complete resolution of pruritus that recurred when doxepin was discontinued. This observation may illustrate a case of central nervous system–mediated pruritus.

pruritus or dysesthesia. However, the authors' experience has been that, when treatment is conducted with a long-term view, it is generally possible to find the optimal agent and optimal dose, to resolve the chronic sensory disorder, and then eventually taper off the medication altogether.

Suggested Readings

Fenollosa P, Pallares J, Cerver J, et al. Chronic pain in the spinal cord injured: Statistical approach and pharmacological treatment. Paraplegia 1993;31:722–729.

Gaston L, Lassone M, Bernier-Buzzanga J, et al. Role of emotional factors in adults with atopic dermatitis. Int J Dermatol 1987;17:82–86.

Ginsburg IH, Prystowsky JH, Kornfeld DS, et al. Role of emotional factors in adults with atopic dermatitis. Int J Dermatol 1993;32:65–66.

Koblezer, CS. Psychocutaneous disease. Orlando, FL, Grune & Stratton, 1987, pp. 77–78, 117.

Koo JYM. Psychoderamtology: A practice manual for clinicians. Cur Prob Dermatol 1995;6:204–232.

Koo JYM. Psychotropic agents in dermatology. Dermatol Clin 1993;11:215–224.

Koo JY. Skin disorders. In: Kaplan HI, Saduch BJ, eds. Comprehensive textbook of psychiatry, ed 6. Baltimore, Williams & Wilkins, 1995.

Koo JY, Pham CT. Psychodermatology: Practical guidelines on pharmacotherapy. Arch Dermatol 1992;128: 381–388.

Medansky RS, Handler RM. Dermatopsychosomatics: Classification, physiology and therapeutic approaches. J Am Acad Dermatol 1981;5:125–136.

Rasmussen SA, Eisen JL. Treatment strategies for chronic and refractory obsessive-compulsive disorder. J Clin Psychiatry 1997;58(Suppl 13):9–13.

Stein DJ, Mullen L, Islam MN, Cohen L, et al. Compulsive and impulsive symptomatology in trichotillomania. Psychopathology 1995;28:208–213.

Zanol K, Slaughter J, Hall R. An approach to the treatment of psychogenic parasitosis. Int Dermatol 1998; 37:56–63.

SECTION III

INFECTIOUS DISEASES IN THE SKIN

CHAPTER 21

Dermatologic Bacteriology

John C. Hall

Bacteria exist on the skin as normal nonpathogenic resident flora or as pathogenic organisms. The pathogenic bacteria cause primary, secondary, and systemic infections. For clinical purposes it is justifiable to divide the problem of bacterial infection into three classifications (Table 21-1). Some of the diseases listed are of dubious bacterial etiology, but they appear bacterial, may have a bacterial component, can be treated with antibacterial agents, and are, therefore, included in this chapter.

With an alteration in immune capabilities in a person, bacteria and other infectious agents can have erratic be-

havior. Ordinary nonpathogens can act as pathogens, and pathogenic agents can act more aggressively.

Primary Bacterial Infections (Pyodermas)

The most common causative agents of the primary skin infections are the coagulase-positive micrococci (staphylococci) and the β-hemolytic streptococci. Superficial or deep bacterial lesions can be produced by these organisms. In managing the pyodermas, certain general principles of treatment must be initiated.

195

TABLE 21-1 ■ Classification of Bacterial Infection

Primary Bacterial Infections

Impetigo
Ecthyma
Folliculitis
  Superficial folliculitis
  Folliculitis of the scalp
    Superficial—acne miliaris necrotica
    Deep scarring—folliculitis decalvans
  Folliculitis of the beard
  Stye
Furuncle
Carbuncle
Sweat gland inflammations
Erysipelas

Secondary Bacterial Infections

Cutaneous diseases with secondary infection
Infected ulcers
Infectious eczematoid dermatitis
Bacterial intertrigo

Systemic Bacterial Infections

Scarlet fever
Granuloma inguinale
Chancroid
Mycobacterial infections
  Tuberculosis of the skin
  Leprosy
Gonorrhea
Rickettsial diseases
Actinomycosis

- *Improve bathing habits:* More frequent bathing and the use of bactericidal soap, such as Dial, or Lever 2000, are indicated. Any pustules or crusts should be removed during the bathing to facilitate penetration of the local medications. In rare instances when these infections are recalcitrant to standard therapies, I use ½ to 1 cup of bleach in a full tub of water to soak daily as long as indicated.
- *General isolation procedures:* Clothing and bedding should be changed frequently and cleaned. The patient should have a separate towel and washcloth.
- *Systemic drugs:* The patient should be questioned regarding ingestion of drugs that can cause lesions that mimic or cause pyodermas, such as iodides, bromides, testosterone, corticosteroids, progesterone, and lithium.

- *Diabetes:* In chronic skin infections, particularly recurrent boils, diabetes should be ruled out by history and laboratory examination.
- *Immunosuppressed patients:* A history of abnormal findings should alert the physician to the increasing number of patients now who are on chemotherapy for cancer, are posttransplant, or have the acquired immunodeficiency syndrome (AIDS).

Impetigo

Impetigo is a common superficial bacterial infection seen most often in children; it is the "infantigo" every parent respects.

Primary Lesions

The lesions vary from small vesicles to large bullae that rupture and discharge a honey-colored serous liquid (Fig. 21-1; see also Fig. 3-1A). New lesions can develop in a matter of hours.

Secondary Lesions

Crusts form from the discharge and appear to be lightly stuck on the skin surface. When removed, a superficial erosion remains, which may be the only evidence of the disease. In debilitated infants, the bullae may coalesce to form an exfoliative type of infection called *Ritter's disease* or *pemphigus neonatorum.*

Distribution

The lesions occur most commonly on the face but may be anywhere.

Contagiousness

It is not unusual to see brothers or sisters of the patient and, rarely, the parents similarly infected.

SAUER'S NOTES

Body piercing has frequently been associated with localized staphylococcal infection and pseudomonas infection and rarely bacteremia and endocarditis. Tuberculosis, hepatitis C and B, and even HIV may have been transmitted in this way. Noninfectious complications are keloids and allergic dermatitis. This fad should not be recommended, especially in tongue, lips, navels, nipples, and genitalia.

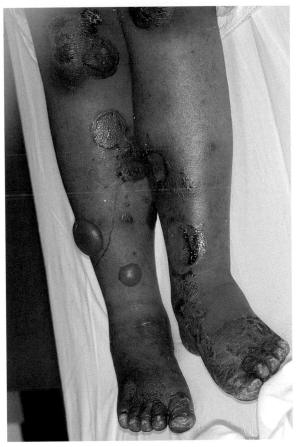

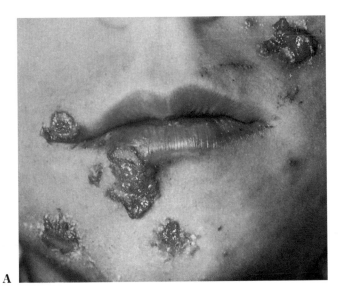

A   B

FIGURE 21-1 ■ **(A)** Impetigo of the face. The honey-colored crusts are typical. *(Courtesy of Abner Kurtin, Folia Dermatologica, No. 2. Geigy Pharmaceuticals.)* **(B)** Bullous impetigo on the legs of a young child.

Differential Diagnosis

- *Contact dermatitis* due to poison ivy or oak: Linear blisters; does not spread as rapidly; itches (see Chap. 9).
- *Tinea of smooth skin:* Fewer lesions; spread slowly; small vesicles in annular configuration, which is an unusual form for impetigo; fungi found on scraping; culture is positive (see Chap. 25).
- *Toxic epidermal necrolysis:* In infants and rarely in adults, massive bullae can develop rapidly, particularly with staphylococcal infection. The severe form of this infection is known as the *staphylococcal scalded skin syndrome,* which is a type of toxic epidermal necrolysis (see Chap. 18).

Treatment

1. Outline the general principles of treatment. Emphasize the removal of the crusts once or twice a day during bathing with an antibacterial soap such as Lever 2000 or chlorhexidine (Hibiclens) skin cleanser.

2. Mupirocin (Bactroban) or gentamicin (Garamycin) ointment or Polysporin ointment q.s. 15.0

   Sig: Apply t.i.d. locally for 10 days. Treat all affected family members or other affected contacts.

3. Oral antibiotics such as a 10-day course of erythromycin, cephalexin, or clindamycin may be necessary.

4. Methicillin-resistant *Staphylococcus aureus* in the community acquired form (CAMRSA) now occurs in epidemic proportions. *Fortunately it often* is sensitive to sulfamethoxazole (Septra) or tetracycline derivatives. Abcesses are common.

Ecthyma

Ecthyma is another superficial bacterial infection, but it is seen less commonly and is deeper than impetigo. It is usually caused by β-hemolytic streptococci and occurs on the buttocks and the thighs of children (Fig. 21-2).

Primary Lesion

A vesicle or vesiculopustule appears and rapidly changes into the secondary lesion.

Secondary Lesion

This is a piled-up crust, 1 to 3 cm in diameter, overlying a superficial erosion or ulcer. In neglected cases, scarring can occur as a result of extension of the infection into the dermis.

Distribution

Most commonly the disease is seen on the posterior aspect of the thighs and the buttocks, from which areas it can spread. Ecthyma commonly follows the scratching of chigger bites.

Age Group

Children are affected mainly.

Contagiousness

Ecthyma is rarely found in other members of the family.

Differential Diagnosis

- *Psoriasis:* Unusual in children; whitish, firmly attached scaly lesion, also in scalp, on knees, and elbows (see Chap. 14)
- *Impetigo:* Much smaller crusted lesions, not as deep (see preceding section)

Treatment

1. The general principles of treatment are listed earlier in the chapter. The crusts must be removed daily. Response to therapy is slower than with impetigo, but the treatment is the same for both conditions.

2. *Systemic antibiotics:* Commonly with extensive ecthyma in children, but only rarely with impetigo, there is a low-grade fever and evidence of bacterial infection in other

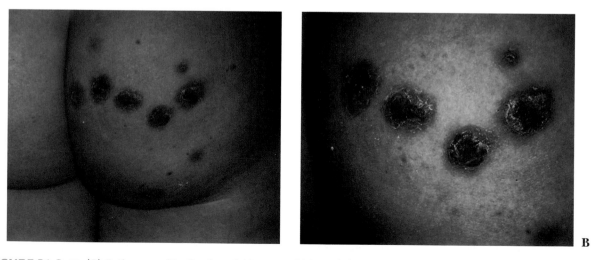

FIGURE 21-2 ■ **(A)** Ecthyma of buttocks of 13-year-old boy. **(B)** Close-up of lesions. *(Courtesy of Burroughs Wellcome Co.)*

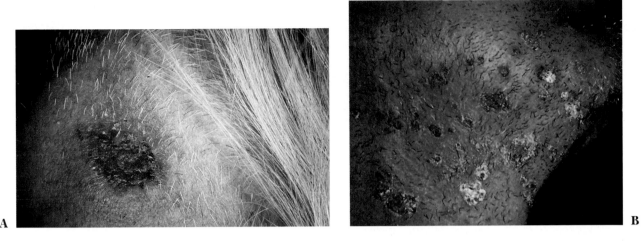

A   B

FIGURE 21-3 ■ (A) Folliculitis of the scalp. **(B)** Folliculitis of the beard area *(Courtesy of Burroughs Wellcome Co.)*

organs, due to sepsis. If so, one of the antibiotic syrups or tablets can be given orally q.i.d. for 10 days.

Folliculitis

Folliculitis is a common pyogenic infection of the hair follicles, usually caused by coagulase-positive staphylococci (Fig. 21-3). Seldom does a patient consult the physician for a single outbreak of folliculitis. The physician is consulted because of recurrent and chronic pustular lesions. The patient realizes that the present acute episode clears with the help of nature, but seeks medicine and advice to prevent recurrences. For this reason, the general principles of treatment listed, particularly the drug history and the diabetes investigation, are important. Some physicians believe that a focus of infection in the teeth, tonsils, gallbladder, or genitourinary tract should be ruled out when pyodermas are recurrent.

The folliculitis may invade only the superficial part of the hair follicle, or it may extend down to the hair bulb. Many variously named clinical entities based on the location and the chronicity of the lesions have been carried down through the years. A few of these entities bear presentation here, but most are defined in the Dictionary–Index.

Superficial Folliculitis

The physician is rarely consulted for this minor problem, which is most commonly seen on the arms, scalp, face, and buttocks of children and adults with the acne–seborrhea complex. A history of excessive use of hair oils, bath oils, or suntan oils can often be obtained. The use of these oily agents should be avoided. Culture for *Staphylococcus* or *Streptococcus* may be negative and then the same therapeutic regiments as for acne are used.

Folliculitis of the Scalp (Superficial Form)

A superficial form has the appellation *acne necrotica miliaris*. This is an annoying, pruritic, chronic, recurrent folliculitis of the scalp in adults. The scratching of the crusted lesions occupies the patient's evening hours.

Treatment.

1. Follow the general principles of treatment.
2. Selenium sulfide (Selsun, Head & Shoulders Intensive Treatment) suspension shampoo 120.0

   Sig: Shampoo twice a week as directed on the label.
3. Other shampoos such as T-Sal and sulfur washes such as Ovace and Plexion used as a shampoo, can be tried.
4. Antibiotic and corticosteroid cream mixture q.s. 15.0

   Sig: Apply to scalp h.s.

SAUER'S NOTES

My routine for *chronic* folliculitis cases includes the following:

1. Sulfur ppt. 5%
   Hydrocortisone 1%
   Bactroban cream q.s. 15.0
   Sig: Apply b.i.d. locally.
2. Long-term low-dose antibiotic therapy can be used, such as erythromycin, 250 mg, q.i.d. for 3 days then two or three times a day for months.
3. Lichenified papules of excoriated folliculitis respond to superficial liquid nitrogen applications or intralesional corticosteroid injections.

Folliculitis of the Scalp (Deep Form)

The deep form of scalp folliculitis is called *folliculitis decalvans.* This is a chronic, slowly progressive folliculitis with an active border and scarred atrophic center. The end result, after years of progression, is patchy, scarred areas of alopecia, with eventual burning out of the inflammation. It is not a true infection and bacterial cultures are negative.

Differential Diagnosis

- *Chronic discoid lupus erythematosus:* Redness, hypopigmentation, and hyperpigmentation; enlarged hair follicles with follicular plugs (see Chap. 25).
- *Alopecia cicatrisata* (pseudopelade of Brocq): Rare; no evidence of inflammation. Some authors think this is burnt out lichen planus of the scalp (see Chap. 27).
- *Tinea of the scalp:* It is important to culture the hair for fungi in any chronic infection of the scalp; *Trichophyton tonsurans* group can cause a subtle noninflammatory clinical picture (black dot tinea in children, which is endemic in large urban areas in African-American children who braid their hair) (see Chap. 25).
- *Excoriated folliculitis:* Chronic thickened excoriated papules or nodules (can be called *prurigo nodularis*), usually seen on posterior scalp, posterior neck, anus, and legs. When allowed to heal, whitish scars remain. The infection can last for years. Liquid nitrogen applied to the papules is effective, as are intralesional corticosteroids. Occasionally these patients can be treated with a drug to decrease obsessive–compulsive behavior, such as a selective serotonin reuptake inhibitor.

Treatment. Results of treatment may be disappointing. Long-term antibiotics, especially tetracycline derivatives, may be helpful. Occasionally intralesional corticosteroids may be palliative.

Folliculitis of the Beard

This is the familiar "barber's itch," which in the days before antibiotics was resistant to therapy. This bacterial infection of the hair follicles is spread rather rapidly by shaving.

Differential Diagnosis

- *Contact dermatitis* caused by shaving lotions: History of new lotion applied; general redness of the area with some vesicles (see Chap. 9).

- *Tinea of the beard:* Very slowly spreading infection; hairs broken off; usually a deeper nodular type of inflammation (Majocchi's granuloma); culture of hair produces fungi (see Chap. 25).
- *Ingrown beard hairs* (pseudofolliculitis barbae): Hair circling back into the skin with resultant chronic inflammation; a hereditary trait, especially in African Americans. Close shaving aggravates the condition. Local antibiotics rarely help, but locally applied depilatories may help. Other local therapy to consider is Retin-A gel and Benzashave. Permanent hair removal by electrolysis or laser can be helpful. Vaniqa applied twice a day after hair removal can be used to reduce rate of regrowth of hair. Growing a beard or mustache eliminates the problem. Hairs may also become ingrown in axillae, pubic area, or legs, especially when closely shaved in places with curly hair.

Treatment.

1. Follow the general principles of treatment, stressing the use of Dial or other antibacterial soap for washing of the face.
2. Shaving instructions:
   a. Change the razor blade daily or sterilize the head of the electric razor by placing it in 70% alcohol for 1 hour.
   b. Apply the following salve very lightly to the face before shaving and again after shaving. *Do not shave closely.*
3. Antibiotic and hydrocortisone cream mixture q.s. 15.0
   Sig: Apply to face before shaving, after shaving, and at bedtime.
   Comment: For stubborn cases, add sulfur 5% to the cream.
4. Oral therapy with erythromycin, 250 mg (can also use cephalexin on clindamycin)
   Sig: 1 capsule q.i.d. for 7 days, then 1 capsule b.i.d. for 7 days.

Sty (Hordeolum)

A *sty* is a deep folliculitis of the stiff eyelid hairs. A single lesion is treated with hot packs of 1% boric acid solution and an ophthalmic antibiotic ointment. Recurrent lesions may be linked with the blepharitis of seborrheic dermatitis (dandruff). For this type, sulfacetamide ophthalmic ointment, or cleansing the eyelashes with Johnson's Baby Shampoo is indicated.

Furuncle

A furuncle, or boil (Fig. 21-4), is a more extensive infection of the hair follicle, usually due to *Staphylococcus*. A boil can occur in any person at any age, but certain predisposing factors account for most outbreaks. An important factor is the acne–seborrhea complex (oily skin, dark complexion, and history of acne and dandruff). Other factors include poor hygiene, diabetes, local skin trauma from friction of clothing, and maceration in obese persons. One boil usually does not bring the patient to the physician, but recurrent boils do.

Differential Diagnosis

Single Lesion

- *Primary chancre-type diseases:* See list in Dictionary–Index.

Multiple Lesions

- *Drug eruption from iodides or bromides:* See Chap. 9.
- *Hidradenitis suppurativa:* See later in this chapter.

Treatment

Case Example. A young man has had recurrent boils for 6 months. He does not have diabetes, is not obese, is taking no drugs, and bathes daily. He now has a large boil on his buttocks.

1. Burow's solution hot packs.

    Sig: 1 packet of Domeboro powder to 1 quart of hot water. Apply hot wet packs for 30 minutes twice a day.

2. Incision and drainage: This should be done only on "ripe" lesions where a necrotic white area appears at the top of the nodule. Drains are not necessary unless the lesion has extended deep enough to form a fluctuant abscess.

3. Oral antistaphylococcal penicillin, such as dicloxacillin or cephalexin, should be prescribed for 5 to 10 days. (Bacteriologic culture and sensitivity studies are helpful in determining which antibiotic to use.)

4. For recurrent form:

    a. Follow general principles of treatment use of an antibacterial soap.

    b. Rule out focus of infection in teeth, tonsils, genitourinary tract, and so on.

    c. Begin oral therapy with erythromycin, 250 mg, which is very effective in breaking the cycle of recurrent cases.

    Sig: 4 capsules a day for 10 days.

    Cultures should be done to determine sensitivity and antibiotic choices altered as indicated.

Carbuncle

A carbuncle is an extensive infection of several adjoining hair follicles that drains with multiple openings onto the skin surface (Fig. 21-5). Fatal cases were not unusual in the preantibiotic days. A common location for a carbuncle is the posterior neck region. Large, ugly, criss-cross scars in this area in an older patient demonstrate the outdated treatment for this disease, namely, multiple bold incisions. Because a carbuncle is, in reality, a multiple furuncle, the same etiologic factors apply. Recurrences are uncommon.

Treatment. Treatment is the same as for a boil (see preceding section) but with greater emphasis on systemic antibiotic therapy.

Sweat Gland Inflammations

Although not true infections, inflammations of the sweat gland are included here because of similar clinical appearance (Fig. 21-6) and similar treatment. Primary eccrine sweat gland or duct infections are very rare. However, prickly heat, a sweat-retention disease, frequently develops secondary bacterial infection. Primary apocrine gland inflammation is rather common. Two types of inflammation exist:

- *Apocrinitis* denotes inflammation of a single apocrine gland, usually in the axilla, and is commonly associated with a change in deodorant. It responds to the therapy listed for furuncles. In addition, a lotion containing an antibiotic aids in keeping the

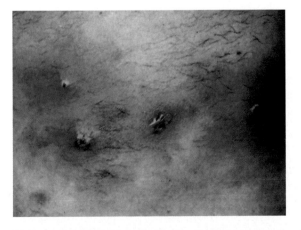

FIGURE 21-4 ■ Multiple furuncles (boils) on the chest. *(Courtesy of Abner Kurtin, Folia Dermatologica, No. 2. Geigy Pharmaceuticals)*

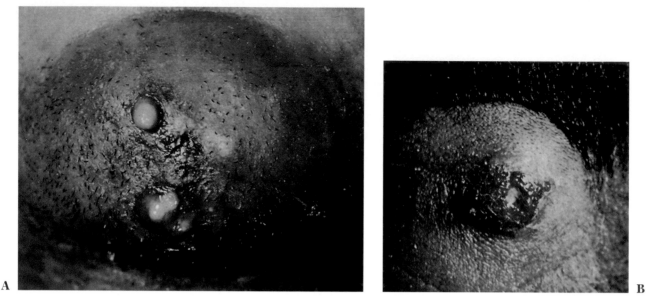

FIGURE 21-5 ■ **(A)** Carbuncle on the chin. Notice the multiple openings. *(Courtesy of Abner Kurtin, Folia Dermatologica, No. 2. Geigy Pharmaceuticals.)* **(B)** Carbuncle on the back of the neck. *(Courtesy of J. Lamar Callaway, Folia Dermatologica, No. 4. Geigy Pharmaceuticals.)*

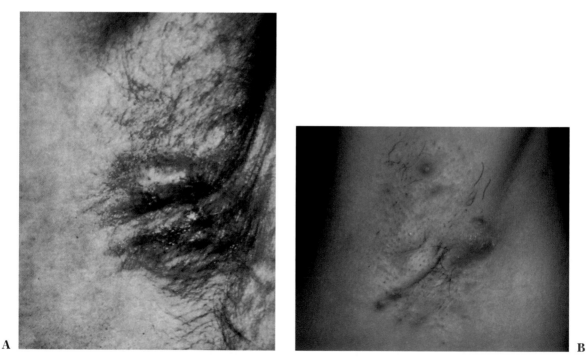

FIGURE 21-6 ■ **(A)** Sweat gland inflammation of the axilla (hidradenitis suppurativa). *(Courtesy of Abner Kurtin, Folia Dermatologica, No. 2. Geigy Pharmaceuticals.)* **(B)** Hidradenitis suppurativa of axilla of 6 years' duration. *(Courtesy of Burroughs Wellcome Co.)*

area dry, such as an erythromycin solution (A/T/S, Erymax, EryDerm, Erycette, T-Stat, Staticin).

■ The second form of apocrine gland inflammation is *hidradenitis suppurativa.* This chronic, recurring inflammation is characterized by the development of multiple nodules, abscesses, draining sinuses, and eventual hypertrophic bands of scars. The most common location is in the axillae, but it can also occur in the groin, perianal, submammary, and suprapubic regions. It does not occur before puberty. Etiologically, there appears to be a hereditary tendency in these patients toward occlusion of the follicular orifice and subsequent retention of the secretory products. Two other diseases are related to hidradenitis suppurativa and may be present in the same patient: (1) a severe form of acne called *acne conglobata* and (2) *dissecting cellulitis of the scalp.*

Treatment

The management of these cases is difficult. In addition to the general principles mentioned previously, hot used packs locally and an oral antibiotic, especially tetracycline, should be given for several weeks.

Plastic surgery or a marsupialization operation is indicated in severe cases. When draining canals or sinuses are present, the marsupialization operation is curative and can be done in the office. After the bridge over the canal has been trimmed away, bleeding is controlled by electrosurgery. Laser therapy has its advocates. Isotretinoin (Accutane) can be tried for 5 to 10 months (see Chap 13). Do not give if chance of pregnancy.

Erysipelas

Erysipelas is an uncommon β-hemolytic streptococcal infection of the subcutaneous tissue that produces a characteristic type of cellulitis (Fig. 21-7), with fever and malaise. Recurrences are frequent.

Primary Lesion

A red, warm, raised, brawny, sharply bordered plaque enlarges peripherally. Vesicles and bullae may form on the surface of the plaque. Multiple lesions of erysipelas are rare.

Distribution

Most commonly lesions occur on the face and around the ears (following ear piercing), but no area is exempt. Some authors now think the legs are the most common site.

Course

When treated with systemic antibiotics, response is rapid. Recurrences are common in the same location and may lead to lymphedema of that area, which eventually can become irreversible. The lips, cheeks, and legs are particularly prone to this chronic change, which is called *elephantiasis nostras* or when the area develops a more warty appearance, *elephantiasis nostra verrucosa.*

Subjective Complaints

Fever and general malaise can precede the development of the skin lesion and persist until therapy is instituted. Elderly patients may present with altered sensorium and somnolence. Pain at the site of the infection can be severe.

Differential Diagnosis

■ *Cellulitis:* Lacks a sharp border; recurrences rare
■ *Contact dermatitis:* Sharp border absent; fever and malaise absent; eruption predominantly vesicular and very pruritic rather than painful (see Chap. 9)

Treatment

1. Institute bed rest and direct therapy toward reducing the fever. If the patient is hospitalized, semi-isolation procedures should be initiated. Blood cultures should be considered to rule out sepsis.
2. Give an appropriate systemic antibiotic, such as erythromycin or a penicillin derivative, for 10 days.
3. Apply local, cool, wet dressing, as necessary for comfort.

Erythrasma

Erythrasma is an uncommon bacterial infection of the skin that clinically resembles regular tinea or tinea versicolor (Fig. 21-8). It affects the crural area, axillae, and webs of the

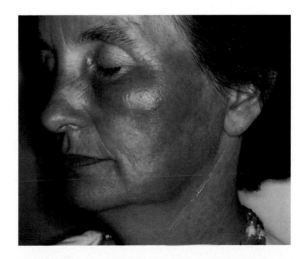

FIGURE 21-7 ■ Erysipelas of cheek. *(Courtesy of Burroughs Wellcome Co.)*

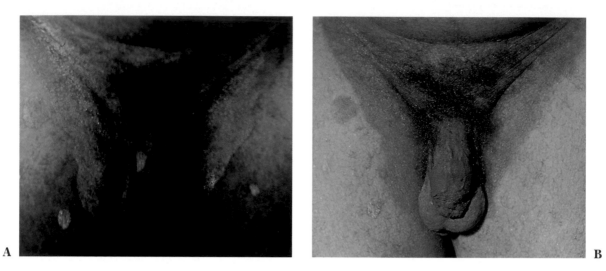

FIGURE 21-8 ■ Erythrasma of crural area with fluorescence under Wood's light (**A**) and in natural light (**B**). *(Courtesy of Burroughs Wellcome Co.)*

toes with flat, hyperpigmented, fine, scaly patches. If the patient has not been using an antibacterial soap, these patches fluoresce a striking coral reddish orange under Wood's light. The causative agent is a diphtheroid organism called *Corynebacterium minutussimum.*

The most effective treatment is erythromycin, 250 mg, q.i.d. for 5 to 7 days. Locally the erythromycin lotions are quite effective (e.g., Staticin, T-Stat, EryDerm, and A/T/S lotion). They are applied twice daily for 10 days.

Secondary Bacterial Infections

Secondary infection develops as a complicating factor on a preexisting skin disease. The invasion of an injured skin surface with pathogenic streptococci or staphylococci is enhanced in skin conditions that are oozing and of long duration.

SAUER'S NOTES

Any type of skin lesion, such as hand dermatitis, poison weed dermatitis, atopic eczema, chigger bites, fungus infection, traumatic abrasion, and so on, can become secondarily infected.

The treatment is usually simple: An antibacterial agent is added to the local treatment one would ordinarily use for the dermatosis in question. For extensive secondary bacterial infection, the appropriate systemic antibiotic is indicated, based on bacterial culture and sensitivity studies.

Cutaneous Diseases With Secondary Infection

Failure in the treatment of many common skin diseases can be attributed to the physician's not recognizing the presence of the secondary bacterial infection.

Infected Ulcers

Ulcers are deep skin infections owing to injury or disease that invade the subcutaneous tissue and, on healing, leave scars. Ulcers can be divided into primary and secondary ulcers, but most become secondarily infected with bacteria.

Primary Ulcers

Primary ulcers from infection result from the following causes: gangrene owing to pathogenic streptococci, staphylococci, and *Clostridium* species; syphilis; chancroid; tuberculosis; diphtheria; fungi; leprosy; anthrax; cancer; and lymphomas.

Secondary Ulcers

Secondary ulcers can be related to the following diseases: vascular disorders (arteriosclerosis, thromboangiitis obliterans, Raynaud's phenomenon, phlebitis, thrombosis); neurologic disorders (spinal cord injury with bedsores or decubiti, central nervous system syphilis, spina bifida, poliomyelitis, syringomyelia); diabetes; trauma; ulcerative colitis; Crohn's disease; immunosuppression; allergic local anaphylaxis; and other conditions. Finally, there is a group of secondary ulcers called *phagedenic ulcers*, variously described under many different names, that arise in diseased skin or on the apparently normal skin of debilitated persons. These ulcers undermine the skin in large areas, are notoriously chronic, and are resistant to therapy.

Treatment

1. For primary ulcers, specific therapy is indicated, if available. The response to therapy is usually quite rapid.

2. For secondary ulcers, appropriate therapy should be directed toward the primary disease. The response to therapy is usually quite slow. This is especially true for the decubitus ulcer of the immobile, incontinent person.

3. The basic rules of local therapy for ulcers can be illustrated best by outlining the management of a patient with a stasis leg ulcer (see Stasis Dermatitis and Stasis Ulcers in Chap. 12).

   a. Rest of the affected area: If rest in bed is not feasible, then an Ace elastic bandage, 4 inches wide, should be worn. This bandage is applied over the local medication and before getting out of bed in the morning. A more permanent support is a modification of an Unna boot (Dome-Paste bandage, Gelocast, or an easy-to-apply and effective adhesive flexible bandage). This boot can be applied for 1 week or more at a time if secondary infection is under control.

   b. Elevation of the affected extremity: This should be carried out in bed and can be accomplished by placing two bricks, flat surface down, under both feet of the bed. (Arteriosclerotic leg ulcers should not be elevated.)

   c. Burow's solution wet packs

   Sig: 1 packet of Domeboro powder to 1 quart of warm water. Apply wet dressings of gauze or sheeting for 30 minutes t.i.d.

   d. If debridement is necessary, this can be accomplished by enzymes, such as Debrisan, Santyl (collagenase) ointment, Acuzyme, Panafil, or Elase ointment, applied twice a day and covered with gauze.

   e. Gentian violet 1%

   Distilled water q.s. 15.0

   Sig: Apply to ulcer b.i.d. with applicator.

   Comment: A liquid is usually better tolerated on ulcers than a salve. If the gentian violet solution becomes too drying, the following salve can be used alternately for short periods.

   f. Bactroban or other antibiotic ointment q.s. 15.0

   Sig: Apply to ulcer and surrounding skin b.i.d.

   g. Long-term erythromycin or cephalexin therapy: 250 mg, 1 capsule q.i.d. for 14 or more days, then 1 capsule b.i.d. for weeks, is helpful for chronic pyogenic ulcers. Other systemic antibiotics may be used.

   h. Low-dose oral corticosteroid therapy: prednisone, 10 mg

   Sig: 1 or 2 tablets every morning for 3 to 4 weeks, then 1 tablet every other morning for months. When this is added to the above routine many indolent ulcers heal.

   Comment: The best treatment for one ulcer does not necessarily work for another ulcer. Many other local medications are available and valuable.

4. Surgical management, such as excision and grafting, may be indicated.

5. Various surgical dressings may be beneficial, such as OpSite, Duoderm, Tegaderm, or Polymem; Johnson & Johnson makes an inexpensive surgical wound dressing.

Infectious Eczematoid Dermatitis

The term *infectious eczematoid dermatitis* or *auto eczematous dermatitis* is more often used incorrectly than correctly. Infectious eczematoid dermatitis is an uncommon disease characterized by the development of an acute eruption around an infected exudative primary site, such as a draining ear, mastitis, a boil, or a seeping ulcer (Fig. 21-9). Widespread eczematous lesions can develop at a distant site from the primary infection, presumably owing to an immune phenomenon, and *autoeczemtous dermatitis* or an *id reaction* is the better term.

Primary Lesions

Vesicles and pustules in circumscribed plaques spread peripherally from an infected central source. Central healing usually does not occur, as in ringworm infection.

Secondary Lesions

Crusting, oozing, and scaling predominate in widespread cases.

Distribution

Mild cases may be confined to a small area around the exudative primary infection, but widespread cases can cover the entire body, obscuring the initial cause.

SAUER'S NOTES

The primary factor in the management of an ulcer is to not let it happen. This is especially appropriate for decubitus ulcers.

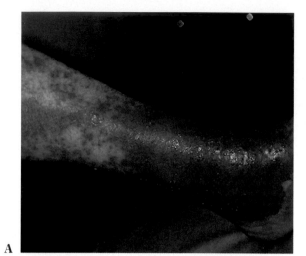

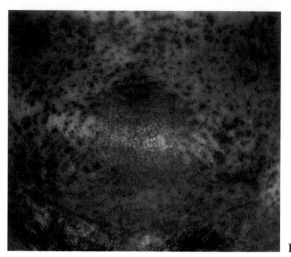

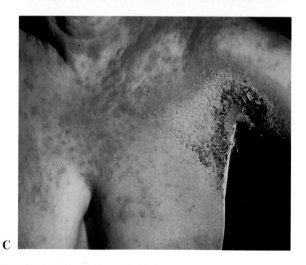

FIGURE 21-9 ■ Bacterial infections of skin. *(Burroughs Wellcome Co.)* Infectious eczematoid dermatitis (**A**) from stasis dermatitis of legs with spread to body (**B**). (**C**) Infectious eczematoid dermatitis in axilla.

Course

The course depends on the extent of the eruption. Chronic cases respond poorly to therapy. Recurrences are common even after the primary source is healed.

Subjective Complaints

Itching is usually present.

Cause

Coagulase-positive staphylococci are frequently isolated.

Contagiousness

Despite the strong autoinoculation factor, passage of the infective material to another person rarely elicits a reaction.

Differential Diagnosis

- *Contact dermatitis with secondary infection:* No history or finding of primary exudative infection; history of contact with poison ivy, new clothes, cosmetics, or dishwater; responds faster to therapy (see Chap. 9)
- *Nummular eczema:* No primary infected source; coin-shaped lesions on extremities; clinical differentiation of some cases difficult (see Chap. 9)
- *Seborrheic dermatitis:* No primary infected source; seborrhea–acne complex, with greasy, scaly eruption in hairy areas (see Chap. 13)
- *Eczematous psoriasis:* A recently described skin ailment with the appearance of diffuse severe nummular eczema, but with a response to therapy mimicking that of psoriasis

Treatment

Case Example. An 8-year-old boy presents with draining otitis media and pustular, crusted dermatitis on the side of face, neck, and scalp.

1. Treat the primary source—the ear infection, in this case.
2. Apply Burow's solution wet packs

    Sig: 1 packet of Domeboro powder to 1 quart of warm water. Apply wet sheeting or gauze to area for 20 minutes t.i.d.

3. Apply antibiotic and corticosteroid cream, such as

    Bactroban ointment 15.0
    Triamcinolone 0.1% cream 15.0
    Sig: Apply t.i.d. locally, after the wet packs are removed.

A patient with a widespread case might require hospitalization, daily mild soap baths, oral antibiotics, or corticosteroid systemic therapy.

Bacterial Intertrigo

The presence of friction, heat, and moisture in areas where two opposing skin surfaces contact each other leads to a secondary bacterial, fungus, or yeast infection.

Primary Lesion

Redness from friction and heat of opposing forces and maceration from inability of the sweat to evaporate freely leads to an eroded patch of dermatitis.

Secondary Lesion

The bacterial infection may become severe enough to result in fissures and cellulitis.

Distribution

The inframammary region, axillae, umbilicus, pubic, crural, genital, and perianal areas as well as the areas between the toes may be involved.

Course

In certain persons intertrigo tends to recur each summer.

Causes

The factors of obesity, diabetes, and prolonged contact with urine, feces, and menstrual discharges predispose to the development of intertrigo. AIDS may present with recurrent bullous groin impetigo.

Differential Diagnosis

- *Candidal intertrigo:* Scaling at border of erosion with an overhanging fringe of epidermis; presence of surrounding small satellite lesions; scraping and culture reveals *Candida albicans* (see Chap. 25)
- *Tinea:* Scaly or papulovesicular border; scraping and culture are positive for fungi (see Chap. 25)
- *Seborrheic dermatitis:* Greasy red scaly areas, also seen in scalp; bacterial intertrigo may coexist with seborrheic dermatitis (see Chap. 13)

Treatment

Case Example. A 6-month-old infant presents with red, fistular dermatitis in diaper area, axillae, and folds of neck.

1. Bathe child once a day in lukewarm water with antibacterial soap. Dry affected areas thoroughly.
2. Double rinse diapers to remove all soap or use disposable diapers.
3. Change diapers as frequently as possible and apply a powder each time, such as

    Talc, unscented (Zeasorb) 45.0
    Sig: Place in powder can.

4. Hydrocortisone 1%

    Bactroban ointment q.s. 15.0
    Sig: Apply to affected areas t.i.d. Continue local therapy for at least 1 week after dermatitis is apparently clear—"therapy-plus." Allow only two refills of this salve to avoid atrophy of the skin.

Systemic Bacterial Infections

Scarlet Fever

Scarlet fever is a less common streptococcal infection characterized by a sore throat, high fever, and a scarlet rash. Decreased incident in recent decades is probably related to different "phase" type streptococci. The eruption develops after a day of rapidly rising fever, headache, sore throat, and various other symptoms. The rash begins first on the neck and the chest but rapidly spreads over the entire body, except for the area around the mouth. Close examination of the pale scarlet eruption reveals it to be made up of diffuse pinhead-sized, or larger, macules. In untreated cases the rash reaches its peak on the 4th day, and scaling commences around the 7th day and continues for 1 or 2 weeks. "Strawberry tongue" is seen at the height of the eruption.

The presence of petechiae on the body is a grave prognostic sign. Complications are numerous and common in untreated cases. Nephritis, in mild or severe form, and rheumatic heart disease are serious complications.

Differential Diagnosis

- *Measles:* Early rash on face and forehead; larger macular rash; running eyes; photophobia; cough (see Chap. 23)
- *Drug eruption:* Lack of high fever and other constitutional signs; atropine and quinine can cause eruption clinically similar to scarlet fever (see Chap. 9)

Treatment

Penicillin or a similar systemic antibiotic is the therapy of choice. Complications should be watched for and should be treated early.

Granuloma Inguinale

Before the use of antibiotics, particularly streptomycin and tetracycline, this disease was one of the most chronic and resistant afflictions of humans. Formerly, it was a rather common disease. Granuloma inguinale should be considered a venereal disease, although other factors may have to be present to initiate infection.

Primary Lesion

An irregularly shaped, bright red, velvety appearing, flat ulcer with rolled border is seen (Fig. 21-10).

Secondary Lesions

Scarring may lead to complications similar to those seen with lymphogranuloma venereum. Squamous cell carcinoma can develop in old, chronic lesions.

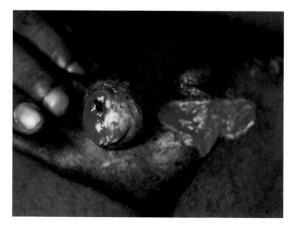

FIGURE 21-10 ■ Granuloma inguinale of penis and crural area. *(Courtesy of Derm-Arts Laboratories.)*

Distribution

Genital lesions are most common on the penis, the scrotum, the labia, the cervix, or the inguinal region.

Course

Without therapy, the granuloma grows slowly and persists for years, causing marked scarring and mutilation. Under modern therapy, healing is rapid, but recurrences are not unusual.

Cause

Granuloma inguinale is due to *Calymmatobacterium granulomatis,* which can be cultured on special media.

Laboratory Findings

Scrapings of the lesion reveal Donovan bodies, which are dark-staining, intracytoplasmic, cigar-shaped bacilli found in large macrophages. The material for the smear can be obtained best by snipping off a piece of the lesion with a small scissors and rubbing the tissue on several slides. Wright or Giemsa stains can be used.

Differential Diagnosis

- *Granuloma pyogenicum:* Small lesion; history of injury, usually; short duration; rarely on genitalia; no Donovan bodies
- *Primary syphilis:* Short duration; inguinal adenopathy; serology may be positive; spirochetes (see Chap. 16)
- *Chancroid:* Short duration; lesion small, not red and velvety; no Donovan bodies (see next section)
- *Squamous cell carcinoma:* More indurated lesion with nodule; may coexist with granuloma inguinale; biopsy specific

Treatment

Tetracycline, 500 mg q.i.d., is continued until all the lesions are healed.

SAUER'S NOTES

Syphilis must be considered in any patient with a penile lesion. It can be ruled out by darkfield examination (there is rarely anyone qualified to accurately do this test so its usefulness has been greatly reduced) or blood serology tests. The serology should be repeated in 6 weeks if clinical suspicion is high because the initial serology in primary syphilis may be negative.

Chancroid

Chancroid is a venereal disease with a very short incubation period of 1 to 5 days. It is caused by *Haemophilus ducreyi.*

Primary Lesion

Small, superficial or deep erosion occurs with surrounding redness and edema (Fig. 21-11). Multiple genital or distant lesions can be produced by autoinoculation.

Secondary Lesions

Deep, destructive ulcers form in chronic cases, which may lead to gangrene. Marked regional adenopathy, usually unilateral, is common and eventually suppurates in untreated cases.

Course

Without therapy most cases heal within 1 to 2 weeks. In rare cases, severe local destruction and draining lymph nodes (buboes) result. Early therapy is effective.

Laboratory Findings

The organisms arranged in "schools of fish" can often be demonstrated in smears of clean lesions.

Differential Diagnosis

- *Primary or secondary syphilis genital lesions:* Longer incubation period; more induration; *Treponema pallidum* found on darkfield examination; serology positive in late primary and secondary stage (see Chap. 22)
- *Herpes simplex progenitalis:* Recurrent multiple painful blisters or erosions; mild inguinal adenopathy; initial episode may have systemic symptoms (see Chap. 23)
- *Lymphogranuloma venereum:* Primary lesion rare; Frei test positive (see Chap. 23)
- *Granuloma inguinale:* Chronic, red velvety plaque; Donovan bodies seen on tissue smear (see preceding section)

Treatment

The therapy for chancroid is a sulfonamide such as sulfisoxazole, 1 g q.i.d. for 2 weeks, or erythromycin, 2 g/d for 10 to 15 days. Third-generation cephalosporins are also effective. A fluctuant bubo should never be incised but should be aspirated with a large needle.

Tuberculosis

Skin tuberculosis (Fig. 21-12; see also Fig. 3-1B) is rare in the United States; however, a text on dermatology would not be complete without some consideration of this infection. Although the incidence has been decreasing in the United States and leveled off worldwide since 1992, it is still a significant disease worldwide, and multidrug-resistant tuberculosis, especially in AIDS patients, is a particularly difficult problem. For this purpose the most common cutaneous tuberculosis infection, lupus vulgaris, is discussed. A classification of skin tuberculosis is given in Table 21-2.

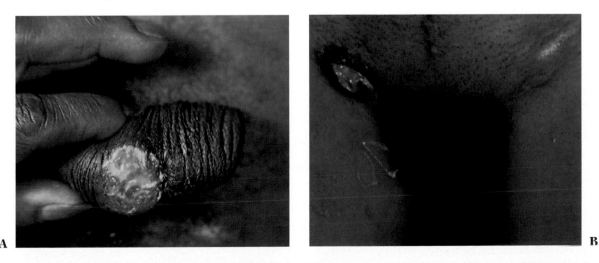

A　　　　　　　　　　　　　　　　　　　　　　　　　　**B**

FIGURE 21-11 ■ **(A)** Chancroid of penis. **(B)** Chancroid buboes in inguinal area. *(Courtesy of Derm-Arts Laboratories.)*

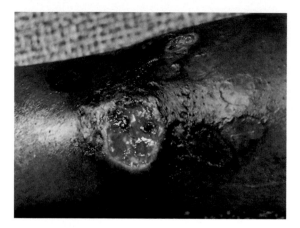

FIGURE 21-12 ■ Tuberculosis ulcer of leg. *(Courtesy of Derm-Arts Laboratories.)*

Presentation and Characteristics

Lupus vulgaris is a chronic, granulomatous disease characterized by the development of nodules, ulcers, and plaques arranged in any conceivable configuration. Scarring in the center of active lesions or at the edge, in severe, untreated cases, leads to atrophy and contraction, resulting in mutilating changes.

Distribution

Facial involvement is most common.

Course

The course is often slow and progressive, in spite of therapy.

Laboratory Findings

The histopathology shows typical tubercle formation with epithelioid cells, giant cells, and peripheral zone of lymphocytes. The causative organism, *Mycobacterium tuberculosis,* is not abundant in the lesions. The 48-hour tuberculin test is usually positive.

Differential Diagnosis

Other granulomas, such as those associated with syphilis, leprosy, sarcoidosis, deep fungus disease, and neoplasm, are to be ruled out by appropriate studies (see Chap. 16).

Treatment

Early localized lesions can be treated by surgical excision. For more widespread cases, long-term systemic therapy offers high hopes for cure. Isoniazid is usually prescribed

TABLE 21-2 ■ **Classification of Cutaneous Tuberculosis**

True Cutaneous Tuberculosis (Lesions Contain Tubercle Bacilli)

1. *Primary tuberculosis* (no previous infection; tuberculin-negative in initial stages)
   a. Primary inoculation tuberculosis; Ttuberculosis chancre (exogenous implantation into skin producing the primary complex)
   b. Miliary tuberculosis of the skin (hematogenous dispersion)
2. *Secondary tuberculosis* (lesions develop in person already sensitive to tuberculin as result of prior tuberculous lesion; tubercle bacilli difficult or impossible to demonstrate)
   a. Lupus vulgaris (inoculation of tubercle bacilli into the skin from external or internal sources)
   b. Tuberculosis verrucosa cutis (inoculation of tubercle bacilli into the skin from external or internal sources)
   c. Scrofuloderma (extension to skin from underlying focus in bones or glands)
   d. Tuberculosis cutis orificialis (mucous membrane lesions and extension onto the skin near mucocutaneous junctions)

Tuberculids (Allergic Origin; No Tubercle Bacilli in Lesions)

1. *Papular forms*
   a. Lupus miliaris disseminatus faciei (purely papular)
   b. Papulonecrotic tuberculid (papules with necrosis)
   c. Lichen scrofulosorum (follicular papules or lichenoid papules)
2. *Granulomatous, ulceronodular forms*
   a. Erythema induratum (nodules or plaques subsequently ulcerating; may be a nonspecific vasculitis)

along with other antituberculous drugs, such as rifampin and ethambutol (Myambutol). Multidrug-resistant tuberculosis is an increasing problem in AIDS patients.

Leprosy

Leprosy, or Hansen's disease, is to be considered in the differential diagnosis of any skin granulomas. It is endemic in the southern part of the United States and in semitropical and tropical areas the world over.

Presentation and Characteristics

Two definite types of leprosy are recognized: tuberculoid (Fig. 21-13) and lepromatous (Fig. 21-14). In addition,

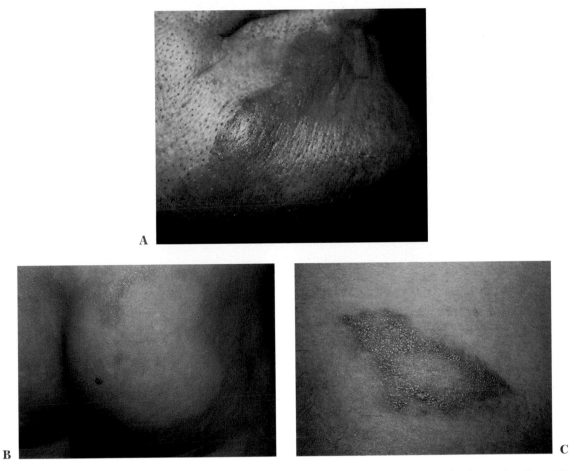

FIGURE 21-13 ■ **(A)** Tuberculoid leprosy of the chin. **(B)** Tuberculoid leprosy on the buttocks. *(A and B courtesy of Drs. W. Schorr and F. Kerdel-Vegas.)* **(C)** Tuberculoid leprosy on the chest. *(Courtesy of Dr. M. Rico, Durham, NC.)*

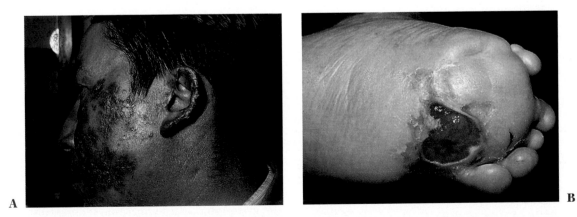

FIGURE 21-14 ■ **(A)** Lepromatous leprosy. *(Courtesy of Dr. A. Gongalez-Ochoa, Mexico.)* **(B)** Lepromatous leprosy on the foot. *(Courtesy of Dr. M. Rico, Durham, NC.)*

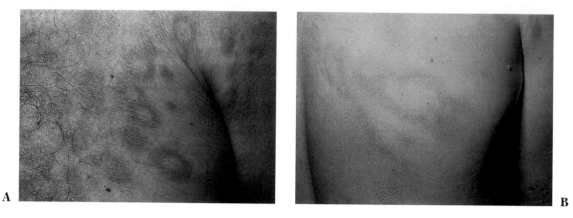

FIGURE 21-15 ■ **(A)** Dimorphic leprosy on the chest. *(Courtesy of Dr. R. Caputo, Atlanta, GA.)* **(B)** Dimorphic leprosy on the back. *(Courtesy of Dr. M. Rico, Durham, NC.)*

there are cases, called *dimorphic leprosy* (Fig. 21-15), that cannot presently be classified in either of these two categories but eventually develop either lepromatous or tuberculoid leprosy.

Tuberculoid leprosy is generally benign in its course because of considerable resistance to the disease on the part of the host. This is manifested by a positive lepromin test, histology that is not diagnostic, cutaneous lesions that are frequently erythematous with elevated borders, and minimal effect of the disease on the general health.

Lepromatous leprosy is the malignant form, which represents minimal resistance to the disease, with a negative lepromin reaction, characteristic histologic appearance, infiltrated cutaneous lesions with ill-defined borders, and progression to death, usually from secondary amyloidosis, unless treated.

Early symptoms of the lepromatous type include reddish macules with an indefinite border, nasal obstruction, and nosebleeds. Erythema nodosum–like lesions occur commonly. The tuberculoid type of leprosy is diagnosed early by the presence of an area of skin with impaired sensation, polyneuritis, and skin lesions with a sharp border and central atrophy.

Cause

The causative organism is *Mycobacterium leprae*.

Contagiousness

The source of infection is believed to be from patients with the lepromatous form. Infectiousness is of a low order.

Laboratory Findings

The bacilli are usually discovered in the lepromatous type but seldom in the tuberculoid type. Smears should be obtained from the tissue exposed by a small incision made into the dermis through an infiltrated lesion.

The lepromin reaction, a delayed reaction test similar to the tuberculin test, is of value in differentiating the lepromatous form from the tuberculoid form of leprosy, as stated. False-positive reactions do occur.

Biologic false-positive tests for syphilis are common in patients with the lepromatous type of leprosy.

Differential Diagnosis

Consider any of the granulomatous diseases, such as

■ *syphilis,*
■ *tuberculosis,*
■ *sarcoidosis,* and
■ *deep fungal infections.*

See also Chap. 16.

Treatment

Dapsone (diaminodiphenylsulfone), rifampin, and isoniazid are all effective.

Other Mycobacterial Dermatoses

Mycobacteria are pathogenic and saprophytic. *Mycobacterium marinum* can cause swimming pool granuloma and also granulomas in fishermen and those involved with fish tanks. Minocycline and combinations of ethambutol and rifampin, clarithromycin, and levofloxacin have been used as treatments.

Mycobacterium avium-intracellulare is seen in patients with AIDS, but skin lesions are rare.

Gonorrhea

Gonorrhea is considerably more prevalent than syphilis. Skin lesions with gonorrheal infection are rare, but a statement is due here on the therapy for uncomplicated gonorrhea. The therapy suggested by the Centers for Disease Control and Prevention is ceftriaxone, 250 mg, intramuscularly, one dose, or spectinomycin, 2 g, intramuscularly, one dose. Untreated or inadequately treated infection due to *Neisseria gonorrhoeae* can involve the skin through metastatic spread (Fig. 21-16). Primary cutaneous infection with multiple erosions at the site of the purulent discharge is very rare.

Metastatic complications include a bacteremia, in which there is an intermittent high fever, arthralgia, and skin lesions. The skin lesions are characteristic hemorrhagic vesiculopustules, most commonly seen on the fingers. Treatment with intravenous penicillin for 10 days at 5 to 10 million units per day is indicated.

The rarer septicemic form, with very high fever and meningitis or endocarditis, may have purpuric skin lesions similar to those seen in meningococcemia.

Rickettsial Diseases

The most common rickettsial disease in the United States is Rocky Mountain spotted fever, which is spread by ticks of various types. The skin eruption occurs after 3 to 7 days of fever and other toxic signs and is characterized by pur-

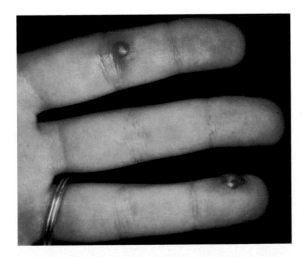

FIGURE 21-16 ■ Gonococcal septicemia with hemorrhagic vesicles. *(Courtesy of Derm-Arts Laboratories.)*

puric lesions on the extremities, mainly the wrists and the ankles, which then become generalized. The Weil-Felix test using *Proteus* OX19 and OX2 is positive. Tetracycline and chloramphenicol are effective.

The typhus group of rickettsial diseases includes epidemic or louse-borne typhus, Brill's disease, and endemic murine or flea-borne typhus. Less common forms include scrub typhus (tsutsugamushi disease), trench fever, and rickettsialpox, which is produced by a mite bite. The mite ordinarily lives on rodents. Approximately 10 days after the bite a primary lesion develops in the form of a papule that becomes vesicular. After a few days fever and other toxic signs are accompanied by a generalized eruption that resembles chickenpox. The disease subsides without therapy.

Ehrlichiosis is another rickettsial disease well known in dogs and now seen in humans. It is transmitted by tick bite. The nonspecific symptoms are similar to those of Rocky Mountain spotted fever, but only 20% of the patients have a rash.

Actinomycosis

Actinomycosis is a chronic, granulomatous, suppurative infection that characteristically causes the formation of a draining sinus. The most common location of the draining sinus is in the jaw region, but thoracic and abdominal sinuses do occur.

Primary Lesion

A red, firm, nontender tumor in the jaw area slowly extends locally to form a "lumpy jaw." It mimics a draining dental sinus from an infected tooth.

Secondary Lesions

Discharging sinuses become infected with other bacteria and, if untreated, may develop into osteomyelitis.

Course

General health is usually unaffected unless extension occurs into bone or deeper neck tissues. Recurrence is unusual if treatment is continued long enough.

Cause

Actinomyces israelii, which is an anaerobic bacterium that lives as a normal inhabitant of the mouth, particularly in persons who have poor dental hygiene, is the causative agent. Injury to the jaw or a tooth extraction usually precedes the development of the infection. Infected cattle are not the source of human infection. The disease is twice as common in men as in women.

Laboratory Findings

Pinpoint-sized "sulfur" granules, which are colonies of the organism, can be seen grossly and microscopically in the draining pus. A Gram stain of the pus shows masses of interlacing gram-positive fibers with or without club-shaped processes at the tips of these fibers. The organism can be cultured anaerobically on special media.

Differential Diagnosis

- *Pyodermas*
- *Tuberculosis*
- *Draining dental abscess*
- *Neoplasm*

Treatment

1. Penicillin, 2.4 million units intramuscularly, is given daily, until definite improvement is noted. Then oral penicillin in the same dosage should be continued for 3 weeks after the infection apparently has been cured. In severe cases, 10 million or more units of penicillin given intravenously, daily, may be necessary.
2. Incision and drainage is performed of the lumps and the sinuses.
3. Good oral hygiene is required.
4. In resistant cases, broad-spectrum antibiotics can be used alone or in combination with the penicillin.

Suggested Reading

Aly R, Maibach H. Atlas of the infections of the skin. Philadelphia, WB Saunders, 1998.

Drugs for sexually transmitted infections. Med Lett Drugs Ther 1999;41:85–90.

Epstein ME, Amodio-Groton M, Sadick NS. Antimicrobial agents for the dermatologist: I. β-Lactam antibiotics and related compounds. J Am Acad Dermatol 1997;37:2.

Epstein ME, Amodio-Groton M, Sadick NS. Antimicrobial agents for the dermatologist: II. Macrolides, fluoroquinolones, rifamycins, tetracyclines, trimethoprim-sulfamethoxazole, and clindamycin. J Am Acad Dermatol 1997;37:3.

Lesher JL. An atlas of microbiology of the skin. London, Parthenon Publishing Group, 2000.

Modlin RL, Rea TH. Leprosy: New insight into an ancient disease. J Am Acad Dermatol 1987;17:1.

Parish LC, Witkowksi JA, Crissey JT. The decubitus ulcer in clinical practice. New York, Springer, 1997.

Sanders CV. Skin and infection: A color atlas and text. Baltimore, Williams & Wilkins, 1995.

Sehgal VN, Sooneita AW. Cutaneous tuberculosis. Int J Dermatol 1990;23:237.

Spach DH, Liles WC, Campbell GL, et al. Tick-borne diseases in the United States: Review article. N Engl J Med 1993;329:936.

CHAPTER 22

Spirochetal Infections

John C. Hall

Two spirochetal diseases are discussed in this chapter: syphilis and Lyme disease.

Syphilis

When Gordon C. Sauer was stationed at the West Virginia State Rapid Treatment Center, from 1946 to 1948, the average admittance was 30 patients a day with venereal disease. Approximately one third of these patients had infectious syphilis. In 1949, the center was closed because of the patient census. The incidence of reported syphilis has risen again to alarming heights. Many patients with acquired immunodeficiency syndrome (AIDS) also have syphilis. Because of this resurgence, it is imperative for all physicians to have a basic understanding of this polymorphous disease.

Cutaneous lesions of syphilis occur in all three stages of the disease. Under what circumstances will the present-day physician be called on to diagnose, evaluate, or manage a patient with syphilis?

1. The cutaneous manifestations, such as a penile lesion or a rash that could be secondary syphilis, may bring a patient to the office.
2. A positive blood test found on a premarital examination or as part of a routine physical examination may be responsible for a patient's being seen by the physician.
3. Syphilis may be seen in conjunction with AIDS. The problem becomes complicated because the serologic test for syphilis (STS) may not be positive in patients with AIDS and routine antibiotic dosage regimens may be ineffective.
4. Cardiac, central nervous system, or other organ disease may be a reason for a patient to consult a physician.

To manage these patients properly a thorough knowledge of the natural untreated course of the disease is essential.

> ### SAUER'S NOTES
>
> 1. To diagnose syphilis, the physician must have a high index of suspicion for it.
> 2. Syphilis is the great imitator and can mimic many other conditions.

Primary Syphilis

The first stage of acquired syphilis usually develops within 2 to 6 weeks (average 3 weeks) after exposure. The *primary chancre* most commonly occurs on the genitalia (Figs. 22-1 and 22-2), but extragenital chancres are not rare and are often misdiagnosed. Without treatment the chancre heals within 1 to 4 weeks, depending on the location, the amount of secondary infection, and host resistance.

The blood STS may be negative in the early days of the chancre but eventually becomes positive. The spirochete, *Treponema pallidum*, is readily found with darkfield examination. This test is of limited value since there are few people with the expertise to interpret the test reliably. A cerebrospinal fluid examination during the primary stage reveals invasion of the spirochete in approximately 25% of cases.

Clinically, the chancre may vary in appearance from a single small erosion to multiple indurated ulcers of the genitalia. It is usually painless. Primary syphilis commonly goes unnoticed in the female patient. Bilateral or unilateral regional lymphadenopathy is common. Malaise and fever may be present.

Early Latent Stage

Latency, manifested by positive serologic findings and no other subjective or objective evidence of syphilis, may occur between the primary and the secondary stages.

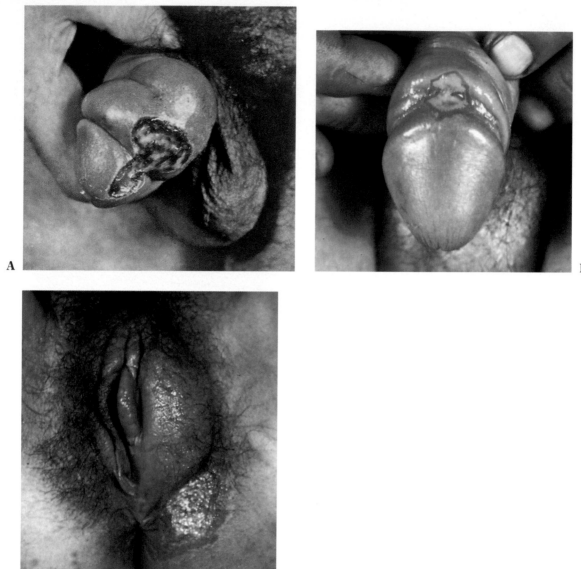

FIGURE 22-1 ■ Primary syphilis with primary chancres of the genitalia. **(A)** Chancre of the penis is accompanied by marked edema of the penis. **(B)** Penile chancre. **(C)** Vulvar chancre with edema of the labia majora. *(Courtesy of J.E. Moore and The Upjohn Company.)*

Secondary Syphilis

Early secondary lesions may develop before the primary chancre has healed or after latency of a few weeks (Figs. 22-3, 22-4, and 22-5). *Late secondary lesions* are more rare and usually are seen after the early secondary lesions have healed. Both types of secondary lesions contain the spirochete *T. pallidum,* which can be easily seen with the darkfield microscope. The STS is positive (an exception is in some patients with AIDS), and approximately 30% of the cases have abnormal cerebrospinal fluid findings.

Clinically, the early secondary rash can consist of macular, papular, pustular, squamous, or eroded lesions or combinations of any of these lesions; papulosquamous is the most common with oval lesions and fine dry adherent scale. This can easily be confused with pityriasis rosea. Palm and sole involvement is characteristic. The entire body may be involved or only the palms and the soles, the mouth, or the genitalia. A "moth-eaten" scalp alopecia may develop in the late secondary stage.

Condylomata lata is the name applied to the flat, moist, warty lesions teeming with spirochetes found in the

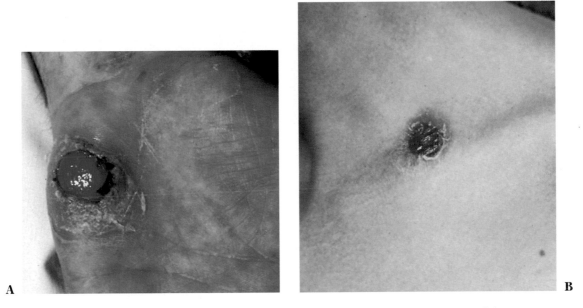

FIGURE 22-2 ■ Primary syphilis with extragenital chancres. (**A**) Chancre of the palm. (**B**) Chancre over the clavicle. *(Courtesy of The Upjohn Company.)*

groin and the axillae (see Figs. 22-4 and 22-5). Mucous patches are white elevated verrucous skin usually on the oral mucous membranes.

The late secondary lesions are nodular, squamous, and ulcerative and are distinguished from the tertiary lesions only by the time interval after the onset of the infection and by the finding of the spirochete in superficial smears of serum from the lesions. Annular and semiannular configurations of late secondary lesions are common.

Generalized lymphadenopathy, malaise, fever, and arthralgia occur in many patients with secondary syphilis.

Early Latent Stage

Following the secondary stage, many patients with untreated syphilis have only a positive STS. After 4 years of infection, the patient enters the late latent stage.

Late Latent Stage

This time span of 4 years arbitrarily divides the early infectious stages from the later noninfectious stages, which may or may not develop.

Tertiary Syphilis

This late stage is manifested by subjective or objective involvement of any of the organs of the body, including the skin (Figs. 22-6 and 22-7; see also Fig. 3-1A). Tertiary changes may be precocious but most often develop 5 to 20 years after the onset of the primary stage. Clinically, the skin lesions are characterized by nodular and gummatous ulcerations. Solitary multiple annular and nodular lesions are common. Subjective complaints are rare unless considerable secondary bacterial infection is present in a gumma. Scarring, on healing, is inevitable in the majority of the tertiary skin lesions. Larger texts should be consulted for the late changes seen in the central nervous system, the cardiovascular system, the bones, the eyes, and the viscera. Approximately 15% of the patients who acquire syphilis and receive no treatment die of the disease.

Late Latent Stage

Another latent period may occur after natural healing of some types of benign tertiary syphilis.

Congenital Syphilis

Congenital syphilis is acquired *in utero* from an infectious mother (Fig. 22-8; see also Fig. 36-4C). The STS required of pregnant women by most states has lowered the incidence of this unfortunate disease. Stillbirths are not uncommon from mothers who are untreated. After the birth of a live infected child, the mortality rate depends on the duration of the infection, the natural host resistance, and the rapidity of initiating treatment. Early and late lesions are seen in these children, similar to those found in the adult cases of acquired syphilis. Blistering can occur.

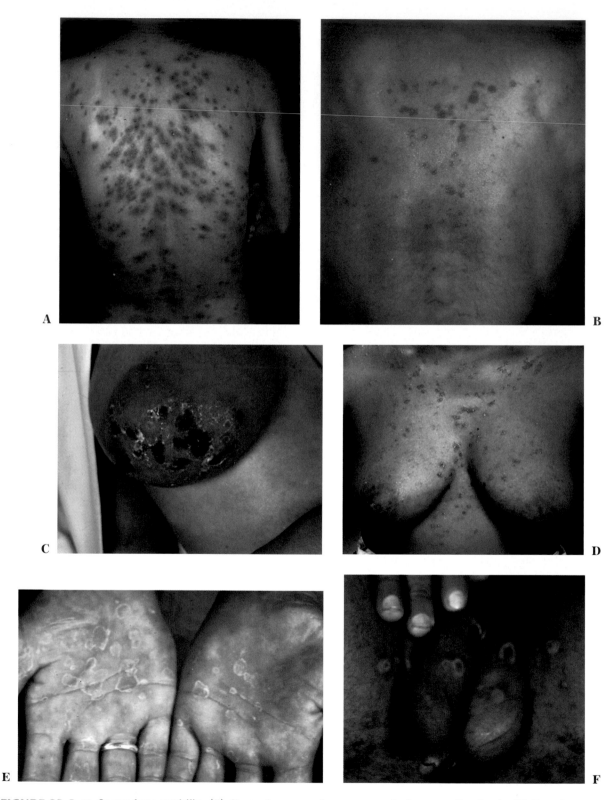

FIGURE 22-3 ■ Secondary syphilis. (**A**) Secondary papulosquamous lesions on the back. (**B**) Papulosquamous lesions on the back. (**C**) Crusted lesions on the breast. (**D**) Papular lesions on the chest. *(Courtesy of K.U.M.C.)* (**E**) Papulosquamous lesions on the palms. (**F**) Late secondary annular lesions on penis and scrotum.

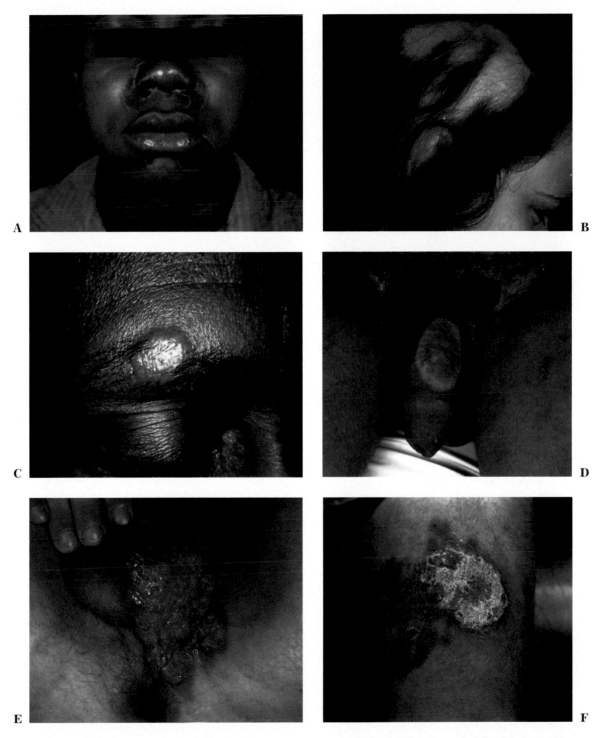

FIGURE 22-4 ■ Late secondary syphilis. (**A**) Annular lesions. (**B**) Syphilitic alopecia. (**C**) Nodular lesion on eyebrow. (**D**) Annular lesion on penis. (**E**) Condylomata lata in groin area. (**F**) Psoriatic-type lesion on leg.

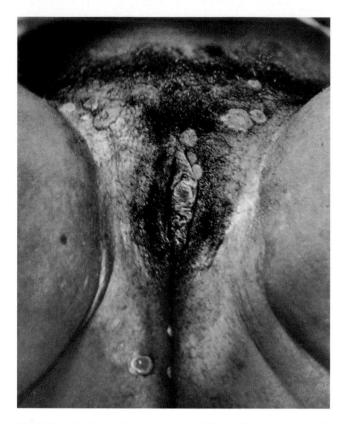

FIGURE 22-5 ■ Secondary syphilis with *condylomata lata* of the vulva. *(Courtesy of J. E. Moore and The Upjohn Company.)*

Laboratory Findings

Darkfield Examination

The etiologic agent, *T. pallidum,* can be found in the serum from the primary or secondary lesions. However, a darkfield microscope is necessary, and very few physician's offices or laboratories have this instrument. A considerable amount of experience is necessary to distinguish *T. pallidum* from other *Treponema* species.

Serologic Test for Syphilis

The STS is simple, readily available, and has several modifications. The rapid plasma reagin (RPR) test and the Venereal Disease Research Laboratories (VDRL) flocculation test are used most commonly. Treponemal tests such as the fluorescent treponemal antibody absorption (FTA-ABS) test and modifications are more difficult to perform in the laboratory and therefore are used primarily when the RPR and VDRL tests are "reactive."

When a report is received from the laboratory that the STS is positive (RPR or VDRL reactive), a second blood specimen should be submitted to obtain a quantitative report. In many laboratories this repeat test is not necessary, because a quantitative test is run routinely on all positive blood specimens. A dilution of 1:2 is only weakly positive and might be a biologic false-positive reaction. A test positive in a dilution of 1:32 is strongly positive. In evaluating the response of the STS to treatment, one must remember that a change in titer from 1:2 to 1:4 to 1:16 to 1:32 to 1:64, or downward in the same gradations, is only a change in one tube, in each instance. Thus a change from 1:2 to 1:4 is of the same magnitude as a change from 1:32 to 1:64. Quantitative tests enable the physician to

- evaluate the efficacy of the treatment,
- discover a relapse before it becomes infectious,
- differentiate between a relapse and a reinfection,
- establish a reaction as a seroresistant type, and
- differentiate between true and biologic false-positive serologic reactions.

In most laboratories it is now routine to do an FTA-ABS test on all patients with reactive RPR and VDRL tests. With rare exceptions, a positive FTA-ABS test means that the patient has or had syphilis and is not a biologic false-positive reactor. The STS may not be positive in patients with AIDS.

Tissue Examination

A direct fluorescent antibody test for *T. pallidum* can be performed on lesion exudate or on biopsy tissue.

Cerebrospinal Fluid Test

As has been stated, the cerebrospinal fluid is frequently positive in the primary and secondary stages of the disease. Invasion of the central nervous system is an early manifestation, even though the perceptible clinical effects are a late manifestation. The cerebrospinal fluid should be examined at least once during the course of the disease. However, in actual practice primary or secondary disease is usually treated without a cerebrospinal fluid exam but with antibiotic doses that are sufficient to eliminate the treponeme from the cerebrospinal fluid. Cerebrospinal fluid examination is appropriate for all patients with syphilis who are at a high risk for human immunodeficiency virus (HIV) infection. The best routine is to perform a cerebrospinal fluid test before treatment is initiated and repeat the test as indicated. If the cerebrospinal fluid is negative in a patient who has had syphilis for 4 years, central nervous system syphilis will not occur, and future cerebrospinal fluid tests

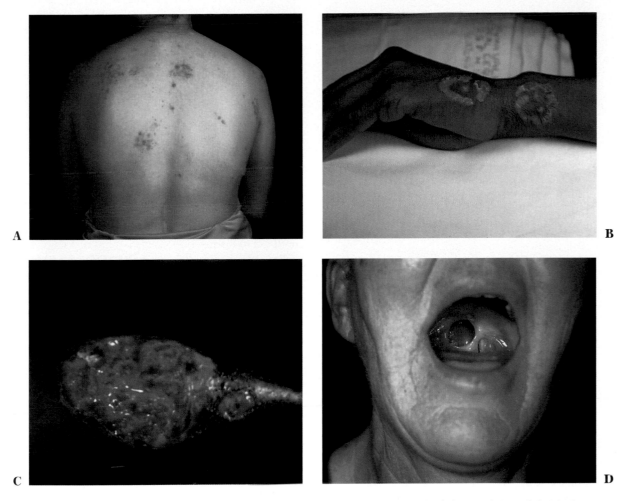

FIGURE 22-6 ■ Tertiary syphilis. (**A**) Grouped papular lesions on the back. (**B**) Annular nodular lesions on hand. (**C**) Gumma on the leg. (**D**) Perforation from old gumma of soft palate.

are not necessary. If the test is positive, repeat tests should be done every 6 months for 4 years. The following three tests are run on the cerebrospinal fluid:

- *Cell count:* The finding of four or more lymphocytes or polymorphonuclear leukocytes per cubic millimeter is positive. The cell count is the most labile of the tests. It becomes increased early in the infection and responds fastest to therapy. Therefore, it is a good index of activity of the disease. The cell count must be done within an hour after the fluid is withdrawn.
- *Total protein:* Measured in milligrams per deciliter, it normally should be below 40.
- *Nontreponemal flocculation test:* Presently, the most common test performed is the qualitative and quantitative VDRL. This test is the last to turn positive and the slowest to return to negativity. In some cases, therapy causes a decrease in the titer, but slight positivity or "fastness" can remain for the lifetime of the patient.

Differential Diagnosis

- *Primary syphilis:* From chancroid, herpes simplex, fusospirochetal balanitis, granuloma inguinale, and any of the *primary chancre-type diseases* (see Dictionary–Index).
- *Secondary syphilis:* From any of the papulosquamous diseases (especially pityriasis rosea), fungal diseases, drug eruption, and alopecia areata.
- *Tertiary skin syphilis:* From any of the granulomatous diseases, particularly tuberculosis, leprosy, sarcoidosis, deep mycoses, and lymphomas.

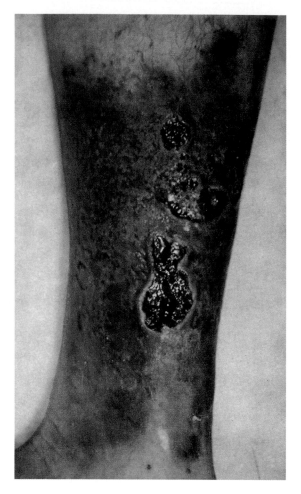

FIGURE 22-7 ■ Tertiary syphilis with a gumma of the leg. This resembles a stasis ulcer. *(Courtesy of J.E. Moore and The Upjohn Company.)*

■ *Congenital syphilis:* From atopic eczema, diseases with lymphadenopathy, hepatomegaly, and splenomegaly.

A true-positive syphilitic serology is to be differentiated from a biologic false-positive reaction. This serologic differentiation is accomplished best by using the FTA-ABS test, or its modifications, along with a good history and a thorough examination of the patient. Many patients with biologic false-positive reactions develop one of the collagen diseases at a later date.

Treatment

Case Example. A 22-year-old married man presents with a sore 1 cm in diameter on his glans penis of 5 days' duration. Three weeks previously he had extramarital intercourse, and 10 days before this office visit he had marital intercourse. The patient knows his extramarital sexual contact only as "Jane," and he cannot remember which bar she presided over.

First Visit.

1. Perform a darkfield examination of the penile lesion. Treatment can be started if *T. pallidum* is found. If you cannot perform a darkfield examination, refer the patient to the local health department or another facility that can perform a darkfield examination.
2. If a darkfield examination cannot be performed or is negative, obtain a blood specimen for an STS.
3. While waiting for the STS report, advise the patient to soak the site in saline solution for 15 minutes twice a day. The solution is made by placing 1/4 teaspoon of salt in a glass of water.

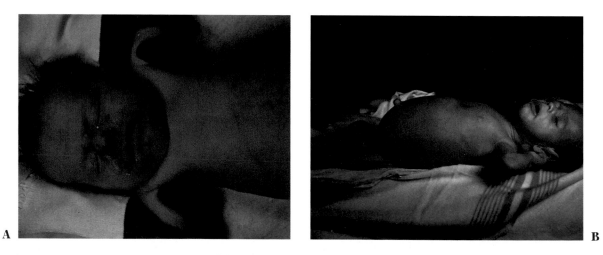

A **B**

FIGURE 22-8 ■ Congenital syphilis. (**A**) Scaly and erosive lesions with large liver (fatal). (**B**) Massively enlarged liver and spleen.

4. Advise the patient against sexual intercourse until the reports are completed.
5. Explain to the patient the seriousness of treating him for syphilis if he does not have it. The "syphilitic" label is one he should not want, if it is at all possible to avoid it.

Second Visit. Three days later the lesion is larger and the STS report is "nonreactive."

1. Obtain blood specimen for a second STS.
2. Antibiotic ointment 15.0

    Sig: Apply t.i.d. locally after soaking in saline solution.

3. Explain again why you are delaying therapy until a definite diagnosis is made.

Third Visit. Three days later the sore is smaller, but the STS report is "reactive." The diagnosis is now known to be "primary syphilis."

1. The patient is reassured that present-day therapy is highly successful but that he must follow your instructions closely.
2. His wife should be brought in for examination and a blood test. If the blood test is negative, it should be repeated weekly for 1 month. However, some syphilologists believe that therapy is indicated for the marital partner in the presence of a negative STS if the husband has infectious syphilis and is being treated. A single injection of 2.4 million units of a long-acting type of penicillin is used. This prevents "ping-pong" syphilis, which is a cycle of reinfection from one marital partner to another.
3. The patient's contact should be found. The patient's findings, including his contact with an unidentified sexual partner, should be reported to the local health department. This is usually done automatically by the laboratory where the blood tests were done but this does not relieve the physician of the responsibility of reporting the patient to the health department.
4. A cerebrospinal fluid specimen should be obtained. (The report was returned as normal for all three tests.)
5. Penicillin therapy should be begun. Here, two factors are important:
   a. The dose must be adequate.
   b. The effective blood levels of medication must be maintained over 10 to 14 days.

Dosage

Primary and Secondary Syphilis

1. Administer 2.4 million units of benzathine penicillin G, half in each buttock, single session.

2. Consult larger texts or relevant literature for other treatment schedules.

Latent (Both Early and Late) Syphilis

1. If no cerebrospinal fluid examination, administer 7.2 million units benzathine penicillin G divided into three weekly injections.
2. If cerebrospinal fluid examination is nonreactive, give 2.4 million units in single dose.

Neurosyphilis or Cardiovascular Syphilis

1. Administer 9 to 12 million units of a long-acting penicillin.
2. For other routines or complicated cases, consult larger texts for therapy and care.
3. HIV-infected patients with neurosyphilis should be treated for 10 days at least with aqueous crystalline penicillin G in a dosage of 2 to 4 million units IV every 4 hours.

Benign Late Syphilis

Treatment is the same as for neurosyphilis.

Congenital Syphilis

1. Early congenital syphilis
   a. Younger than 6 months of age: Aqueous procaine penicillin G, 10 daily IM doses totaling 100,000 to 200,000 units/kg.
   b. Six months to 2 years of age: As above, *or* benzathine penicillin G, 100,000 units/kg IM in one single dose.
2. Late congenital syphilis
   a. Ages 2 to 11 years, or weighing less than 70 pounds: Same as for 6 months to 2 years.
   b. Twelve years or older, and weighing more than 70 pounds: Same treatment as for adult-acquired syphilis, with comparable time and progression of infection.

Lyme Disease

Originally described as Lyme arthritis, Lyme disease is caused by a spirochete that is transmitted by several species of *Ixodes* tick. Early removal of the tick (<24 hours) usually prevents disease transmission. The disease has been reported from most states and on every continent except Antarctica. Endemic areas include the northeastern United States and the upper Midwestern states. Clinical manifestations include erythema chronicum migrans (ECM) skin lesions, flu-like

SAUER'S NOTES: SYPHILIS

1. Any patient treated for gonorrhea should have a STS 4 to 6 weeks later.
2. Persons with HIV infection acquired through sexual contact or IV drug abuse should be tested for syphilis.
3. Seventy-five percent of the persons who acquire syphilis suffer no serious manifestations of the disease.
4. Syphilis does not cause vesicular or bullous skin lesions, except in infants with congenital infection.

PRIMARY STAGE

1. Syphilis should be ruled in or out in the diagnosis of any penile or vulvar sores.
2. Multiple primary chancres are moderately common.

SECONDARY STAGE

1. The rash of secondary syphilis, except for the rare follicular form, does not usually itch.
2. Secondary syphilis should be ruled in or out in any patient with a generalized, nonpruritic rash especially when it is papulosquamous. A high index of suspicion is necessary.

LATENT STAGE

The diagnosis of "latent syphilis" cannot be made for a particular patient unless cerebrospinal fluid tests have been done and are negative for syphilis.

TERTIARY STAGE

1. Tertiary syphilis should be considered in any patient with a chronic granuloma of the skin, particularly if it has an annular or circular configuration.
2. Invasion of the central nervous system occurs in the primary and secondary stages of the disease. A cerebrospinal fluid test is indicated during these stages.
3. If the cerebrospinal fluid tests for syphilis are negative in a patient who has had syphilis for 4 years, central nervous system syphilis usually will not occur and future spinal punctures are not necessary.
4. Twenty percent of patients with late asymptomatic neurosyphilis have a negative STS.

CONGENITAL SYPHILIS

An STS should be done on every pregnant woman to prevent congenital syphilis of the newborn.

SEROLOGY

1. The STS may be negative in the early days of the primary chancre. The STS is always positive in the secondary stage; an exception to this is in patients with AIDS.
2. A quantitative STS should be done on all syphilitic patients to evaluate the response to treatment or the development of relapse or reinfection.
3. The finding of a low-titer STS in a patient not previously treated for syphilis calls for a careful evaluation to rule out a biologic false-positive reaction.

symptoms, and possible neurologic, cardiac, and rheumatologic involvement.

Late cutaneous manifestations of Lyme disease are borrelia lymphocytoma, acrodermatitis chronica atrophicans and, although controversial, possibly in some cases (especially in Europe) morphea (localized scleroderma).

Presentation and Characteristics

Primary Lesion

The erythematous circular rash appears at the site of the tick bite and enlarges with central clearing, but multiple ECM eruptions can occur. The rash typically develops from 2 to 30 days after the bite. The bite area can become necrotic.

Secondary Lesion

Multiple ECM eruptions can develop.

Distribution

Usually ECM begins at the site of the tick bite.

Season

The disease occurs from late May through early fall.

Course

In untreated patients the ECM lesions may last only 10 to 14 days, they may persist for months, or they may come and go over a year's time. The bite papule and ECM fade rapidly after therapy is begun. Late-stage cutaneous lesions include acrodermatitis chronic atrophicans and borrelia lymphocytoma (see Chap. 33).

Subjective Symptoms

Flulike symptoms, with fever, chills, myalgia, and headache, appear with the rash. Later other organs may be affected.

Cause

The spirochete *Borrelia burgdorferi* is transmitted by *Ixodes* species of ticks and possibly by the hard-bodied ticks. The white-tailed deer and white-footed mouse are preferred hosts of the tick.

Diagnosis

High index of suspicion, history of tick bite (patient is not always aware of bite), previous "ringworm-type" rash, and, later, positive Lyme disease antibody titer may be present (but these tests are not reliable).

Histologic findings are not specific and culture of the spirochete is often not practical. Polymerase chain reaction may be helpful on biopsy tissue in a qualified laboratory.

Differential Diagnosis

Cutaneously, the ECM rash can resemble an allergic reaction or tinea. See *figurate erythemas* in the Dictionary–Index. Systemically, many diseases can be considered, with fever, myalgia, cardiac, joint, or neurologic manifestations.

Treatment

Because diagnosis of Lyme disease is difficult, treatment may be indicated, especially in endemic areas, based on history and clinical findings. Early therapy for this disease is doxycycline, 100 mg, b.i.d. for 21 days, or amoxicillin, 500 mg, t.i.d. for 21 days. Early tick removal (in less than 24 hours) probably prevents disease transmission. Removing deer and mice habitats such as brush, leaves, stonewalls, and woodpiles may be helpful.

For late stages of the disease with cardiac or neurologic manifestations, treatment is ceftriaxone, 2 to 4 g/d IM or IV for 14 days. Because efficacy of therapy is difficult to evaluate, the literature is replete with other therapeutic regimens. Lyme vaccination is effective and should be considered in people at high risk in endemic areas. It takes 12 months to confer immunity.

Lymephobia is a term coined to describe a common psychological problem owing to the nonspecific nature of symptoms and the lack of specific tests. Well-meaning physicians can fall into the trap of long-term antibiotics for multiple vague systemic complaints. Permethrin 5% applied to clothing is a helpful tick repellant.

Suggested Reading

Abele DC, Anders KH. The many faces and phases of borreliosis: I. Lyme disease. J Am Acad Dermatol 1990; 23:167.

Abele DC, Anders KH. The many faces and phases of borreliosis: II. J Am Acad Dermatol 1990;23:401.

Baum EW, et al. Secondary syphilis, still the great imitator. JAMA 1983;249:3069.

Bennet ML, Lynn AW, Klein LE. Congenital syphilis: Subtle presentation of fulminant disease. J Am Acad Dermatol 1997;36:2.

Burlington DB. FDA public health advisory: Assays for antibodies to *Borrelia brugdorferi*: Limitations, use, and interpretation for supporting a clinical diagnosis of Lyme disease. FDA, July 7, 1997.

Don PC, Rubenstein R, Christie S. Malignant syphilis (lues maligna) and concurrent infection with HIV. Int J Dermatol 1995;34:403.

Drugs for sexually transmitted infections. Med Lett 1999;41:1062.

Stere AC, Taylor E, McHugh GL, et al. The overdiagnosis of Lyme disease. JAMA 1993;269:1812.

Treatment of Lyme disease. Med Lett Drugs Ther 1997; 39:47–48.

Trevisan G, Cinco M. Lyme disease. Int J Dermatol 1990; 29:1.

CHAPTER 23

Dermatologic Virology

Jashin J. Wu, David B. Huang, Stephen K. Tyring

Viral diseases of the skin are exceedingly common. The various clinical entities are distinct, and, because we have no specific antiviral drug, the treatment varies for each entity. The following list contains the virus diseases that are discussed here:

- Herpes simplex virus 1 and 2
- Varicella-zoster virus
- Human papillomavirus
- Molluscum contagiosum virus
- Lymphogranuloma venereum
- Measles (rubeola)
- German measles (rubella)
- Erythema infectiosum
- Coxsackievirus infections
- Herpangina
- Echovirus exanthema

Herpes Simplex Virus 1

Herpes simplex virus 1 (HSV-1) is the usual cause of herpes labialis as well as the cause of 30% of first episode genital herpes. Approximately 90% of people between 20 to 40 years of age have antibodies against HSV-1. The primary infection typically occurs early in life, with viral latency established in neural ganglia. Reactivation can occur due to several different triggers, including immunosuppression, physical trauma, psychological stress, or sun exposure. Transmission of HSV-1 occurs with viral shedding during the asymptomatic and symptomatic periods through direct contact with infected secretions (i.e., saliva).

Presentation and Characteristics

Asymptomatic primary infection is the rule. For some, prodromal symptoms may occur first, such as burning, itching, or tingling. The mouth and lips are the most common areas of primary infection (Figs. 23-1 and 23-2). Lesions start as erythematous vesicles that develop into ulcerations and crusts. Recurrent episodes present often

as three to five vesicles at the vermilion border of the lip, which last at least 48 hours. The recurrent episodes are less severe than the primary if the primary episode has symptoms.

Treatment

Oral acyclovir and oral famciclovir are effective for the treatment of herpes labialis. Oral acyclovir is taken at 400 mg five times daily for 5 days. It reduces duration of pain by 36% and time to loss of crust by 27%. Famciclovir is taken 500 mg three times a day for 5 days. Valacyclovir, is also effective against HSV-1; episodic therapy for recurrent herpes labialis is 2 g twice daily for 1 day.

Herpes Simplex Virus 2

Herpes simplex virus 2 (HSV-2) is one of the most widespread sexually transmitted diseases (STDs) in the world. It causes 70% of primary genital herpes and over 95% of recurrent genital herpes (Fig 23-3). In the United States, the prevalence of genital herpes is 40 to 60 million, and the incidence is 500,000 to 1,000,000 cases/year. Similar to HSV-1, HSV-2 causes primary, latent, and recurrent infections, and is transmitted during both asymptomatic and symptomatic phases, typically through sexual contact. HSV-2 can also cause neonatal herpes, with the highest risk occurring when the mother has primary genital herpes during delivery. In addition to cutaneous lesions, the infected neonate may develop multiorgan involvement, which carries a high mortality rate.

Presentation and Characteristics

Up to 90% of patients infected with HSV-2 become infected with asymptomatic viral shedding. Genital herpes infection is typically asymptomatic, because the lesions may be painless and inapparent. The first clinically recognized lesions of genital herpes may be either true primary or a first episode nonprimary. True primary genital herpes usually

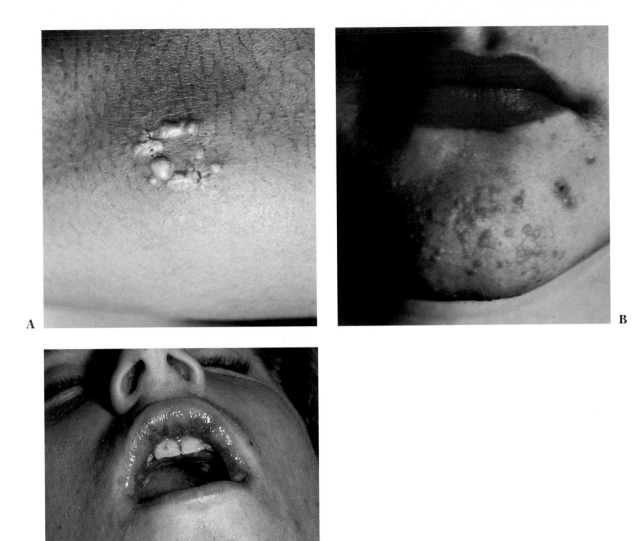

FIGURE 23-1 ■ ■ Herpes simplex on arm (**A**), chin (**B**), and true primary infection on lips and mouth (interoral). *(Courtesy of Dermik Laboratories, Inc.)*

develops after 2 to 14 days of HSV exposure. There may be widespread vesicles and ulcers on the genitalia with inguinal adenopathy, and the patient may complain of discharge, dysuria, fever, lethargy, myalgias, and photophobia.

More than half of patients with the first recognized signs and symptoms of genital herpes have a first episode nonprimary, which occurs when the initial episode is asymptomatic. This may occur weeks, months, or even years after initial HSV infection. A strong immune response may prevent the infection from becoming clinically recognizable. The initial immune response does attenuate the severity of first episode nonprimary genital herpes. Lesions are often less extensive and systemic symptoms are less common and severe compared to that of true primary genital herpes.

Treatment

Because there is no cure for genital herpes, therapy is aimed at controlling the signs and symptoms of an outbreak. In 2002, the Centers for Disease Control and Prevention (CDC) recommended therapy for individuals with a first clinical episode of genital herpes; episodic development of genital herpes; and suppressive therapy for recurrent genital herpes (Table 23-1). Therapies used for genital herpes are

- acyclovir,
- valacyclovir,
- famciclovir,
- cidofovir,

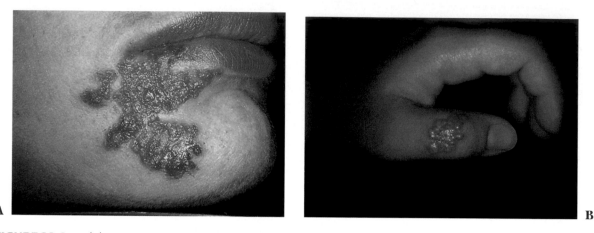

FIGURE 23-2 ■ **(A)** Recurrent herpes simplex on chin with secondary bacterial infection. **(B)** Recurrent herpes simplex on a thumb. *(Courtesy of Dermik Laboratories, Inc.)*

- fomivirsen,
- foscarnet, (especially in cases in HIV patients) and
- penciclovir.

Varicella-Zoster Virus

Varicella-zoster virus (VZV) causes primary varicella (chickenpox) and herpes zoster (shingles), which is a reactivation of the primary varicella infection. Primary varicella is usually a self-limited disease in immunocompetent children. There are more than 11,000 hospitalizations each year in the United States due to complications of varicella infection in children who are often otherwise healthy. Susceptible adults typically develop more profuse skin lesions, more frequent complications, and worse constitutional symptoms, such as prolonged fever.

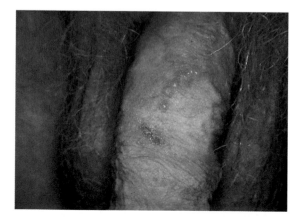

FIGURE 23-3 ■ Recurrent herpes simplex on the penis. *(Courtesy of Dermik Laboratories, Inc.)*

Following primary VZV infection, the virus resides in a latent state in the sensory ganglia. With aging or a weakened immune system, the VZV may be reactive as shingles. With the highest incidence of all neurologic diseases, it occurs annually in more than 1,000,000 people in the United States and during the lifetime in 20% of the population.

Presentation and Characteristics

Two weeks after exposure, primary varicella may start with 2 to 3 days of prodromal symptoms such as low-grade fever, chills, headache, malaise, nausea, and vomiting. The rash appears as crops of small red macules on the face and scalp, which spreads to the trunk with sparing of the distal upper and lower extremities. Over 12 hours, the macules progress to 1- to 3-mm papules, vesicles, and then pustules. Crusting occurs within a few days, and complete healing in approximately 1 week.

More than 90% of patients with zoster have a prodrome of intense pain in the involved single sensory ganglion (dermatome) preceding the zoster rash (Fig. 23-4). The appearance of the characteristic dermatomal rash (erythematous vesicles with subsequent crusting) is accompanied by severe pain. Shingles is typically localized to a dermatome, does not usually extensively cross the midline of the body, and occurs at the site which was most severely affected during primary varicella infection. Although any dermatome can be affected, the most common regions of involvement are the ophthalmic (V1) and midthoracic to upper lumbar (T3 to L2) dermatomes. The rash heals within 2 to 4 weeks, but the pain associated with herpes zoster is its most distressing symptom. Pain that persists after cutaneous healing is called postherpetic neuralgia

TABLE 23-1 ■ **Treatments for Genital Herpes**

First Clinical Episode of Genital Herpes	Episodic Therapy for Recurrent Genital Herpes	Suppressive Therapy for Recurrent Genital Herpes
Acyclovir 400 mg PO t.i.d. for 7–10 days	Acyclovir 400 mg PO t.i.d. for 5 days	Acyclovir 400 mg PO b.i.d.
Acyclovir 200 mg PO 5 times a day for 7–10 days	Acyclovir 200 mg PO 5 times a day for 5 days	Famciclovir 250 mg PO b.i.d.
Famciclovir 250 mg PO t.i.d. for 7–10 days	Acyclovir 800 mg PO b.i.d. for 5 days	Valacyclovir 500 mg PO q.d. (≤9 outbreaks/year)
Valacyclovir 1 g PO b.i.d. for 7–10 days	Famciclovir 125 mg PO b.i.d. for 5 days	Valacyclovir 1 g PO q.d. (>9 outbreaks/year)
	Valacyclovir 500 mg PO b.i.d. for 3–5 days	
	Valacyclovir 1 g PO q.d. for 5 days	

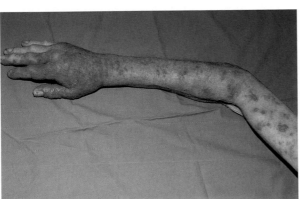

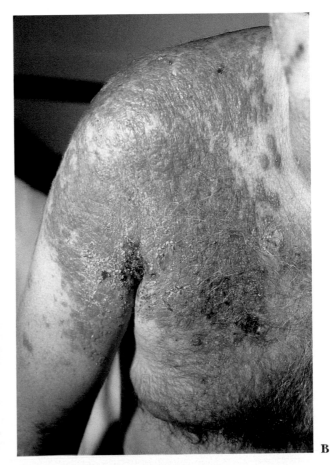

A   B

FIGURE 23-4 ■ Herpes zoster in a lymphoma patient. (**A**) Right upper extremity. (**B**) Right chest.

(PHN), a chronic neuropathic pain syndrome that can last for months or even years.

Treatment

Primary varicella in immunocompetent children is self-limited and treated symptomatically. However, if the rash has appeared within 24 to 72 hours of medical attention, primary varicella in children may be treated with 20 mg/kg q.i.d. up to 800 mg/dose for 5 to 7 days. Systemic antiviral treatment is recommended in primary varicella in adults and in immunocompromised patients. Although valacyclovir and famciclovir have anti-VZV activity, there are no clinical trials reporting their efficacy in primary varicella, but both antiviral agents are used at the shingles dose for therapy or primary VZV in adults.

Both oral and IV acyclovir have an important role in the treatment of herpes zoster. Oral acyclovir in immunocompetent patients leads to an accelerated healing of lesions and reduction in acute pain, but it has only modest effects on the incidence or duration of PHN. IV administration (500 mg/mL every 8 hours for 10 days) is indicated for the treatment of severe complications in immunocompetent patients and the treatment of zoster in immunosuppressed patients. Adverse effects with acyclovir are rare and include headache, nausea, diarrhea, and renal toxicity (especially in dehydrated elderly patients).

Valacyclovir, the orally administered prodrug of acyclovir, is effective in reducing time to crusting, the appearance of new zoster lesions, and time to 50% healing. The typical dose is 1 g t.i.d. for 7 days. Valacyclovir, when compared to acyclovir, decreased the median duration of pain from 60 days to 40 days. It has a similar adverse event profile with acyclovir but with no reports of nephropathy or neurotoxicity.

Famciclovir, the prodrug of penciclovir, is at least equal to acyclovir in promoting cutaneous healing and decreasing the duration of acute pain. The typical dose is 500 mg t.i.d. for 7 days. Its efficacy and safety are equivalent to that of valacyclovir. Like all antiviral agents, therapy should be started as soon as possible after the onset of the zoster rash, preferably within 72 hours. However, it has been reported that patients may also benefit if antiviral therapy is started after 72 hours at the onset of the rash, but the upper limit of time for initiation of antiviral therapy has not been determined.

Human Papillomavirus

There are over 100 genotypes of human papillomavirus (HPV), which are DNA viruses that infect the epithelia cells of skin and mucosa and cause warts or benign papillomas. HPV infection in sexually active women is very common, with an incidence of 15% to 40%. HPV types 16 and 18 are considered high risk because they are the primary etiologic agents for cervical cancer and other anogenital cancers, as well as some upper aerodigestive tract and skin cancers. Vaccine to prevent HPV type 16 and 18 is being developed and could prevent cervical cancer.

Presentation and Characteristics

Warts appear as hyperkeratotic papillomas with black dots, which are thrombosed capillaries within the wart. These lesions can manifest on any body site, but specific HPV subtypes may have a tendency to affect a certain anatomic location. HPV-1 infection may cause palmar and plantar warts. HPV-2 causes common warts. HPV-3 and HPV-10 typically cause flat warts. HPV-6 and HPV-11 are the main causes of anogenital warts, or condyloma acuminatum. Cervical warts, or condyloma plata, may be difficult to visualize by examination without application of acetic acid, which cause subclinical lesions to become white.

Treatment

Currently, there is no curative treatment for HPV infections. The 2002 CDC recommendations for HPV therapy include

- treatment with trichloroacetic acid,
- cryotherapy,
- podofilox, and
- surgical removal with laser surgery.

The CDC also recommended imiquimod or interferon, which stimulates the host's immune response against infected cells. Other less commonly used treatments include

- 5-fluorouracil,
- electrosurgery,
- retinoids,
- bleomycin (intralesional and systemic), and
- salicylic acid.

The therapy with the lowest recurrence rate following a complete response is imiquimod. This can be used after any other therapy to prevent reoccurrence.

Molluscum Contagiosum Virus

Molluscum contagiosum (Fig. 23-5), caused by the molluscum contagiosum virus of the DNA poxvirus group, is a benign skin infection that affects children and young adults worldwide. Molluscum contagiosum commonly affects immunocompromised patients, and the prevalence of molluscum contagiosum infection among HIV-infected patients ranges from 5% to 18%. Because the infection is limited to the epidermis, most lesions regress spontaneously within 9 to 12 months, and molluscum contagiosum has not been reported to progress to malignancy.

The prevalence in the general population is unknown; the molluscum contagiosum virus has not been cultured.

In the United States, it is estimated that the incidence of genital molluscum contagiosum is relatively low compared to other STDs (1 case per 42 to 60 cases of gonorrhea), and the age distribution of patients with genital molluscum contagiosum is similar to that of other STDs. Outbreaks of molluscum contagiosum may be spread between family members from casual contact.

Presentation and Characteristics

Molluscum contagiosum lesions present as small, smooth, umbilicated papules. In sexually active young adults, these lesions are primarily on the inner thighs, genitalia, and pubic areas.

Treatment

Molluscum contagiosum is treated with similar therapies available for warts to control transmission and for cosmetic reasons. Effective therapies are

- imiquimod,
- cryotherapy,
- cantharidin,
- electrosurgery, and
- cold steel surgery.

Less commonly used therapies are

- topical cidofovir,
- lasers,
- podofilox,
- trichloroacetic acid, and
- retinoids.

Lymphogranuloma Venereum

Lymphogranuloma venereum is an uncommon venereal disease characterized by a primary lesion on the genitals and secondary changes involving the draining lymph channels and glands.

Presentation and Characteristics

The primary erosion or blister is rarely seen, especially on the female patient. Within 10 to 30 days after exposure, the

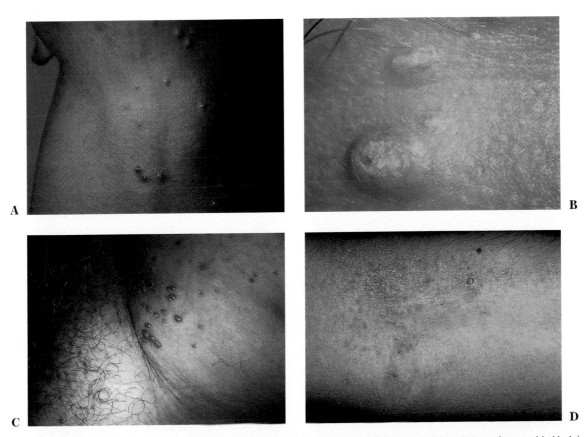

FIGURE 23-5 ■ Molluscum contagiosum on neck (**A**), in close-up (**B**) *(Drs. L. Calkins, A. Lemoine, and L. Hyde)*, of vulvar area (**C**), and with atopic eczema of cubital fossae (**D**). *(Courtesy of Glaxo Dermatology.)*

inguinal nodes, particularly in the male patient, enlarge unilaterally. This inguinal mass may rupture if treatment is delayed. In the female patient the lymph drainage most commonly is toward the pelvic and the perirectal nodes, and their enlargement may be overlooked. Low-grade fever, malaise, and generalized lymphadenopathy frequently occur during the adenitis stage. Scarlatina-like rashes and erythema nodosum lesions also may develop. The later manifestations of lymphogranuloma venereum occur as the result of scaring of the lymph channels and fibrosis of the nodes. These changes result in rectal stricture, swelling of the penis or the vulva, and ulceration.

Lymphogranuloma venereum is caused by the obligate intracellular parasite *Chlamydia trachomatis*, serotypes L_1, L_2, and L_3.

Diagnosis

A complement fixation test (LGV-CFT) becomes positive 3 to 4 weeks after the onset of the disease in 80% to 90% of the patients.

Treatment

Tetracycline 500 mg q.i.d., and minocycline 100 mg b.i.d. are the drugs of choice. These are most effective in the early stages and should be continued for at least 3 weeks. Fluctuant inguinal nodes should be aspirated to prevent rupture.

Measles (Rubeola)

Measles is a very common childhood disease. The characteristic points are as follows: the incubation period averages 14 days before the appearance of the rash. The prodromal stage appears around the 9th day after exposure and consists of fever, conjunctivitis, running nose, Koplik spots, and even faint red rash. The Koplik spots measure from 1 to 3 mm in diameter, are bluish-white on a red base, and occur bilaterally on the mucous membrane around the parotid duct and on the lower lip. With increasing fever and cough, the "morbilliform" rash appears first behind the ears and on the forehead and then spreads over face, neck, trunk, and extremities. The fever begins to fall as the rash comes out. The rash is a faint, reddish, patchy eruption, occasionally papular. Scaling occurs in the end stage. Complications include secondary bacterial infection and encephalitis.

Differential Diagnosis

- *German measles:* Postauricular nodes; milder fever and rash; no Koplik spots (see following section)
- *Scarlet fever:* Circumoral pallor; rash brighter red and confluent (see Chap 21)
- *Drug eruption:* History of new drugs; usually no fever (see Chap 9)
- *Infectious mononucleosis:* Rash similar; characteristic blood picture; high titer of heterophile antibodies

Treatment

Prophylactic

Measles virus vaccine, live, attenuated, can be administered.

Active

Supportive therapy for the cough, bed rest, and protection from bright light are measures for the active disease. The antibiotics have eliminated most of the bacterial complications. Corticosteroids are of value for the rare but serious complication of encephalitis.

German Measles (Rubella)

Although German measles is a benign disease of children, it is serious if it develops in a pregnant woman during the first trimester because it causes anomalies in a low percentage of newborns.

The incubation period is around 18 days, and, as in measles, there may be a short prodromal stage of fever and malaise. The rash also resembles measles, because it occurs first on the face then spreads. However, the redness is less intense and the rash disappears within 2 to 3 days. Enlargement of the cervical and the postauricular nodes is a characteristic finding. Serious complications are rare.

Differential Diagnosis

- *Measles:* Koplik spots; the fever and the rash are more severe; no postauricular nodes
- *Scarlet fever:* High fever; perioral pallor; rash may be similar (see Chap 21)
- *Drug eruption:* Get new drug history; usually no fever (see Chap 9)

Treatment

Prophylactic

Rubella virus vaccine, live, attenuated, can be administered.

Active

Active treatment is usually unnecessary. Immune globulin given to an exposed pregnant woman in the first trimester of pregnancy may prevent the disease.

Congenital Rubella Syndrome

Infants born to mothers who had rubella in the first trimester of pregnancy can have multiple system abnormalities. The skin lesions include

- thrombocytopenic purpura;
- hyperpigmentation of the navel, forehead, and cheeks;
- acne;
- seborrhea; and
- reticulated erythema of the face and extremities.

Erythema Infectiosum

Also known as "fifth disease," erythema infectiosum occurs in epidemics and is believed to be caused by parvovirus B19. It affects children primarily, but in a large epidemic many causes are seen in adults.

Presentation and Characteristics

The incubation period varies from 1 to 7 weeks. In children the prodromal stage lasts from 2 to 4 days and is manifested by low-grade fever and occasionally by joint pains. When the red macular rash develops, it begins on the arms and the face and then spreads to the body. The rash in children is measle-like on the body, but on the face it looks as though the cheeks have been slapped. On the arms and the legs the rash is more red and confluent on the extensor surfaces. A low-grade fever persists for a few days after the onset of the rash, which lasts for approximately 1 week. In adults, the rash on the face (the "slap") is less conspicuous, joint complaints are more common, and itching is present.

Differential Diagnosis

- *Drug eruption:* See Chapter 9
- *Measles:* Coryza, eruption begins on face and behind ears
- *Other measle-like eruptions*

Treatment

Treatment usually is not necessary.

Coxsackievirus Infections

Coxsackievirus infections are identified by type-specific antigens that appear in the blood 7 days or so after the onset of the disease.

Differential Diagnosis

- Measles,
- German measles,
- scarlet fever,
- infectious mononucleosis, and
- drug eruption.

Treatment

No treatment is necessary except to reduce the high fever.

Herpangina

Herpangina is an acute febrile disease that occurs mainly in children in the summer months. The first complaints are fever, headache, sore throat, nausea, and stiff neck. Blisters are seen in the throat that are approximately 2 mm in size and surrounded by an intense erythema. These lesions may coalesce and some may ulcerate. The course is usually 7 to 10 days.

The cause of herpangina is primarily coxsackievirus A, but echovirus types have also been isolated from sporadic cases.

Differential Diagnosis

- Aphthous stomatitis,
- drug eruption,
- primary herpes gingivostomatitis, and
- hand–foot–mouth disease (another related viral condition).

Treatment

Soothing mouthwashes and antipyretics are used.

Echovirus Exanthem

ECHO is an acronym for *entire cytopathic human orphan,* the label given to the virus before it was know to be causative of any disease. Symptoms include fever, nausea, vomiting, diarrhea, sore throat, cough, and stiff neck. A measle-like eruption occurs in one third of cases. Small erosions may develop on the mucous membranes of the cheek. Echoviruses 9 and 4 have been isolated from most cases with skin lesions.

Treatment

Treatment is symptomatic. The infection usually lasts 1 to 2 weeks.

Suggested Reading

Beutner KR, Antivirals in the treatment of pain. J Geriatr Dermatol 1994;6(2suppl):23A–28A.

Brown ST, Nalley JF, Kraus SJ. Molluscum contagiosum. Sex Transm Dis 1981;8:227–334.

Brown TJ, Yen-Moore A, Tyring SK. An overview of sexually transmitted disease, Part I. J Am Acad Dermatol 1999;41:511–29.

Decroix J, Partsch H, Gonzalex R, et al. Factors influencing pain outcome in herpes zoster: an observational study with valaciclovir. Valaciclovir International Zoster Assessment Group (VIZA). J Eur Acad Dermatol Venereol 2000;14:23–33.

Donohue JG, Choo PW, Manson JE, Platt R. The incidence of herpes zoster. Arch Intern Med 1995;155:1605–1609.

Margolis S. Genital warts and molluscum contagiosum. Urol Clin North Am 1984;11:163–170.

Pereira FA. Herpes simplex: evolving concepts. J Am Acad Dermatol 1996;35:503–520.

Sexually transmitted diseases treatment guidelines 2002. Centers for Disease Control and Prevention. MMWR Recomm Rep 2002;51:1–78.

Spruance SL, Stewart JC, Rowe NH, et al. Treatment of recurrent herpes simplex labialis with oral acyclovir. J Infect Dis 1990;161:185–190.

Ting PT, Dytoc MT. Therapy of external anogenital warts and molluscum contagiosum: A literature review. Dermatol Ther 2004;17:68–101.

Tyring SK. Belanger R, Bezwoda W, et al. A randomized, double-blind trial of famciclovir versus acyclovir for the treatment of localized dermatomal herpes zoster in immunocompromised patients. Cancer Invest 2001;19:13–22.

Tyring SK, Beutner KR, Tucker BA, et al. Antiviral therapy for herpes zoster: Randomized, controlled clinical trial of valacyclovir and famciclovir therapy in immunocompetent patients 50 years and older. Arch Fam Med 2000;9:863–869.

Wu JJ, Huang DB, Pan KR, Tyring SK. Vaccines and immunotherapies for the prevention of infectious diseases having cutaneous manifestations. J Am Acad Dermatol 2004;50:495–528.

Yeung-Yue KA, Brentjens MH, Lee PC, Tyring SK. Herpes simplex viruses 1 and 2. Dermatol Clin 2002;20:249–266.

CHAPTER 24

Cutaneous Diseases Associated With Human Immunodeficiency Virus

Mary M. Feldman, MD, and Clay J. Cockerell, MD

Cutaneous signs and symptoms may herald the presence of systemic disease, and often this is the case with human immunodeficiency virus (HIV) infection. A number of skin conditions are characteristically associated with such infection or the resultant acquired immunodeficiency syndrome (AIDS). In many instances, the manifestations of common dermatologic disorders are modified in HIV-infected individuals and thus differ in severity, prevalence, morphology, or response to therapy. The astute clinician is aware of these variations and thereby better able to accurately diagnose and manage disease in the infected patient. Equally important, knowledge of these conditions may facilitate an initial diagnosis of HIV seropositivity in a previously undiagnosed individual.

Although the health implications of cutaneous disease are of primary concern, the profound impact on quality of life issues should not be forgotten. Skin changes are by nature highly visible and therefore cosmetically distressing to the patient. Myriad reports have been published documenting the importance of physical appearance in all facets of life, from self-esteem and interpersonal relationships to ability to obtain employment. This is particularly relevant to HIV-infected individuals who may fear becoming stigmatized by characteristic processes such as Kaposi's sarcoma (KS).

Epidemiology

HIV is a blood-borne enveloped RNA retrovirus acquired through both homo- and heterosexual unprotected sex, sharing of "dirty" needles by IV drug users, vertically from mother to unborn child, or, historically, via transfusion of contaminated blood products. The virus infects CD4 helper T lymphocytes and monocytes–macrophages. As the disease progresses CD4 cells decrease in number. AIDS, by definition, begins when the count falls below 200/mm^3. The virus also alters the immune profile by suppressing the Th1 subset of helper T cells and creating a predominance of Th2-type cells. This may in part explain the unique profile of cutaneous disease associated with HIV.

The number of people infected with HIV has grown steadily since the onset of the epidemic in the early 1980s. An estimated 39.4 million people worldwide are infected with HIV, and 3.1 million deaths resulted in 2004. Currently in North America 1 million people are living with HIV. Each year, an additional 40,000 people in the United States and 4.9 million globally join these ranks. Sub-Saharan Africa is disproportionately affected, with an estimated 25.4 million cases.

The face of the AIDS epidemic has changed greatly over the past decade in developed parts of the world after the introduction of the life-prolonging highly active antiretroviral therapy (HAART). Death rates have dropped to just over 16,000 per annum in the United States. Other changes include an increasing number of infections among heterosexual women and people of color. Because many conditions are secondary to immunosuppression (and correlated with CD4 level), the incidence of HIV-related skin disease has diminished with the advent of improved therapy. HAART has also improved quality of life with regard to HIV-associated skin disease.

Infections and Infestations

Viral Infections

Acute infection with HIV results in a flulike illness 2 to 6 weeks after exposure to the virus in more than half of patients. A morbilliform eruption resembling a typical viral exantham or a medication reaction occurs in 40% to 80%. In high-risk individuals who present with a vague illness accompanied by rash, testing with the core antigen (p24) assay or a plasma viral load assay is indicated. Western blot and the standard enzyme immunoassay, by contrast, are not reliable in early infection. Treatment is supportive until the transient symptoms resolve.

Molluscum contagiosum is a large DNA poxvirus that infects epithelial cells. Resultant lesions are flesh colored or slightly pearly papules measuring 2 to 6 mm in diameter with a central dell or umbilication (Fig. 24-1). The condition in healthy adults is uncommon, limited in severity, and generally restricted to the genital area or lower abdomen. In HIV-infected patients, however, hundreds of lesions may simultaneously develop and often occur on the face. In addition, "giant mollusca" become greater than 1 cm and as large as 6 cm in diameter. Destructive modalities are employed for therapy.

Human papillomavirus (HPV), a double-stranded circular DNA virus, is responsible for verrucae, or "warts," in genital and nongenital locations (Fig. 24-2). Over 80 strains of HPV have been identified. Several of these, including types 16, 18, 31, and 33, confer higher risk for squamous cell carcinoma (SCC) of the cervix and perianal region. HIV-infected individuals have a higher prevalence of HPV infection than the general population.

Treatment

Therapy is accomplished with destructive modalities such as cryotherapy or topical immunomodulators. (imiquimod)

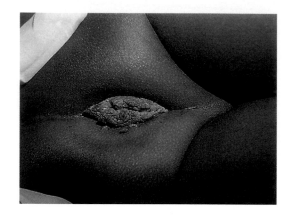

FIGURE 24-2 ■ Condyloma acuminata. Fungating perianal warts in a child infected with HIV. *(Courtesy of Drs. J. Rico and N. Prose.)*

Herpes Virus Infections

The herpes viruses are a group of double stranded DNA viruses that cause frequent opportunistic infection in people with HIV.

Herpes Simplex Virus

Herpes simplex virus (HSV) presents as clustered vesicles on or near mucosal surfaces. HSV-1 is classically associated with herpes labialis, or "cold sores," and HSV-2 is the cause of sexually transmitted genital disease. However, the subtypes are not strictly limited to these anatomic sites, and some crossover is observed. Transmission is via direct contact. HSV lesions tend to be more severe, chronic, and resistant to treatment in HIV-infected patients.

Treatment. First-line therapy is oral acyclovir, famciclovir, or valacyclovir. IV acyclovir or IV foscarnet for acyclovir-resistant disease may be necessary.

Varicella Zoster Virus

Varicella zoster virus is the causative agent in chicken pox and is acquired via inhalation of respiratory droplets or through direct contact. After the primary infection, the virus remains latent in the dorsal root ganglia and can reactivate years later as herpes zoster, or "shingles," when cell-mediated immunity is compromised (Fig. 24-3). HIV-infected individuals have a greatly increased risk of developing herpes zoster, which can become disseminated with potentially fatal systemic involvement.

Treatment. Treatment with antivirals is necessary.

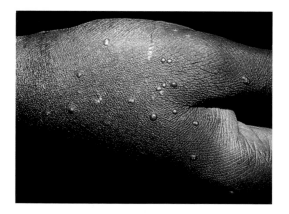

FIGURE 24-1 ■ Molluscum contagiosum. Multiple firm white papules scattered over the dorsal hand and forearm in a Haitian man with AIDS. *(Courtesy of Drs. J. Rico and N. Prose; Owen/Galderma.)*

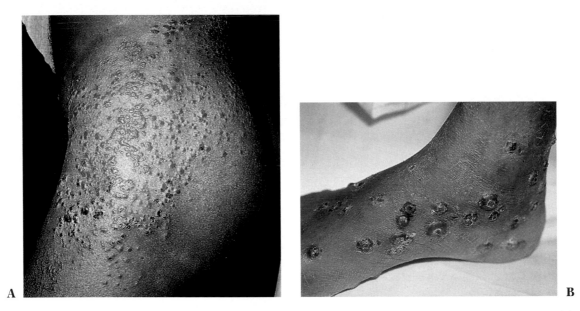

A **B**

FIGURE 24-3 ■ **(A)** Herpes zoster. Umbilicated vesicles in a dermatomal distribution in a man with AIDS. *(Courtesy of Drs. J. Rico and N. Prose; Owen/Galderma.)* **(B)** Ecthymatous herpes varicella-zoster. Crusted erosions and blisters on the foot of a patient with AIDS. *(Courtesy of Drs. J. Rico and N. Prose; Owen/Galderma.)*

Epstein-Barr Virus

Oral hairy leukoplakia, caused by the Epstein-Barr virus (EBV), is nearly exclusive to HIV-infected patients. EBV infects the epithelial cells on the lateral aspects of the tongue. This results in hyperkeratotic, verrucous white plaques that do not scrape away (Fig. 24-4).

Treatment. Topical treatment with podophyllin is generally effective. EBV can also lead to non-Hodgkin's lymphoma.

Other Viruses

Cytomegalovirus viremia is associated with advanced immunosuppression. Skin disease, although uncommon, can manifest as papules, vesicles, morbilliform eruptions, hyperpigmented plaques, or painful perianal ulcers.

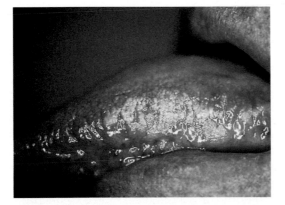

FIGURE 24-4 ■ Oral hairy leukoplakia. Filamentous white papules on the sides of the tongue. *(Courtesy of Drs. J. Rico and N. Prose; Owen/Galderma.)*

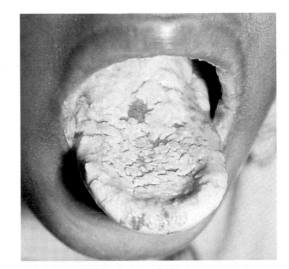

FIGURE 24-5 ■ Oral candidiasis. White plaques on the tongues of a child with AIDS. *(Courtesy of Drs. J. Rico and N. Prose.)*

Human herpes virus 8 (HHV-8) is also known as KS-associated herpes virus. Infection with HHV-8 has been demonstrated in over 95% of AIDS-associated KS.

Bacterial Infections

Staphylococcus aureus

Most bacterial skin infections in HIV patients are caused by *Staphylococcus aureus.* This gram-positive organism can produce folliculitis, impetigo, abscesses, cellulitis, and even necrotizing fasciitis in immunocompromised patients. Although infection usually responds to standard antibiotic therapy, recurrence is often a problem.

Bacillary angiomatosis most commonly presents as one or several vascular proliferations clinically and histologically similar to pyogenic granuloma. The causative organism is either *Bartonella henselae* or *B. quintana.*

Treatment. Erythromycin and doxycycline have been effective for treatment.

Mycobactria

Systemic mycobacterial infections in immunosuppressed patients can involve the skin in a number of ways including papules, pustules, abscesses, ulcerations, or nodules. *Mycobacterium avium-intracellulare* and *M. haemophilum* are the most commonly encountered mycobacteria in the setting of HIV infection, but the overall frequency has greatly diminished with improved therapy and the use of prophylactic antibiotics.

Fungal Infections

Dermatophyte

Dermatophyte infection is more common in HIV patients than in the immunocompetent population. The presence of superficial pnoximal white onychomycosis in one or few digits a specific type of dermatophytosis, should raise suspicion for HIV infection. Like many conditions, dermatophyte infections may be atypical or more severe, widespread, and difficult to treat in the immunosuppressed patient.

Treatment. Treatment is similar to that in healthy patients, including topical or oral antifungals.

Candida

Candida infection occurs with a decline in immune function and can be the initial manifestation of HIV disease. Oral candidiasis or *thrush* (Fig. 24.5) is the most prevalent type, and presents on the tongue and buccal mucosa as white plaques that can be scraped away. Other conditions include esophagitis, chronic vaginitis, urethritis, paronychia, intertrigo, or the rare, usually fatal disseminated candidiasis.

Treatment. Topical or oral *-azole* antifungals are therapeutic.

Systemic

A subset of opportunistic fungal disease is acquired via inhalation of spores from contaminated soil or bird droppings. When CD4 levels drop below 200/mm^3, dissemination from the primary pulmonary infection can occur and involves the skin in 10% to 20% of infected individuals. Tissue should be obtained for both routine formalin fixation and for culture if a fungal process is suspected clinically (Table 24-1).

Infestations

Scabies is an intensely pruritic and highly contagious eruption caused by the ectoparasitic mite *Sarcoptes scabiei* var. *hominis.* The common presentation includes small, discrete, crusted papules as well as burrows with a predilection for the interdigital spaces, wrists, periumbilicus, and genital region. In patients with compromised immunity, findings may be more severe and can progress to Norwegian scabies, in which a single patient may harbor thousands to millions of mites. Pediculosis pubis or "crabs," caused by *Phthirus pubis,* occurs in HIV-infected patients but not in greater frequency relative to the general population. *Demodex* mites are resident flora of the pilosebaceous units in the highly sebaceous head and neck region. They can produce a rosacea-like papular eruption, which has been reported in HIV-infected patients.

Treatment

The initial treatment of choice for ectoparasitic infestation is topical permethrin cream, but oral ivermectin may become necessary in refractory cases.

Parasitic Infections

Skin lesions of *Pneumocystis carinii* are found in the external auditory canal or nares and present as abscesses, bluish cellulitic plaques or as papules similar in appearance to molluscum contagiosum. Retrograde spread from the lungs through the Eustachian tubes is postulated.

Leishmaniasis is a condition caused by protozoa from the genus *Leishmania.* The parasite is transmitted from sand flies in endemic parts of the world: Mexico, Brazil, the Mediterranean, East Africa, Sudan, Iraq and India.

TABLE 24-1 ■ Systemic Fungal Diseases

Disease Entity	Causative Organism	Organism Characteristics	Mode of Transmission/ Reservoir	Clinical Findings
Blastomycosis	*Blastomyces dermatitidis*	Broad-based budding yeast	Endemic areas	Verrucous papules, nodules, and plaques
Coccidiomycosis	*Coccidiodes immitis*	Dimorphic fungus; encapsulated endospores in tissue	Endemic to Southwestern United States	Leukocytoclastic vasculitis, painful erythema of the buttocks, papulopustules, ulcers, abscesses, and nodules
Cryptococcosis	*Cryptococcus neoformans*	Encapsulated yeast	Contaminated soil and bird droppings; pigeons	Papules, pustules, nodules, ulcers; may simulate molluscum contagiosum
Histoplasmosis	*Histoplasma capsulatum*	Dimorphic fungus	Bird or bat excrement; endemic to Ohio and Mississippi River Valleys	Cutaneous and mucosal ulcerations, macules, patches, papules, nodules, pustules, verrucous plaques, and fistulae
Sporotrichosis	*Sporothrix schenckii*	Dimorphic fungus	Lives on grasses and shrubs; primary inoculation from rose bushes	Ulcers, papules, nodules, plaques, and putules

Disseminated leishmaniasis is a systemic illness, likely a reactivation of previous infection, which involves the skin in the form of ulcerated nodules on the extremities.

The intestinal helminthe *Strongyloides stercoralis* is endemic to subtropical and tropical areas as well as some regions of the United States. The classic cutaneous manifestation is larva currens, a rapidly migrating serpiginous eruption resulting from penetration of the skin by larvae. This is often modified in immunosuppressed individuals and can present as urticaria, localized purpura, or livedo reticularis.

Amebae from the genus *Acanthamoeba,* often part of the normal oral flora, have very rarely caused cutaneous acanthamebiasis. Cutaneous findings are usually deep dermal or subcutaneous nodules. Prognosis for AIDS patients is extremely poor with mortality rates of 75% to 100%.

Sexually Transmitted Diseases

HIV is itself a sexually transmitted disease (STD). Preexistent ulcerative genital disease (such HSV infected) creates a greater risk of HIV infection by providing a portal of entry for the virus. Table 24-2 summarizes the ulcerative STDs. STDs are also associated with known HIV disease because of shared risk factors or compromised immunity.

Other sexually transmitted cutaneous conditions previously discussed include HPV, HHV-8, pediculosis pubis, scabies, and molluscum contagiosum.

Treatment

Current treatment recommendations are periodically published by the Centers for Disease Control and Prevention.

Inflammatory Disorders

Pruritic Disorders

Noninfectious inflammatory disorders may be more prevalent or more severe in the context of underlying HIV. One such disorder is seborrheic dermatitis, which presents as erythema and greasy scaling on the scalp, face, and anterior chest (Fig. 24-6). It may also present in unusual sites such as the back, axillae, and groin. The condition affects up to 85% of HIV-positive patients and worsens with decline in immune status. Psoriasis, although not more common in HIV infection, is more severe and recalcitrant to treatment, and the development of psoriatic arthritis is more likely in these patients. Reiter's syndrome, a disease closely related to psoriasis but with the additional triad of urethritis, conjunctivitis, and arthritis, is associated with HIV infection

TABLE 24-2 ■ Ulcerative Sexually Transmitted Diseases

Condition	Causative Organism	Organism Characteristics	Diagnosis	Clinical Presentation
Genital herpes	HSV-2, less commonly HSV-1	DNA virus	Culture or Tzanck prep	Painful clustered genital and perianal vesicles and ulcerations; often large and/or chronic
Syphilis	*Treponema pallidum*	Spirochete	Serology or darkfield examination	*Primary:* painless chancre; *secondary:* papulosquamous eruption most common; *Tertiary:* neurologic and cardiac symptoms
Chancroid	*Haemophilus ducreyi*	Gram-negative bacterium	Culture	"Punched out," painful ulcerations with ragged edges
Lymphogranuloma venereum	*Chlamydia trachomatis*	Gram-negative bacterium	Serology	*Primary:* painless genital vesicle or erosion; *Secondary:* inguinal adenopathy; *Tertiary:* rectal
Granuloma inguinale	*Calymmatobacterium granulomatis*	Gram-negative bacterium	Intracytoplasmic Donovan bodies visualized on microscopic exam	Beefy red nontender granulomatous ulceration

(Fig. 24-7). A sudden flare of preexisting skin disease or resistance to treatment can be a clue to HIV infection.

Pruritic diseases are particularly troublesome for HIV patients and pose a therapeutic challenge. Eosinophilic folliculitis is an eruption composed of multiple sterile eosinophilic pustules distributed over the trunk, head, neck and proximal extremities. This is often confused clinically

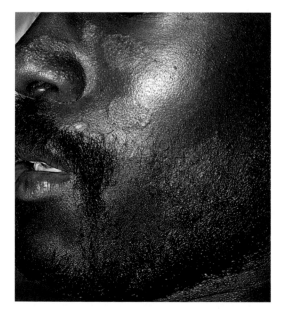

FIGURE 24-6 ■ Seborrheic dermatitis. Annular scaling plaques on the nasolabial fold and cheeks. *(Courtesy of Drs. J. Rico and N. Prose.)*

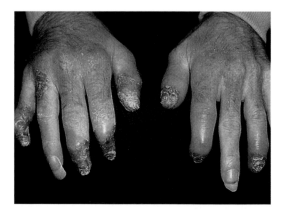

FIGURE 24-7 ■ Reiter's disease. Psoriasiform dermatitis involving the distal fingers. Note the joint changes owing to active arthritis. *(Courtesy of Drs. J. Rico and N. Prose; Owen/Galderma.)*

with bacterial folliculitis, but is distinguished by the intense pruritus and failure to respond to oral antibiotics. Another similar condition, pruritic papular eruption, is characterized by multiple intensely pruritic nonfollicular papules. The cause is unknown but thought to be a hypersensitivity response to unidentified antigens. Both conditions are indicative of poor immune status. Xerosis or acquired ichthyosis occurs in nearly one third of HIV-positive patients and can lead to exacerbation of underlying atopic dermatitis. Prurigo nodularis and lichen simplex chronicus are end-stage processes caused by persistent rubbing, picking, or scratching regardless of underlying etiology. The HIV-associated pruritic conditions are chronic and difficult to manage.

Treatment

Various treatment modalities have been employed to treat the pruritic diseases of HIV, including topical antipruritics, steroids, and immune modulators; oral antihistamines, opiate antagonists, and antidepressants; and ultraviolet phototherapy.

Photosensitivity Disorders

HIV patients are at greater risk of developing eruptions in sun-exposed sites. Known photosensitive disorders include porphyria cutanea tarda (PCT), photo-exacerbated drug reactions, and actinic reticuloid. The higher incidence of PCT, a blistering disorder owing to elevated porphyrins in the blood, may be related to higher rates of hepatitis or other liver disease in this high-risk population.

Treatment

Management of photosensitivity should include sun avoidance, protective clothing, and sunscreens.

Neoplastic Disorders

Cutaneous Carcinomas

Cutaneous neoplasms occur with greater frequency in immunosuppressed patients. In a manner analogous to cervical intraepithelial neoplasia, epithelial cells are subject to metaplasia and eventual transformation to SCC as a result of infection with oncogenic HPV (-16, -18, -31, or -33) strains. This presents most commonly on anogenital skin as premalignant warty growths, epidermodysplasia verruciformis, or as Bowenoid papulosis (SCC in situ), which is clinically similar to condyloma acuminata. A giant form of verrucous carcinoma (giant condyloma acuminate of Buschke-Lowenstein) can also evolve. Basal cell carcinoma (BCC) can be more aggressive in HIV patients and occur in

sun-protected areas. BCC has rarely been reported to metastasize to local lymph nodes or to lung. Malignant melanoma, in some cases aggressive, has been observed in the setting of HIV. Cases of multiple primary nevoid melanomas have been reported.

Lymphomas

HIV patients are at risk for developing lymphoreticular malignancies. The most common are non-Hodgkin's B-cell lymphomas, half of which are related to EBV infection. Lymphoma in HIV has a younger age of onset, higher grade of atypia, and the propensity to involve extranodal sites, including the skin, at presentation. Lesions present as pink to violaceous papules on the skin in severely immunocompromised patients. Cutaneous T-cell lymphoma, HTLV-1–associated lymphoma and Hodgkin's lymphoma also occur in the HIV-positive population. Children with HIV are at higher risk of developing mucosa-associated lymphoid tissue (MALT) lymphomas.

Kaposi's Sarcoma

KS was one of the first recognized and most characteristic manifestations of AIDS early in the epidemic. AIDS-related KS appears to be caused by HHV-8, which is most likely transmitted sexually between homosexual men. Lesions occur on the upper body, face, and oral mucosal surfaces (Fig. 24-8). They appear as violaceous papules or plaques, sometimes along skin cleavage lines. Because KS regresses with the recovery of immune function, the condition is now relatively uncommon in populations with access to HAART.

Treatment

If treatment is desired, it can be accomplished with destructive modalities, intralesional chemotherapy, or topical retinoids.

Medication-Related Side Effects

The development of an HIV-related lipodystrophy syndrome has occurred in many patients within months after initiation of HAART. This is characterized by a redistribution of fat similar to a Cushingoid pattern with truncal obesity, referred to as a *protease paunch* or *crix belly*; dorsocervical lipohypertrophy or buffalo hump; and simultaneous wasting of subcutaneous fat on the central face and extremities. Patients also exhibit disturbances in lipid and glucose metabolism. Unfortunately, the severity of disfigurement can lead to noncompliance with therapy.

A reactivation phenomenon has been observed with reinstitution of immune function in patients on HAART. Certain conditions such as varicella zoster, leprosy, and

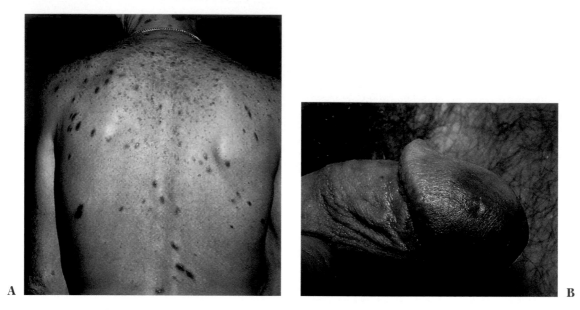

FIGURE 24-8 ■ (**A**) Disseminated KS: Multiple red to brown papules and plaques distributed along the skin tension lines in a man with AIDS. (**B**) KS: an ill-defined purple plaque on the glans penis of a man with AIDS. *(Courtesy of Drs. J. Rico and N. Prose.)*

M. avium paradoxically worsen with improvement in immune function.

HIV-infected patients have a propensity to develop cutaneous reactions to oral antimicrobials. Trimethoprim–sulfamethoxazole is the most problematic, with a morbilliform eruption affecting 50% to 60% of those treated (Fig. 24-9). This can often be controlled by slow reintroduction with induction of tolerance. Stevens-Johnson syndrome or even frank toxic epidermal necrolysis can occur.

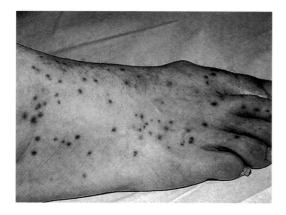

FIGURE 24-9 ■ Leukocytoclastic vasculitis. Palpable purpura on the foot. This patient developed vasculitis after receiving trimethoprim–sulfamethoxazole. *(Courtesy of Drs. J. Rico and N. Prose.)*

Foscarnet is associated with ulceration because the drug, excreted in the urine, is toxic to the genital mucosa. Zidovudine causes a hyperpigmentation of the nails and lichen planus–like reactions; interferon A is associated with a peculiar lengthening of the eyelashes.

Suggested Reading

Aftergut K, Cockerell CJ. Update on the cutaneous manifestations of HIV infection. Dermatol Clin 1999;17: 445–471.

Bolognia JL, Jorizzo JL, Rapini RP, et al, eds. Dermatology. Philadelphia, Elsevier Limited, 2003.

Czelusta A, Yen-Moore A, Van der Straten M, et al. An overview of sexually transmitted disease. Part III. Sexually transmitted diseases in HIV-infected patients. J Am Acad Dermatol 2000;43:409–432.

Daar ES, Little S, Pitt J, et al. Diagnosis of primary HIV-1 infection. Ann Intern Med 2001;134:25–29.

De Moore GM, Hennessey NP, Kunz NM, et al. Kaposi's sarcoma: *The Scarlet Letter* of AIDS, the psychological effects of a skin disease. Psychosomatics 2000;41:360–363.

Elder DE, et al, eds. Lever's histopathology of the skin, ed 9. Philadelphia, Lippincott, Williams &Wilkins, 2005.

Eng W, Cockerell CJ. Histological features of Kaposi sarcoma in a patient receiving highly active antiviral therapy. Am J Dermatopathol 2004;26:127–132.

Garman ME, Tyring SK. The cutaneous manifestations of HIV infection. Dermatol Clin 2002;20:193–208.

Joint United Nations Programme on HIV/AIDS (UNAIDS) and the World Health Organization (WHO). AIDS Epidemic Update: December 2004. Available: http://www.unaids.org. Accessed July 2005.

Lifson AR, Hessol NA, Buchbinder SP, et al. The association of clinical conditions and serologic tests with CD4 lymphocyte counts in HIV-infected subjects without AIDS. AIDS 1991;5:1209–1215.

Majewski S, Jablonsda S. Human papillomavirus-associated tumors of the skin and mucosa. J Am Acad Dermatol 1997;36:659–685.

Majors MJ, Cockerell CJ, Cruz PD. Pruritus in HIV-infected patients: An algorithmic approach and review of selected pruritic eruptions. Immunol Allergy Clin North Am 1997;17:239–251.

Mirmirani P, Maurer TA, Berger TG, et al. Skin related quality of life in HIV-infected patients on highly active antiretroviral therapy. J Cutan Med Surg 2002;6:10–15.

Myskowski PL, Ahkami R. Dermatologic complications of HIV infection. Med Clin North Am 1996;80:1415–1435.

Soeprono FF, Schinella RA, Cockerell CJ, et al. Seborrheic-like dermatitis of acquired immunodeficiency syndrome: A clinicopathologic study. J Am Acad Dermatol 1986;14:242.

Trent JT, Kirsner RS. Cutaneous manifestations of HIV: A primer. Adv Skin Wound Care 2004;17:116–129.

CHAPTER 25

Dermatologic Mycology

John C. Hall

Fungi can be present as part of the normal flora of the skin or as abnormal inhabitants. Dermatologists are concerned with the abnormal inhabitants, or pathogenic fungi. However, so-called nonpathogenic fungi can proliferate and invade immunosuppressed persons. Pathogenic fungi have a predilection for certain body areas; most commonly they infect the skin, but the lungs, the brain, and other organs can also be infected. Pathogenic fungi can invade the skin superficially or deeply and are thus divided into these two groups.

Superficial Fungal Infections

The superficial fungi live on the dead horny layer of the skin and elaborate an enzyme that enables them to digest keratin, causing the superficial skin to scale and disintegrate, nails to crumble, and hairs to break off. The deeper reactions of vesicles, erythema, and infiltration are presumably owing to the fungi liberating an exotoxin. Fungi are also capable of eliciting an allergic or id reaction.

When a skin scraping, hair, or culture growth is examined with the microscope in a wet preparation (see Chap. 2 and Fig. 2-1), the two structural elements of the fungi are seen: the spores and the hyphae.

- *Spores* are the reproducing bodies of the fungi. Sexual and asexual forms occur. Spores are rarely seen in skin scrapings except in tinea versicolor.
- *Hyphae* are threadlike, branching filaments that grow out from the fungus spore. The hyphae are the identifying filaments seen in skin scrapings in potassium hydroxide (KOH) solution.
- *Mycelia* are matted clumps of hyphae that grow on culture plates.

Culture media vary greatly in content, but modifications of Sabouraud's dextrose agar are used to grow the superficial fungi (see Fig. 2-2). Sabouraud's agar and corn meal agar are both used to identify the deep fungi. Hyphae and spores grow on the media, and identification of the species of fungi is established by the gross appearance of the mycelia, the color of the substrate, and the microscopic appearance of the spores and the hyphae when a sample of the growth is placed on a slide (lactophenol cotton blue stain). Some media show a color change when pathogenic fungi are isolated.

Classification

The latest classification divides the superficial fungi into three genera: *Microsporum*, *Epidermophyton*, and *Trichophyton*. Only *Microsporum* and *Trichophyton* invade the hair. As seen in a KOH preparation, *Microsporum* species cause an ectothrix infection of the hair shaft, whereas *Trichophyton* species cause either an ectothrix or an endothrix infection. The ectothrix fungi cause the formation of an external spore sheath around the hair, whereas the endothrix fungi do not. The filaments of mycelia penetrate the hair in both types of infection.

The species of fungi is correlated with the clinical diseases in Table 25-1. The organism causing tinea versicolor is not included in this table because it does not liberate a keratolytic enzyme.

Clinical Classifications

Superficial fungal infections of the skin affect various sites of the body. The clinical lesions, the species of fungi, and the therapy vary for these different sites. Therefore, fungal diseases of the skin are classified, for clinical purposes, according to the location of the infection. These clinical types are as follows:

- Tinea of the feet (tinea pedis)
- Tinea of the hands (tinea manus)
- Tinea of the nails (onychomycosis)
- Tinea of the groin (tinea cruris)
- Tinea of the smooth skin (tinea corporis)
- Tinea of the scalp (tinea capitis)

SAUER'S NOTES

Since the discovery of specific systemic antifungal agents many physicians have believed that (1) these agents are indicated for every fungus infection and (2) most skin diseases are caused by a fungus, so they should treat the patient with the antifungal agent and make a diagnosis later. Both of these assumptions are erroneous.

1. Correct diagnosis of a fungal infection is necessary. An oral antifungal drug should not be prescribed for a patient if the diagnosis has not been confirmed. Systemic antifungal agents are of no value in treating atopic eczema, contact dermatitis, psoriasis, pityriasis rosea, and so on.
2. Except for tinea of the scalp and nails, true fungal infections are noticeably improved after only 1 to 2 weeks of oral antifungal therapy. If there is no improvement, the diagnosis of the dermatosis as a fungus disease is erroneous and the therapy should be stopped.
3. An adequate dosage is necessary, including (1) the correct daily dose for the particular type of fungal infection and (2) the correct duration of such dosage.
4. In general, systemic antifungal therapy should not be used to treat tinea of the feet. The recurrence rate after completion of therapy is very high.
5. Candidal infections should not be treated with oral griseofulvin. Very commonly, candidal intertrigo of the groin or candidal paronychias are erroneously treated with griseofulvin. Griseofulvin is of no value in these conditions. Because it is a penicillin-related drug, it usually aggravates the candidiasis.
6. Tinea versicolor does not respond to oral griseofulvin therapy.
7. So-called fungal infection of the ear does not respond to oral antifungal therapy. Most external ear diseases are not caused by a fungus (see External Otitis, Chap. 11).

- Tinea of the beard (tinea barbae)
- Dermatophytid
- Tinea versicolor (see Chap. 15)
- Tinea of the external ear (see Chap. 11).

There is a predilection for certain sites of tinea in which the frequency varies with the age of the patient. This is outlined in Table 25-2.

Tinea of the Feet

Tinea of the feet (athlete's foot, fungal infection of the feet, ringworm of the feet) is a very common skin infection (Figs. 25-1 and 25-2). Many persons have the disease and are not even aware of it. The clinical appearance varies.

Primary Lesions

Acute Form. Blisters occur on the soles and the sides of feet or between the toes.

Chronic Form. Lesions are dry and scaly.

Intertriginous Form. Especially between 4th and 5th toes with macerated, fissured skin.

Secondary Lesions

Bacterial infection of the blisters is very common; maceration and fissures are also seen.

Course

Recurrent acute infections can lead to a chronic infection. If the toenails become infected, a cure is highly improbable, because this focus is very difficult to eradicate.

The species of fungus influences the response to therapy. Most vesicular, acute fungal infections are due to *T. mentagrophytes* and respond readily to correct treatment. The chronic scaly type of infection is usually due to *T. rubrum* and is exceedingly difficult, if not impossible, to cure.

Contagiousness

Experiments have shown that there is a susceptibility factor necessary for infection. Men are much more susceptible than women, even when exposed.

Laboratory Findings

KOH-ink preparations of scrapings and cultures on Sabouraud's media serve to demonstrate the presence of fungi and the specific type. A KOH preparation is a very simple office procedure and should be resorted to when the diagnosis is uncertain or the response to therapy is slow (see Chap. 2).

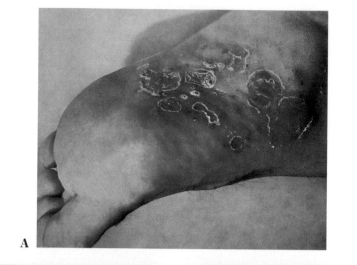

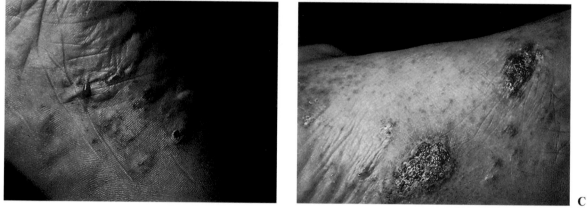

FIGURE 25-1 ■ Tinea of the foot. (**A**) This dry, scaly form of fungus infection is usually due to *T. rubrum. (Courtesy of Smith Kline & French Laboratories.)* (**B**) Acute tinea of foot with secondary bacterial infection. (**C**) Acute tinea of sole of foot of *T. mentagrophytes* type. *(Courtesy of Schering Corp.)*

Differential Diagnosis

- *Contact dermatitis:* From shoes, socks, gloves, foot powder usually on dorsum of feet or hands; history of new shoes or new foot powder; fungi not found (see Chap. 9)
- *Atopic eczema:* Especially on dorsum of toes in children; quite chronic; usually in winter; very pruritic; atopic family history; on dorsum of toes; fungi not found (see Chap. 9 and Fig. 36-24)
- *Psoriasis:* Affects soles and palms; rarely pustular, thickened, well-circumscribed lesions; psoriasis elsewhere on body; fungi not found (see Chap. 14)
- *Pustular bacterid:* Pustular lesions only; chronic; resistant to local therapy; fungi not found; may be associated with a focus of infection, as in tonsil, teeth, or gallbladder

- *Hyperhidrosis of feet:* Can be severe and cause white, eroded maceration of the soles, accompanied by a foul odor; Zeasorb AF powder is helpful, as is Drysol solution
- *Symmetric lividity of the soles* (Fig. 25-3): Rather common condition of the soles of the feet characterized by the presence of patches of macerated, whitish, sharply defined, odoriferous skin associated with hyperhidrosis
- *Pitted keratolysis* (keratolysis plantare sulcatum): Produces circular areas of erosions with a punched-out appearance on the soles of the feet; associated with hyperhidrosis; filamentous, gram-positive, branching microorganisms are found on skin scrapings caused by corynebacterium; topical or systemic erythromycin is usually beneficial

TABLE 25-1 ■ Relationship of Fungi to Body Areas

Fungus	Feet and Hands	Nails	Groin	Smooth Skin	Scalp	Beard
Microsporum species						
M. audouini	0	0	0	Uncommon	Uncommon	0
M. canis	0	0	0	Common	Uncommon	Rare
M. gypseum	0	0	0	Rare	Rare	0
Epidermophyton species						
E. floccosum	Moderately common	Rare	Common	Moderately common	0	0
Trichophyton species						
Endothrix species						
T. schoenleini	0	Rare	0	Rare	(Favus) rare, especially tropics	0
T. violaceum	0	Rare	0	0	Rare	Rare
T. tonsurans	0	Rare	0	Rare	Common	0
Ectothrix species						
T. mentagrophytes	Common	Moderately common	0	Common	Rare	Moderately common
T. rubrum	Common	Common	Moderately common	Common	0	Rare

SAUER'S NOTES

A favorite medication of mine for tinea of the feet and body is

Sulfur, ppt.	5%
Hydrocortisone	1%
Antifungal cream q.s. 30.0	

Treatment

Case Example: Acute Infection. An acute vesicular, pustular fungal infection of 2 weeks' duration is present on the soles of the feet and between the toes in a 16-year-old boy. This clinical picture is usually caused by *T. mentagrophytes*.

First Visit.

1. The fear of the infectiousness of athlete's foot should be minimized but normal cleanliness emphasized, including the wearing of slippers over bare feet, wiping the feet last after a bath (not the groin last), and changing socks daily (white socks are not necessary).
2. Debridement: The physician or the patient should snip off the tops of the blister with small scissors.

This enables the pus to drain out and allows the medication to reach the organisms. The edges of any blister should be kept trimmed, because the fungi spread under these edges. Debridement is followed by a foot soak.

3. Burow's solution soak

   Sig: 1 packet of Domeboro powder to 1 quart of warm water. Soak feet for 10 minutes b.i.d. Dry skin carefully afterward.

4. Antifungal cream 15.0

   Miconazole (Monistat-Derm, Micatin), clotrimazole (Lotrimin, Mycelex), econazole (Spectazole), ketoconazole (Nizoral), ciclopirox (Loprox), oxiconazole (Oxistat), naftifine (Naftin), terbenifine (Lamisil), butenafine (Mentax), and tolnaftate (Tinactin) (see Table 19-3 for detailed list of antifungal agents).
   Sig: Apply b.i.d. locally to feet after soaking.
   Sig: Apply b.i.d. locally for long term.

5. Rest at home for 2 to 4 days may be advisable, if severe.
6. Place small pieces of cotton sheeting or cotton between the toes when wearing shoes.

Five days later, the secondary infection and blisters should have decreased.

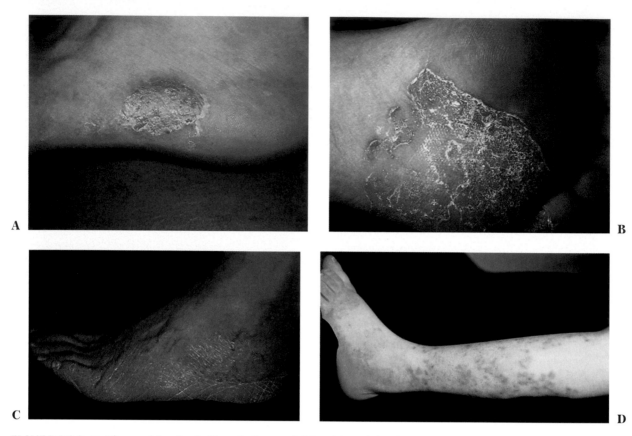

FIGURE 25-2 ■ Tinea of the foot. Chronic tinea of side of foot (**A**), of the sole due to *T. rubrum* (**B**), in a patient on corticosteroids, with extensive spread (**C**), and extending up the leg (**D**). *(Courtesy of Schering Corp.)*

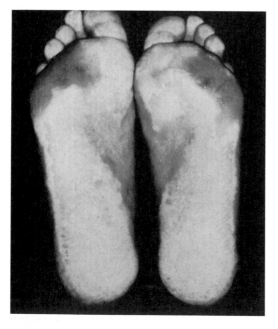

FIGURE 25-3 ■ Symmetric lividity of the soles associated with hyperhidrosis.

TABLE 25-2 ■ **Sites of Tinea in Relationship to Age Groups**

Tinea Site	Children (0–16 y)	Adults
Tinea capitis (scalp)	Common	Very rare
Tinea corporis (body)	Common	Fairly common
Tinea cruris (groin)	Rare	Common (esp. men)
Tinea pedis (feet)	Rare (mimics eczema)	Very common
Onychomycosis (nails)	Very rare	Very common

Subsequent Visits

1. The soaks may be continued for another 3 days or stopped if no marked redness or infection is present.
2. The previously described salve is continued or the following salves are substituted: A combination of an antifungal cream and a corticosteroid, as in Lotrisone cream, is beneficial. Antifungal solutions, such as Lotrimin, Mycelex, or Loprox, are quite effective. Apply a few drops on affected skin and rub in.
3. Antifungal powder q.s. 45.0

   Zeasorb AF, Micatin, Tinactin, and Desenex.
   Sig: Supply in powder can. Apply small amount to feet over the salve and to the shoes in the morning.
4. Systemic antifungal therapy: These forms of oral treatment are not recommended for acute tinea of the feet because (1) response to oral agents is slow for these acute and rather disabling cases; (2) the recurrence rate is very high; and (3) the cost and potential side effects of oral therapy is much greater than that of the more rapidly effective local therapy.

Case Example: Chronic Infection. A patient presents with chronic, scaly, thickened fungal infection of 4 years' duration. In the past week a few small tense blisters on the sole of the feet had developed. This type of clinical picture probably is caused by *T. rubrum*.

First Visit

1. The patient is told that the acute flare-up (the blisters) can be cleared but that it will be difficult and time consuming to cure the chronic infection. If the toenails are found to be infected, the prognosis for cure is even poorer (see Tinea of the Nails later in this chapter).
2. The blisters are debrided and trimmed with manicure scissors.
3. Any of the antifungal creams

   Sig: Apply locally to soles b.i.d., *or*
   Antifungal solution 10.0
   Sig: Rub in a few drops b.i.d.

Subsequent Visits

1. Systemic antifungal therapy: This type of oral therapy is not recommended for chronic tinea of the feet, but the patient may have heard or read about the "pill for athlete's feet," so it would be wise for you to discuss this with the patient. If you mention that you cannot guarantee a cure, even after months of taking a large quantity of rather expensive pills, most patients are content with keeping the chronic infection in an innocuous state with sporadic local therapy.

2. However, if after you have explained about the poor results and the expense of therapy, the patient still wants to try oral therapy, then consider the systemic antifungal agents listed in the following section on Tinea of the Hands and in Table 25-3. Long-term therapy is indicated, with appropriate monitoring of the patient.

Tinea of the Hands

A primary fungal infection of the hand or hands is quite rare. In spite of this fact, the diagnosis of "fungal infection of the hand" is commonly applied to cases that in reality are contact dermatitis, atopic eczema, pustular bacterid, or psoriasis. The best differential point is that tinea of the hand usually is seen only on one hand, not bilaterally (Fig. 25-4).

Primary Lesions

Acute Form. Blisters on the palms and the fingers are seen at the edge of red areas.

Chronic Form. Lesions are dry and scaly; usually there is a single patch, not separate patches.

Secondary Lesions

Bacterial infection is rather unusual.

Course

This gradually progressive disease spreads to fingernails. It usually is nonsymptomatic.

Laboratory Findings

KOH-ink preparations reveal mycelia, or cultures on Sabouraud's media grow the fungus (see Chap. 2).

Differential Diagnosis

- *Contact dermatitis of hands:* From soap, detergents, and other irritants; usually bilateral, periodic, more vesicular, and less frequently chronic; fungi not found (see Chap. 9)
- *Atopic eczema:* History of atopy in patient or family; bilateral; periodic; fungi not found (see Chap. 9)
- *Psoriasis:* Thick patch or patches in palms of menopausal women, usually bilateral; occasionally see psoriasis elsewhere; fungi not found (see Chap. 14)
- *Pustular bacterid:* Pustular lesions only; periodic and chronic; resistant to local therapy; fungi not found
- *Dyshidrosis of palms:* Recurrent; seasonal incidence; mainly vesicular on the sides of the fingers; not scaly; bilateral; related to atopic eczema; fungi not found

TABLE 25-3 ▪ **Antifungal Agents**

Antifungal Agent	Route of Administration	Organism Responsive	Side Effects
Allylamines			
Naftifine (Naftin)	Cream, gel	Dermatophytes	Rare
Terbinafine (Lamisil)	Cream, spray, oral	Dermatophytes, tinea versicolor	Oral, rarely liver toxicity
Benzylamines			
Butenafine HCl (Mentax, Lotrimin Ultra Cream)	Cream	Dermatophytes	Rare
-Azoles			
Clotrimazole (Mycelex, Lotrimin cream, solution Troches suppositories)	Cream	Dermatophytes, tinea versicolor, Candida	Rare
Econazole (Spectazole)	Cream	Dermatophytes, tinea versicolor, gram(+) bacteria	Rare
Fluconazole (Diflucan)	Oral	Dermatophytes, tinea versicolor, cryptococcosis, Candida	Rare
Itraconazole (Sporanox)	Oral (with food)	Dermatophytes, tinea versicolor, Candida, sporotrichosis, some deep fungi	Rare liver toxicity
Ketoconazole (Nizoral)	Cream shampoo	Dermatophytes, some deep fungi Candida, tinea versicolor	Liver toxicity
Miconazole (Micatin, Monistat, Zeasorb AF)	Cream, powder spray, suppositories	Dermatophytes, tinea versicolor, Candida	Rare
Oxiconazole (Oxistat)	Cream	Dermatophytes, tinea versicolor, Candida	Rare
Sertaconazole (ertaczol)	Cream	Dermatophytes, tinea versicolor, Candida	Rare
Polyenes			
Amphotericin B (Fungizone, Abelcet)	Intravenous	Deep fungi sepsis, Candida sepsis	Common renal toxicity thrombophlebitis, hypokalemia
Nystatin (Mycostatin)	Cream, ointment, powder, oral (not absorbed), pastilles, with triamcinolone (Mycolog II cream, ointment)	Candida	Rare
Miscellaneous			
Flucytosine (Ancobon)	Oral, usually given with amphotericin B	Deep fungi sepsis, Candida sepsis	Liver, renal, bone marrow toxicity, gastrointestinal
Ciclopirox (Loprox, Penlac) Nail lacquer	Gel, cream, shampoo, suspensions	Dermatophytes, Candida	Rare
Griseofulvin (Gris-Peg, Fulvicin, Grifulvin)	Oral (evening with fatty dermatophytes meal) tablets, suspension		Rare

(continued)

TABLE 25-3 ■ *(Continued)*

Antifungal Agent	Route of Administration	Organism Responsive	Side Effects
Selenium sulfide (Selsun, Head & Shoulders Intensive Treatment)	Shampoo (sometimes used as lotion)	Tinea versicolor	Irritation
Saturated solution of potassium iodide (SSKI)	Oral	Sporotrichosis	Gastrointestinal toxicity, bitter taste, goiter if long-term
Tolnaftate (Tinactin)	Cream	Dermatophytes	Rare
Undecylenic acid (Desenex)	Cream	Dermatophytes	Rare
Capsofungin (Candidas)	Intravenous	Candidiasis sepsis, Aspergillosis sepsis	Common, fever, headache thrombophlebitis, rash
Micafungin (Mycoviral)	Intravenous	Candidiasis sepsis, esophagitis	Common, headaches, rash, fever, bone marrow thrombophlebitis
Vericonazole (Ufend)	Intravenous, oral	Candida sepsis, esophageal, Aspergillosis sepsis, Fusariesis sepsis	Visceral impairment, liver toxicity, fever, cardiac toxicity

Treatment

Case Example. A man presents with scaly thickening of one palm of 8 years' duration. His fingernails are not involved. Itching is noted slightly at times.

1. Antifungal creams, especially naftifine (Naftin), terbinafine (Lamisil) cream, or butenafine (Mentax) may control or occasionally cure the tinea of the hand.
2. Systemic therapy (see Table 25-3): The following medicines are all expensive, especially because therapy must be continued, as for hand tinea, for several months. Appropriate monitoring of the patient during therapy is necessary. There are also drug interactions that can occur.

   a. Griseofulvin (Gris-Peg, 250 mg; Fulvicin P/G, 330 mg; Grisactin, 330 mg; Grifulvin, 330 mg)

   Sig: 1 tablet t.i.d after meals for at least 8 weeks, and probably for 4 to 6 months.
   Comment: Griseofulvin commonly causes headaches in the first few days of therapy. It is a penicillin derivative.

   b. Ketoconazole, 200 mg (rarely 400 mg)

   Sig: 1 tablet once a day for 3 to 4 months.
   Comment: Hepatotoxicity has been rarely reported with ketoconazole therapy, also impotence.

   c. Itraconazole (Sporanox) capsule, 100 mg. 200 mg b.i.d. for 7 days, repeated once a month for 3 to 4 months. Monitoring for rare liver toxicity must be done. Drug interactions are numerous.

   d. Fluconazole (Diflucan) has not been approved for superficial dermatophyte therapy. It may be effective in doses of 200 mg per week for 1 to 3 months. Drug interactions are numerous. It is expensive.

   e. Terbinafine (Lamisil) 250 mg.

   Sig: 1 tablet each day for 1 to 3 months. It is expensive.

Tinea of the Nails

Tinea of the toenails is very common, but tinea of the fingernails is uncommon. Tinea of the toenails is almost inevitable in patients who have recurrent attacks of tinea of the feet. Once developed, the infected nail serves as a resistant focus for future skin infection.

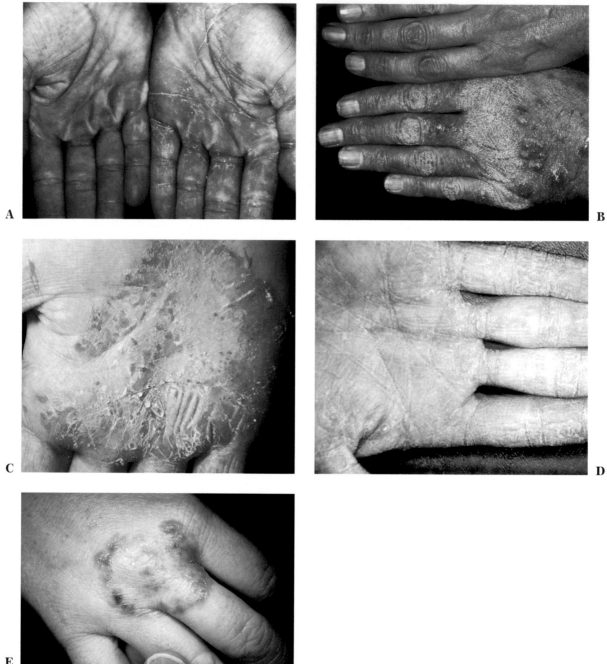

FIGURE 25-4 ■ Tinea of the hand usually affects only one hand but both feet. Thus, it is called "one-hand, two-foot syndrome." (**A**) Tinea of the left palm only, caused by *T. mentagrophytes*. (**B**) Deep tinea of left hand, caused by *T. mentagrophytes*. (**C**) Tinea of the palm, due to *T. rubrum*. (**D**) Tinea of the palm, of dry, scaly type, caused by *T. rubrum*. (**E**) Tinea on the back of the hand. *(Duke Laboratories, Inc.)*

Primary Lesions

Distal and lateral detachment of the nail occurs with subsequent thickening and deformity (Fig. 25-5).

Secondary Lesions

Bacterial infection can result from the pressure of shoes on the deformed nail and surrounding skin. Ingrown toenails are another undesirable consequence.

Distribution

The infection usually begins in the fifth toenail and may remain there or spread to involve the other nails.

Course

Tinea of the toenails can rarely be cured. Aside from the deformity, ingrown toenail (especially in cases of diabetes mellitus and marked vascular or neurologic compromise to the feet) and an occasional mild flare-up of acute tinea, treatment is not necessary. Progression is slow, and spontaneous cures are rare. Tinea of the fingernails can be treated, but the treatment usually takes months.

Cause

This type of tinea is usually due to *T. rubrum* and, less importantly, to *T. mentagrophytes*.

Laboratory Findings

These organisms can be found in a KOH preparation of a scraping and occasionally can be grown on culture media.

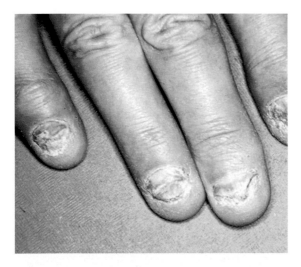

FIGURE 25-5 ■ Tinea of fingernails caused by *T. rubrum*. *(Courtesy of Duke Laboratories, Inc.)*

The material should be gathered from the most proximal debris under the nail plate. It is often difficult to obtain a positive test. Better yield on diagnosis is partial removal of nail plate sent to pathology for PAS stain.

Differential Diagnosis

See also Chap. 29, Diseases Affecting the Nails.

- *Nail injury:* A history of the injury must be obtained (Jogger's nails or pseudoonychomycosis), although tinea infection often starts in an injured nail; fungi are absent
- *Psoriasis of fingernails:* Pitting, red areas occur under nail with resulting detachment; psoriasis is elsewhere, usually; no fungi are found (see Chap. 14)
- *Psoriasis of toenails:* This may be impossible to differentiate from tinea, because many psoriatic nails have some secondary fungal invasion
- *Candidiasis of fingernails:* Common in people who frequently wash their hands; paronychial involvement common; *Candida* found (see later in this chapter)
- *Green nails:* This fingernail infection yields *C. albicans* and *P. aeruginosa* most commonly. Clinically, there is a distal detachment of the nail plate, with underlying greenish black debris. For cure, complete debridement of the detached part of the nail is necessary, plus local antiyeast therapy.

Treatment

Case Example: Tinea of the Fingernails. A young salesman presents with a fungal infection in three fingernails of his left hand of 9 months' duration. The surrounding skin shows mild redness and scaling.

1. Griseofulvin therapy (see earlier and Table 25-3). Griseofulvin ultrafine type, 250 to 330 mg or equivalent

   Sig: 1 tablet b.i.d. or t.i.d. for 9 months
   Comment: Therapy is stopped when there is no clinical evidence of infection (crumbling, thickening of nail plate, or subungual debris) and no cultural or KOH-ink mount evidence of fungi.

2. Ketoconazole therapy: If the patient and the physician are aware of the possibility of liver and other toxicity, then a 200-mg tablet once a day for 9 months might be curative. Close patient monitoring is necessary. There are many drug interactions, and it is very expensive.

3. Itraconazole therapy has been reported to be curative, 200 mg b.i.d. for 7 days, repeated monthly for 4

to 6 months. Available as a Pulse Pack. Many drug interactions. Check liver toxicity.

4. Terbinafine (Lamisil) 250 mg a day for 3 months. Very expensive. Check liver toxicity. Can also use 250 mgs q.day for 7 days every 3 months for 1 year. Cheaper and less liver toxicity.

5. Loprox nail lacquer (Penlac). Apply 2 times q.week.

Case Example: Tinea of the Toenails. A 45-year-old woman presents with three infected toenails on the right foot and two on the left foot. These are causing mild pain when she wears certain tight-fitting shoes. Scaliness of soles of feet is also evident.

1. Griseofulvin or ketoconazole therapy: This oral therapy is not effective or indicated for tinea of the toenails. Apparently some dermatologists have cured cases after oral therapy was continued for several years or when oral therapy was combined with evulsion of the toenails. The only time such therapy for toenails is prescribed, in our practice, is when the patient understands the problem but still wants to attempt a cure or a cosmetic improvement. At least 12 months of griseofulvin therapy is necessary. Women respond to this therapy better than men.

2. Itraconazole may be used. A dosage of 200 mg b.i.d. for 7 days, repeated monthly for 4 to 8 months, has been suggested. A Pulse Pack is available. Drug interactions must be watched for. Monitoring of the patient is necessary for rare liver toxicity. Very expensive.

3. Terbinafine (Lamisil) 250 mg a day for 3 or 4 months. Very expensive. Can also use 250 mgs q.day for 7 days every 3 months for 1 year. Cheaper and less liver toxicity.

4. Antifungal solution, 15 mL: For the patient who wants to "do something," applications two to four times a day for months might help some mild cases. One can combine this therapy with debridement of the nails. These solutions include Fungi-Nail, Fungoid, and Loprox.

5. Debriding of thick nails by patient, dermatologist, or podiatrist offers obvious relief from discomfort. This can be accomplished by the use of nail clippers or filing or picking away with a scalpel blade or a motor-driven drill.

6. Surgical evulsion of the toenail is rarely curative. As stated, this surgical approach can be combined with oral systemic therapy with probable enhancement of the end result.

7. Loprox nail lacquer (Penlac). Apply 2 times q.week.

Tinea of the Groin

Tinea of the groin is a common, itching, annoying fungal infection appearing usually in men and often concurrently with tinea of the feet (Fig. 25-6). Home remedies often result in a contact dermatitis that adds "fuel to the fire."

Primary Lesions

Bilateral, fan-shaped, red, scaly patches with a sharp, slightly raised border occur. Small vesicles may be seen in the active border.

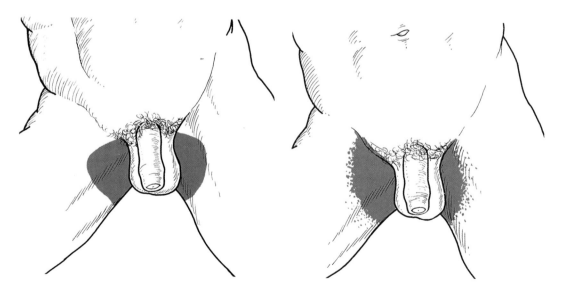

FIGURE 25-6 ■ Dermagrams for comparison of tinea of crural area and candidiasis of crural area. (*Left*) Tinea of crural area. Note sharp border of lesions. (*Right*) Candidiasis of crural area. Note indefinite border with satellite pustule-like lesions as edge. Candidiasis can also involve the scrotum.

Secondary Lesions

Oozing, crusting, edema, and secondary bacterial infection are evident. In chronic cases lichenification may be marked. Lichen simplex chronicus can develop.

Distribution

The infection affects the crural fold, extending to involve the scrotum, penis, thighs, perianal area, and buttocks.

Course

The type of fungus influences the course, but most acute cases respond rapidly to treatment. Other factors that affect the course and recurrences are obesity, hot weather, sweating, and chafing garments.

Cause

Tinea of the groin is commonly caused by the fungi of tinea of the feet, *T. rubrum*, and *T. mentagrophytes*, as well as *E. floccosum*.

Contagiousness

This is minimal, even between husband and wife.

Laboratory Findings

The organism is found in KOH preparations of scrapings and can be grown on culture. Material is taken from the active border (see Chap. 2).

Differential Diagnosis

- *Candidiasis:* No sharp border; fine scales, oozing, redness, satellite pustule-like lesions at edges; more common in obese females; *Candida* found (see later in this chapter)
- *Contact dermatitis:* Often coexistent but can be separate entity; new contactant history; no fungi found; no active border (see Chap. 9)
- *Prickly heat:* Pustular, papular; no active border, no fungi; may also be present with tinea
- *Lichen simplex chronicus:* Unilateral, usually; may have resulted from old chronic tinea; no fungi (see Chap. 11)
- *Psoriasis:* Usually unilateral; may or may not have raised border; psoriasis elsewhere; no fungi (see Chap. 14)
- *Erythrasma:* Faint redness, fine scaling with no elevated border, also seen in axilla and webs of toes; coral reddish fluorescence under Wood's light;

caused by a diphtheroid organism called *Corynebacterium minutissimum* (see Chap. 21)
- *Bowen's Disease or Extramammary Paget's Disease:* Consider these diagnoses if unilateral and recalcitrant to therapy; biopsy necessary to make these diagnoses

Treatment

Case Example. A young man presents with an oozing, red dermatitis with sharp border occurring in the crural area.

1. Because the infection usually comes from chronic tinea of the feet, to prevent recurrences, advise the patient to dry the feet last and not the groin area last when taking a bath.
2. Vinegar wet packs
    Sig: ½ cup of white vinegar to 1 quart of warm water. Wet the sheeting or thin toweling and apply to area for 15 minutes twice a day.
3. Antifungal cream 15.0
    Sig: Apply b.i.d. locally (see Table 19-3).
4. Griseofulvin oral therapy
    Griseofulvin ultrafine types, 250 to 330 mg
    Sig: 1 tablet b.i.d. for 6 to 8 weeks for extensive case.
5. Ketoconazole, itraconazole, or terbinafine therapy may also be used.

Tinea of the Smooth Skin

The familiar ringworm of the skin is most common in children partially because of their intimacy with animals and other children (Fig. 25-7; see also Fig. 36-30C). The lay public believes that *most* skin conditions are "ringworm," and many physicians erroneously agree with them.

Primary Lesions

Round, oval, or semicircular scaly patches have a slightly raised border that commonly is vesicular. Rarely, deep,

---

SAUER'S NOTES

An effective therapy for tinea of the groin is:

Sulfur, ppt.	5%
Hydrocortisone	1%
Antifungal cream q.s.	15.0

Sig: Apply b.i.d. locally, and continue for 7 days after apparently clear ("therapy-plus" routine).

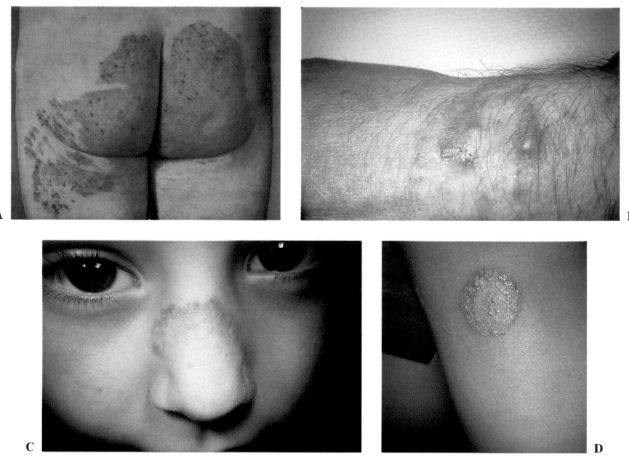

FIGURE 25-7 ■ Tinea of the smooth skin. **(A)** This infection on the buttocks had spread from the crural region. *(Courtesy of Smith Kline & French Laboratories.)* **(B)** Majocchi granulomas on flexor wrist. **(C)** Tinea faciei on young girl caught from cat. **(D)** Tinea corporis on arm. *(Ortho Pharmaceutical Corp.)*

ulcerated, granulomatous lesions (Majocchi's granuloma) are caused by superficial fungi.

Secondary Lesions

Bacterial infection, particularly at the advancing border, is common in association with certain fungi, such as *M. canis* and *T. mentagrophytes.*

Course

Infection is short lived, if treated correctly. It seldom recurs unless treatment is inadequate.

Cause

This disorder is most commonly caused by *M. canis* from kittens and puppies and less commonly by *E. floccosum* and *T. mentagrophytes* from groin and foot infections.

Contagiousness

The incidence is high.

Laboratory Findings

This is the same as for previously discussed fungal diseases.

Differential Diagnosis

- *Pityriasis rosea:* History of herald patch; sudden shower of oval lesions; fungi not found (see Chap. 14)
- *Impetigo:* Vesicular, honey-colored, crusted; most commonly on face; no fungi found (see Chap. 15)
- *Contact dermatitis:* No sharp border or central healing; may be coexistent with ringworm worsened by overtreatment (see Chap. 9)

Treatment

Case Example. A child has several 2- to 4-cm scaly lesions on his arms of 1 week's duration. He has a new kitten that he holds and plays with.

1. Examine the scalp, preferably with a Wood's light, to rule out scalp infection.
2. Advise the mother regarding moderate isolation procedures in relation to the family and others.
3. Antifungal salve q.s. 15.0

    Sig: Apply b.i.d. locally (see Table 19-3).

Subsequent Visit of Resistant Case or a New Widespread Case: Griseofulvin Oral Therapy. Griseofulvin (ultrafine types) can be given in tablet or oral suspension form. The usual dose for children is 165 mg b.i.d., but the pharmaceutical company's product information sheet should be consulted. Therapy should be maintained for 3 to 6 weeks or until lesions are gone. Occasionally, a higher dose is needed in deeper forms of infection.

Tinea of the Scalp

Tinea of the scalp is the most common cause of patchy hair loss in children (Fig. 25-8; see also Fig. 36-30AB). Endemic cases are with us always, but epidemics, usually due to the human type, were the real therapeutic problem, until the discovery of griseofulvin. Oral griseofulvin finds its greatest therapeutic usefulness and triumph in the management of tinea of the scalp. Before griseofulvin, children with the human type of scalp tinea had to be subjected to traumatic shampoos and salves for weeks or months, or they had to be epilated by x-ray. Often they were kept out of school for this entire period of therapy.

Ketoconazole, terbinafine, or itraconazole systemic therapy is available for griseofulvin-resistant cases, if these truly occur in tinea of the scalp.

Tinea capitis infections can be divided into two clinical types: noninflammatory and inflammatory. The treatment, cause, and course vary for these two types.

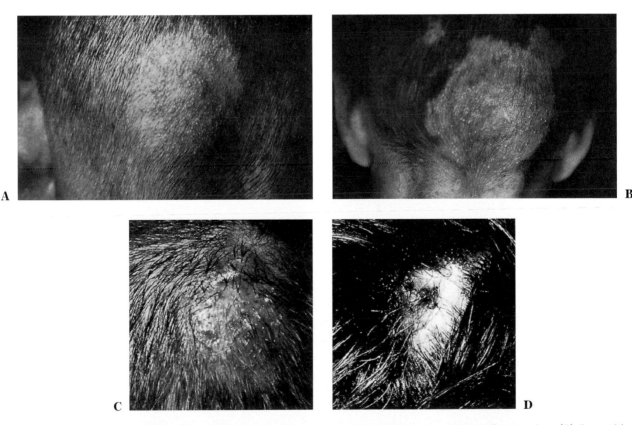

FIGURE 25-8 ■ Tinea of the scalp. (**A**) Caused by *M. audouini*. Note absence of visible inflammation. (**B**) Caused by *T. tonsurans*. Wood light examination revealed no fluorescence. (**C**) Caused by *T. mentagrophytes*. Note inflammation. (**D**) Favus, caused by *T. shoenleini*, of 11 years' duration.

Noninflammatory Type

Primary Lesions. Grayish, scaly, round patches with broken-off hairs are seen, causing balding areas. The size of the areas varies.

Secondary Lesions. Bacterial infection and id reactions are rare. A noninflammatory patch can become inflamed spontaneously or as the result of strong local treatment. Scarring almost never occurs. "Black dot" hairs (short broken-off hairs) are seen with *T. tonsurans* infection.

Distribution. The infection is most common in the posterior scalp region. Body ringworm from the scalp lesions is common, particularly on the neck and the shoulders.

Course. The incubation period in and on the hair is short, but clinical evidence of the infection cannot be expected less than 3 weeks after inoculation. Parents often do not notice the infection for another 3 weeks to several months, particularly in girls. Spontaneous cures are rare in 2 to 6 months, but after that time occur with greater frequency. Some cases last for years if untreated. Recurrence of the infection after the cure of a previous episode is possible because adequate immunity does not develop.

Age Group. Infection of the noninflammatory type is most common between the ages of 3 and 8 years and is rare after the age of puberty. This adult resistance to infection is attributed in part to the higher content of fungistatic fatty acids in the sebum after puberty. This research laboratory finding had great therapeutic significance, and the direct outgrowth was the development of Desenex and other fatty-acid ointments and powders.

T. tonsurans infection is seen mainly in African-American urban preadolescent children (often those who braid their hair). Spontaneous cures at puberty do not always occur.

Cause. The noninflammatory type of scalp ringworm is caused most frequently by *T. tonsurans* and occasionally by *M. canis* and *M. audouini*. *M. audouini* and *T. tonsurans* are anthropophilic fungi (human-to-human passage only),

whereas *M. canis* is a zoophilic fungus (animals are the original source, mainly kittens and puppies).

Contagiousness. The case can be a part of a large urban epidemic.

Laboratory Findings. Wood's light examination of the scalp hairs is an important diagnostic test, but hairs infected with *T. tonsurans* do not fluoresce. The Wood's light is a specially filtered long-wavelength ultraviolet light. The hairs infected with *M. audouini* and *M. canis* fluoresce with a bright yellowish green color (see Fig. 36-30). The bright fluorescence of fungus-infected hairs is not to be confused with the white or dull yellow color emitted by lint particles or sulfur-laden scales.

Microscopic examination of the infected hairs in 20% KOH solution shows an ectothrix arrangement of the spores when caused by the *Microsporum* species and endothrix spores when caused by *T. tonsurans*. Culture is necessary for species identification (see Fig. 2-2). The cultural characteristics of the various fungi can be found in many larger dermatologic or mycologic texts and are not presented here.

Treatment

Prophylactic

1. Hair is washed after every haircut by a barber or beautician.
2. Parents and teachers are educated on methods of spread of disease, particularly during an epidemic.
3. Suggestions should be given for provision for individual storage of clothing, particularly caps, in school and home.

Active

1. Griseofulvin oral therapy: The ultrafine types of griseofulvin (Fulvicin U/F, Fulvicin P/G, Gris-Peg, Grifulvin V, and Grisactin) can be administered in tablet form or liquid suspension (not all brands are available in liquid form). The usual dose for a child aged 4 to 8 is 250 mg b.i.d., but some require a larger dose. The duration of therapy is usually 6 to 8 weeks. Both dose and duration have to be individualized and based on clinical, Wood's light, or culture response.
2. Ketoconazole, terfinafine, itraconazole, or fluconozale oral therapy. This type of therapy is usually not indicated or necessary, but regimens are effective and preferred by some.
3. Selenium sulfide (Selsun) shampoo is sporicidal and may help to decrease the spread of infection.

4. Manual epilation of hairs: Near the end of therapy, the remaining infected and fluorescent hairs can be plucked out, or the involved area can be shaved closely. This eliminates the infected distal end of the growing hair.

Inflammatory Type

Primary Lesions. Pustular, scaly, round patches with broken-off hairs are found, resulting in bald areas.

Secondary Lesions. Bacterial-like infection is common. When the secondary reaction is marked, the area becomes swollen and tender. This inflammation is called a *kerion*. Minimal scarring sometimes remains.

Distribution. Any scalp area is involved. Concurrent body ringworm infection is common.

Course. Duration is much shorter than the noninflammatory type of infection. Spontaneous cures will result after 2 to 4 months in many cases, even if untreated, except for the *T. tonsurans* type.

Cause. The inflammatory type of scalp ringworm is most commonly caused by *T. tonsurans* and *M. canis* and rarely by *M. audouini*, *M. gypseum*, *T. mentagrophytes*, and *T. verrucosum*. *T. tonsurans*, *M. audouini*, and *T. mentagrophytes* are anthropophilic (coming from humans); *M. canis* and *T. verrucosum* are zoophilic (passed from infected animals); and *M. gypseum* is geophilic (coming from the soil).

Contagiousness. The incidence is high in children and farmers. It is mainly endemic, except for cases caused by *M. audouini*.

Laboratory Findings. Microscopic examination of the infected hairs in 20% KOH solution shows an ectothrix arrangement of the spores, but *T. tonsurans* shows endothrix

spores. The hairs infected with *M. canis* and *M. audouini* fluoresce with a bright yellowish green color under the Wood's light.

Differential Diagnosis
See Table 25-4.

Treatment

Prophylactic. This is the same as for noninflammatory cases.

Active

1. Griseofulvin oral therapy (as under noninflammatory type).
2. Local therapy: For some mild cases of the inflammatory type, or where drug expense is a factor, local therapy can be used with good results.

   Bactroban ointment 15.0
   Sig: Apply locally b.i.d. The scalp and the hair should be shampooed nightly.

3. If kerion is severe, with or without griseofulvin therapy:

   a. Burow's solution wet packs.

   Sig: 1 Domeboro packet to 1 pint of warm water. Apply soaked cloths for 15 minutes twice a day.

   b. Oral antibiotic therapy helps to eliminate secondary bacterial infection.

Tinea of the Beard

Fungal infection is a rare cause of dermatitis in the beard area (Fig. 25-9). Farmers occasionally contract it from infected cattle. Any presumed bacterial infection of the beard that does not respond readily to proper treatment should be examined for fungi.

Primary Lesions

Follicular, pustular, or sharp-bordered ringworm-type lesions or deep, boggy, inflammatory masses are seen.

TABLE 25-4 ■ Differential Diagnosis of Scalp Dermatoses

Dermatosis	Wood's Light	Scales	Redness	Hair Loss	Remarks
Tinea Capitis	±	Dry or crusted	Uncommon	Yes	Back of scalp, child
Alopecia areata	Neg	None	No	Yes	Exclamation point hairs at edges
Seborrheic dermatitis	Neg	Greasy	Yes	No	Diffuse scaling
Psoriasis	Neg	Thick and dry	Yes	No	Look at elbows, knees and nails
Trichotillomania	Neg	None	No	Yes	Psychoneurotic child
Pyoderma	Neg	Crusted	Yes	Occasional	Poor hygiene

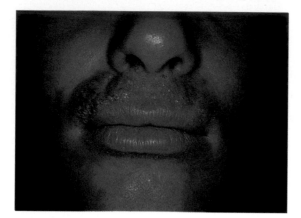

FIGURE 25-9 ■ Tinea of the beard caused by *T. mentagrophytes*.

Secondary Lesions

Bacterial infection is common. Scarring is unusual.

Cause

See Table 25-1.

Differential Diagnosis

■ *Bacterial folliculitis:* Acute onset, rapid spread; no definite border; responds rather rapidly to antibiotic therapy; no fungi found on examination of hairs or culture (see Chap. 21)

Treatment

Case Example. A farmer presents with a quarter-sized, boggy, inflammatory, pustular mass on his chin of 3 weeks' duration.

1. Have veterinarian inspect cattle if farmer is not aware of source of infection.
2. Burow's solution wet packs
   Sig: 1 Domeboro packet to 1 pint of hot water. Apply wet cloths to area for 15 minutes t.i.d.
3. Antifungal cream q.s. 15.0
   Sig: Apply locally b.i.d.
4. Griseofulvin oral therapy: The usual dose of griseofulvin, ultrafine type, for an adult is 250 to 330 mg b.i.d. for 6 to 8 weeks or longer, depending on clinical response or negative Sabouraud's culture.
5. Other oral antifungals can be used.

Dermatophytid

During an acute episode of any fungal infection, an id eruption can develop over the body. This is a manifestation of an allergic reaction to the fungal infection. The most common id reaction occurs on the hands during an acute tinea infection on the feet. To assume a diagnosis of an id reaction, the following criteria should be followed:

1. The primary focus should be acutely inflamed or infected with fungi, not chronically infected;
2. The id lesions must not contain fungi; and
3. The id eruption should disappear or wane after adequate treatment of the acute focus.

Primary Lesions

Vesicular eruption of the hands (primary lesion on the feet) and papulofollicular eruption on body (primary lesion commonly is scalp kerion) are found; pityriasis rosea-like id eruptions and others are seen less commonly.

Secondary Lesions

Excoriation and infection occur, when itching is severe, which is unusual.

Treatment

1. Treat the primary focus of infection.
2. For a vesicular id reaction on the hands:
   Burow's solution soaks
   Sig: 1 Domeboro packet to 1 quart of cool water. Soak hands for 15 minutes b.i.d.
3. For an id reaction on the body that is moderately pruritic:
   Aveeno oatmeal bath
   Sig: 1 packet of Aveeno to 6 to 8 inches of cool water in a tub, once daily.
   Hydrocortisone 1% lotion 120.0
   Sig: Apply locally b.i.d.
   Comment: Menthol 0.25%, phenol 0.5%, or camphor 2% could be added to this lotion.
4. For a severely itching, generalized id eruption:
   Prednisone, 10 mg, or related corticosteroid tablets #30
   Sig: 1 tablet q.i.d. for 2 days, then 2 tablets every morning for 7 days (or longer if necessary).

Deep Fungal Infections

Those fungi that invade the skin deeply and go into living tissue are also capable of involving other organs. Only the skin manifestations of these deeply invading fungi are discussed here.

The following diseases are included in this group of deep fungal infections (other, rarer, deep mycotic diseases are found in the Dictionary–Index and in Chap. 38):

- Candidiasis
- Sporotrichosis (see Fig. 38-18)
- North American blastomycosis (see Fig. 25-15)

Systemic fungus infections that were extremely rare are now being seen more frequently in patients who are immunocompromised, such as patients on chemotherapy, organ transplant recipients, and those with the acquired immunodeficiency syndrome.

Candidiasis

Candidiasis (moniliasis) is a fungal infection caused by *Candida albicans* that produces lesions in the mouth, vagina, skin, nails, lungs, or gastrointestinal tract, and occasionally a septicemia (Figs. 25-10, 25-11, and 25-12; see also Figs. 24-5, 36-4AB, and 36-18). The latter condition is seen in patients who are on long-term, high-dose antibiotic therapy and in those who are immunosuppressed. Because *C. albicans* exists commonly as a harmless skin inhabitant, the laboratory findings of this organism are not adequate proof of its pathogenicity and etiologic role. *Candida* or-

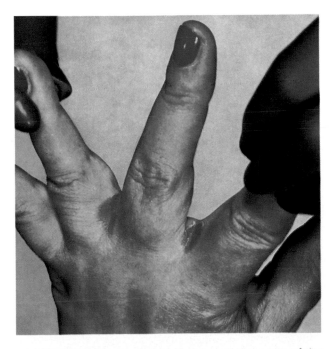

FIGURE 25-10 ■ Candidal intertrigo of the webs of the fingers. *(Smith Kline & French Laboratories.)*

ganisms commonly seed preexisting disease conditions. Concern here is with the cutaneous and the mucocutaneous candidal diseases. The following classification is helpful.

Cutaneous Candidiasis

Localized Diseases

Candida Paronychia. This common candida infection is characterized by the development of painful, red swellings of the skin around the nail plate. In chronic infections the nail becomes secondarily thickened and hardened. Candidal paronychia is commonly seen in housewives and those persons whose occupations predispose to frequent immersion of the hands in water.

This nail involvement is to be differentiated from superficial tinea of the nails (the candidal infection usually does not cause the nail to lose its luster or to become crumbly, and debris does not accumulate beneath the nail, except in chronic mucocutaneous candidiasis) and from bacterial paronychia (this is more acute in onset and throbs with pain and may drain pus).

Candida Intertrigo. This moderately common condition is characterized by red, eroded patches, with scaly, pustular or pustulovesicular lesions, with an indefinite border of satellite pustules (see Figs. 25-6, 25-11, and 25-12). The most common sites are axillae, inframammary areas, umbilicus, genital area, anal area, and webs of toes and fingers. Obesity, diabetes, and systemic antibiotics predispose to the development of this intertriginous type.

Candida intertrigo is to be differentiated from superficial tinea infections, which are not as red and eroded, and from seborrheic dermatitis or psoriasis.

Generalized Cutaneous Candidiasis. This rare infection (see Figs. 36-4 and 36-18) involves the smooth skin, mucocutaneous orifices, and intertriginous areas. It follows in the wake of general debility, as seen in immunosuppressed patients, and was very resistant to treatment before the discovery of ketoconazole and, more recently, fluconazole and itraconazole.

Mucous Membrane Candidiasis

Oral Candidiasis (Thrush and Perlèche). Thrush is characterized by creamy white flakes on a red, inflamed mucous membrane (Fig. 25-13). The tongue may be smooth and atrophic, or the papillae may be hypertrophic, as in the condition labeled "hairy tongue." Therapy with nystatin (Mycostatin) pastilles (lozenges) or Mycelex troches is

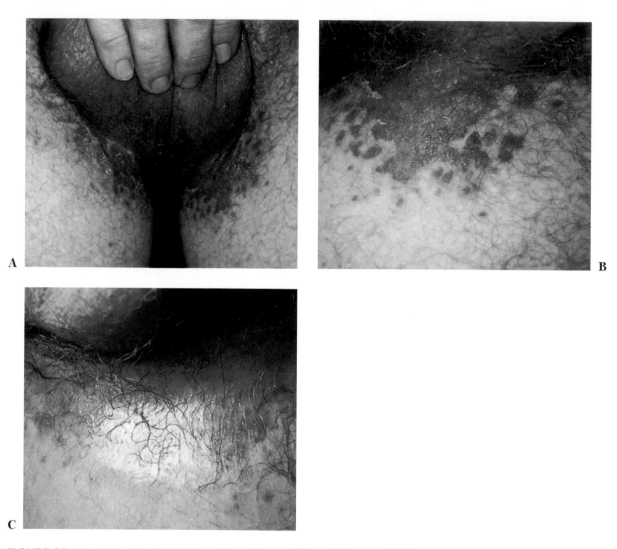

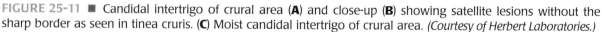

FIGURE 25-11 ■ Candidal intertrigo of crural area (**A**) and close-up (**B**) showing satellite lesions without the sharp border as seen in tinea cruris. (**C**) Moist candidal intertrigo of crural area. *(Courtesy of Herbert Laboratories.)*

effective. Perlèche is seen as cracks or fissures at the corners of the mouth and is usually associated with candidal disease elsewhere and rarely a dietary deficiency (usually B_{12} deficiency). Thrush is seen commonly in immunosuppressed patients.

A noncandida, clinically similar condition is commonly seen in elderly persons with ill-fitting dentures in whom the corners of the mouth override. Oral candidiasis is also to be differentiated from allergic conditions, such as those caused by toothpaste or mouthwash.

Candida Vulvovaginitis. The clinical picture is an oozing, red, sharply bordered skin infection surrounding an inflamed vagina that contains a buttermilk-like discharge.

This type of candida infection is frequently seen in pregnant women, diabetics, and those who have been on antibiotics systemically. It is to be differentiated from an allergic condition or from trichomonal or chlamydial vaginitis.

Laboratory Findings. Skin or mucous membrane scrapings placed in 20% KOH solution and examined with the high-power microscope lens reveal small, oval, budding, thin-walled, yeast-like cells with occasional mycelia. Culture on Sabouraud's media produces creamy dull-white colonies in 4 to 5 days. Further cultural studies on corn meal agar are necessary to identify the species as *C. albicans*.

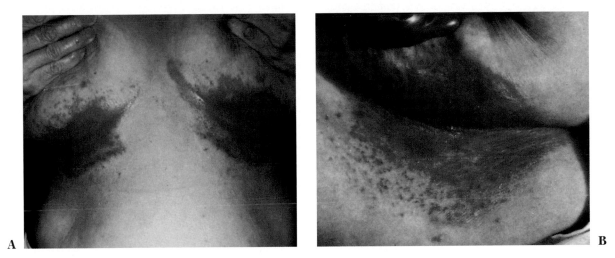

FIGURE 25-12 ■ **(A)** Candida intertrigo under breasts. **(B)** Note the lack of a definite border to the eruption, which distinguishes it from a tinea infection. *(Courtesy of Smith Kline & French Laboratories.)*

Treatment

> **SAUER'S NOTE**
>
> Do not treat a candidal infection with oral griseoful-vin. This intensifies the candidal infection.

Case Example. Candidal paronychia of two fingers is seen in a 37-year-old male bartender.

1. Advise the patient to avoid exposure of his hands to soap and water by wearing cotton gloves under rubber gloves, hiring a dishwasher, and so on.

2. Antifungal imidazole-type solution (Lotrimin or Mycelex solution 1%) 15.0

   or Fungi-Nail 15.0
   Sig: Apply to base of nail q.i.d. Continue treatment for several weeks.

3. At night, apply:

   Mycolog cream 15.0
   Sig: Apply locally h.s.

Case Example. Candidal intertrigo of inframammary and crural region is seen in an elderly obese woman.

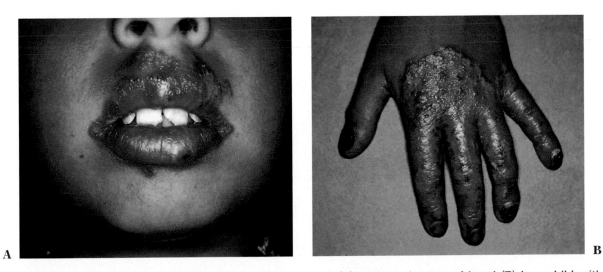

FIGURE 25-13 ■ Extensive candidiasis around the mouth **(A)** and on dorsum of hand **(B)** in a child with Addison's disease. *(Herbert Laboratories.)*

1. Advise the patient to wear pieces of cotton sheeting under breasts to keep the apposing tissues drier. Frequent bathing with thorough drying is helpful. Use of antibacterial soap should be avoided.

2. Sulfur, ppt. 5%

   Hydrocortisone 1%
   Mycostatin cream q.s. 30.0
   Sig: Apply locally t.i.d.

3. Powder can be used over cream:

   Mycostatin dusting powder q.s. 15.0
   Sig: Apply locally t.i.d.

Case Example. Candida vulvovaginitis is found in a woman who is 6 months pregnant.

1. Mycostatin vaginal tablets, 100,000 units #20

   Sig: Insert 1 tablet b.i.d. in vagina.

2. Monistat-Derm lotion, or

   Sulfur, ppt. 5%
   Hydrocortisone 1%
   Mycostatin cream q.s. 30.0
   Sig: Apply locally b.i.d. to vulvar skin.

3. Fluconazole

   150 mg tablet. Single dose p.o. Can repeat for resistant cases.

Ketoconazole, Itraconazole, or Fluconazole Therapy. This systemic therapy is rarely indicated for routine candidal infections. For chronic mucocutaneous candidiasis, ketoconazole and fluconazole can heal dramatically. Dosage information is provided in the package insert. The patient must be monitored carefully.

Sporotrichosis *(see Chap. 38)*

Sporotrichosis is a granulomatous fungal infection of the skin and the subcutaneous tissues (Fig. 25-14; see Fig. 38-18). Characteristically, a primary chancre precedes more extensive skin involvement. Invasion of the internal viscera is rare (see Chap. 38).

Primary Lesion

A sporotrichotic chancre develops at the site of skin inoculation, which is commonly the hand and less commonly the face or the feet. The chancre begins as a painless, movable, subcutaneous nodule that eventually softens and breaks down to form an ulcer.

Secondary Lesions

Within a few weeks subcutaneous nodules arise along the course of the draining lymphatics and form a chain of tumors that develop into ulcers. This is the classic clinical picture, of which there are variations.

Course

The development of the skin lesions is slow and rarely affects the general health.

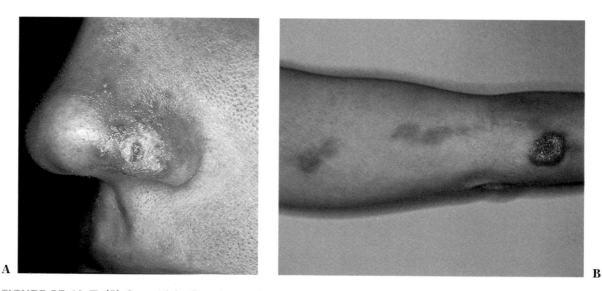

FIGURE 25-14 ■ **(A)** Sporotrichotic primary lesion on the nose. **(B)** Sporotrichotic chancre on arm with subcutaneous nodules. *(Courtesy of Stiefel Laboratories.)*

Cause

The causative agent is *Sporothrix schenckii,* a fungus that grows on wood and in the soil. It invades open wounds and is an occupational hazard of farmers (especially sphagnum moss), gardeners (especially roses), laborers, and miners.

Laboratory Findings

Cultures of the purulent material from unopened lesions readily grow on Sabouraud's media. The organism is difficult to see, even with special stains or tissue examination from a biopsy.

Differential Diagnosis

Any of the skin granulomas should be considered, such as

- *Pyodermas*
- *Syphilis*
- *Tuberculosis*
- *Sarcoidosis*
- *Leprosy*

An ioderma or bromoderma can cause a similar clinical picture.

Treatment

1. Saturated solution of potassium iodide, 60.0 mL

   Sig: On the first day, 10 drops t.i.d., p.c. added to milk or water; second day, 15 drops t.i.d.; third day, 20 drops t.i.d. and increase until 30 to 40 drops t.i.d. are given.

   Comment: The initial doses may be smaller and the increase more gradual if one is concerned about tolerance. Gastric irritation and ioderma should be watched for. There is a very bitter taste. This very specific treatment must be continued for 1 month after apparent cure.

2. Ketoconazole, 200 mg

   Sig: 2 tablets a day for 8 weeks.

   Comment: Some cases are not helped. The patient must be monitored closely.

3. Itraconazole, 100 mg

   Sig: 1 tablet daily for 4 to 6 weeks.

   Comment: Patient should be monitored for rare liver toxicity.

North American Blastomycosis

Two cutaneous forms of this disease are seen: primary cutaneous blastomycosis and secondary localized cutaneous blastomycosis.

Primary cutaneous blastomycosis occurs in laboratory workers and physicians after accidental inoculation (Fig. 25-15). A primary chancre develops at the site of the inoculation, and the regional nodes enlarge. In a short time the primary lesion and nodes heal spontaneously and the cure is complete.

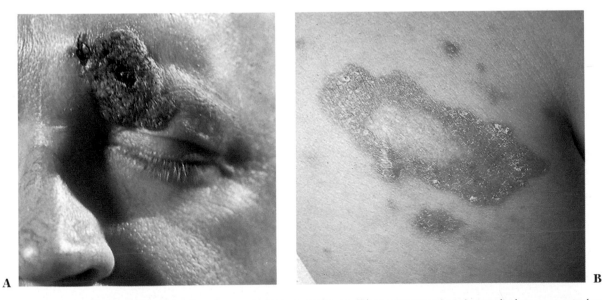

A   B

FIGURE 25-15 ■ **(A)** Blastomycotic primary lesion of eyebrow. **(B)** Blastomycotic primary lesion on scapular area. *(Courtesy of Stiefel Laboratories.)*

The following discussion is confined to the secondary cutaneous form. Systemic blastomycosis is rarer than the cutaneous forms but is seen occasionally in immunosuppressed patients.

Primary Lesion (Secondary, Localized, Cutaneous Form)

The lesion begins as a papule that ulcerates and slowly spreads peripherally, with a warty, pustular, raised border. The face, hands, and feet are involved most commonly.

Secondary Lesion

Central healing of the ulcer occurs gradually, with resultant thick scar.

Course

A large lesion develops over several months. Therapy is moderately effective on a long-term basis. Relapses are common.

Cause

The fungus *Blastomyces dermatitidis* is believed to invade the lungs primarily and the skin secondarily as a metastatic lesion. High native immunity prevents the development of more than one skin lesion. This immunity is low in the rare systemic form of blastomycosis in which multiple lesions occur in the skin, bones, and other organs. This fungal disease affects adult men most frequently.

Laboratory Findings

The material for a 20% KOH solution mount is collected from the pustules at the border of the lesion. Round, budding organisms can be found in this manner or in a culture mount. A chest roentgenogram is indicated in every case.

Differential Diagnosis

Consider any of the granuloma-producing diseases, such as

- *Tuberculosis*
- *Syphilis*
- *Iodide* or *bromide drug eruption*
- *Pyoderma*
- *Neoplasm*

Treatment

1. Surgical excision and plastic repair of early lesions is effective.
2. Amphotericin B suppresses the chronic lesion more effectively than any other drug. It is administered by IV infusion, daily, in varying schedules, which are described in larger texts or reviews. Amphotericin (Abelcet) is a safer more effective form of this drug.
3. Ketoconazole or itraconazole therapy on a long-term basis is also beneficial. Higher than normal dosages for a longer period of time are necessary for immunosuppressed patients.

Suggested Reading

Drake LA, Dinehart SM, et al. Guidelines of care for superficial mycotic infections of the skin: Mucocutaneous candidiasis. J Am Acad Dermatol 1996;34:287.

Gupta AK, Hofstader SLR, et al. Tinea capitis: An overview with emphasis on management. Pediatr Dermatol 1999;16:171–189.

Mooney MA, Thomas I, Sirois D. Oral candidiasis. Int J Dermatol 1995;34:759.

Odom R. Pathophysiology of dermatophyte infections. J Am Acad Dermatol 1993;28:S2.

Onychomycosis. Int J Dermatol 1999;38(Suppl 2).

Proceedings of the International Summit on Cutaneous Antifungal Therapy and Mycology Workshop, San Francisco, CA. J Am Acad Dermatol Suppl 1994;31.

Proceedings of a symposium, Onychomycosis: Issues and Observations, Chicago, IL. J Am Acad Dermatol Suppl 1995;35:3.

Radentz WH. Opportunistic fungal infections in immunocompromised hosts. J Am Acad Dermatol 1989;20:989.

Sehgal VN, Jain S. Onychomycosis: Clinical perspective. Int J Dermatol 2000;39:241–249.

Smith EB. Topical antifungal drugs in the treatment of tinea pedis, tinea cruris, and tinea corporis. J Am Acad Dermatol 1993;28:S24.

Sugar AM, Lyman CA. A practical guide to medically important fungi and the diseases they cause. Philadelphia, Lippincott–Raven Publishers, 1997.

Systemic antifungal drugs. Med Lett 1997;39:1009.

Update on dermatophytosis. J Am Acad Dermatol 2000;43:2000.

SECTION IV

TUMORS OF THE SKIN

CHAPTER 26

Tumors of the Skin

John C. Hall

Classification

A patient comes into your office for care of a tumor on his skin. What kind is it? What is the best treatment? This complex process of diagnosing and managing skin tumors is not learned easily. As an aid to the establishment of the correct diagnosis, all skin tumors (excluding warts, which are caused by a virus) are classified

1. as to their histologic origin (Table 26-1),
2. according to the patient's age group (Table 26-2),
3. by location (Table 26-3), and
4. on the basis of clinical appearance (Table 26-4).

A complete histologic classification is found at the end of this chapter; only the more common tumors are classified and discussed here. This histologic classification is divided into epidermal tumors, mesodermal tumors, nevus cell tumors, lymphomas, and myeloses. In making a clinical diagnosis of any skin tumor, one should apply a histopathologic label. Whether the label is correct or not depends on the clinical acumen of the physician and whether the tumor, or a part of it, has been examined microscopically.

SAUER'S NOTES

1. A histologic examination should be performed on every malignant skin tumor.
2. Similarly, a biopsy should be performed on any tumor when a malignancy cannot be definitely ruled out clinically.

TABLE 26-1 ■ Histologic Classification of Tumors of the Skin

Epidermal Tumors

Tumors of the Surface Epidermis

1. *Benign tumors:* defined as neoplasms that probably arise from arrested embryonal cells

    a. Seborrheic keratosis
    b. Pedunculated fibroma (skin tag, fibroepithelial polyp, acrochordon)
    c. Cysts
        • Epidermal cyst
        • Trichilemmal (pilar or sebaceous cyst)
        • Milium
        • Dermoid cyst
        • Mucous cyst

2. Precancerous tumors

    a. Actinic keratosis and cutaneous horn
    b. Arsenical keratosis
    c. Leukoplakia
    d. Porokeratosis

3. *Carcinoma:* squamous cell carcinoma

Tumors of the Epidermal Appendages

1. Basal cell carcinoma
2. Sebaceous gland hyperplasia
3. Numerous other types benign and malignant, usually classified by appendage of origin

Mesodermal Tumors

Tumors of Fibrous Tissue

1. Histiocytoma and dermatofibroma

2. Keloid

Tumors of Vascular Tissue

1. Hemangiomas

Nevus Cell Tumors

Nevi

1. Junctional (active) nevus
2. Intradermal (resting) nevus
3. Dysplastic nevus syndrome (familial atypical mole–melanoma syndrome or sporadic atypical mole–melanoma syndrome)

Malignant Melanoma

Lymphoma and Myelosis

Monomorphous Group
Polymorphous Group

1. Mycosis fungoides (cutaneous T-cell lymphoma)

Modified from Lever WF, Schaumberg-Lever G. Histopathology of the skin, ed 8. Philadelphia, Lippincott, 1997.

TABLE 26-2 ■ Age-Based Classification of Tumors of the Skin

Age Group	Possible Tumor Types*
Children	1. Warts (viral), very common
	2. Nevi, junctional type, common
	3. Molluscum contagiosum (viral)
	4. Hemangiomas
	5. Café-au-lait spot
	6. Granuloma pyogenicum
	7. Mongolian spot
	8. Xanthogranulomas
Adults	1. Warts (viral), plantar-type common
	2. Nevi
	3. Cysts
	4. Pedunculated fibromas (skin tags, acrochordons)
	5. Sebaceous gland hyperplasias
	6. Histiocytomas (dermatofibromas, sclerosing hemangiomas)
	7. Keloids
	8. Lipomas
	9. Granuloma pyogenicum
Older Adults**	1. Seborrheic keratoses
	2. Actinic keratoses
	3. Capillary hemangiomas (cherry angiomas, senile angiomas)
	4. Basal cell carcinomas
	5. Squamous cell carcinomas
	6. Leukoplakia

*The most common tumors are listed first.
**In addition to tumors of adults.

An age group classification is helpful from a differential diagnostic viewpoint. Viral warts are considered in this classification because of the frequent necessity of differentiating them from other skin tumors.

The clinical appearance of any tumor is a most important diagnostic factor. Some tumors have a characteristic color and growth that is readily distinguishable from any other tumor, but a large number, unfortunately, have clinical characteristics common to several similar tumors. A further hindrance to making a correct diagnosis is that the same histopathologic lesion may vary in clinical appearance. The following generalizing classification should be helpful, but, if in doubt, the lesion should be examined histologically.

Seborrheic Keratoses

It is a rare elderly patient who does not have any seborrheic keratoses. These are the unattractive "moles" or "warts"

TABLE 26-3 ■ Classification of Tumors Based on Location

Location	Possible Tumor Type	Location	Possible Tumor Type
Scalp	Seborrheic keratosis		Warty dyskeratoma
	Epidermal cyst (pilar cyst)		Atypical fibroxanthoma
	Nevus		Angiolymphoid hyperplasia with eosinophilia
	Actinic keratosis (bald males)		
	Wart		Blue nevus
	Trichilemmal cyst		Pedunculated fibroma
	Basal cell carcinoma	Eyelids	Seborrheic keratosis
	Squamous cell carcinoma		Milium
	Nevus sebaceous		Syringomas
	Proliferating trichilemmal tumor		Basal cell carcinoma
	Cylindroma		Xanthoma
	Syringocystadenoma papilliferum		Pedunculated fibroma
	Seborrheic keratosis	Neck	Seborrheic keratosis
Ear	Actinic keratoses		Epidermal cyst
	Basal cell carcinoma		Keloid
	Nevus		Fordyce's disease
	Squamous cell carcinoma	Lip and mouth	Lentigo
	Keloid		Venous lake (varix)
	Epidermal cyst		Mucous retention cyst
	Chondrodermatitis nodularis helicis		Leukoplakia
	Venous lakes (varix)		Pyogenic granuloma
	Gouty tophus		Squamous cell carcinoma
Face	Seborrheic keratosis		Granular cell tumor (tongue)
	Sebaceous gland hyperplasia		Giant cell epulis (gingivae)
	Actinic keratosis		Verrucous carcinoma
	Lentigo		White sponge nevus
	Milium		Acral lentiginous melanoma
	Nevi		Pedunculated fibroma
	Basal cell carcinoma	Axilla	Epidermal cyst
	Squamous cell carcinoma		Molluscum contagiosum
	Lentigo maligna melanoma		Lentigo (multiple lentigo in axillae neurofibromatosis called Crowe's sign)
	Flat wart		
	Trichoepithelioma		
	Dermatosis papulosa nigra (African American women)	Chest and back	Seborrheic keratosis
			Angioma
	Fibrous papule of the nose		Nevi
	Colloid milium		Ephelides
	Dilated pore of Winer		Actinic keratosis
	Keratoacanthoma		Lipoma
	Pyogenic granuloma		Basal cell carcinoma
	Spitz nevus		Epidermal cyst
	Ephelides		Keloid
	Hemangioma		Lentigo
	Adenoma sebaceum		Café-au-lait spot
	Apocrine hydrocystoma		Squamous cell carcinoma
	Eccrine hydrocystoma		Melanoma
	Trichilemmoma		Hemangioma
	Trichofolliculoma		Histiocytoma
	Merkel cell carcinoma		Steatocystoma multiplex
	Angiosarcoma (elderly men)		Eruptive vellus hair cyst
	Nevus of Ota		Blue nevus

(Continued)

TABLE 26-3 ■ (Continued)

Location	Possible Tumor Type	Location	Possible Tumor Type
	Nevus of Ito		Ganglion
	Becker's nevus		Common blue nevus
Groin and crural areas	Pedunculated fibroma		Acral lentigines melanoma
	Seborrheic keratosis		Giant cell tumor of tendon sheath
	Molluscum contagiosum		Pyogenic granuloma
	Wart		Acquired digital fibrokeratoma
	Bowen's disease		Recurrent infantile digital fibroma
	Extramammary Paget disease		Traumatic fibroma
	Wart		Xanthoma
Genitalia	Molluscum contagiosum		Dupuytren contracture
	Squamous intraepithelial lesions	*Feet*	Wart
	Epidermal cyst		Nevi
	Angiokeratoma (scrotum)		Blue nevus
	Pearly penile papules (around edge of glans)		Acral lentigines melanoma
	Squamous cell carcinoma		Seborrheic keratosis
	Seborrheic keratosis		Verrucous carcinoma
	Erythroplasia of Queyrat		Eccrine poroma
	Bowen's disease	*Arms and legs*	Seborrheic keratosis
	Median raphe cyst of penis		Lentigo
	Verrucous carcinoma		*Wart*
	Hidradenoma papilliferum (labia majora)		*Histiocytoma*
Hands	Wart		*Actinic keratosis*
	Seborrheic keratosis		*Squamous cell carcinoma*
	Actinic keratosis		*Melanoma*
	Lentigo		*Lipoma*
	Myxoid cyst (proximal nail fold)		*Xanthoma*
	Squamous cell carcinoma		*Clear cell acanthoma (legs)*
	Glomus tumor (nail bed)		*Kaposi's sarcoma (legs, classic type)*

that perturb the elderly patient, occasionally become irritated, but are benign (Fig. 26-1).

Dermatosis papulosa nigra is a form of seborrheic keratosis of African Americans that occur on the face, mainly in women. These small, black, multiple tumors can be removed, but there is the possibility of causing keloids or hypopigmentation. Stucco keratoses are numerous white 1- to 3-mm seborrheic keratoses mainly over feet, ankles, and lower legs. A very large seborrheic keratosis is sometimes referred to as a *melanoacanthoma*.

Presentation and Characteristics

Description

The size of seborrheic keratoses varies up to 3 cm for the largest, but the average diameter is 1 cm. The color may be flesh-colored, tan, brown, or coal black. They are usually oval in shape, elevated, and have a greasy, warty sensation to touch. White, brown, or black pinhead-sized keratotic areas called *pseudohorned cysts* are commonly seen within this tumor. There is an appearance of being superficial and "stuck on" the skin. Pruritus is common and sudden appearance may occur. Numerous lesions coming on rapidly can be a marker of underlying cancer (sign of Leser-Trélat).

Distribution

The lesions appear on the face, neck, scalp, back, and upper chest, and less frequently on arms, legs, and the lower part of the trunk.

Course

Lesions become darker and enlarge slowly. However, sometimes they can enlarge rapidly and this can be accompanied by bleeding and inflammation, which is very frightening to the patient. Trauma from clothing occasionally results in

TABLE 26-4 ■ **Classification of Skin Tumors Based on Clinical Appearance**

Appearance	Possible Tumor Type
Flat, skin-colored tumors	1. Flat warts (viral) 2. Histiocytomas 3. Leukoplakia
Flat, pigmented tumors	1. Nevi, usually junctional type 2. Lentigo 3. Café-au-lait spot 4. Histiocytomas 5. Mongolian spot 6. Melanoma (superficial spreading type)
Raised, skin-colored tumors	1. Warts (viral) 2. Pedunculated fibromas (skin tags) 3. Nevi, usually intradermal type 4. Cysts 5. Lipomas 6. Keloids 7. Basal cell carcinomas 8. Squamous cell carcinoma 9. Molluscum contagiosum (viral) 10. Xanthogranuloma (yellowish, usually children)
Raised, brownish tumors	1. Warts (viral) 2. Nevi, usually compound type 3. Actinic keratoses 4. Seborrheic keratoses 5. Pedunculated fibromas (skin tags) 6. Basal cell epitheliomas 7. Squamous cell carcinoma 8. Malignant melanoma 9. Granuloma pyogenicum 10. Keratoacanthomas
Raised, reddish tumors	1. Hemangiomas 2. Actinic keratoses 3. Granuloma pyogenicum 4. Glomus tumors 5. Senile or cherry angiomas
Raised, blackish tumors	1. Seborrheic keratoses 2. Nevi 3. Granuloma pyogenicum 4. Malignant melanomas 5. Blue nevi 6. Thrombosed angiomas or hemangiomas

infection and bleeding, and this prompts the patient to seek medical care. Any inflammatory dermatitis around these lesions causes them to enlarge temporarily and become more evident, so much so that many patients suddenly note them for the first time. Malignant degeneration of seborrheic keratoses is doubted.

Cause

Heredity is the biggest factor, along with old age.

Differential Diagnosis

- *Actinic keratoses:* See Table 26-5
- *Pigmented nevi:* Longer duration, smoother surface, softer to touch; may not be able to differentiate clinically (see later in this chapter)
- *Flat warts:* In younger patients; acute onset, with rapid development of new lesions, colorless and flat topped without pseudohorned cysts; tiny black thrombosed capillaries may be seen usually smaller; may Koebnerize (see Chap. 23)
- *Malignant melanoma:* Less common, usually with rapid growth, indurated; examination histologically with biopsy may be necessary (see later)

Treatment

Case Example. A 58-year-old woman requests the removal of a warty, tannish, slightly elevated 2- × 2-cm lesion of the right side of her forehead.

1. The lesion should be examined carefully. The diagnosis usually can be made clinically, but if there is any question, a scissors biopsy (see Chap. 2) can be performed. It would be ideal if all of these seborrheic keratoses could be examined histologically, but this is not economically feasible or necessary.
2. An adequate form of therapy is curettement, with or without local anesthesia, followed by a light application

---

SAUER'S NOTES

1. For many benign lesions, it often is best cosmetically to err on the side of surgical undertreatment rather than overtreatment. You can always remove any remaining growth later, but you cannot put back what you took off.
2. Scarring should be kept to a minimum.
3. After any surgical procedure, I hand out a "Surgical Notes" sheet that indicates postoperative care. Skin surgery sites usually heal without any complication. However, there are always questions and concerns from the patient about aftercare.

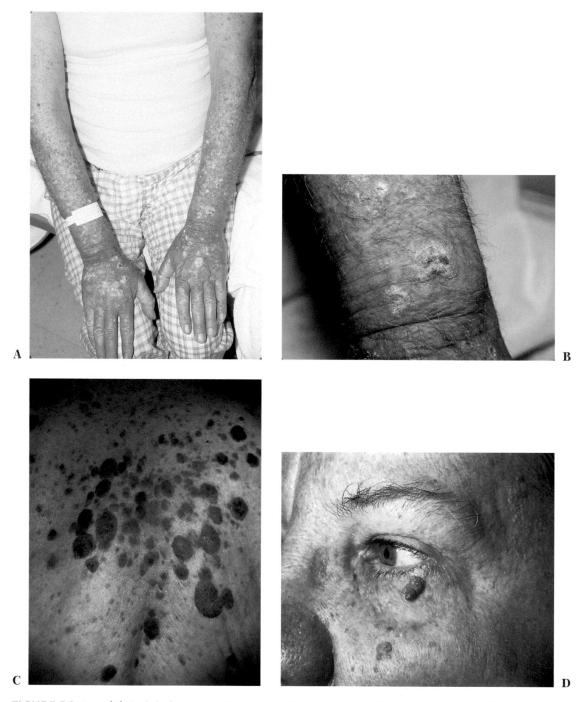

FIGURE 26-1 ■ (**A**) Actinic keratoses in an oil refinery worker. (**B**) Hyperkeratotic actinic keratoses. (**C**) Seborrheic keratoses on back. (**D**) Pedunculated seborrheic keratosis of eyelid. *(Courtesy of Stiefel Laboratories, Inc.)*

SURGICAL NOTES FOR THE PATIENT

Minor surgery has been performed for the removal or biopsy of a skin lesion.

If liquid nitrogen was used to remove the growth, a blister or peeling at the growth site will develop in 24 hours; if electrosurgery, laser, or burning was used, a crust and scab will form; if a biopsy was made, there will be a crust or suture(s).

The sites treated heal better if they are covered with a dressing with Polysporin ointment underneath during the day for 5 to 7 days and left uncovered at night and while bathing. Do not pick at the spot and try to avoid accidentally hitting the area.

You can wash over the area lightly.

A certain amount of redness and swelling around the surgery site is to be expected. Also you might have a small amount of drainage and crusting. A mild amount of redness and infection can be treated with Polysporin ointment locally three times a day.

If more drainage or infection develops, apply a wet dressing with sheeting, or soak the area. Oral antibiotics can be given. Use a solution made with 1 teaspoon of salt to 1 pint of cool water or Domeboro compresses and apply for 20 minutes three times a day. Make a fresh solution every day.

If the infection becomes excessive, call the office or go to a hospital emergency department.

If the scab is knocked off prematurely, bleeding may occur. This can be stopped by applying firm pressure with gauze or cotton for 10 minutes by the clock, and then releasing pressure gradually.

Depending on the size of the surgery site, healing takes from 1 to 8 weeks. Some scarring or loss of pigment at the surgery site is possible. A few individuals have a tendency to form thick or keloidal scars, which is not predictable.

If a biopsy was done, you may receive a separate bill for the pathology study from the laboratory. Call the office in 7 days for this report.

Return to the office for further care or follow-up as directed.

of trichloroacetic acid. The resulting fine atrophic scar will hardly be noticeable in several months.

3. Electrosurgery can be used, but this usually requires anesthesia.
4. Liquid nitrogen freezing therapy works well, if available. It is the therapy of choice of most dermatologists. Do not freeze excessively.
5. Laser therapy has been used recently by some authors.
6. Surgical excision is an unnecessary and more expensive form of removal.

Pedunculated Fibromas (Skin Tags, Acrochordons)

Multiple skin tags are common on the neck and the axillae of middle-aged, usually obese, men and women (Fig. 26-2). The indications for removal are two-fold: cosmetic, as desired and requested by the patient, and to prevent the irritation and the secondary infection of the pedicle that frequently develops from trauma of a collar, necklace, or other article of clothing. May be part of metabolic syndrome.

Presentation and Characteristics

Description

Pedunculated pinhead-sized to pea-sized soft tumors of normal skin color or darker are seen. The base may be inflamed from injury and the lesion may thrombose and turn black if twisted. This can cause alarm in the patient.

Distribution

The lesions occur on the neck, axillae, or groin, or less frequently on any area.

Course

These fibromas grow very slowly. They may increase in size during pregnancy. Some become infected or thrombosed and drop off.

Differential Diagnosis

- *Filiform wart:* Digitate projections, more horny; also seen on chin area (see Chap. 23)
- *Pedunculated seborrheic keratosis:* Larger lesion, darker color, warty or velvety appearance (see preceding section)
- *Neurofibromatosis:* Lesions seen elsewhere; larger; can be pushed back into skin; also café-au-lait spots; hereditary; single lesions do not indicate systemic disease (see Chaps. 33 and 35)

Treatment

Case Example. A 42-year-old woman has 20 small pedunculated fibromas on her neck and axillae that she wants removed. This could be done by electrosurgery. Without anesthesia, gently grab the small tumor in a thumb forceps and stretch the pedicle. Touch this pedicle with the electrosurgery needle and turn on the current for a split second. The tumor separates from the skin, and no bleeding occurs. The site heals in 4 to 7 days.

TABLE 26-5 ■ Differential Diagnosis of Keratoses

Parameter	Actinic or Senile Keratosis	Seborrheic Keratosis
Appearance	Flat, brownish, reddish, or tan scale firmly attached to skin, poorly demarcated	Greasy, elevated, Brown, black, flesh-colored, warty scale and can be easily scratched away at times, "stuck on," well demarcated
Location	Sun-exposed areas	Face, back
Complexion	Blue eyes, light hair, dry skin	Brown eyes, dark hair, oily skin
Symptoms	Some burning and stinging	Occasional itching
Precancerous	Yes	No
Cause	Sun	Inherited

For very small lesions, a short spark with the electrosurgical needle suffices. Scissor excision with or without local anesthetic is commonly done.

Cysts

The three common types are

- epidermal cyst;
- trichilemmal (pilar), or sebaceous cyst; and
- milium.

An *epidermal cyst* (Fig. 26-3A,B) has a wall composed of true epidermis and probably originates from an invagination of the epidermis into the dermis and subsequent detachment from the epidermis, or it can originate spontaneously. The most common locations for epidermal cysts are the face, ears, neck, back, and scalp, where tumors of varying size can be found. A central pore may be seen over the surface.

Trichilemmal cysts, formerly known as *wens* and *pilar* or *sebaceous cysts* (Fig. 26-3C), are less common than epi-

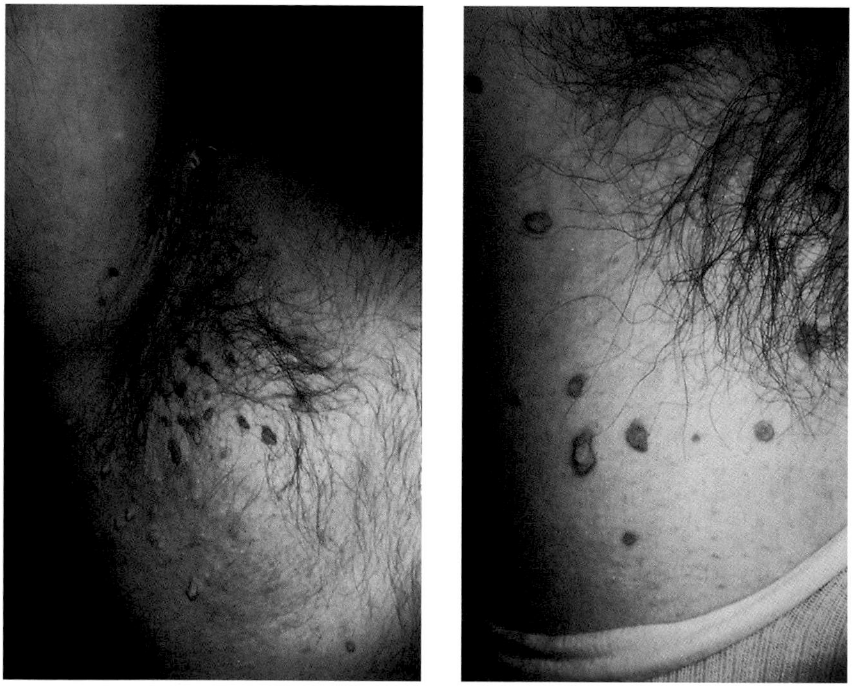

FIGURE 26-2 ■ (A, B) Pedunculated fibromas in axilla. *(Courtesy of Stiefel Laboratories, Inc.)*

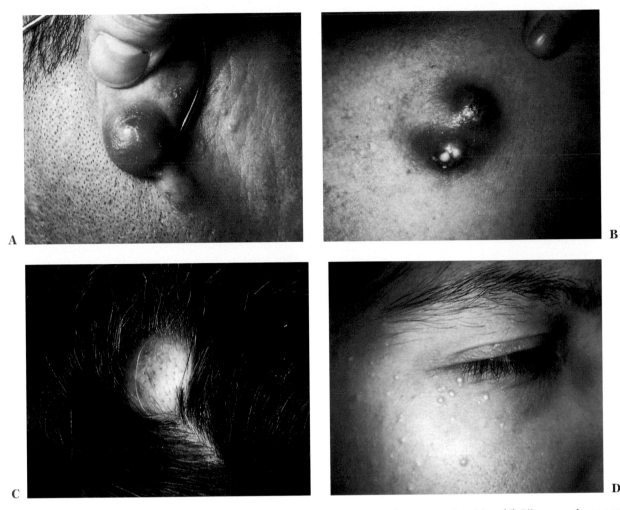

FIGURE 26-3 ■ **(A)** Epidermal cyst of earlobe. **(B)** Infected epidermal cyst on shoulder. **(C)** Pilar or sebaceous cyst of scalp. **(D)** Milia on upper cheek of 21-year-old woman. *(Courtesy of Texas Pharmacal.)*

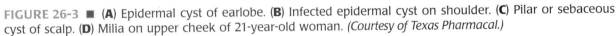

dermal cysts, occur mainly on the scalp, usually are multiple, and show an autosomal-dominant inheritance. The sac wall is thick, smooth, and whitish and can be quite easily enucleated.

Milia (Fig. 26-3D) are very common, white, pinhead-sized, firm lesions that are seen on the face. They are formed by proliferation of epithelial buds following trauma to the skin (dermabrasion for acne scars), following certain dermatoses (pemphigus, epidermolysis bullosa, and acute contact dermatitis), or from no apparent cause. Occurrence with porphyria cutanea tarda, after 5-fluorouracil therapy, in areas of corticosteroid induced atrophy, after burns and after radiation therapy, are other causes.

They can occur spontaneously at any age including newborns. Treatment consists of opening with a No. 11 Bard Parker blade and expression with a comedone extractor. This is done for cosmetic reasons only.

Differential Diagnosis of Epidermal and Trichilemmal Cysts

- *Lipoma:* Difficult to differentiate clinically; more firm, no central pore, lobulated; no cheesy material extrudes on incision; removal is by complete excision or by liposuction; clinically similar to hibernoma

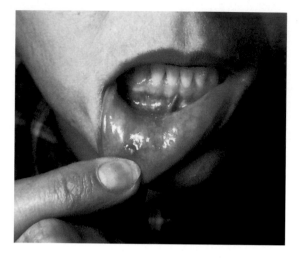

FIGURE 26-4 ■ Mucous cyst on lower lip. *(Courtesy of Texas Pharmacal.)*

- *Dermoid cyst:* Clinically similar; can also be found internally; usually a solitary skin tumor; histologically, contains hairs, eccrine glands, and sebaceous glands
- *Mucous cysts* (Fig. 26-4): Translucent pea-sized or smaller lesions on the lips, treated by cutting off top of the lesion and carefully lightly cauterizing the base with a silver nitrate stick or light electrosurgery; laser therapy can also be used
- *Synovial cysts (myxoid cysts) of the skin* (Fig. 26-5): Globoid, translucent, pea-sized swellings around the joints of fingers and toes that drain a syrupy clear liquid and is most common at base of nail on proximal nail fold

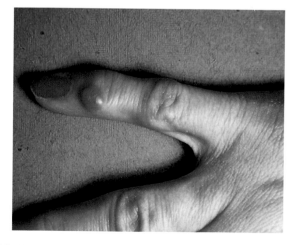

FIGURE 26-5 ■ Synovial cyst on finger. *(Courtesy of Texas Pharmacal.)*

Treatment of Epidermal and Trichilemmal Cysts

Several methods can be used with success. The choice depends on the ability of the operator and the site and the number of cysts. Cysts can regrow after even the best surgical care, because of incomplete removal of the sac.

1. A single 3-cm cyst on the back should be removed by surgical excision and suturing. This can be done in two ways: either by incising the skin and skillfully removing the intact cyst sac or by cutting straight into the sac with a small incision, shelling out the evacuated lining by applying strong pressure to the sides of the incision, and suturing the skin. The latter procedure is simpler, requires a smaller incision, and is quite successful.
2. A patient with several cysts in the scalp can be treated in another simple way. A 3- to 4-mm incision can be made directly over and into the cyst. The cheesy, foul-smelling contents can be evacuated by pressure and the use of a small curette. The sac can then be popped out of the hole with very firm pressure, or the sac can be grasped with a small hemostat and pulled out of the opening. No suturing or only a single suture is necessary. The resulting scar is imperceptible after a short time.
3. If, during incision by any technique, a solid tumor is found instead of a cyst, the lesion should be excised completely and the material studied histologically. This diagnostic error is common because of the clinical similarity of cysts, lipomas, and other related tumors.

Treatment of Milia

1. Simple incision of the small tumors with a scalpel or a Hagedorn needle and expression of the contents by a comedone extractor is sufficient.
2. Another procedure is to remove the top of the milia lightly with electrodesiccation.
3. An 11 Bard Parker blade can be used to open the top and then an acne stylette used to express the contents.

Precancerous Tumors

Precancerous types of tumors include actinic keratosis and cutaneous horn, arsenical keratosis, and leukoplakia.

Actinic Keratosis

Actinic keratosis is a common skin lesion of light-complexioned older persons that occurs on the skin surfaces exposed to sunlight (Fig. 26-6). A small percentage of these lesions develop into squamous cell carcinomas (approximately 5-10%). Because of the popularity of sunbathing, these

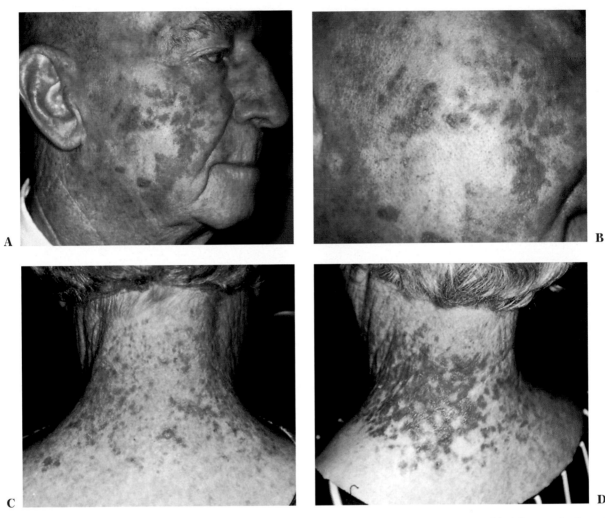

FIGURE 26-6 ■ Actinic keratoses. **(A)** Multiple actinic keratoses on face of 80-year-old, fair-complexioned farmer. **(B)** Close-up. Actinic keratoses of back of neck showing lesions before **(C)** and normal accentuation after **(D)** therapy with 5-fluorouracil for 2 weeks. *(Courtesy of Dermik Laboratories, Inc., and Owen Laboratories, Inc.)*

lesions (probably 5–10%) are seen also in persons in the 30- to 50-year-old age group.

SAUER'S NOTES

1. Patients with actinic keratoses should be advised to return every 6 to 12 months for examination; this is especially important if they have extensive actinic damage.
2. All patients with actinic keratoses should be told to use a sunscreen lotion or cream to lessen the occurrence of future keratoses. Wear protective clothing and avoid sun exposure between 10.00 am and 4:00 pm.

Description

Lesions are usually multiple, flat or slightly elevated, pink, brownish or tan colored, scaly and adherent, measuring up to 1.5 cm in diameter, and often arising on an ill-defined base (Fig. 26-7). There is a dark variant called a superficial pigmented actinic keratosis (SPAK). Individual lesions may become confluent. A *cutaneous horn* may be a proliferative, hyperkeratotic form of actinic keratosis that resembles a horn (Fig. 26-8). A cutaneous horn can also originate from a seborrheic keratosis, wart, squamous cell carcinoma, basal cell carcinoma, keratoacanthoma, and most commonly an actinic keratosis. If a biopsy is done, enough of the base of the lesion must be removed to obtain an accurate histologic diagnosis.

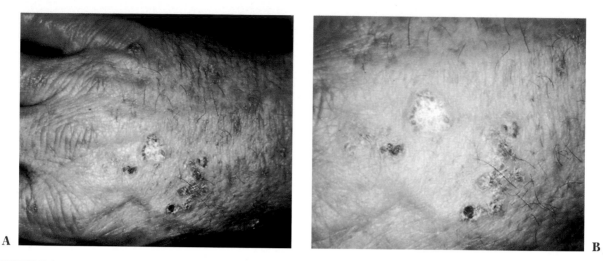

FIGURE 26-7 ■ Actinic keratoses. (**A**) Lesions on dorsum of hands. (**B**) Close-up in 44-year-old, blue-eyed outdoor worker. *(Courtesy of Dermik Laboratories, Inc., and Owen Laboratories, Inc.)*

Distribution

Areas of skin exposed to sunlight, such as face, ears, neck, and dorsum of hands, are involved.

Course

The lesion begins as a faint red, slightly scaly patch that enlarges slowly, peripherally and deeply, over many years. A sudden spurt of growth, increased thickness, or surrounding induration could indicate a change to a squamous cell carcinoma.

Subjective Symptoms

Patients often complain that these lesions are sensitive or they burn and sting.

Cause

Heredity and sun exposure are the two main causative factors. The blue-eyed, thin-skinned, light-haired person with a family history of such lesions is the best subject for multiple actinic keratoses.

Sex Incidence

The disorder is most commonly seen in men.

Differential Diagnosis

■ *Seborrheic keratosis:* see Table 26-5
■ *Squamous cell carcinoma:* Any thickened lesion that has grown rapidly should undergo biopsy (see later in this chapter)

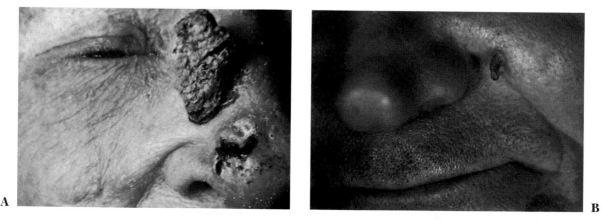

FIGURE 26-8 ■ (**A**) Cutaneous horn with basal cell carcinomatous degeneration of the base. *(Courtesy of Texas Pharmacal).* (**B**) Cutaneous horn, on cheek. *(Courtesy of Syntex Laboratories, Inc.)*

- *Arsenical keratosis:* Mainly on palms and soles; history of arsenic ingestion
- *Porokeratosis:* Mainly on legs in women; thread-like keratotic border (cororail lamellae) that sharply demarcates tumor from surrounding skin.

Treatment

Case Example. A 60-year-old farmer has three small actinic keratoses on his face. The lesions should be examined carefully. If there is any evidence of induration or marked inflammation, the lesion should undergo biopsy (see Chap. 2). There are two methods of removal of these keratoses. For a single lesion, or only three or four lesions, a one-visit surgical treatment is usually preferable, especially if the lesion is relatively thick.

Surgical Method. Liquid nitrogen, if available, applied very lightly to the lesion is an effective and rapid method of removal. This is the therapy of choice of dermatologists.

Curettement, followed by destruction of the base by acid or electrosurgery, is satisfactory. Local anesthesia is usually necessary. Firmly scrape the lesion with the dermal curette, which removes the mushy, scaly keratosis and exposes the more fibrous normal skin. Experience provides the necessary "feel" of abnormal versus normal tissue. Some of the bleeding can be controlled by pressure or use of either one of the two following procedures:

1. application with a cotton-tipped applicator of a saturated solution of trichloroacetic acid, aluminum chloride solution, or Monsel solution cautiously to the bleeding site; or
2. electrocoagulation of the bleeding base.

Small lesions heal in 7 to 14 days. No bandage is required. Laser is also an acceptable form of therapy used by some dermatologists.

Fluorouracil Method. For the patient with multiple superficial actinic keratoses, fluorouracil therapy is effective and eliminates for some months or years the early damaged epidermal cells. Thus, this fluorouracil therapy is really a cancer-prevention routine.

Several preparations and strengths of solutions and creams are available, but the two most commonly indicated are as follows:

1. Fluoroplex 1% solution, or cream 30.0
2. Efudex 2% solution or Efudex 5% cream 10.0

    Sig: Apply with fingers to area to be treated twice a day.
    Comment: It is wise to treat only a small area on the face at a time. Give instructions carefully and warn the patient that it is natural for the skin to get quite red and irritated and sore after 4 to 5 days. Most commonly the course of therapy is for 2 weeks. Some patients must stop therapy sooner, and some need more time to get the desired effect.

After completion of the course of therapy, the skin usually heals rapidly. A corticosteroid cream may be prescribed to hasten healing.

Another form of administration of fluorouracil is the pulse method. Here the medication is applied twice a day for only 2 to 4 consecutive days of each week, for a total duration of 3 or 4 months of therapy.

This therapy may have to be repeated in several months or years. If some keratoses are too thick to be removed by this fluorouracil method, then the liquid nitrogen or surgical method, as described, is indicated for these lesions.

Imiquimod (Aldara) can be used twice a day for 2 weeks or as a pulse therapy three times a week for 3 months. Unlike fluorouracil therapy, it does not cause a more severe reaction in the sun but topical steroids should not be used to lessen the reaction because they may decrease the benefit.

Treatment of a Cutaneous Horn

The same surgical technique as for actinic keratosis is used. To rule out cancer, most cutaneous horns should be sent with intact base for histopathologic examination. The incidence of squamous cell carcinomatous change in the base of a cutaneous horn is appreciable.

Arsenical Keratosis

Prolonged ingestion of inorganic arsenic (*e.g.*, Fowler's solution, Asiatic pills, well water that is high in arsenic) can result in the formation many years later of small, punctate keratotic lesions, mainly seen on the palms and the soles. Progression to a squamous cell carcinoma can occur but is unusual. These patients have an increased risk of underlying solid tumor malignancies.

Treatment

Small arsenical keratoses can be removed by electrosurgery; larger lesions can be excised and skin grafted if necessary.

Leukoplakia

Leukoplakia is an actinic keratosis of the mucous membrane (Fig. 26-9).

Description

A flat, whitish plaque occurs localized to the mucous membranes of lips, mouth, vulva, and vagina. Single or multiple lesions may be present.

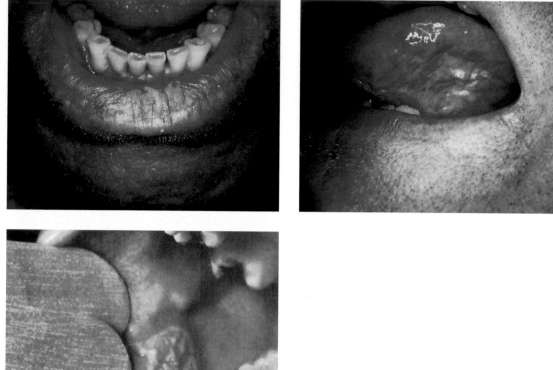

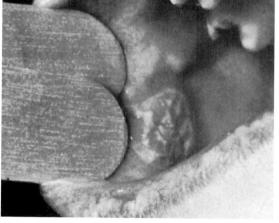

FIGURE 26-9 ■ **(A)** Leukoplakia on lower lip, mild. **(B)** Leukoplakia on tongue, from chronic biting. *(Courtesy of Westwood Pharmaceuticals.)* **(C)** Biopsy-proven leukoplakia on the mucous membrane of the cheek. This was erroneously diagnosed, clinically, as lichen planus.

Course

Progression to squamous cell carcinoma occurs in 20% to 30% of chronic cases. Squamous cell cancer of the mucous membrane is more aggressive with 40% to 50% metastasis versus only 4% to 5% on the skin.

Cause

Smoking, sunlight, ethanol ingestion, chewing tobacco, snuff, and chronic irritation are the important factors in the development of leukoplakia. Recurrent actinic cheilitis may precede leukoplakia of the lips. The vulvar form may develop from presenile or senile atrophy of this area.

Differential Diagnosis

■ *Lichen planus:* A lacy network of whitish lesions, mainly on the sides of the buccal cavity; when on lips, it may clinically resemble leukoplakia; lichen planus elsewhere on body (see Chap. 15); biopsy is often indicated; ulcerative lichen planus in the oral mucous membranes may have an increased risk of squamous cell carcinoma

■ *Pressure calluses* from teeth or dentures: Evidence of irritation; differentiation may be possible only by biopsy

■ On the vulva, *lichen sclerosus et atrophicus* or *kraurosis vulvae:* No induration, as in leukoplakia of this area; can extend onto skin of inguinal folds and perianal region; pruritus may or may not be present and can be severe with dyspareunia; biopsy is helpful; up to 5% of lichen sclerosis et atrophicus may develop a squamous cell cancer

Treatment

Case Example. Small patch of leukoplakia is seen on lower lip of man who smokes considerably.

1. The lesion should be examined carefully. Perform a biopsy on any questionable area that shows inflammation and induration. If a squamous cell carcinoma is present, the patient should receive surgical or radiation therapy by a physician who is an expert in this form of treatment.
2. Advise against use of tobacco products. The seriousness of continued smoking or other use of tobacco must be pointed out to the patient. Many early cases of leukoplakia disappear when smoking is stopped.
3. Eliminate any chronic irritation from teeth or dentures.
4. Protect the lips from sunlight with a sunscreen stick.
5. Electrosurgery, preceded by local anesthesia, is excellent for small, persistent areas of leukoplakia. The coagulating current is effective. Healing is usually rapid. Laser therapy or a surgical lip shave are used by some dermatologists.
6. Liquid nitrogen freezing is also effective.
7. If alcohol abuse is present, cessation is advisable.
8. Topical 5FU or aldara can be used.

Epitheliomas and Carcinomas

Basal Cell Carcinoma

Basal cell carcinoma is the most common malignancy of the skin (Fig. 26-10, and see Figs. 26-8 and 3-1C). Fortunately, a basal cell epithelioma or carcinoma is almost never a metastasizing tumor, and the cure rate can be close to 100% if these lesions are treated early and adequately.

Description

There are four clinical types of basal cell carcinoma:

1. noduloulcerative,
2. pigmented,
3. fibrosing (sclerosing, morphea-like), and
4. superficial.

Noduloulcerative basal cell carcinoma is the most common type. It begins as a small waxy nodule that enlarges slowly over the years. A central depression usually forms that eventually progresses into an ulcer surrounded by a pearly or waxy border. The surface of the nodular component has a few telangiectatic vessels, which are highly characteristic. Upon stretching the skin, a gray translucent appearance may aid in diagnosis.

SAUER'S NOTES

Whenever the clinical appearance of a skin tumor suggests a basal cell carcinoma, the lesion should be studied histologically.

The *pigmented type* is similar to the noduloulcerative form, with the addition of brown or black pigmentation. The pigmentent may be in small (1-2m) dots over the tumor surface.

The *fibrosing type* is extremely slow growing, is usually seen on the face, and consists of a whitish, scarred plaque with an ill-defined border, which rarely becomes ulcerated. This type is difficult to treat since borders are difficult to determine.

The *superficial form* may be single or multiple, is usually seen on the back and the chest, and is characterized by slowly enlarging red, scaly areas that, on careful examination, reveal a nodular border with telangiectatic vessels. A healed atrophic center may be present. Ulceration is superficial when it develops.

Distribution

Over 90% of the basal cell carcinomas occur on the head and the neck, with the trunk next in frequency. On the trunk and extremities the tumors may appear pink and flat without ulcerations. These tumors are rarely found on the palms or the soles.

Course

The tumor is very slow growing, but sudden rapid growth periods do occur. Bleeding is common. Destructive forms of this tumor can invade cartilage, bone, blood vessels, or large areas of skin surface and result in death. There are rare reports of metastasizing basal cell carcinomas; these are usually very large tumors.

Cause

Basal cell carcinomas develop most frequently on the areas of the skin exposed to sunlight and in blond or red-haired persons. Trauma and overexposure to radium and x-radiation can cause basal cell carcinomas. Long-term ingestion of inorganic arsenic can lead to formation of superficial basal cell carcinomas. It can be part of the basal cell nevus syndrome. Most authors believe that a basal cell tumor is a carcinoma of the basal cells of the epidermis. Lever and Schaumberg-Lever (see Suggested Reading) and others believe it not to be a carcinoma but a nevoid tumor (epithelioma) derived from incompletely differentiated embryonal cells.

Age Group

This tumor can occur from childhood to old age but is seen most frequently in men older than age 50 years.

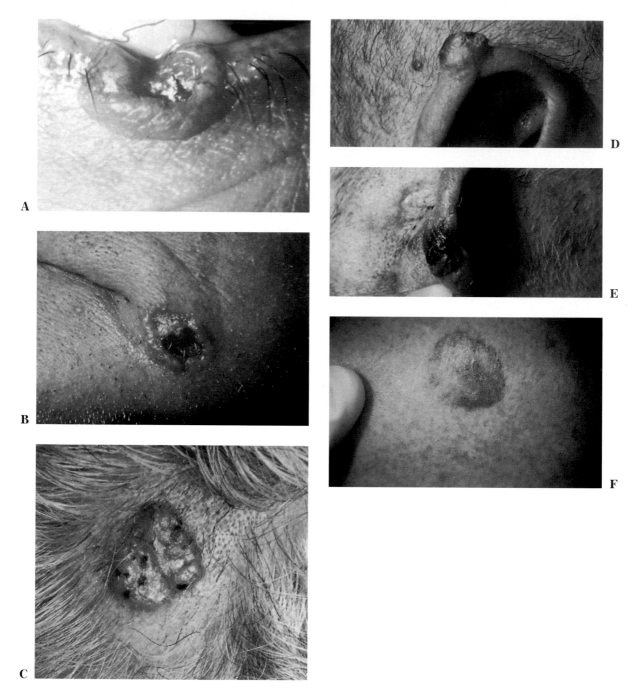

FIGURE 26-10 ■ Basal cell carcinomas. (**A**) Of the lower eyelid. Note telangiectasia on the rolled edge of the ulcer. *(Courtesy of Drs L. Calkins and A. Lemoine.)* (**B**) Ulcerated lesion on chin. *(Courtesy of K.U.M.C.)* (**C**) Basal cell carcinomatous change in a syringocystadenoma papilliferum nevus on the scalp. (**D**) On helix of the ear. (**E**) Hemorrhagic lesion on helix of ear. (**F**) Superficial basal cell carcinoma on the back. *(Courtesy of Texas Pharmacal.)*

Differential Diagnosis

- *Squamous cell carcinoma:* More rapid growth, firm, scaly papule or nodule, more inflammation, no pearly telangiectatic border; biopsy is necessary
- *Sebaceous hyperplasias:* Very common, with a central dell and fine telangiectasia, but on stretching the skin appears slightly yellow or orange and sebaceous gland lobules may be seen
- *Keratoacanthomas*
- *Sebaceous adenomas*
- *Large comedones*
- *Warts*
- *Nevi*
- *Small cysts*
- *Scarring from injury or radiation*

Superficial basal cell carcinomas can resemble lesions of psoriasis, seborrheic dermatitis, lupus vulgaris, and Bowen's disease.

If multiple basal cell carcinomas are found, one should consider the basal cell nevus syndrome. This is a rare, hereditary condition characterized by multiple genetically determined basal cell carcinomas, cysts of the jaws, peculiar pits of the hands and feet, and developmental anomalies of the ribs, spine, and skull.

Treatment

Case Example. A 48-year-old woman has an 8- × 8-mm basal cell carcinoma on her forehead.

1. Inform the patient that she has a cancer of the skin that needs to be removed. Tell the patient that this tumor usually does not spread into the body, but if it is not treated it can spread on the skin. State that removal of the lesion is almost 100% effective but periodic examinations are necessary to check for any regrowth. If this tumor recurs, it will regrow only at its previous site. Tell the patient that a scar will result from the treatment.
2. If the diagnosis of the lesion is not definite clinically, a biopsy (see Chap. 7) can be done safely. Further treatment depends on the laboratory report.
3. Surgical excision of a basal cell carcinoma is the only method of treatment that should not be attempted by the physician who only occasionally is confronted with these tumors. (Some criticism will arise from this statement, but it is our belief that a great amount of experience is necessary to remove these tumors adequately by curettement, chemocautery, electrosurgery, cryosurgery, radiation, laser, or any combination of these methods. If the operator believes that he or she is qualified in these procedures, then this statement is not meant for him or

her.) To excise the lesion, the area is anesthetized, an elliptical incision is made with a scalpel to include a border of 3 to 4 mm around the tumor, one side of the excised skin is tagged with a piece of suture, the incision is closed, and the specimen is submitted for careful histologic examination (see Chap. 7). If the pathologist states that the tumor extends up to the edge of the excision, a further, more radical excision should be performed.
4. The patient should return for a checkup on a definite schedule, such as in 4 months, then every 6 months for four visits, then yearly, for a total of 5 years. Ten-year follow-up is being suggested by some authors.
5. Topical imiquimod (5% cream) is an available option for superficial lesions. Typical courses of therapy would be a thin coat b.i.d. Mondays, Wednesdays, and Fridays for 3 months. Because of inflammation, rest periods of a week or two may have to be initiated and repeat therapy may be necessary. This is a popular treatment in superficial lesions where scarring is to be avoided.

Treatment of recurrent, deeply ulcerated, fibrosing, or large superficial basal cell carcinomas should be in the domain of the competent dermatologist, surgeon, or radiologist. Mohs'-type surgery for these more difficult lesions is microscopically controlled and, unless the tumor is massive, results in a very high cure rate.

Squamous Cell Carcinoma

This rather common skin malignancy can arise primarily or from an actinic keratosis or leukoplakia. The grade of malignancy and metastasizing ability varies histoligically from grade I (low, well differentiated) to grade IV (high, poor differentiated).

Description

The most common clinical picture is a rapidly growing nodule that soon develops a central ulcer and an indurated raised border with some surrounding redness (Fig. 26-11). This type of lesion is the most malignant. The least malignant form has the clinical appearance of a warty, piled-up growth, which may not ulcerate. However, it is important to realize that the grade of malignancy can vary in the same tumor from one section to another, particularly in the larger lesions. This variation demonstrates the value of multiple histologic sections.

> ### SAUER'S NOTES
>
> Whenever the clinical appearance of a skin tumor suggests a squamous cell carcinoma, the lesion should be studied histologically.

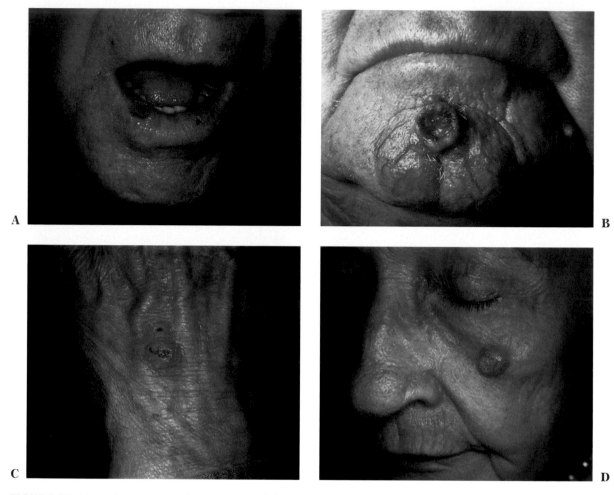

FIGURE 26-11 ■ Squamous cell carcinomas. (**A**) Squamous cell carcinoma of lower lip. (**B**) Squamous cell carcinoma of chin. (**C**) Squamous cell carcinoma on dorsum of hand. (**D**) Squamous cell carcinoma on cheek. *(Courtesy of Westwood Pharmaceuticals.)*

Distribution

The lesion can occur on any area of the skin and mucous membrane but most commonly on the face, particularly the lower lip and ears, tongue, and dorsa of the hands. Chronic trauma associated with certain occupations can lead to formation of this cancer on unusual sites. Any chronic ulcer can develop a squamous cell carcinoma.

Course

The course varies with the grade of malignancy of the tumor. Lymph node metastases (4% to 5% incidence) may occur early in the development of the tumor or may never occur. The cure rate can be very high when the lesions are treated early and with the best indicated modality.

Cause

As in basal cell carcinomas, many factors contribute to provide the soil for growth of a squamous cell carcinoma. A simple listing of factors is sufficient:

- hereditarily determined type of skin;
- age of patient (elderly);
- trauma from chemicals (tars, oils), heat, wind, sunlight, x-radiation, psoralen plus long wave ultraviolet light (PUVA) therapy, and severe burns;
- skin diseases that form scars, such as discoid lupus erythematosus, lupus vulgaris, burns (Majocchi granuloma) and chronic ulcers;
- ingestion of inorganic arsenic; and
- in the natural course of xeroderma pigmentosum.

Immunosuppressed patients, such as organ transplant patients and patients with the acquired immunodeficiency syndrome, have an increased incidence of basal cell and squamous cell carcinoma.

Age and Sex Incidence

Most tumors are seen in elderly men, but exceptions are not rare.

Differential Diagnosis

- *Basal cell carcinoma:* Slower growth, pearly border with telangiectasis, less inflammation; biopsy may be necessary to differentiate (see preceding section)
- *Actinic keratosis:* Slow-growing, flat, pink, constantly peeling, scaly lesions; no induration; little surrounding erythema (see preceding section)
- *Pseudoepitheliomatous hyperplasia:* Primary chronic lesion, such as old stasis ulcer, bromoderma, deep mycotic infection, syphilitic gumma, lupus vulgaris, basal cell carcinoma, and pyoderma gangrenosum; differentiation is often impossible clinically and very difficult histologically
- *Keratoacanthoma* (Fig. 26-12): Very fast-growing single or, more rarely, multiple lesions; clinically, this is a firm, raised, symmetric nodule with a central crater; it should be studied histologically; it may disappear spontaneously. On the other hand, a few keratoacanthomas can be highly destructive locally. Histologically, a keratoacanthoma can be

difficult to distinguish from a squamous cell carcinoma. Rapid growth over days to weeks is the most distinguishing clinical characteristic.

Treatment

Because of the rapid locally invasive nature of squamous cell carcinomas, intensive surgical or radiation therapy, or both, is indicated. A discussion of such procedures is beyond the scope of this text (see Chap. 7 for an overview).

Histiocytoma and Dermatofibroma

Histiocytomas and dermatofibromas are common, usually single, flat or only slightly elevated, tannish, reddish, or brownish nodules, less than 1 cm in size, that occur mainly on the extremities (Fig. 26-13). These tumors have a characteristic clinical appearance and firm button-like feel that establishes the diagnosis. They often dimple when firm pressure is applied from both sides. They occur in adults and are nonsymptomatic and unchanging.

The histologic picture varies with the age of the lesion. The younger lesions are called *histiocytomas,* the older ones *dermatofibromas.* If the nodule contains many blood vessels, it is histologically labeled a *sclerosing hemangioma.*

Differential Diagnosis

- *Fibrosarcoma:* Active growth with invasion of subcutaneous fat; any questionable lesions should be excised and examined histologically

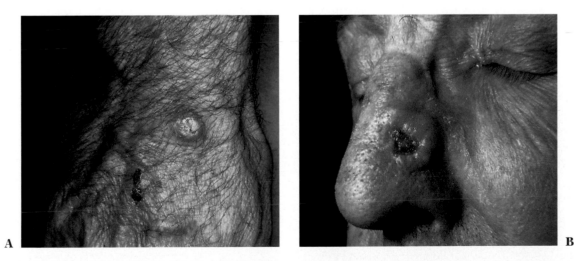

FIGURE 26-12 ■ Keratoacanthomas. **(A)** Keratoacanthoma on dorsum of hand. **(B)** Keratoacanthoma, on nose that healed without therapy, except for biopsy. *(Courtesy of Syntex Laboratories.)*

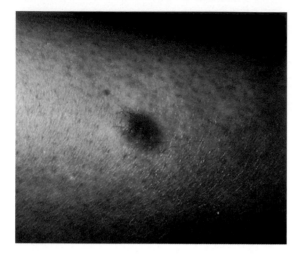

FIGURE 26-13 ■ Histiocytoma, on leg. *(Courtesy of Syntex Laboratories, Inc.)*

Treatment

No treatment is indicated. If there is any doubt as to the diagnosis, surgical excision and histologic examination are indicated.

For the female patient who shaves her legs and hits this lesion, liquid nitrogen applied to the papule flattens it.

Keloid

A keloid is a tumor resulting from an abnormal overgrowth of fibrous tissue following injury in certain predisposed persons (Fig. 26-14). Unusual configurations can occur, depending on the site, extent, and variety of the trauma. This tendency occurs so commonly in African Americans that one should think twice before attempting a cosmetic procedure on a dark-skinned person or on any other person with a history of keloids. The

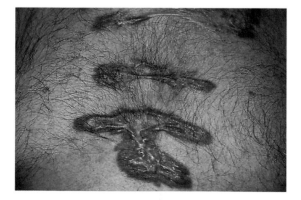

FIGURE 26-14 ■ Keloids on chest (common).

> ### SAUER'S NOTES
>
> Before any surgical procedure, the patient should be warned that a hypertrophic scar or keloid could follow the procedure. This is especially frequent following surgery on the chest or upper back.

back and the upper chest areas are especially prone to this proliferation.

Differential Diagnosis

- *Hypertrophic scar:* Initially same clinically and histologically as a keloid; flattens spontaneously in most cases after 1 or several years and does not extend beyond the original site of trauma

Treatment

Therapy is unsatisfactory. Intralesional corticosteroids after cryospray or massaging with a corticosteroid ointment for 60 seconds daily after bath or shower can be tried. Occasionally, combined procedures using excision on laser and intralesional corticosteroid injections or interferon α-2b (Intron A) injections have been successful. Silicone sheeting therapy has its advocates. Excision should be done cautiously because recurrence of a larger tumor may occur. If removal is done, intralesional corticosteroids should be used to attempt to prevent a recurrence.

Hemangiomas

Hemangiomas are vascular abnormalities of the skin (Fig. 26-15). Heredity is not a factor in the development of these lesions. There are nine types of hemangiomas, which vary as to depth, clinical appearance, and location:

- Superficial hemangioma
- Cavernous hemangioma
- Mixed hemangioma (when both superficial and cavernous elements are present)
- Spider hemangioma
- Port wine hemangioma
- Nuchal hemangioma
- Capillary hemangioma
- Venous lake
- Angiokeratoma

Superficial and Cavernous Hemangiomas

This familiar, bright-red, raised "strawberry" tumor has been seen by all physicians (see Figs. 3-2E and 36-12).

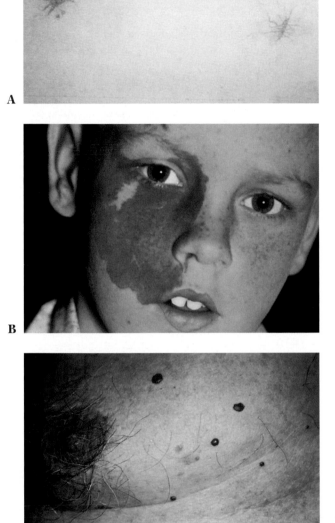

A

B

C

FIGURE 26-15 ■ (**A**) Two spider hemangiomas on the arm of a pregnant woman. (**B**) Port wine stain on the face of a boy. (**C**) Capillary (cherry, senile) angiomas on the chest near the nipple. *(Courtesy of Ortho Pharmaceutical Corp.)*

Strawberries have to grow, and they start from a small beginning. Parents are usually the first to notice the small, red, pinhead-sized, flat lesions. They are noticed at, or soon after, birth. These red tumors can occur on any area of the body and can begin as small lesions and stay that way, remaining as superficial hemangiomas, or they can enlarge and extend into the subcutaneous tissue, forming

a cavernous type. The enlargement can occur rapidly or slowly. Occasionally there can be multiple lesions.

Two aspects of the larger hemangiomas can be disturbing. First, the mere presence of the lesion or lesions causes concern to parents. If the lesion is on an exposed area of the body, this causes additional concern and comment by relatives, neighbors, and other well-meaning persons, which can be most disconcerting.

Second, if the lesion is large and near an eye, urogenital area, neck, rectum, nose, or mouth, it can, by its physical size, cause an obstructive problem. Systemic corticosteroids, arterial embolization, cryosurgery, laser surgery, compression, and interferon have been used successfully. Surgery may be indicated. However, even some massive hemangiomas in these areas can be left alone and resolve amazingly over a period of several months.

Treatment

The treatment of hemangiomas that are not of the obstructive type has been the subject of considerable discussion. To begin with, the size, depth, and location of the hemangiomas, and the pressure on the physician from parents and relatives, are factors that must be considered in every case.

There are those who favor treating almost every superficial or cavernous hemangioma, and there are others who believe that all hemangiomas should be left alone to involute spontaneously. The latter group stands behind the studies of our English colleagues, Bowers, Simpson, and others, who showed that around 85% of hemangiomas disappeared without any appreciable scar by the age of 7 years. They also found that the hemangiomas usually stopped growing by the age of 1 year. We advocate the treatment of some hemangiomas, and we leave others alone. Let us illustrate with two case histories.

Case Example 1. A 6-week-old child is brought in by her parents. She has a 4- × 4-mm slightly raised red lesion on her cheek. The parents first noticed it when she was 3 weeks of age, when it was of pinhead size.

1. Reassure the parents that this birthmark is not hereditary and that it will not turn into a cancer.
2. Inform them that this lesion should be treated because it probably will enlarge and could become a significant deformity. If one wishes, one can explain that the lesion, if left alone, might or might not enlarge, and if it does enlarge it will probably disappear without much of a mark in 5 to 7 years. However, treatment at this time is suggested to possibly abort any further growth.
3. A simple form of therapy is cryosurgery with liquid nitrogen.

Case Example 2. An 8-month-old girl is brought in by her parents. They state that she has a birthmark on her cheek that began at the age of 3 weeks. Their physician was consulted and stated that the lesion should be watched, because "a lot of them just go away."

At the age of 3 months, the lesion had grown further, but the physician still advised them to wait and watch.

Now at the age of 8 months the red hemangioma measures 12 × 12 × 5 mm and has a bluish mass at the base. It is a mixed hemangioma.

1. Reassure the parents that the lesion is not hereditary and that it will not turn into a cancer.
2. Because the child is now 8 months of age, and the lesion has in all probability reached its maximum growth, no treatment is indicated. The parents must be told in no uncertain terms why no treatment is necessary. They are told that you believe it will not enlarge further and that you know from your experience, and that of others, that it will probably be gone by the age of 2 or 3 years and almost certainly by the age of 5 to 7. You can almost predict that the residual mark will be insignificant. However, if it does not disappear completely by that age, the remaining, usually insignificant lesion can be excised.

To summarize, the advantages of early treatment of small superficial or cavernous hemangiomas are as follows: (1) The lesion is eliminated completely, or almost completely; (2) it is not left to chance the fact that it might or might not enlarge considerably; (3) apprehension on the part of the parents and relatives regarding the course of the lesion is alleviated; and (4) with properly applied cryotherapy no mark is left, or only a slight one that would be no worse than that resulting from leaving the hemangioma alone. Other treatments that may be beneficial are high-dose systemic or intralesional corticosteroids, surgery, interferon α-2b, embolization, lasers, and pentoxifylline.

The advantages of not treating one of these hemangiomas are as follows:

■ The residuum after 5 to 7 years may be better cosmetically than if the lesion had been treated.
■ The cost of therapy and trauma to the patient is saved.

Spider Hemangioma

A spider hemangioma consists of a small pinpoint- to pinhead-sized central red arteriole with radiating smaller vessels like the spokes of a wheel or the legs of a spider (see Fig. 26-15A). These lesions develop for no apparent reason or may develop in association with pregnancy or chronic liver disease. The most common location is on the face. The reason for removal is cosmetic.

Differential Diagnosis

■ *Venous stars:* Small, bluish, telangiectatic veins, usually seen on the legs and the face but may appear anywhere on the body; these can be removed, if desired, by the same method as for spider hemangioma
■ *Hereditary hemorrhagic telangiectasis* (Rendu-Osler-Weber disease) (see Fig. 30-3): Small, red lesions on any organ of the body that can hemorrhage and are numerous on lips and oral mucous membranes as well as far into the gastrointestinal tract; get family history

Treatment

Case Example. A spider hemangioma is present on the cheek of a young woman who is 6 months postpartum. This lesion developed during her pregnancy and has persisted unchanged.

Electrosurgery or laser are the treatments of choice. The fine epilating needle is used with either a very low coagulating sparking current or a low cutting current. The needle is stuck into the central vessel and the current turned on for 1 or 2 seconds until the vessel blanches. No anesthetic is necessary in most patients. The area forms a scab and heals in about 4 days, leaving an imperceptible scar. Rarely, a second treatment is necessary to eliminate the central vessel. If the radiating vessels are large and persistent, they can be treated in the same manner as the central vessel. For laser therapy, see Chapter 6.

Port Wine Hemangioma

The port wine hemangioma is commonly seen on the face as a reddish purple, flat, disfiguring facial mark (see Fig. 26-15B). It can occur elsewhere in a less extensive form. Faint reddish lesions are often found on infants on the sides of the face, forehead, eyelids, and extremities. The color increases with crying and alarms the mother, but most of these faint lesions disappear shortly after birth. When located above the palpebral tissue it can be associated with underlying hemangioma at the meninges occasionally in association with seizures (Sturge–Weber syndrome).

SAUER'S NOTES

It is advisable to tell the patient that it will be difficult to remove every vessel in a spider hemangioma. To attempt to do so might cause a scar.

Treatment

Case Example. An extensive port wine hemangioma is present on the left side of a man's face.

1. Laser beam (flash lamp–pulse dye laser) is an effective form of therapy.
2. Cosmetics, such as Dermablend or Covermark, or any good pancake type of makeup, are effective to a certain degree.

Nuchal Hemangioma

Nuchal hemangioma is a common, persistent, faint red patch on the posterior neck region, at or below the scalp margin. It does not disappear with aging, and treatment is not effective or necessary. Because the posterior neck area is also the site of the common lichen simplex chronicus, it is well to remember that following the cure of the lichen simplex a redness that persists could be a nuchal hemangioma that was present for years and not noticed previously.

Capillary Hemangioma

Capillary or cherry hemangiomas are also called *senile hemangiomas*, but this term obviously should not be used in discussing the lesion with the patient who is in the 30- to 60-year-old age group (see Fig. 26-15C). These pinhead-sized or slightly larger, bright red, flat or raised tumors are present in many young adults and in practically all elderly persons. They cause no disability except when they are injured and bleed. They tend to be inherited.

Treatment is usually not desired, but if it is, light electrosurgery or laser is effective.

Venous Lake (Varix)

Another vascular lesion that occurs in older persons is a *venous lake.* Clinically, it is a soft, compressible, flat or slightly elevated, bluish-red, 3- to 6-mm lesion, usually located on the lips or the ears. Lack of induration and rapid growth distinguish it from a melanoma. Lack of pulsation distinguishes a venous lake on the lower lip from a tortuous segment of the inferior labial artery.

Treatment is usually not desired, only reassurance concerning its nonmalignant nature.

Angiokeratomas

Three forms of angiokeratoma are known:

- *Mibelli's form* occurs on the dorsa of the fingers, the toes, and the knees;
- *Fabry's form* occurs over the entire trunk in an extensive pattern; and
- the *Fordyce form* occurs on the scrotum.

The lesions are dark-red, pinhead-sized papules with a somewhat warty appearance. Treatment is not indicated for Mibelli form and the Fordyce form. The Fabry form (angiokeratoma corporis diffusum), however, is the cutaneous manifestation of a systemic phospholipid storage disease in which phospholipids are deposited in the skin, as well as in various internal organs. Death usually occurs in the fifth decade from the result of such deposits in the smooth muscles of the blood vessels, in the heart, and in the kidneys (see Chap. 33).

Nevus Cell Tumors

Nevus cell tumors can be classified as melanocytic nevi or as malignant melanoma. Nevi, in turn are classified as

- Junctional or active nevus
- Intradermal or resting nevus
- Dysplastic nevus syndrome

Nevi are discussed here, but malignant melanoma is discussed separately, in Chapter 27.

Melanocytic Nevi

Nevi are pigmented or nonpigmented tumors of the skin that contain nevus cells (Fig. 26-16). Nevi are present on every adult, but some persons have more than others. There are two main questions concerning nevi or moles: When and how should they be removed? What is the relationship between nevi and malignant melanomas?

Histologically, it is possible to divide benign nevi into *junctional* or *active nevi* and *intradermal* or *resting nevi.* Combinations of these two forms commonly exist and are labeled *compound nevi.*

In the dysplastic nevus syndrome (familial atypical mole–melanoma syndrome), the nevi are more numerous and larger than ordinary (usually 5 to 15 mm in size), have an irregular border, and show a haphazard mixture of tan, brown, pink, and black. There is a propensity for this type of nevus, especially when familial, to develop into malignant melanomas.

Clinically, one never can be positive with which histopathologic type of nevus one is dealing, but certain criteria are helpful in establishing a differentiation between the forms.

Description

Clinically, nevi can be pigmented or nonpigmented, flat or elevated, hairy or nonhairy, warty, papillomatous, or

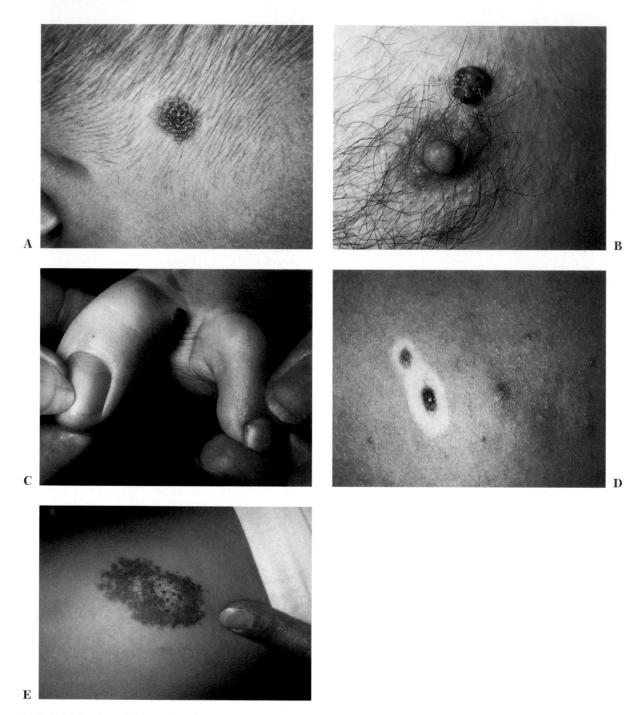

FIGURE 26-16 ■ (**A**) Junctional nevus in scalp of 12-year-old child. (**B**) Compound nevus, on chest above nipple. (**C**) Junctional nevus on web of toe of 8-year-old child. (**D**) Halo nevus, or leukoderma acquisitum centrifugum, on the back. (**E**) Giant pigmented nevus on thigh. *(Courtesy of The Upjohn Company.)*

pedunculated. They can have a small or a wide base. The brown- or black-pigmented, flat or slightly elevated, non-hairy nevi are usually junctional nevi. The nonpigmented or pigmented, elevated, hairy nevi are more likely to be the intradermal nevi.

A nevus with a depigmented area surrounding it is called a *halo nevus, Sutton's nevus* or *leukoderma acquisitum centrifugum* (Fig. 26-17). The nevus in the center of the halo that histologically has an inflammatory infiltrate around it usually involutes in several months in contradistinction to the rarer noninflammatory halo nevus which may not involute. Excision of the halo nevus is usually not indicated unless the central nevus has the appearance of melanoma.

Distribution

Nevi are very prevalent on the head and the neck but may be on any part of the body. The nevi on the palms, the soles, and the genitalia are usually junctional nevi.

Course

A child is born with no, or relatively few, nevi, but with increasing age, particularly after puberty, nevi slowly become larger, can remain flat or become elevated, and may become hairy and darker. A change is also seen histologically with age. A junctional-type active nevus, although it may remain as such throughout the life of the person, more commonly changes slowly into an intradermal or resting nevus. Some nevi do not become evident until adult or later life, but the precursor cells for the nevus were present at birth. A malignant melanoma can originate from a junctional nevus, compound nevus, very rarely an intradermal nevus, and from dysplastic nevi, particularly

in relationship to ultraviolet exposure. Most melanomas arise *de novo*. A benign junctional nevus in a child can histologically look like a malignant melanoma. Known as a *Spitz nevus*, this poses a difficult diagnostic and management problem. It is usually a dome-shaped reddish-brown tumor and rarely can occur in adults.

Histogenesis

The origin of the nevus cell is disputed, but the most commonly accepted theory is that it originates from melanocytes.

Differential Diagnosis

In Childhood

- *Warts:* Flat or common warts not on the hands or the feet may be difficult to differentiate clinically; should see warty growth with black "seeds" (the capillary loops), rather acute onset, and rapid growth (see Chap. 23)
- *Freckles:* On exposed areas of the body; many lesions; fade in winter; not raised
- *Blue nevus:* Flat or elevated, soft, dark bluish, steel-gray or black nodule
- *Granuloma pyogenicum:* Rapid onset of reddish or blackish vascular tumor, usually at site of injury and often with history of bleeding
- *Molluscum contagiosum:* One, or usually more, crater-shaped, waxy tumors (see Chap. 23)
- *Urticaria pigmentosa:* Single, or multiple slightly elevated, yellowish to brown papules that urticate with trauma (Darier's sign)(see Chap. 33)

In Adulthood

- *Warts:* Usually rather obvious; black "seeds" (see Chap. 23)
- *Pedunculated fibromas:* On neck and axillae (see earlier in this chapter)
- *Histiocytoma* (see Fig. 26-13): On extremities; flat, button-like in consistency (see earlier in this chapter) that indents upon squeezing

Other epidermal and mesodermal tumors are differentiated histologically.

In Older Adults

- *Actinic or senile keratosis:* On exposed areas; scaly surrounding skin usually thin and dry; not a sharply demarcated lesion (see earlier in this chapter)
- *Seborrheic keratosis:* Greasy, waxy, warty tumor, "stuck on" the skin; however, some are difficult to

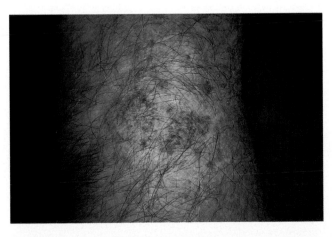

FIGURE 26-17 ■ Speckled lentigines nevus on forearm (nevus spilus).

differentiate clinically from nevus or malignant melanoma (see earlier in this chapter)

- *Lentigo:* Flat, tan or brown spot, usually on exposed skin surface, sometimes appears as a small splotchy, splash of flat black color (solar ink-spot lentigo)
- *Malignant melanoma* (Fig. 26-18): Seen at site of junction nevus or can arise from skin that appears normal, shows a change in pigmentation either by spreading, becoming spotty, or turning darker; may bleed, form a crust, or ulcerate (see following section)
- *Basal cell and squamous cell carcinomas:* If there is any question of malignancy, a biopsy is indicated (see earlier in this chapter)

Treatment

Case Example 1. A mother comes into your office with her 5-year-old son, who has an 8- × 8-mm flat, brown nevus on the forehead. She wants to know if this "mole" is dangerous and if it should be removed.

1. Examine the lesion carefully. This lesion shows no sign of recent growth or change in pigmentation. (If it did, it should be excised and examined histologically.)
2. Reassure the mother that this mole does not appear to be dangerous and that it would be unusual for it to become dangerous. If any change in the color or growth appears, the lesion should be examined again.
3. Tell the mother that it is best to leave this nevus alone at this time. The only treatment would be surgical excision, and you are quite sure that her boy would not sit still for this procedure unless he was given a general anesthetic. When the boy is 10 years of age or older, the lesion can be examined again and possibly removed at that time by a simpler method under local anesthesia.

Case Example 2. A 25-year-old woman desires a brown, raised, hairy nevus on her upper lip removed. There has been no recent change in the tumor.

1. Examine the lesion carefully for induration, scaling, ulceration, and bleeding. None of these signs is present. (If the diagnosis is not definite, a scissor biopsy may be performed safely and the base gently coagulated by electrosurgery or Monsel solution applied. Further treatment depends on the biopsy report.)
2. Tell the patient that you can perform a biopsy and remove the mole safely but that there will be a residual, very slightly depressed scar and that probably the hairs will have to be removed separately after the first surgery has healed.
3. Surgical excision with tissue examination is the best method of removal. However, hairy, raised, pigmented nevi have been removed by shave excision with biopsy for years with no proof that this form of removal has caused a malignant melanoma.
4. First, following local anesthesia, perform a shave biopsy. Then electrosurgery can be done with the coagulating or cutting current or with cautery or applying aluminum chloride or Monsel solution. The site should not be covered and will heal in 7 to 14 days, depending on the size. If the hairs regrow, they can be removed later by electrosurgical epilation (see Chap. 6).

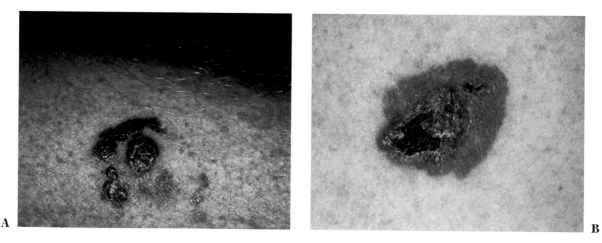

FIGURE 26-18 ■ **(A)** Malignant melanoma, on arm. **(B)** Malignant melanoma in a nevus present since birth, on the scapular area. *(Courtesy of The Upjohn Company.)*

SAUER'S NOTES

DO'S AND DON'TS REGARDING NEVI

1. Don't remove a nevus in a child by destructive methods. Remove only by surgical excision and submit nevus for histopathologic examination.
2. Do remember that in a child a benign junctional nevus may resemble a malignant melanoma histologically (Spitz nevus). Don't alarm the parents unnecessarily, because these nevi are no threat to life. A second pathology opinion can be helpful in equivocal cases.
3. Don't perform a radical deforming surgical procedure on a possible malignant melanoma until the biopsy report has been returned. Many of these tumors can turn out to be seborrheic keratoses, granuloma pyogenicum, and so on.

Malignant Melanoma
(see Chap. 27)

The incidence of malignant melanoma has increased considerably in the past 2 decades. Predisposing factors for the development of malignant melanoma include heredity, complexion (fair skin, red or blonde hair, blue eyes), ultraviolet exposure (the incidence of melanoma in the United States is increased in those states nearer the equator or with milder winters where people are outside more with less clothing), and the presence of large bathing trunk congenital nevi (greater than 20 cm). The person with hereditary dysplastic nevi is more prone to develop a malignant melanoma. An appreciable percentage of melanomas arise from preexisting nevi. Although melanomas make up only 1% of all skin cancers, they account for over 60% of the deaths owing to skin cancer in the United States. The incidence of malignant melanoma is increasing faster than any other cancer. The best chance for a cure lies in early diagnosis and prompt adequate treatment of the primary lesion.

There are four major types of malignant melanomas (Fig 26-18; see Chap. 27). They differ in terms of mode of onset, course, prognosis, and incidence.

- The most common melanoma is the superficial spreading melanoma, which develops from an *in situ* lesion. It grows slowly with a resulting good prognosis.
- Nodular melanomas grow quite rapidly and have a poorer prognosis.
- Acral lentigines melanoma, the least frequent type, occurs, as the title signifies, on the palms, soles, and around the nails as well as perioral and

perirectal; is the most common type seen in people of color or dark-skinned Caucasians; ulcerates; and metastasizes rapidly, so that it has a poor prognosis.
- Lentigo maligna melanoma develops from a lentigo maligna, occurs on the exposed areas of the body in the elderly, mainly on the forearms and face, grows slowly peripherally, and has a high survival rate.

Presentation and Characteristics

Description

The classic malignant melanoma is a black or purple nodule, but it may be flat or pedunculated and may be pink, red, tan, brown, or black or have no color (amelanotic).

The changes in a recent or longstanding skin lesion that should arouse suspicion include change in the size or shape, change in pigmentation (particularly the development of pseudopodia or areas of satellite pigmentation or leakage of pigment into surrounding skin), erythema surrounding the lesion, induration, friability with easy bleeding tendency, and ulceration.

Distribution

The site of predilection for a melanoma varies with the type of lesion. The superficial spreading melanoma is seen most commonly on the backs of men and the legs of women, in areas of sunburns. The nodular melanoma is seen in any location, more frequently in men. The acral type is seen, as indicated, on the palms and soles, and the lentigo maligna melanoma occurs mainly on face and arms in areas of chronic sun exposure.

Course

The greater the depth of involvement of the growth, the worse the prognosis. Clark has defined five levels of invasion; Breslow measured the tumor thickness with a micrometer placed in the eyepiece of the microscope. Risk groups have been defined using these measurements. For instance, a melanoma less than 0.76 mm thick and not invading the reticular dermis is in a low-risk group. Regional lymph node involvement or distant metastases gravely affect the prognosis. The most common sites of distant metastases to other organs are the lung, liver, brain, and bowel.

Histopathology

The histopathologic diagnosis of melanoma can be difficult at times. An adequate biopsy or, better yet, an initial complete excisional biopsy provides the most information.

Differential Diagnosis

■ *Benign nevus:* No recent change in lesion, not black, border smooth, single color, symmetrical, no bleeding; hairy nevi are most frequently benign, but if there is any question as to the diagnosis, a biopsy, preferably by complete excision, is indicated

The other lesions to be thought of in the differential diagnosis are the same as under nevi (see earlier section), with the addition of a pigmented basal cell epithelioma (biopsy indicated for diagnosis) and a subungual hematoma (history of recent injury; if in doubt, perform a biopsy, especially in a light-skinned person).

Treatment

Rapid and adequate therapy is indicated after the diagnosis and staging are completed. The procedures include wide surgical excision, lymph node dissection (often involving sentinel lymph node biopsy involving gamma probe guidance as the initial step), chemotherapy, and immunotherapy.

Lymphomas

The classification system for lymphomas is given in Table 26-6.

Mycosis Fungoides (Cutaneous T-Cell Lymphoma)

This polymorphous lymphoma involves the skin only, except in some rare cases that terminally invade the lymph nodes and the visceral organs. As is true with most lymphomas, the histologic type may change gradually to another form of lymphoma, with progression of the disease. However, most cases of mycosis fungoides begin as such and terminate unchanged.

Mycosis fungoides is a thymus-derived (T)-helper cell lymphocyte malignancy. The name *cutaneous T-cell lymphoma* (CTCL) is preferred by many.

Monoclonal antibodies and gene rearrangement studies may help in the histologic diagnosis of this disease.

Associations with human T-cell lymphotrophic virus types I and II and Epstein-Barr virus are found in some patients with mycosis fungoides.

Most cases are CD4 positive with clonal arrangements of the T-cell receptor. There is a rare, very aggressive subtype that is CD3 positive that expresses a different T-cell receptor.

Description

The clinical picture of this disease is classic and is divided into three stages: the erythematous stage, the plaque stage, and the tumor stage. The course usually proceeds in order, but all stages may be evident at the same time, or the first two stages may be bypassed (the d'emblée type of mycosis fungoides).

TABLE 26-6 ■ Classification of Lymphomas of Skin

	T-cell Lymphoma	B-cell Lymphoma
Indolent	Mycosis fungoides Mycosis fungoides-associated follicular mucinosis Pagetoid reticulosis CD30⁺ cutaneous large T-cell (anaplastic; immunoblastic; pleomorphic) Lymphomatoid papulosis	Follicle center cell lymphoma Immunocytoma (marginal zone B-cell lymphoma)
Intermediate	—	Large B-cell lymphoma of the leg
Aggressive	Sézary syndrome CD30-negative cutaneous large T-cell lymphoma (immunoblastic; pleomorphic)	—
Provisional	Granulomatous slack skin Cutaneous T-cell lymphoma, small/medium-sized Subcutaneous panniculitis-like T-cell lymphoma	Intravascular large B-cell lymphoma Plasmacytoma

Chan JKC. Is the REAL Classification for Real? Do We Need a Separate Classification for Cutaneous Lymphomas? Advances in Anatomic Pathology 1997; 4:6.

- *Erythematous stage:* Commonly seen are scaly, red, rather sharply defined patches that resemble atopic eczema, psoriasis, or parapsoriasis. The eruption may become diffuse as an *exfoliative dermatitis.* Itching is usually quite severe.
- *Plaque stage:* The red scaly patches develop induration and some elevation, with central healing that result in ring-shaped lesions. This stage is to be differentiated from tertiary syphilis, psoriasis, erythema multiforme perstans, mycotic infections, and other lymphomas.
- *Tumor stage:* This terminal stage is characterized by nodular and tumor growths of the plaques, often with ulceration and secondary bacterial infection. These tumors are to be differentiated from any of the granulomas (see Chap. 16). Prognosis is poor.

Course

The early stages may progress slowly, with exacerbations and remissions over many years, or the disease may be rapidly fulminating. Once the tumor stage is reached, the eventual fatal outcome is more imminent. Gene rearrangement studies may help make the diagnosis in skin lesions and may help predict the prognosis of positive lymphadenopathy.

Treatment

The combined services of a dermatologist, an oncologist, a radiologist, and an internist or a hematologist are required for the management of this sometimes fatal disease.

Locally, for early cases, a tar cream (LCD 5% in a water-washable base or in a corticosteroid cream) plus ultraviolet B therapy is quite beneficial. PUVA therapy (see Chap. 6) is also temporarily effective in resolving lesions. Narrow-band UVB (311 nm) is considered to be safer by some authors and often as effective. Local nitrogen mustard solution or ointment on the erythematous- and plaque-stage lesions has proved to be effective for some cases. BCNU is also reported to be efficacious topically.

Use of systemic therapy depends on the stage and extent of the disease. Most therapists believe that one should treat the symptoms and signs only as they appear. Corticosteroids are quite helpful, especially for the first two stages. Radiation therapy for the superficial type is effective for plaque and small tumor lesions; electron beam radiation therapy can be administered to the total body, either early or late in the disease.

Systemic chemotherapeutic agents enter into the therapy routine in the plaque and tumor stages of mycosis fungoides but are usually unsuccessful. These include the alkylating agents cyclophosphamide (Cytoxan), chlorambucil (Leukeran), and nitrogen mustard; the plant alkaloid vincristine (Oncovin); the antimetabolite methotrexate; the antibiotic doxorubicin (Adriamycin); and the antibiotic derivative bleomycin (Blenoxane). Monoclonal antibodies are also being used for therapy, as is interferon *a*-2a. Extracorporeal photophoresis therapy and systemic retinoids are other recent therapeutic modalities. Bexarotene (a retinoid, Targretin, it is an RXR receptor agonist) can be used topically and systemically. Fludarabine can be used systemically. Advanced recalcitrant disease can be treated with allogenic and hematopoietic stem cell transplant. A recombinant fusion protein (Ontak) can be beneficial in severe disease that is CD25 positive.

Complete Histologic Classification

A histologic classification of tumors of the skin is listed here. Those tumors discussed in the first part of this chapter are marked with an asterisk. The rarer tumors listed are defined or can be found in the Dictionary–Index. This classification is modified from Lever and Schaumberg-Lever (1997).

I. **EPIDERMAL TUMORS**

  A. **Tumors of the Surface Epidermis**

    1. Benign tumors

      a. Linear epidermal nevus (Fig. 26-19): A rather common tumor usually present at birth, consisting of single or multiple lesions in various forms that give rise to several clinical designations, such as hard nevus, nevus verrucous, nevus unius lateris, and, when systematized (more generalized), ichthyosis hystrix. No nevus cells are present.

      *b. Seborrheic keratosis and dermatosis papulosa nigra

      *c. Fibroma

      d. Cysts

        *1) Epidermal cyst

        *2) Trichilemmal, pilar, or sebaceous cyst

        3) Steatocystoma multiplex: A dominantly inherited condition with small, moderately firm, cystic nodules adherent to the

---

SAUER'S NOTES

A histologic examination of tissue is indicated for a definite diagnosis of most growths of the skin.

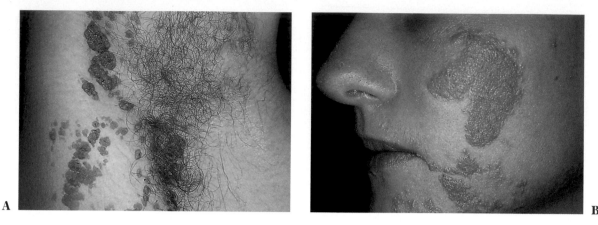

FIGURE 26-19 ■ **(A)** Linear epidermal nevus in axilla. **(B)** Nevus unius lateris of face. *(Courtesy of Owen/ Galderma.)*

overlying skin, which on incision yield an oily fluid

*4) Milium

*5) Dermoid cyst

*6) Mucous retention cyst

  e. Clear cell acanthoma: A rare, usually single, slightly elevated, flat, pale red, scaling nodule less than 2 cm in diameter, nearly always located on the lower extremities.

  f. Warty dyskeratoma: A solitary warty lesion with a central keratotic plug, most commonly seen on the scalp, face, and neck. Histology is characteristic.

*g. Keratoacanthoma

2. Precancerous tumors

*a. Senile or actinic keratosis and cutaneous horn

*b. Arsenical keratosis

*c. Leukoplakia

3. Epitheliomas and carcinomas

*a. Basal cell carcinoma

*b. Squamous cell carcinoma

  c. Bowen's disease and erythroplasia of Queyrat: Bowen's disease is a single red scaly lesion with a sharp but irregular border that grows slowly by peripheral extension. Histologically, it is an intraepidermal squamous cell carcinoma (Fig. 26-20). Erythroplasia of Queyrat represents Bowen's disease of the mucous membranes and occurs on the glans penis and rarely on the vulva. The lesion has a bright red, velvety surface.

  d. Paget's disease: A unilateral scaly red lesion resembling a dermatitis, usually present on the female nipple, but the lesion can be extra-mammary. The early lesion on the nipple is an intraductal carcinoma that also involves the mammary ducts and deeper connective tissue. In the perirectal area it can be associated with underlying bowel cancer.

B. Tumors of the Epidermal Appendages

1. Nevoid tumors

  a. Organic nevi or hamartomas

    1) Sebaceous nevi

      a) Nevus sebaceous (Jadassohn) (Fig. 26-21): Seen on the scalp or face as a single lesion present from birth, slightly

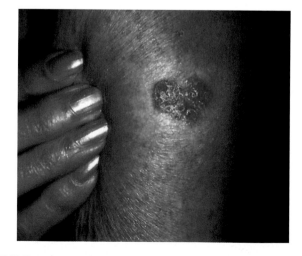

FIGURE 26-20 ■ Bowen's disease, on arm. *(Courtesy of Syntex Laboratories, Inc.)*

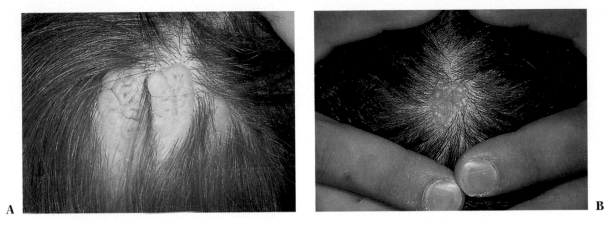

FIGURE 26-21 ■ **(A)** Nevus sebaceous of Jadassohn on scalp. **(B)** Nevus sebaceous on scalp. *(Courtesy of Owen/ Galderma.)*

raised, firm, hairless, yellowish, with furrowed surface. Large examples may be associated with a "neurocutaneous syndrome" of epilepsy and mental retardation. Basal cell and squamous cell carcinomas can develop within these growths in approximately 10% of cases.

b) Adenoma sebaceum (Pringle's disease): Part of a triad of epilepsy, mental deficiency, and the skin lesions of adenoma sebaceum. This is called *tuberous sclerosis.* The skin lesions occur on the face and consist of yellowish brown, papular, nodular lesions with telangiectases. Histopathology shows an angiofibroma (see Chap. 33).

c) Sebaceous hyperplasia (Fig. 26-22): Very common on the face in older persons and consists of one or several small, yellowish, translucent, slightly umbilicated nodules.

d) Fordyce's disease (see Chap. 30): A rather common condition of pinpoint-sized yellowish lesions of the vermilion border of the lips or the oral mucosa that represent ectopic sebaceous glands.

b. Adenomas or organoid hamartomas

1) Sebaceous adenoma: A very rare solitary tumor of the face or the scalp, smooth, firm, elevated, often slightly pedunculated, and measuring less than 1 cm in diameter;

may be associated with an adenocarcinoma of the bowel (Muir-Torre syndrome).

2) Apocrine adenomas

a) Syringocystadenoma papilliferum (Fig. 26-23): This adenoma of the apocrine ducts appears as a single verrucous plaque, usually seen on the scalp. Basal cell epitheliomatous change occasionally does occur and may arise in sebaceous nevi.

b) Hidradenoma papilliferum: This adenoma of the apocrine glands occurs almost exclusively on the labia majora and the perineum of women as a single, intracutaneous, benign tumor covered by normal epidermis.

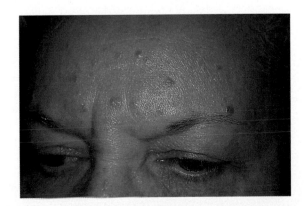

FIGURE 26-22 ■ Sebaceous gland hyperplasia (common).

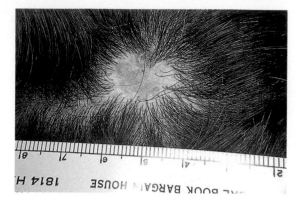

FIGURE 26-23 ■ Syringocystadenoma papilliferum. *(Courtesy of Owen/Galderma.)*

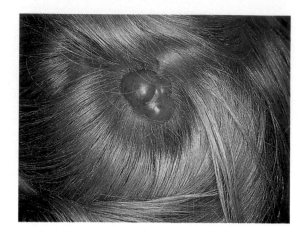

FIGURE 26-24 ■ Cylindroma of the scalp.

3) Eccrine syringofibroadenoma (ESFA): Solitary or multiple nodules with the following subtypes:

a) Solitary ESFA.

b) Multiple ESFAs with hidrotic ectodermal dysplasia.

c) Multiple ESFA.

d) Nonfamilial linear ESFA.

e) Reactive ESFA associated with inflammatory or neoplastic dermatoses usually seen on the lower extremities and easily confused with squamous cell carcinoma.

c. Benign epitheliomas or suborganoid hamartomas

1) Apocrine epitheliomas

a) Syringoma: This is characterized by the appearance of pinhead-sized soft, yellowish nodules at the age of puberty in women, developing around the eyelids, the chest, the abdomen, and the anterior aspects of the thighs.

b) Cylindroma (Fig. 26-24): These appear as numerous smooth, rounded tumors of various size on the scalp in adults and resemble bunches of grapes or tomatoes. These tumors may cover the entire scalp like a turban and are then referred to as *turban tumors*. It can be multiple and autosomal dominant with associated trichoepitheliomas and eccrine spiradenomas.

c) Multiple lesions can occur in the vulva and be extremely pruritic.

2) Hair epitheliomas

a) Trichoepithelioma (Fig. 26-25): Also known as epithelioma adenoides cysticum and multiple benign cystic epithelioma when multiple. This begins at the age of puberty, frequently on a hereditary basis, and is characterized by the presence of numerous pinhead- to pea-sized, rounded, yellowish or pink nodules on the face and occasionally on the upper trunk. May also appear as a single lesion that can be confused with a basal cell cancer histologically.

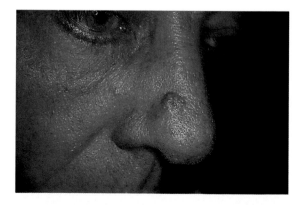

FIGURE 26-25 ■ Trichoepithelioma on nose. *(Courtesy of Owen/Galderma.)*

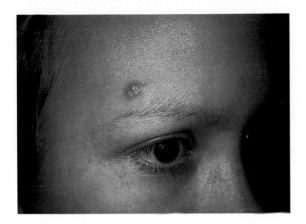

FIGURE 26-26 ■ Rarer tumors of the skin. Calcifying epithelioma of Malherbe on forehead. *(Courtesy of Owen/Galderma.)*

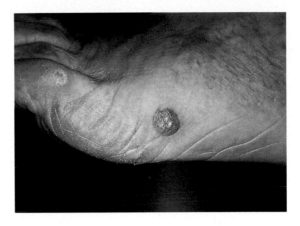

FIGURE 26-28 ■ Eccrine poroma on foot.

b) Calcifying epithelioma of Malherbe (Fig. 26-26) or pilomatrixoma (see Fig. 30-6): Hand, nodular, nondescript 0.5 to 1.0 cm tumors especially on the scalp and face. Malignant degeneration is very rare. There is a perforating form.

c) Microcystic adnexal carcinoma: Relatively rare often extensive and invasive with perineural invasion. Up to 25% misdiagnosed on initial biopsy. Slow growing and 5- to 10-year follow-up needed. Mohs surgery may be the best therapy.

3) Eccrine epitheliomas

a) Eccrine spiradenoma (Fig. 26-27): A rare, usually solitary, intradermal, firm, tender nodule

b) Clear cell hidradenoma: A rare, well-circumscribed, often encapsulated tumor of dermis and subcutaneous tissue

c) Eccrine poroma (Fig. 26-28): This occurs as an asymptomatic solitary tumor on the soles and the palms.

2. Carcinomas of sebaceous glands and eccrine and apocrine sweat glands (rare)

C. Metastatic Carcinoma of the Skin

This occurs frequently from carcinoma of the breast and melanoma but rarely from other internal carcinomas. Metastatic carcinoid nodules may appear in the skin, as well as in lymph nodes and the liver. The primary tumor and the metastases produce excess 5-hydroxytryptamine (serotonin), which in turn produces attacks of flushing of the skin.

II. MESODERMAL TUMORS

A. Tumors of Fibrous Tissue

*1. Histiocytoma and dermatofibroma

*2. Keloid

*3. Fibrosarcomas

a. True fibrosarcoma: A rare tumor that starts most commonly in the subcutaneous fat, grows rapidly, causes the overlying skin to appear purplish, and finally ulcerates

b. Dermatofibrosarcoma protuberans: A tumor that grows slowly in the corium and spreads by the development of adjoining reddish or bluish nodules that may coalesce to form a plaque that can eventually ulcerate. Margins are very difficult to evaluate making recurrence

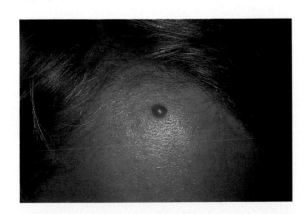

FIGURE 26-27 ■ Eccrine spiradenoma of forehead.

common. Mohs' surgery and positive CD34 immunohistochemical staining are helpful.

B. Tumors of Mucoid Tissue

1. Myxoma: Clinically seen as fairly well circumscribed, rather soft intracutaneous tumors with normal overlying epidermis
2. Myxosarcoma: Subcutaneous tumors that eventually ulcerate the skin
*3. Synovial cyst of the skin

C. Tumors of Fatty Tissue

1. Nevus lipomatosus superficialis: A rare, circumscribed nodular lesion, usually in the gluteal area
2. Lipoma: A rather common tumor that can be multiple or single, lobulated, of varying size, and in the subcutaneous tissue
3. Hibernoma: A form of lipoma composed of embryonic type of fat cells
4. Liposarcoma
5. Malignant hibernoma

D. Tumors of Nerve Tissue and Mesodermal Nerve Sheath Cells

1. Neuroma: Rare, single or multiple small reddish or brown nodules that are usually tender as well as painful.
2. Neurofibroma: Benign flesh-colored soft tumor that is frequently single, but when multiple it is associated with neurofibromatosis; when very large it is called a *plexiform neuroma*. Can have sarcomatous degeneration.
3. Neurofibromatosis (see Figs. 33-14, 35-7, and 36-6): Also known as von Recklinghausen's disease, this hereditary disease classically consists of pigmented patches (café-au-lait spots), pedunculated skin tumors, and nerve tumors. All of these lesions may not be present in a particular case.
4. Neurilemoma
5. Granular cell schwannoma or myoblastoma: From neural sheath cells, this appears usually as a solitary tumor of the tongue, the skin, or the subcutaneous tissue. Also, multiple, nodular, or plaque like.
6. Malignant granular cell schwannoma or myoblastoma

E. Tumors of Vascular Tissue

*1. Hemangioma
2. Granuloma pyogenicum (Fig. 26-29): This is a rather common (especially in pregnancy on gums)

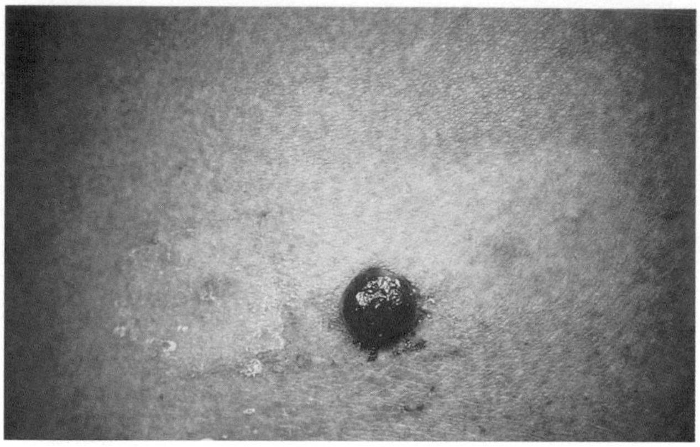

FIGURE 26-29 ■ Pyogenic granuloma of 0.75 cm size on the back. *(Courtesy of Syntex Laboratories, Inc.)*

end result of an injury to the skin that may or may not have been apparent. Vascular proliferation, with or without infection, produces a small red tumor that bleeds easily. It is to be differentiated from a malignant melanoma. Biopsy and mild electrocoagulation are curative.
3. Osler's disease: See Rendu-Osler-Weber disease in the Dictionary–Index.
4. Lymphangioma: A superficial form, lymphangioma circumscriptum, appears as a group of thin-walled vesicles on the skin surface, whereas the deeper variety, lymphangioma cavernosum, causes a poorly defined enlargement of the affected area, such as the lip or the tongue. Large lymphatic cisternae may underlie apparently superficial tumors.
5. Glomus tumor: A rather unusual small, deep-seated, red or purplish nodule that is tender and may produce severe paroxysmal pains. The solitary lesion is usually seen under a nail plate, on the fingertips, or elsewhere on the body and may erode underlying bone.
6. Hemangiopericytoma
7. Kaposi's sarcoma (multiple idiopathic hemorrhagic sarcoma) (Fig. 26-30 and see Figs. 24-4 and 24-8): Kaposi's sarcoma–associated herpes virus (HHV8) is associated with all forms. Most commonly seen on the feet and the ankles as multiple bluish red or dark brown nodules and plaques associated with visceral lesions. It is most prevalent in elderly men of Mediterranean or Jewish origin. Sarcomatous malignant degeneration can occur.

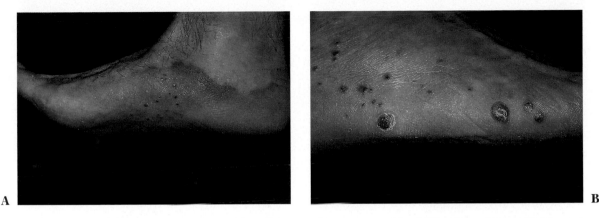

FIGURE 26-30 ■ **(A)** Kaposi's sarcoma of foot. **(B)** Kaposi's sarcoma of foot. *(Courtesy of Owen/Galderma.)*

a. Kaposi's sarcoma is also seen as part of the acquired immunodeficiency syndrome (see Chap. 24). In this complex, the sarcoma lesions are small, oval, red or pink papules that occur on any area of the body.

b. There is an endemic African form often associated with reticuloendothelial cancer.

c. An immunosuppressive drug related form often seen in transplant patients that may dissipate after immunosuppression is decreased.

8. Hemangioendothelioma
9. Postmastectomy lymphangiosarcoma (Stewart–Treves syndrome)
10. Glomangiomas: Large dilated vessels lined with glomus cells as in a glomus tumor but are larger tumors that mimic large venous malformations clinically. Deep blue or purple, poorly compressible and usually on the face. They can be large, disfiguring, inherited as an autosomal dominant.

F. Tumors of Muscular Tissue

1. Leiomyoma: Solitary leiomyomas may be found on the extremities and on the scrotum, whereas multiple leiomyomas occur on the back and elsewhere as pinhead- to pea-sized, brown or bluish, firm, elevated nodules. Both forms are painful and sensitive to pressure, particularly as they enlarge. They may have a butterfly shape.
2. Leiomyosarcoma: Very rare
3. Multiple leiomyomas may be associated with uterine leiomyomas and renal cancer as a familial syndrome.

G. Tumors of Osseous Tissue

1. Osteoma cutis

a. Primary: The primary form of osteoma cutis develops from embryonal cell rests; these may be single or multiple.

b. Secondary: Secondary bone formation may occur as a form of tissue degeneration in tumors, in scar tissue (such as acne), in scleroderma lesions (see CREST syndrome), and in various granulomas.

H. Tumors of Cartilaginous Tissue

1. Nodular chondrodermatitis of the ear: A painful, benign, hyperkeratotic nodule, usually on the inner rim of the helix of the ear of elderly men. Trauma may be the inciting cause. Often awakens the patient at night when pressure applied. Can treat by excision or sometimes intralesional corticosteroids.

III. NEVUS CELL TUMORS

A. Melanocytic Nevi

*1. Junctional (active) nevus
*2. Intradermal (resting) nevus
*3. Dysplastic nevus syndrome
4. Lentigines: These are to be differentiated from freckles (ephelides). A freckle histologically shows hyperpigmentation of the basal layer but no elongation of the rete pegs and no increase in the number of clear cells and dendritic cells. Juvenile lentigines (lentigo simplex) begin to appear in childhood and occur on all parts of the body. Senile lentigines,

(solar lentigo) also known as "liver spots," occur in elderly persons on the dorsa of the hands, the forearms, and the face and are related to sun exposure. Solar ink-spot lentigo is commonly seen on sun-exposed areas and has a characteristic black, splotchy, reticulated pattern. Lentigo maligna melanoma (Hutchinson's Freckle) (see Fig. 36-8) is a dark brown or black macular, malignant lesion, usually on the face or arms of elderly persons, that has a slow peripheral growth (see under Malignant Melanoma earlier). Lentigines can be caused by ionizing radiation, a tanning bed, a sunlamp, PUVA therapy, and, most commonly, from sun exposure.

5. Mongolian spots (see Fig. 36-8): These are seen chiefly in Asian or African-American infants, usually around the buttocks. They disappear spontaneously during childhood. Related bluish patchy lesions are the nevus of Ota, seen on the side of the face (may have scleralpigment), and the nevus of Ito, located in the supraclavicular, scapular, and deltoid regions. Laser therapy may be beneficial.

*6. Blue nevus: Clinically, the blue nevus appears as a slate blue or bluish black, sharply circumscribed, flat or slightly elevated nodule, occurring on any area of the body. It originates from mesodermal cells. The common blue nevus is always benign. Cellular blue nevus is larger, especially on buttocks and can degenerate into malignant melanoma.

*B. **Malignant Melanoma**

IV. LYMPHOMAS (SEE CHAP. 31)

A. **Monomorphous Group**

1. The non-Hodgkin's lymphomas are referred to as *monomorphous lymphomas* because, in contrast to Hodgkin's disease, they lack a significant admixture of inflammatory cells and are composed almost entirely of lymphoma cells largely derived from B or T lymphocytes. A classification of cutaneous lymphomas follows.

2. Lymphomas may have specific skin lesions containing the lymphomatous infiltrate, or nonspecific lesions may be seen. These latter consist of macules, papules, tumors, purpuric lesions, blisters, eczematous lesions, exfoliative dermatitis, and secondarily infected excoriations.

B. **Polymorphous Group**

1. Hodgkin's disease: Specific lesions are very rare, but nonspecific dermatoses are commonly seen.

> ### SAUER'S NOTES
>
> Sun tanning salons should be strongly discouraged. They are associated with increased risk of malignant melanoma, squamous cell cancer, and basal cell cancer. All aspects of photoaging are increased. Lupus erythematosus, various porphyrias, photo drug reactions, dermatomyositis, actinic keratoses, and solar urticaria are all caused by or worsened by sun tanning salon usage. The false tan or immediate pigment darkening of high-dose UVA given by most sun tanning salons does not protect from future sun burning as the sun-induced tan does.

*2. Mycosis fungoides

a. Sézary's syndrome: This is a very rare form of exfoliative dermatitis (see Chap. 19) that occurs at an early leukemic stage of a CTCL. It is diagnosed by finding unusually large monocytoid cells (so-called Sézary cells) in the blood and in the skin. This cell is indistinguishable from the mycosis cell, both of which are derived from the T cell.

V. MYELOSIS (SEE FIG. 33-2)

A. Leukemia: Refers to circulating abnormal blood cells; may be seen along with lymphomas, but in skin almost always associated with myelosis, such as myeloid leukemia. Cutaneous lesions are quite uncommon but may be specific or nonspecific.

VI. PSEUDOLYMPHOMA OF SPIEGLER-FENDT (SEE DICTIONARY–INDEX, FIG. 2C)

A. A benign, localized erythematous, nodular dermatosis usually on the face, with clinical and histologic features that make a distinction from lymphoma difficult. Some cases may eventually be diagnosed as a lymphoma.

Suggested Reading

Barnhill RL. Color atlas and synopsis of pigmented lesions. New York, McGraw-Hill, 1995.

Bernstein SC, Lim KK, Brodland DG, et al. The many faces of squamous cell carcinoma. Dermatol Surg 1996;22:243.

Bowers RE, Graham EA, Tomlinson KM. The natural history of the strawberry nevus. Arch Dermatol 1960;82:667.

Dalton JA, et al. Cutaneous T-cell lymphoma. Int J Dermatol 1997;36:801.

Drake LA, Ceilley RI, et al. Guidelines of care for actinic keratoses. J Am Acad Dermatol 1995;32:1.

Drake LA, Salasche SJ, Ceilley RI, et al. Guidelines of care for basal cell carcinoma. J Am Acad Dermatol 1992; 26:117.

Drake LA, Ceilley RI, et al. Guidelines of care for nevi: II. Nonmelanocytic nevi, hamartomas, neoplasms, and potentially malignant lesions. J Am Acad Dermatol 1995;32:1.

Drake LA, Chanco Turner ML, Ceilley RI, et al. Guidelines of care for malignant melanoma. J Am Acad Dermatol 1993;28:638.

Drake LA, Salasche S, Ceilley RI, et al. Guidelines of care for cutaneous squamous cell carcinoma. J Am Acad Dermatol 1993;28:628.

Lever WF, Schaumburg-Lever G. Histopathology of the skin, ed 8. Philadelphia, JB Lippincott, 1997.

Zackheim HS. Cutaneous T-cell lymphoma, mycosis fungoides and Sézary syndrome. Boca Raton, FL, CRC Press, 2005.

CHAPTER 27

Melanoma

Robin S. Weiner, MD, and Jaeyoung Yoon, MD, PHD

Melanoma (see malignant melanoma in previous chapter) is defined as a malignant tumor arising from melanocytes, and although it may develop in a preexisting nevus, more than 50% of cases are believed to arise *de novo* without a preexisting lesion. Melanomas lacking pigment are termed *amelanotic melanomas*.

Epidemiology

Cancer of the skin accounts for more than 50% of all cancers, and the majority of skin cancer deaths are attributable to melanoma. The American Cancer Society has estimated that approximately 59,580 new melanomas will be diagnosed in the United States during 2005, with 7700 predicted deaths from this disease. Incidence rates for melanoma have increased steadily over the past several decades, currently rising at a rate of approximately 3% per year. Melanoma has historically affected a younger population than most cancers, with half the patients under age 57.

Risk Factors

Several risk factors have been identified for the development of melanoma:

- *Ultraviolet irradiation,* with intermittent intense exposure and sunburn posing a greater risk than cumulative lifetime exposure, and increasing latitude correlating with decreased incidence of melanoma.
- *Atypical or dysplastic nevi,* especially in families with the so-called dysplastic nevus syndrome.
- *Increased number of benign nevi,* with those having greater than 50 nevi at higher risk of developing melanoma.
- *Large congenital nevi,* defined as greater than 20 cm.
- *Phenotypic features,* including pale or light skin, blonde or red hair, blue or green eyes, a tendency toward freckling, and poor tanning ability.
- *Family history of melanoma*
- *Host immunosuppression*
- *Genetic predisposition,* including defects in the CDKN2A gene and/or the CDK4 gene, and genodermatoses such as xeroderma pigmentosum.

Types of Primary Melanoma

Superficial spreading melanoma (Fig. 27-1) represents the most common clinical subtype, accounting for approximately 70% of cutaneous melanomas. These tumors typically experience a slow horizontal growth phase followed by a rapid vertical growth phase, which may be evident by the development of a papule or nodule. Sites of predilection include the backs of males and the backs and legs of women, although it can occur at any site.

Nodular melanoma accounts for approximately 15% of cutaneous melanomas and has a short radial (horizontal) growth phase, accounting for its rapid invasion. It is seen more frequently in men, and sites of predilection include the trunk, head, and neck. It typically appears as a dark blue-black papule or nodule that develops rapidly and may include a history of ulceration or bleeding. Amelanotic melanoma is often a variant of this subtype.

Acral lentiginous melanoma (Fig. 27-2) represents approximately 10% of cutaneous melanomas, but is the most common type found in darker-complected individuals. Most frequent sites include the palms, soles, or beneath the nail plate. Lesions frequently present as brown to black macules with irregular borders and variations in color, although papules and nodules may be present. This subtype typically has a poor prognosis, which may be related to delayed diagnosis. Therefore, early biopsy of suspected lesions is critical.

Lentigo maligna melanoma is a rare clinical subtype, comprising approximately 5% of cutaneous melanomas. This lesion arises from a lentigo maligna (melanoma *in situ* of sun-exposed skin) and involves dermal invasion. Tumors typically occur in the elderly and arise on sun-damaged skin, including the forearms and the face. These

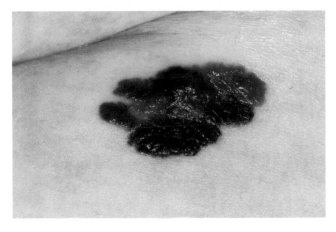

FIGURE 27-1 ■ Superficial spreading melanoma.

lesions present as large, irregularly shaped macules or patches with variations of tan, brown, or black pigment, and may eventually develop a papular or nodular component.

Diagnosis

Early identification and treatment of melanomas are essential as prognosis depends on the stage of disease at diagnosis. Pertinent data should be gathered from the medical history, including personal or family history of melanoma, any change in existing skin lesions including changes in size, shape, or pigmentation, as well as any history of bleeding or ulceration.

Physical examination should include evaluation of all skin, including scalp and mucous membranes, using the American Cancer Society's ABCD mnemonic to identify suspicious lesions. *A* is for asymmetry, *B* for irregular borders, *C* for irregular color, and *D* for diameter, with size >6 mm typically considered suspicious. It has recently

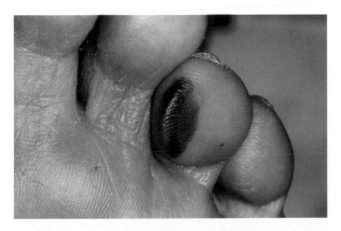

FIGURE 27-2 ■ Acral lentiginous melanoma.

been suggested that the mnemonic be lengthened to include *E* for evolving. Dermatoscopy, also known as *epiluminescence microscopy*, is a noninvasive tool used for magnification and may contribute to diagnosis.

Once identified, suspicious lesions should be evaluated with full-thickness biopsy to allow assessment of lesion thickness. Excisional biopsy should be performed when possible to evaluate the entire lesion; prognosis and treatment are determined by tumor thickness. When excisional biopsy is impractical, such as when the lesion is large, or clinical suspicion is low, punch biopsy technique may be used and should include the most suspicious area of the growth.

Staging and Prognosis

The American Joint Committee on Cancer Staging Manual was revised in 2002 and established the TNM staging system for melanoma given in Table 27-1. Stages I and II represent local disease, stage III represents regional involvement, and stage IV represents distant metastases (Table 27-2).

Important prognostic factors include tumor thickness and ulceration, as well as clinical variables such as anatomic site, sex, and age of the patient. Increased tumor thickness correlates with poorer prognosis and is the most important determinant. Presence of ulceration microscopically is the second most important determinant.

TABLE 27-1 ■ **TNM Staging System for Melanoma**

TX	Primary tumor cannot be assessed
T0	No evidence of primary tumor
Tis	Melanoma *in situ*
T1	Melanoma <1.0 mm in thickness
T2	Melanoma 1.01−2.0 mm in thickness
T3	Melanoma 2.01−4.0 mm in thickness
T4	Melanoma >4.0 mm in thickness
NX	Regional lymph nodes cannot be assessed
N0	No regional lymph node metastasis
N1	Metastasis in one lymph node
N2	Metastasis in 2−3 regional nodes or intralymphatic regional metastasis without nodal metastases
N3	Metastasis in 4 or more regional nodes, or matted metastatic nodes, or in transit metastasis or satellite(s) *with* metastasis in regional node(s)
MX	Distant metastasis cannot be assessed
M0	No distant metastasis
M1	Distant metastasis

TABLE 27-2 ■ Clinical Stage Grouping (AJCC)

Stage 0	Tis	N0	M0
Stage IA	T1a	N0	M0
Stage IB	T1b	N0	M0
	T2a	N0	M0
Stage IIA	T2b	N0	M0
	T3a	N0	M0
Stage IIB	T3b	N0	M0
	T4a	N0	M0
Stage IIC	T4b	N0	M0
Stage III	Any T	N1, N2, or N3	M0
Stage IV	Any T	Any N	M1

Note: a, no ulceration; b, ulceration

Tumor thickness is known as *Breslow's depth,* defined as the distance from the top of the granular cell layer to the deepest point of tumor invasion. Clark's level of invasion may also be described:

- level 1 involves only the epidermis,
- level 2 invades the papillary dermis,
- level 3 fills the papillary dermis,
- level 4 invades the reticular dermis, and
- level 5 involves the subcutaneous fat.

According to Surveillance, Epidemiology and End Results data from 1988–2001, approximately 83% of melanomas are diagnosed at a localized stage. These tumors (Stage I and II) have a 97% 5-year survival rate with appropriate treatment. Melanomas with regional involvement at the time of diagnosis (Stage III) have a 60% 5-year survival rate, and those with distant metastases (Stage IV) have a 5-year survival rate of 16%.

Treatment

Once the diagnosis of melanoma is confirmed, complete excision of the tumor site is performed with margins determined based on Breslow's tumor thickness. Although there is some controversy regarding recommendations for tumors 1 to 2 mm in depth, the American Academy of Dermatology task force recommends the following:

- 0.5 cm margins for *in situ* melanoma,
- 1 cm margins for tumor thickness <2 mm, and
- 2-cm margins for tumors with a thickness >2 mm.

Lymphatic mapping and sentinel lymph node biopsy can be performed as a staging tool and provides prognostic information. The therapeutic value of this procedure awaits further analysis. It is hoped that intense research into chemotherapy, immunotherapy, and cancer vaccinations will improve survival rates, however, the prognosis for advanced melanoma remains grim.

Suggested Reading

Balch CM, Houghton AN, Sober AJ, et al. Cutaneous melanoma, ed 4. St. Louis, Mo., Quality Medical Pub., 2003.

Hearing VJ, Leong SPL. From melanocytes to malignant melanoma. Totowa, NJ, Humana Press, 2005.

Kroon BBR, Morton, DL, Thompson, JF. Textbook of melanoma. London; New York, Martin Dunitz, 2004.

Massi G, LeBoit PE. Histological diagnosis of nevi and melanoma. Darmstadt, Steinkopff, 2004.

Rigel DS, Friedman RJ, Kopf AW, et al. ABCDE—an evolving concept in the early detection of melanoma. Arch Dermatol. 2005 Aug;141(8): 1032–1034.

Riker AI, Glass F, Perez I, et al. Cutaneous melanoma: Methods of biopsy and definitive surgical excision. Dermatol Ther. 2005 Sep-Oct; 18(5):387–393.

Schaffer JV, Rigel DS, Kopf AW, et al. Cutaneous melanoma—past, present, and future. J Am Acad Dermatol. 2004 Jul;51(1 Suppl):S65–S69.

Scottish Intercollegiate Guidelines Network. Cutaneous melanoma: A national clinical guideline/Scottish Intercollegiate Guidelines Network. Edinburgh, Scotland, SIGN, 2003.

SECTION V

STRUCTURES ASSOCIATED WITH THE SKIN

CHAPTER 28

Diseases Affecting the Hair

Thelda M. Kestenbaum, MD

Hair is an extremely important part of an individual's appearance and sense of identity. Loss of hair on the scalp or an excessive amount of unwanted hair on other body parts causes great psychological distress. Our perception of femininity and masculinity is greatly affected by hair quantity, distribution, and styling.

Hair Physiology

There are three types of hairs:

- lanugo,
- vellus, and
- terminal hairs.

Lanugo hairs are long, unmedullated hairs seen *in utero* and are shed during the end of pregnancy and the first several months post partum. *Vellus* (intermediate hairs) are short, nonpigmented hairs produced by follicles that penetrate only into the papillary dermis. *Terminal* hairs are produced by follicles that penetrate into the reticular dermis

307

and are usually medullated (have a medulla) and are wider than the inner root sheath of the follicle that produces them. Hairs on the scalp and beard area are examples of terminal hairs. In the inherited types of balding, some terminal hairs are lost and vellus hairs are seen instead.

Hair growth is not a continuous process. There is an anagen (growth) phase (about 85% to 95% of scalp hairs are in this phase), catagen (regressive) phase (about 1% of scalp hairs are in this phase), and a telogen (resting) phase (about 10% to 15% of scalp hairs are in this phase). The length of the anagen phase determines the length of the hair. The anagen phase for human scalp hair is usually between 2 and 6 years and the hair on the scalp grows about 1 cm per month; therefore, some people can never have very long hair on the scalp even if they never cut their hair. Growth phases of hair on other body parts are much shorter than on the scalp. It is normal to lose between 50 and 100 scalp hairs per day. Plucking the resting hairs from follicles that have already entered anagen can advance the onset of the next anagen phase. Shaving the hair has no effect on the hair cycle. The telogen phase is the period between the completion of follicular regression (catagen) and the onset of the next anagen phase. On the human scalp, the telogen phase lasts about 2 to 4 months. The catagen phase on the human scalp lasts 2 to 4 weeks.

With aging or with the inherited type of hair loss, there is a shortening of the anagen phase and a lengthening of time between telogen and a new anagen phase. Hair cycles are influenced by multiple factors, such as the season and a change in hormonal status as seen in pregnancy. Seasonal changes in hair shedding are usually not that noticeable but are important when conducting studies on treatment of hair loss. During pregnancy, there is an increase in the proportion of follicles in anagen and post partum there is an increase in the proportion of hairs in telogen, resulting in a marked increased shedding, usually 3 months (range, 1 to 5 months) post partum. This problem rectifies itself usually within a year or less.

Hairs vary in diameter and number in different racial groups. The diameter of Asian hair is the widest and is round on cross-section. European hair is round to oval on cross-section; African hair is more elliptical or flattened in cross-section. African hair follicles are spiral in shape. The volume of the hair papilla determines the size of the hair shaft.

Hair amount varies among races with white people (especially those of southern European extraction) generally being hairier than other racial groups. The number of scalp hairs is 10% greater in blonds and 10% less in redheads compared to white brunettes. Black people have significantly fewer hair follicles and more fragile hair than white people.

SAUER'S NOTES

1. Shaving the hair does not increase growth.
2. Frequent shampooing does not damage normal scalp hair.
3. Dandruff does not cause hair loss unless the scalp becomes severely secondarily infected.
4. Excessive brushing of the hair can cause hair breakage and hair loss.

Graying of the hair is a normal process of aging and develops in white people about a decade earlier than in black people. Graying earlier than 20 years of age is considered premature in whites and graying earlier than 30 years of age is considered premature in blacks. By 50 years of age, the average white person is 50% gray. In white people, the age of onset of graying varies from 24 to 44 years of age; in black people the age of onset of graying is from 34 to 54 years of age; and in Asians the age of onset of graying is in the 30s. Premature graying has been associated with pernicious anemia as well as thyroid disease (usually hyperthyroidism; may be seen with hypothyroidism), and a host of unusual inherited syndromes. A frontal white patch of hair may be inherited as an autosomal dominant trait (piebaldism). People with alopecia areata may note regrowing hairs that are light in color. People who are said to have "turned gray overnight" probably are those with "salt and pepper" hair that developed a diffuse form of alopecia areata in which the dark hairs were lost preferentially to the gray hairs.

Many people color their hair. The most common chemical used to dye the hair is paraphenylenediamine, which is sometimes the cause of a contact dermatitis.

Hirsutism and Hypertrichosis

Hirsutism is the excessive growth of terminal hair in an adult male sexual pattern in a female or child. *Hypertrichosis* is hair growth that is abnormal for the age, gender, or race of an individual or for a particular area of the body. Medications can cause either of these problems (Table 28-1).

Hirsutism

Cause and Distribution

The prevalence of hirsutism in women overall is said to vary from 5% to 15%. The most common diagnosis associated with hirsutism is polycystic ovary syndrome (PCOS). About 5% to 15% of cases of hirsutism are idiopathic.

TABLE 28-1 ■ Drugs That Can Cause Hirsutism and Hypertrichosis

	Drug
Hirsutism	Androgens
	Danazol
	Progesterone
Hypertrichosis	Acetazolamide
	Corticosteroids
	Cyclosporine
	Diazoxide
	Interferon
	Latanoprost
	Minoxidil
	Penicillamine
	Phenytoin
	Psoralens
	Streptomycin

Asian and Scandinavian women are generally less hairy than white women of Mediterranean ancestry, so sometimes it is difficult to judge when hair growth in women is abnormal. Also, menopausal women who are not on hormone replacement may note some hirsutism. Androgen excess and drug-induced hirsutism need to be ruled out. Laboratory tests should be guided by the history and physical examination. Certainly other signs of virilization such as severe acne lead one to perform a more aggressive hormonal evaluation.

Laboratory Findings. Sometimes a serum testosterone and 17 α-hydroxyprogesterone may be sufficient, but women with irregular menses and hirsutism should be screened for thyroid dysfunction and prolactin disorders. A DHEAS test is useful for screening for adrenal tumors, but is not reliable for screening late-onset congenital adrenal hyperplasia. The presence of striae, central obesity, and peripheral weakness make the diagnosis of Cushing's syndrome possible, in which case a 24-hour urine free cortisol test is indicated.

Normally, 78% of testosterone in women is bound to sex-hormone binding globulin (SHBG), only 1% to 2% is free (which is the bioactive portion), and 20% is bound to albumin. SHBG may be reduced in amount by obesity, hypothyroidism, and hyperinsulinemia, thereby increasing free testosterone levels and therefore possibly leading to hirsutism.

An early morning follicular phase 17-α progesterone level is one of the better tests to screen for congenital adrenal hyperplasia. There are some rare enzyme deficiencies that can lead to congenital adrenal hyperplasia that might be better done by an endocrinologist.

PCOS has a prevalence of 6% in all women and is the most common diagnosis associated with hirsutism. Stein and Leventhal were the first to describe this syndrome of amenorrhea, obesity, and hirsutism in association with sclerocystic ovaries. PCOS may be better described as chronic anovulation and hyperandrogenism with the exclusion of androgen-secreting tumors, nonclassic adrenal hyperplasia, and hyperprolactinemia. Insulin resistance with compensatory hyperinsulinemia is a prominent feature in many but not all cases of PCOS. Commonly found laboratory abnormalities in PCOS include an elevated total testosterone (about twice normal), an elevated luteinizing hormone level (that is at least twice the value for follicle-stimulating hormone), a slight elevation in prolactin, and a slight elevation in DHEAS. The prostate-specific antigen test may or may not be helpful in distinguishing women with PCOS from those with idiopathic hirsutism.

Treatment

Treatment of hirsutism involves finding the cause and obtaining the help of an endocrinologist in some cases. Oral spironolactone (Aldactone) may be helpful in PCOS and idiopathic hirsutism. Spironolactone interferes with androgen biosynthesis, blocks the action of androgens at the receptor level, and decreases the 5 α-reductase levels in the follicle. Six months of treatment with spironolactone at 100 to 200 mg per day is at least worth a trial. It is important that this not be given to women who are not using adequate contraception because it is teratogenic. Oral contraceptives, flutamide (not approved by FDA), finasteride, cyproterone acetate (this is an ingredient in the contraceptive pill called *Dianette*, which is not available in the United States) are some other treatments that are available. The use of the antihyperglycemic metformin does reduce markers of insulin resistance in PCOS and this may help treat hirsutism. Removal of hair as discussed under treatment of hypertrichosis may be a helpful adjunct to treatments mentioned here.

Hypertrichosis

Hypertrichosis can result from the conversion of vellus hairs to terminal hairs, more hairs being in a prolonged anagen (growth) phase (and therefore a decrease in the number of hairs in the telogen phase), or an increase in hair follicle density.

Presentation and Characteristics

It is helpful to divide hypertrichosis into congenital or acquired and then into generalized and localized types.

Congenital generalized hypertrichosis and congenital hypertrichosis lanuginosa are both very rare inherited disorders; "Dog-faced" or "monkey-faced" people in circus side shows may have had the former diagnosis. Congenital hypertrichosis may be a feature of numerous inherited syndromes such as mucopolysaccharidoses, leprechaunism, and Cornelia de Lange syndrome. Of particular of note is that fetuses exposed to hydantoin (Dilantin) during the first 9 weeks of gestation may have hypertrichosis as part of the fetal hydantoin syndrome. Hypertrichosis may be seen in fetal alcohol syndrome.

Congenital localized hypertrichosis over the vertebral column ("faun tail") may be a marker of an underlying spinal abnormality. Magnetic resonance imaging is strongly recommended in such cases since the underlying problems may require early surgical intervention to prevent neurologic damage. Congenital hypertrichosis of the ears may be seen in the babies of diabetic mothers or in babies with XYY syndrome. Hairy elbows may be present at birth or acquired and may or may not be associated with other abnormalities.

Acquired hypertrichosis may be generalized or localized. Generalized acquired hypertrichosis may be seen as acquired hypertrichosis lanuginosa ("malignant down"), which is a rare, but striking marker of an internal malignancy (usually lung or colon cancer but a multiplicity of underlying tumors have been associated). Multiple normal hair follicles revert to lanugo hair usually starting on the face and progressing caudad. Generalized acquired hypertrichosis may occur in diverse conditions including

- porphyrias,
- dermatomyositis,
- anorexia nervosa,
- mercury intoxication (acrodynia),
- insulin-resistant diabetes,
- hypothyroidism,
- postencephalitis,
- multiple sclerosis,
- head injuries, and
- POEMS syndrome (polyneuropathy, organomegaly, endocrinopathy, M protein and skin changes: hyperpigmentation, hypertrichosis, skin thickening, edema, digital clubbing, and cutaneous angiomas and others).

Multiple drugs can cause hypertrichosis (see Table 28-1). Some cause generalized and some cause localized hypertrichosis. A newer drug in this latter category is one for treatment of glaucoma called *latanoprost*, a prostaglandin $F_{2\alpha}$ analog that causes hypertrichosis and hyperpigmentation of the eyelashes in most (77%) patients using it.

Localized acquired hypertrichosis on the pinnae may be an inherited trait (especially in men from India), or it may be seen with diabetes or with AIDS. Localized hypertrichosis may develop under orthopedic casts or in areas that are chronically traumatized such as lichen simplex chronicus (neurodermatitis), areas in which habitual self inflicted biting occurs, over thrombophlebitis, or over areas of osteomyelitis.

Treatment

Treatment of hypertrichosis may include shaving, depilatories, bleaching, plucking, waxing (a method of plucking of multiple hairs simultaneously), laser, and electrolysis. Electrolysis may require more than one treatment and should be done by someone trained in the procedure who uses sterile patient exclusive needles so as to prevent transmission of blood-borne disease. Shaving, contrary to popular belief, does not increase the amount of hair that regrows. Chemical depilatories and bleaching agents are available over the counter and frequently prove effective but may irritate the skin of some users. Waxing and plucking have the advantage of removing the unwanted hair for longer periods without retreatment than does shaving or chemical removal. Electrolysis can cause scarring and is expensive. Laser may be helpful in selected cases especially dark hair in fair skinned patients. A newer topical cream for treatment of hypertrichosis is eflornithine hydrochloride (Vaniqa), an irreversible inhibitor of ornithine decarboxylase that slows (but does not remove hair) hair growth. This drug is used systemically for treatment of African trypanosomiasis and its side effect of hair loss has been utilized in this cream. It is best not used in pregnant or nursing women and not over vast surface areas.

Alopecia (Hair Loss)

Alopecia of the scalp is of considerable concern to men and women. It is helpful in differentiating among the many causes of alopecia to examine the hair and scalp and observe whether the scalp is scarred or nonscarred and whether the hair loss is diffuse (the most common type) or patchy (Table 28-2). Establishing whether the hair is coming out by the roots or breaking off helps to guide the physician in how best to proceed with the workup. If the hair loss is scarring a scalp biopsy early on will probably prove helpful. If the hair is breaking off, fungal infection, trauma, or hair shaft defects are more likely causes. Loss of up to one half of the scalp hair may occur before the hair loss is clinically obvious on casual inspection.

Nonscarring Diffuse Alopecia

This accounts for the vast majority of people presenting with hair loss. Among the more common causes are

TABLE 28-2 ■ Classification of Alopecia

Nonscarring Hair Loss

Diffuse
   Androgenic* (female pattern; male pattern)
   Telogen effluvium
      Illness
      Post partum
      Sudden weight loss
      Medication
      Toxins
      Post general anesthesia
   Endocrinopathy (hypothyroidism; hyperthyroidism)
   Alopecia areata
   Loose anagen syndrome
Patchy
   Tinea capitis
   Alopecia areata
   Trichotillomania
   Syphilis
   Traumatic (traction)
   Loose anagen syndrome

Scarring Hair Loss

Tinea†
Trauma (traction)
Tumors (malignant or benign)
Skin diseases (such as sarcoid; scleroderma)
Lymphocytic (more common in women)
   Central centrifugal cicatricial alopecia (CCCA)‡
   Discoid lupus§
   Lichen planopilaris
      Frontal fibrosing alopecia
   Pseudopelade of Brocq
Neutrophilic (more common in men)
   Folliculitis decalvans
   Dissecting cellulitis
Mixed
   Acne keloidalis
   Acne necrotica
   Erosive pustular dermatosis

---

*Usually nonscarring; scarring can result in some cases.
†Usually nonscarring.
‡Formerly called "hot comb alopecia" or "follicular degeneration syndrome." CCCA (may include pseudopelade, folliculitis decalvans, and some cases of acne keloidalis and dissecting cellulitis).
§May be seen in SLE; SLE patients may also have diffuse nonscarring hair loss or nonscarring frontal scalp hair loss.

- androgenetic (androgenic; male or female pattern),
- telogen effluvium,
- diffuse alopecia areata, and
- tinea capitis.

A detailed history, past medical history, review of systems, medication history, family history, and social history are helpful; appropriate laboratory testing can then be obtained (Table 28-3). A gradual onset over more than a year is more likely to point to androgenetic hair loss.

Androgenetic Pattern Hair Loss

Androgenetic (androgenic; pattern hair loss; female pattern hair loss; male pattern hair loss; diffuse hormonal alopecia; common baldness) is the most common cause of diffuse nonscarring hair loss in men and in women. It may be that some forms may be scarring but this is still being sorted out (see Scarring Alopecia). Most lay people can diagnose this in men but it is much more difficult to diagnose in women. It is an inherited hair loss induced by androgens in men and in some women who are genetically predisposed. Prevalence is over 50% of men and probably a similar number of women by menopause. People of European ancestry are more likely to have this than other racial groups.

Presentation and Characteristics. In men, androgenetic hair loss is both genetic and androgen dependent and can be inherited from either or both parents. In women with androgenetic hair loss (better termed *female pattern hair loss*), probably only a subset of them that have PCOS are truly the female counterparts of male pattern baldness. Clinically, both men and women with androgenetic hair loss have notable loss of hair on the top of the scalp (vertex, frontal, bitemporal, or mid-scalp). Men have a more severe amount of hair loss than do women generally speaking.

TABLE 28-3 ■ Laboratory Studies to Evaluate Nonscarring Alopecia

Baseline

Complete blood cell count
Ferritin
VDRL with dilutions
Thyroid screening
Microscopic examination of hair
Fungal culture

Other

Scalp biopsy
Antinuclear antibody
Hormones (*e.g.*, dehydroepiandrosterone sulfate, testosterone, androstenedione)
Borate and thallium levels
Heavy metal screens

It used to be thought that in women with female pattern hair loss, the frontal hair line was retained (unlike in men) and this could help distinguish it from telogen effluvium, in which there is often a temporal recession. Olsen has pointed out that many women with female pattern hair loss have a frontal accentuation of hair loss that may encroach on the frontal hair line in a "Christmas tree"–like pattern (with the base of the tree being the frontal hair line).

The inheritance of androgenetic hair loss in men is probably autosomal dominant with variable penetrance and expression, but may not be true for androgenetic hair loss in women (female pattern hair loss), which is a more heterogeneous group. It can be stated that women with female pattern hair loss who are younger than 50 years of age have a positive family history in their mothers and male relatives in over 50% of cases; it is probably polygenic in inheritance.

Severe female pattern hair loss in women may be a marker of insulin resistance and these women are perhaps more likely to have a paternal history of alopecia than women with a milder version of this problem. Female pattern hair loss is the preferred term and its onset may be early (3rd decade) or late (5th decade) with or without androgen excess. It is best to classify it in this way especially when reporting clinical trials of treatment. Most women with female pattern hair loss do not have androgen excess and androgen excess alone does not cause female pattern hair loss.

A workup to exclude other causes of hair loss such as medications, telogen effluvium, diffuse alopecia areata, and loose anagen syndrome is in order (see Table 28-3).

Treatment

Treatment for the inherited types of alopecia includes minoxidil (Rogaine) (2% or 5%) for men or for women, with the exclusion of women of childbearing years who are not using adequate contraception. Only the 2% formulation is approved for use in women but probably the 5% formulation is slightly more effective. Minoxidil is a vasodilator in hypertension; it has a direct mitogenic and morphologic effect on follicular cells and does not have an antiandrogenic effect. Side effects of topical minoxidil include contact or irritant dermatitis (in less than 8%) and facial hypertrichosis in women using it (in at least 3% to 5% of those using the 2% concentration). The absorption of even the 5% concentration minoxidil is well below that necessary to change pulse rate, which is the most sensitive indicator of systemic minoxidil effects. The drug must be used indefinitely to maintain hair growth.

For young men, the use of finasteride (Propecia) 1 mg/d is an additional treatment option in male pattern alopecia. Finasteride is a 5-α-reductase inhibitor. The enzyme 5-α-reductase catalyzes conversion of testosterone to the more potent dihydrotestosterone. Finasteride (Proscar) is used in a higher dose of 5 mg for treatment of benign prostatic hyperplasia. In a study using finasteride in postmenopausal women with female pattern hair loss, it was not helpful for treatment. It is not known for sure if finasteride would or would not be useful in women with female pattern hair loss who are premenopausal or in women in whom there is also androgen treating excess. Finasteride should not be used in pregnant or lactating women; it can lower serum dihydrotestosterone and therefore has a potential risk of causing genital abnormalities in male fetuses exposed in utero. Women who are pregnant or nursing should not even handle finasteride pills (especially crushed or broken pills) to avoid teratogenic problems. Four percent of men aged 18 to 41 years of age taking finasteride may have decreased libido, erectile dysfunction, or a decreased volume of ejaculate. The drug must be taken indefinitely to maintain hair growth.

Although the only FDA-approved treatment for women with female pattern hair loss is 2% minoxidil, it may be that in some women (those with androgen excess would be better suited) that other antiandrogens such as finasteride, spironolactone, cyproterone acetate, and flutamide could prove helpful. I am not advocating these medications be used, but of these medications spironolactone is the most easily available and probably the safest. Flutamide has been associated (rarely) with hepatic deaths. None should be used in pregnant or lactating women.

Telogen Effluvium

Telogen effluvium is another important cause of diffuse non-scarring hair loss. It is the shedding of an abnormal number of hairs in the telogen (resting) phase.

A telogen effluvium may be triggered by

- childbirth,
- major illness,
- high fevers,
- medications (Table 28-4),
- rapid marked weight loss,
- possibly smoking,
- toxin exposure such as heavy metal intoxication, and
- virtually any major insult to the body that causes the ratio of telogen to anagen hairs to increase.

Within 2 or 3 months of the triggering event the person notices an abnormally large number of hairs coming out. It is usually reversible in 4 to 6 months. Some people with telogen effluvium may have a shortening of the

TABLE 28-4 ■ Some Drugs That Can Cause Alopecia

Allopurinol	Interferon
Amiodarone	Isoniazid
Amphetamine	Itraconazole
Anabolic steroids	Levodopa
ACE inhibitors	Lithium
Anticoagulants	Minoxidil (temporary)
Anticonvulsants	MAOI
Antifungals (in high dose)	Nicotinic acid
Antimalarlals	Nitrofurantoin
Antithyroid	NSAID
Benzimidazole	Oral contraceplive
β-Blockers	Progesterone
Bromocriptine	Retinoids
Captopril	Salicylates
Chemotherapeutic drugs	Sulfasalazine
Cholesterol-lowering agents	Tacrolimus
Cimetidine	Terfenadine
Colchicine	Testosterone
Corticosteroids	Tricyclic
Gentamicin	antidepressants
Gold	Vitamin A
Immunoglobulin	

Abbreviations: ACE, angiotensin-converting enzyme; MAOI, monamine oxidase inhibitors; NSAID, nonsteroidal anti-inflammatory drugs.

anagen phase, which leads to shorter hairs in addition. Multiple medications can cause hair loss by inducing a telogen effluvium but some medications such as chemotherapy agents cause an anagen effluvium because they interfere with mitosis. Because about 90% of scalp hairs are in anagen, there is an extremely marked hair loss with chemotherapy. Both hypothyroidism and perhaps low ferritin (less than 40) may trigger a telogen effluvium. There is a chronic telogen effluvium of unclear cause described primarily in middle aged women that affects the entire scalp, starts abruptly, often causes some temporal recession and fluctuates over a prolonged time.

Doing several hair pulls, which involves pulling firmly about 20 hairs between your fingers and extracting more than 2 hairs per pull, suggests a telogen effluvium. Inspecting the hair root under the microscope to make sure it is a telogen hair and not an abnormal anagen hair is important to clinch the diagnosis (and rule out loose anagen syndrome). Of course if a patient has vigorously shampooed and/or brushed their hair prior to seeing you the hair pull may not demonstrate an increased number of easily extractable telogen hairs. On the other hand, if a patient only shampoos and or brushes

their hair very infrequently, their hair pull test may be falsely elevated with excessively large numbers of telogen hairs.

Loose Anagen Syndrome

Loose anagen syndrome is a disorder usually presenting in young blond girls (but can present in adults) that is sporadic or inherited (as autosomal dominant with variable expression and incomplete penetrance) characterized by easily (and painlessly) plucked dystrophic scalp hairs. The plucked hairs have misshapen, irregular, shrunken roots that may have a "mousetail"–like or "loose-sock"–like appearance microscopically. Normal anagen hairs are not pulled out with a firm or gentle pull, but anagen hairs in this syndrome are very easily extracted. In this condition there is a weak adhesion between the hair shaft cuticle and the inner root sheath cuticle. This may present clinically as a diffuse or as a patchy hair loss. It may be associated with other entities such as alopecia areata, Noonan's syndrome, and AIDS. The condition may improve with age.

Alopecia Areata

Usually alopecia areata presents as a patchy hair loss, but sometimes it may present as a diffuse, and sometimes very severely diffuse, hair loss that has a fairly abrupt onset. Because gray or white hairs are lost preferentially to pigmented hair some people who say they "turned gray overnight" may have had salt and pepper hair and developed alopecia areata in which large numbers of their pigmented hairs were lost very rapidly (see alopecia areata discussion under patchy hair loss).

Patchy Nonscarring Alopecia

Patchy nonscarring alopecia is usually caused by

- tinea capitis (especially in children),
- alopecia areata,
- trichotillomania,
- syphilis,
- trauma from cosmetic procedures, and
- loose anagen syndrome.

Certainly a fungal culture and a blood serology to rule out syphilis are important in the proper evaluation of patchy nonscarring hair loss (see Table 28-2).

Tinea Capitis

Tinea capitis may be diagnosed with a KOH examination of the hair and or fungal culture of the hair. It should always be suspected in children with patchy hair loss on the scalp. Oral antifungals are needed to eradicate this problem. Oral griseofulvin is still the "gold standard" of treatment for children but oral terbinafine (Lamisil) or oral itraconazole (Sporanox) may also be used. Monitoring of liver enzymes should be done with these last two mentioned drugs.

Alopecia Areata

Presentation and Characteristics. Alopecia areata has a 0.1% to 0.2% prevalence in the general population. It may account for 1% to 3% of new patient visits to a dermatologist. It is a nonscarring, usually patchy, but sometimes diffuse, hair loss of unclear cause that probably is autoimmune (Fig. 28-1). It has typically an abrupt, asymptomatic onset. Usually the scalp is involved but any hair-bearing area of the body may be affected. At the margin of the bald spots there may be broken off hairs that are thicker distally and thinner proximally near the scalp like the top part of an exclamation point (!) and are very characteristic of this problem. Regrowth may be with white colored hair. In adults regrowth is often in 6 to 12 months.

Factors that bode a poor prognosis are young age at onset, extensive early hair loss (especially if a severe marginal hair loss called *ophiasis*), and associated atopy. If all the scalp hair is lost the term *alopecia totalis* (Fig. 28-2A) is used and if all the body hair is lost the term *alopecia universalis* is used (Fig. 28-2B). Nail pitting, longitudinal ridging, koilonychia, onycholysis, onychomadesis, and a host of other nail dystrophies may be associated in 10% to 66% of patients with alopecia areata and precede, accompany, or follow the hair disorder. An association of alopecia areata may be seen with multiple thyroid abnormalities including goiter, myxedema, and Hashimoto's thyroiditis. Patients are also more likely to have vitiligo, lupus, rheumatoid arthritis, pernicious anemia, inflammatory bowel disease, myasthenia gravis, lichen planus, or HIV infection. Patients with Down's syndrome, Turner's syndrome, and autoimmune polyglandular syndrome have an increased likelihood of developing alopecia areata.

Treatment. Treatments for alopecia areata are primarily

- topical steroids,
- topical anthralin,
- intralesional steroids,

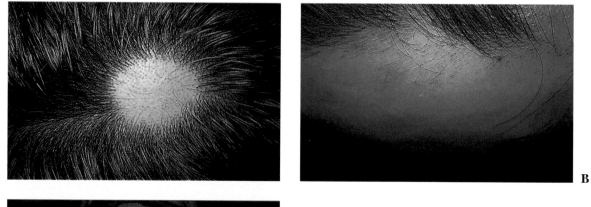

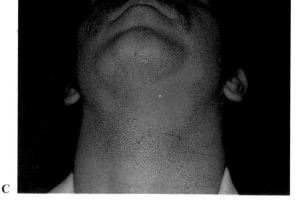

FIGURE 28-1 ■ Hair loss (alopecia) due to alopecia areata. (**A**) Alopecia areata of the scalp. (**B**) Alopecia areata with exclamation point hairs. (**C**) Alopecia areata of beard. *(Courtesy of Neutrogena Skin Care Institute.)*

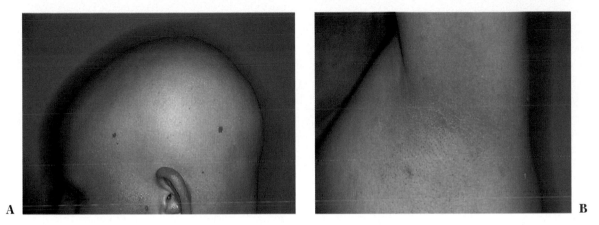

FIGURE 28-2 ■ **(A)** Alopecia areata totalis. **(B)** Alopecia areata universalis (axilla). *(Courtesy of Neutrogena Skin Care Institute.)*

- systemic steroids (not usually warranted),
- ultraviolet light therapy, and
- topical sensitizers (such as squaric acid dibutylester, dinitrochlorobenzene, and diphencyprone).

A hodgepodge of miscellaneous therapies have been used including cryotherapy, aromatherapy, and topical minoxidil. Keep in mind that none of these treatments are formally approved by the FDA and none are resoundingly effective. Topical anthralin (starting with short contact of 30 minutes) and topical steroids are probably the mainstay of therapy. Choosing fairly innocuous agents such as aromatherapy may also be added.

Keep in mind that in most cases regrowth is spontaneous. The National Alopecia Areata Foundation (P. O. Box 150760, San Rafael, CA 94915-0760; telephone 415-472-3780; www.naaf.org) provides support group information and a newsletter that patients may find helpful. Certainly patients with severe, longstanding hair loss may wish help with choosing hair pieces, which this organization can offer.

Trichotillomania

Trichotillomania (hair pulling) is much more common than once thought and may well have a prevalence of at least 1% (based on one survey). In some surveys of students in college, the prevalence is 3.4% of female and 1.5% of male students. These latter figures on prevalence do not fit rigid criteria for DSM-IV criteria. It may be that this disorder is heterogeneous with some patients, probably fitting the criteria for obsessive–compulsive disorder (OCD). Most patients are reluctant to admit to hair pulling because they are ashamed of the problem or afraid they will be viewed as "crazy" by their physician or close family members. The DSM-IV diagnostic criteria for trichotillomania includes:

1. Recurrent pulling out of one's hair resulting in noticeable hair loss (Fig. 28-3).
2. An increasing sense of tension immediately before pulling out the hair or when attempting to resist the behavior.
3. Pleasure, gratification, or relief when pulling out the hair.
4. The disturbance is not better accounted for by another mental disorder and is not due to a general medial condition (*e.g.*, a dermatologic condition).
5. The disturbance provokes clinically marked distress and/or impairment in occupation, social, or other areas of functioning.

Chronic hair pulling has been associated with depression, anxiety, psychosis, and dysthymia. In some young children it may be a transient problem; it also has been described with Sydenham's chorea. Certainly hair pulling may be seen with major mental retardation, schizophrenia, and in those with borderline personality disorder. In those patients in which OCD is suspected, behavioral therapy, oral clomipramine, or oral selective serotonin reuptake inhibitors (gradually going to the highest recommended dosage for at least 12 weeks) may prove helpful. Providing a warm nonjudgmental environment for these patients is invaluable for helping them. The problem tends to be chronic with exacerbations and remissions. If medication is used it should be used probably for at least a year and may have to be utilized again if relapse occurs. Educational material can be provided by the Trichotillomania Learning

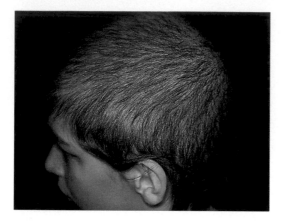

FIGURE 28-3 ■ Alopecia due to trichotillomania. *(Courtesy of Neutrogena Skin Care Institute.)*

Center (telephone: 831-457-1004), which may give these patients further support in dealing with this problem.

Syphilis

Secondary syphilis may cause a patchy or "moth-eaten" alopecia (typically) or it can cause a diffuse nonscarring alopecia. Treatment is discussed elsewhere in this textbook (see Chap. 22).

Trauma

Traumatic hair loss (Fig. 28-4) can result from chemical or physical trauma to the hair from hair grooming procedures such as permanents, relaxers, dyes, hot combs, or pulling the hair in tight braids. Usually this results in hair breakage rather than the hair coming out by the roots as it does in

these other causes of patchy nonscarring hair loss. Sometimes it can lead to a scarring hair loss. Loose anagen syndrome can cause diffuse or a patchy hair loss and has been discussed (see diffuse nonscarring hair loss).

Scarring Alopecia (Cicatricial Alopecia)

The clinical diagnosis of a scarring hair loss (Fig. 28-5) should point the physician toward performing a scalp skin biopsy and a fungal culture. Certainly diagnoses such as metastatic or benign tumors of the scalp, discoid lupus, sarcoid, lichen planopilaris (LPP), or scleroderma can be rapidly diagnosed with a biopsy. There is a larger, murkier group of scarring (cicatricial) alopecias that is undergoing constant renaming as our understanding (or attempts at understanding) these disorders evolves. Overall, scarring hair loss accounts for the minority (about 3.2%) of all hair loss. An excellent discussion by Tan sorts primary cicatricial alopecia into lymphocytic and neutrophilic types. Lymphocytic types are four times as common as neutrophilic types and more common in middle-aged women whereas neutrophilic types are more common in middle-aged men (see Table 28-2).

Lymphocytic Cicatricial Alopecias

Lymphocytic cicatricial alopecias include

- central centrifugal cicatricial alopecia (CCCA) (formerly called "hot comb alopecia" or more recently" follicular degeneration syndrome"),
- discoid lupus erythematosus,
- LPP (and its variant frontal fibrosing alopecia [FFA]), and
- pseudopelade (of Brocq).

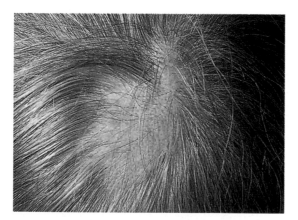

FIGURE 28-4 ■ Traumatic alopecia due to massage. *(Courtesy of Neutrogena Skin Care Institute.)*

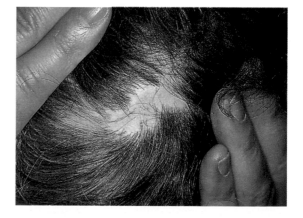

FIGURE 28-5 ■ Alopecia cicatrisata (scarring). *(Courtesy of Neutrogena Skin Care Institute.)*

CCCA probably accounts for most scarring hair loss (certainly in black patients). Discoid lupus is discussed elsewhere in this text (see Chap. 32).

CCCA is usually seen in black women and begins in the crown early on and may be confused with female pattern alopecia (and perhaps it is a scarring variant). Typically it is thought that the inherited types of hair loss are nonscarring, but perhaps this is not entirely true. It is slowly progressive. Certainly, ruling out traumatic alopecia is in order. In earlier days it was called "hot comb alopecia" and its causation attributed to hot comb use. Later on it was appreciated that there were women (as well as some men) who did not use hot combs and had a similar picture and the histology showed premature degeneration of the inner root sheath in many hair follicles.

- LPP presents typically in women as a patchy hair loss with perifollicular erythema, follicular spines, and scarring. About half these patients develop other skin, mucous membrane, or nail changes of lichen planus. Treatments usually include (topical and intralesional) steroids, and antimalarials. Sometimes retinoids, oral griseofulvin, cyclosporine, and methotrexate have been used. Some cases resolve spontaneously, others last for years; the average duration is 18 months.
- FFA*STYLE*, a variant of LPP, is usually seen in women in their 60s as a recession of the frontal and temporal hairline with perifollicular erythema within the marginal hairline that is asymptomatic. There may be loss of eyebrows as well. Histology is that of LPP and the treatment is the same as for LPP.
- Pseudopelade of Brocq is usually in women and presents as a noninflammatory, intermittently progressive, scarring alopecia of unknown cause that starts on the crown and spreads in a pseudopod-like fashion at irregular intervals and has been described as resembling "footprints in the snow" on the affected scalp.

Some people have used *pseudopelade* as an all-encompassing term for an end stage of various types of cicatricial alopecia of unclear cause, but that may be confusing. A "tufted folliculitis" may result as the end stage of multiple types of scarring alopecias. It has the clinical appearance of "doll's hair"–numerous hair shafts exiting out of one aperture in multiple plugs. It is not diagnostic of any one disease, just as *pseudopelade* is not.

Neutrophilic Cicatricial Alopecias

Neutrophilic cicatricial alopecias include folliculitis decalvans and dissecting cellulitis/folliculitis (perifolliculitis capitis abscedens et suffodiens). There is a cicatricial alopecia group in which the inflammatory infiltrate is mixed and this includes acne keloidalis (folliculitis keloidalis), acne (folliculitis) necrotica, and erosive pustular dermatosis.

- Folliculitis decalvans is a scarring folliculitis in which frequently *Staphylococcus aureus* (and sometimes other bacteria) is cultured but response to antibiotics is not always that robust. In addition to giving the appropriate antibacterial agent based on culture and sensitivity, sometimes rifampin at 300 mg twice daily in combination is helpful. In addition to being a good medication to eradicate staphylococci it is effective for gram negative as well as gram positive organisms. It is capable of killing bacteria that are engulfed by phagocytic cells (maybe one of the reasons it works so well in granulomatous diseases such as tuberculosis and leprosy). Rifampin does have numerous drug interactions and stains bodily fluids such as tears, saliva, perspiration, and urine a bright red color. Clindamycin at 300 mg/d can be used with rifampicin if other, safer antibiotics such as doxycycline are not effective but one should be aware of the risk of *Clostridium difficile*–induced diarrhea with clindamycin. Topical fusidic acid, oral zinc sulphate (400 mg/d), and steroids (topical and systemic), may be other considerations for therapy. It has been postulated that the condition is characterized by an altered immunologic response to a variety of organisms and an altered inflammatory foreign body response may play a role as well. Whether or not it is a subtype of CCCA is yet to be determined.
- Dissecting cellulitis is more common in young black men and begins as inflammatory, boggy nodules that drain with purulent drainage. Patients may be more likely to also have hidradenitis suppurativa and acne conglobata (often called the *follicular occlusion triad*). The cause is unknown and it tends to be a chronic problem. Usually it is not symptomatic but the disfiguring scarring and sometimes foul-smelling discharge are very problematic. Bacterial and fungal cultures should be performed. Treatment leaves a lot to be desired and has included various oral antibiotics (sometimes with the addition of rifampicin 600 mg/d to cephalexin or to ciprofloxacin), oral zinc sulphate

400 mg t.i.d. Oral isotretinoin (Accutane) is used in resistant cases for 4 to 5 months.

- The histologically mixed group of cicatricial alopecias includes acne keloidalis primarily. This is more common in young black men and starts as smooth papules and pustules on the occipital scalp and posterior neck that evolve into keloid-like plaques, It may be asymptomatic or may have associated mild burning or itching. In mild cases a topical antibiotic maybe helpful, but usually an oral antibiotic such as tetracycline (500 mg to 1 g total dose per day), doxycycline (100 to 200 m/d), minocycline (100 mg), or erythromycin (500 mg/d to 1 g/d) may prove helpful. Acne necrotica presents usually as papules or necrotic pustules that are on the scalp and perhaps the face, neck, and chest that may lead to varioliform scars. It can be scarring or nonscarring. Oral antibiotics, intralesional or topical steroids, and even oral isotretinoin may be helpful for treatment. Erosive pustular dermatosis is a pustular, necrotic, infundibular folliculitis with crusting that usually appears in older Caucasian women and later on has features of folliculitis decalvans.

Another manner of categorizing scarring hair loss was proffered by Sperling (in 2000) as CCCA (which encompasses pseudopelade, folliculitis decalvans, acne keloidalis, and dissecting folliculitis); LPP (with FFA as a subcategory); and lupus. The exact overlap and exclusivity of these diseases is constantly evolving.

Miscellaneous Hair Diseases

- *Trichorrhexis nodosa* is the most common hair shaft disorder and most commonly is acquired secondary to damage from hair grooming procedures although it may be associated with hypothyroidism and with other rarer syndromes such as argininosuccinicaciduria or Menkes' syndrome. Severe scratching or other trauma as seen with lichen simplex chronicus or trichotillomania may lead to this hair shaft abnormality. Clinically, it presents as tiny white specks on the hair shaft that may superficially look like nits from head lice. When viewed microscopically these specks resemble the bristles of two broom ends interlocked and are the site of fractures. This condition is more likely to occur proximally in black hair and more distally in Caucasian or Asian hair. The resulting breakage may lead to the clinical complaint of the hair not growing very long.

- *Uncombable hair syndrome* ("spun glass hair") is an interesting hair shaft abnormality in which the hair shafts in cross-section are triangular and on electron microscopy there are longitudinal grooves. The onset is usually around 3 years of age when the hair seems particularly wild and unruly. Typically the hair is a silver-blond color and the problem may be generalized (usually) or localized. Spontaneous improvement may occur in childhood. Oral biotin may prove helpful. This same triangular hair-shaft abnormality has been described in loose anagen syndrome and after spironolactone therapy.

- *Acquired progressive kinking* of the hair is an odd entity that usually arises in the teens or early adult years in young white men. Gradually the hair becomes kinky, dry, and more unmanageable. The hair shaft is said to be elliptical with partial twists at irregular intervals. The anagen (growth) phase is said to be diminished. Oral retinoids or local radiation may induce a clinically similar problem. Interestingly, a seemingly converse clinical picture has been described in people of color with the acquired immunodeficiency syndrome who develop softer, silkier hair that replaces previously normal kinky hair. In addition, the color is said to become ashen and the hair becomes sparse.

- *Trichoptilosis* ("split ends") is the longitudinal splitting of the distal hair shaft as a result of weathering and is made more striking by overuse of various cosmetic hair styling and grooming procedures. Hair pulling and scratching may be causative. Various unusual inherited hair shaft defects are more prone to trichoptilosis.

- *Bubble hair* is the result of excessive heat from hair dryers (and perhaps other chemical treatments of the hair) leading to distinctive "bubbles" within the hair shaft. These hairs may appear brittle and broken off. Interestingly with thallium intoxication a bubble-like inclusion can be seen within the hair shaft; typically thallium intoxication leads to massive hair loss.

- *Pseudofolliculitis barbae* is a problem typically seen in the beard area of black men caused by close shaving in curly or kinky hair that may cause the newly emerging hair shaft to grow back into the skin surface or pierce the follicular wall, causing inflammation. Clinically it presents as papulopustules that may lead to hyperpigmentation and scarring. Hair plucking and electrolysis can induce the same type of problem. The best treatment is to avoid shaving or at least avoid close shaving. Topical tretinoin (Retin-A) and or topical eflornithine hydrochloride (used for treatment of hypertrichosis) may prove helpful. A similar problem can be seen with closing shaving in the axillae and in the pubic area.

■ *Green hair* may result from the deposition of copper on light-colored hair from tap water used to shampoo or from water in a swimming pool. Pretreating the hair with some types of conditioners may help prevent the discoloration. Shampooing with a penicillamine-containing mixture may reduce the green color. (Copper intoxication from ingestion in tap water can cause a diffuse alopecia).

■ *Trichomegaly* is the development of abnormally long eyelashes and can be seen in patients with AIDS, underlying malignancy (such as adenocarcinoma), kala-azar, various unusual syndromes in which it is just one feature (such as dwarfism or Cornelia-de-Lange syndrome), or certain medications (α-interferon or latanoprost [which is an analog of prostaglandin $F_{2\alpha}$ used topically for treatment of chronic open-angle glaucoma], and perhaps also with cyclosporine).

Suggested Reading

Abramowicz M. Propecia and Rogaine extra strength for alopecia. Med Lett 1998;40:25.

Bernard J, ed. Ethnic hair and skin: What is the state of the science. J Am Acad Dermatol 2003;48(Suppl 6).

Camacho F, Montagna W. Trichology, diseases of the pilosebaceous follicle. Basel, S. Karger Publisher, 1998.

Dawber R. Disease of Hair and Scalp. Oxford, Blackwell Scicnce, 1997.

Dawber R, Van Neste D. Hair and scalp disorders: Common presenting signs, differential diagnosis and treatment. Philadelphia, Lippincott, 1995.

Headington JT. Telogen effluvium: New concepts and review. Arch Dermatol 1993;129:356.

Hordinsky MK. Alopecias. In Bolognia J, Rapini, RP, Jorizzo JL, eds, Dermatology. New York, Mosby Publishers, 2003, pp. 1033–1050.

Kossard S, Lee MS, Wilkinson B. Postmenopausal frontal fibrosing alopecia: A frontal variant of lichen planopilaris. J Am Acad Dermatol 1997;36:59.

Leung AKC, Robson WLM. Hirsutism. Int J Dermatol 1993;32:773.

Nuss MA, Carlisle D, Hall M, et al. Trichotillomania: A review and case report. Cutis 2003;72:191.

Olsen EA. Disorders of hair growth: Diagnosis and treatment. New York, McGraw-Hill, 2003.

Olsen EA. Female pattern hair loss. J Am Acad Dermatol 2001;45:S70.

Tan E, Martinka M, et al. Primary cicatricial alopecias: Clinicopathology of 112 cases. J Am Acad Dermatol 2004;50:2.

Wendelin DS, Pope DN, Mallory S. Hypertrichosis. J Am Acad Dermatol 2003;48:161.

Whiting DA. Update on hair disorders. Dermatol Clin 1996;14(4).

Whiting DA, Howsden FL. Color atlas of differential diagnosis of hair loss. Cedar Grove, NJ, Canfield Publishing, 1996.

CHAPTER 29

Diseases Affecting the Nail

Adam I. Rubin, MD, and Richard K. Scher, MD

The nail unit is an essential component of the integumentary system and can be affected primarily by dermatologic disorders or can provide the first clue to serious systemic illness. Certain nail disorders, such as subungual melanoma, are life threatening. The nail unit serves a variety of functions, including digit protection, improved agility in handling and picking up of small objects, and enhancing the transmission of delicate sensations. Disorders of the nail unit can be very distressing to patients, because nails often serve as a point of cosmetic enhancement and focus of the digits. This chapter reviews common and serious nail disorders, including those caused by infectious, traumatic, neoplastic, congenital, and primary dermatologic disorders.

When evaluating a patient with a nail disorder, a complete history and physical examination should be performed. A medication history is essential. If the patient has any systemic diseases, this should be noted. The family history can give clues to hereditary nail abnormalities as can be found in the nail–patella syndrome (osteo-onychodysplasia), pachyonychia congenita, or Darier's disease (keratosis follicularis). An occupational history can provide insight into possible allergic or irritant chemical exposures. Treatments to the nails by prior physicians, with home remedies, and at nail salons are important to note and can sometimes be factors contributing to persistent nail disease. All of the nails on the hands and feet should be examined. A magnifying glass and/or dermatoscope can be employed to enhance fine details. A complete skin examination, including the oral mucosa, is important; subtle lesions can give clues as to the cause of a nail disorder in question. Laboratory investigations frequently employed in the evaluation of nail disease include biopsy of the nail plate and nail matrix, fungal cultures, bacterial cultures, and potassium hydroxide preparations. Imaging modalities including x-ray and magnetic resonance imaging, can be helpful in determining the extent of disease that presents in the nail unit.

Anatomy of the Nail Unit

The nail unit is a specialized appendage of the skin, composed of unique structures not found elsewhere in the body. The nail unit consists of the proximal and lateral nail folds, the nail matrix, the nail bed, and the hyponychium (Fig. 29-1). What most people commonly consider the "nail" refers to the nail plate. This is the clear, firm section of the nail that is made of hard keratin. The nail plate is created by the nail matrix, a section of germative cells located proximal to the nail plate. The nail matrix contains a layer of actively dividing keratinocytes that mature and, after death, contribute to the formation of the nail plate. The nail plate is bordered by the proximal nail fold and two lateral nail folds. The lunula is the most distal portion of the matrix and is seen as a white, arched area under the nail plate and bordered by the proximal nail fold. The nail plate sits on top of the nail bed, which is highly vascular. The hyponychium is the section of skin located under the free edge of the nail plate between the nail bed and the distal nail groove.

Fingernails grow constantly at a rate of 0.1 mm per day or 3 mm per month. At this rate, a fingernail can be totally replaced in 4 to 6 months. Toenails, however, grow at about half this rate. It can take 8 to 12 months for a toenail to be totally replaced by a new nail. Certain disease states such as psoriasis, minor trauma, pityriasis rubra pilaris, the brittle nail syndrome, hyperpituitarism, and hyperthyroidism can cause nails to grow at a faster rate than normal. Slower nail growth has been noted in patients with malnutrition, acute infections, peripheral neuropathy, onychomycosis, and hypothyroidism as well as in smokers. Nail growth can be faster or slower secondary to a variety of medications.

Onychomycosis

Onychomycosis refers to fungal infection of the nail. Onychomycosis is the most common nail disorder and accounts for up to half of all nail problems encountered

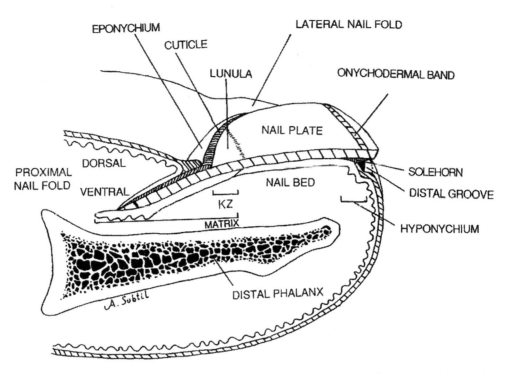

FIGURE 29-1 ■ Anatomy of the nail unit (KZ, keratogenous zone). *(Reprinted from Atlas of Hair and Nails, Hordinsky, Sawaya, and Scher, Chapter: Histology of the Normal Nail Unit, Page 19, Copyright 2000, with permission from Elsevier.)*

in clinical practice. More than 90% of cases of onychomycosis are caused by the dermatophytes *Trichophyton rubrum* and *T. mentagrophytes*. The prevalence of onychomycosis has been shown to be higher in older age groups. Risk factors for developing onychomycosis include smoking, peripheral arterial disease, diabetes mellitus, and HIV infection. Onychomycosis has been classified into five major types:

- distal and lateral subungual onychomycosis,
- superficial onychomycosis,
- endonyx onychomycosis,
- proximal subungual onychomycosis, and
- total dystrophic onychomycosis.

Clinical signs of onychomycosis include

- thickening of the nail bed and nail plate,
- subungual debris,
- onycholysis (separation of the nail plate from the nail bed),
- nail discoloration,
- ridging of the nail, and
- nail pitting.

Diagnosis

Diagnosis of onychomycosis is made by identifying fungal infection of the nail by direct microscopy of nail debris using a potassium hydroxide (KOH) preparation, fungal culture, or histologic examination of the nail plate stained with periodic acid-Schiff (PAS) stain.

Presentation and Characteristics

Distal and lateral subungual onychomycosis are the most common form of onychomycosis (Fig. 29-2). The hyponychium or the lateral nail folds are the first sites of fungal invasion. Onycholysis occurs when subungual keratotic debris separates the nail plate from the nail bed. Beside subungual hyperkeratosis and onycholysis, it has been noted that paronychia can also occur with distal and lateral subungual onychomycosis. Dermatophytes such as *T. rubrum* and *T. mentagrophytes* are the most common fungi to cause distal and lateral subungual onychomycosis. *Candida albicans* and *C. parapsilosis* are less frequently responsible. The most common nondermatophyte mold reported to cause distal and lateral subungual onychomycosis in a multicenter study population is *Scopulariopsis brevicaulis*.

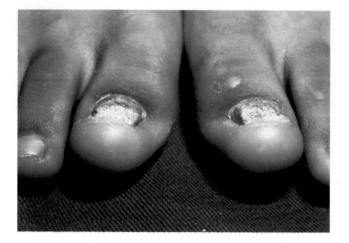

FIGURE 29-2 ■ Distal and lateral subungual onychomycosis.

Superficial onychomycosis can be divided into superficial white onychomycosis and superficial black onychomycosis. Superficial white onychomycosis is also known as *leukonychia trichophytica* and *leukonychia mycotica*. It is usually found on the toenails. The exposed surface of the nail plate is the initial site of fungal invasion. Clinically, it presents on the nail plate as superficial white patches with distinct edges. If left untreated, more developed lesions can have a yellow color. The infectious fungi can often be scraped from the nail plate surface. Superficial white onychomycosis is most often caused by the dermatophyte *T. mentagrophytes*. Molds such as *Aspergillus, Acremonium,* and *Fusarium* spp. can also cause superficial white onychomycosis. Superficial black onychomycosis has a similar clinical presentation to superficial white onychomycosis, with the distinction being that the invading fungi are black in color. This type of onychomycosis has been reported to be caused by *Scytalydium dimidiatum* and *T. rubrum.*

Endonyx onychomycosis is the type of onychomycosis in which both the superficial and deep layers of the nail plate are infected by fungi, without involving the nail bed. Tunnels formed by invading fungi may be present. Clinically, this can appear as a "milky-white" discoloration of the nail plate that is not accompanied by subungual hyperkeratosis or onycholysis. There is lamellar splitting of the nail plate. Endonyx onychomycosis is caused by *T. soudanese* and *T. violaceum.*

Proximal subungual onychomycosis occurs by fungal invasion at the proximal nail fold. It appears clinically as a discoloration of the nail plate extending from the proximal nail fold and involving the area of the lunula. The distal end of the nail plate appears normal in early infection. It is most often caused by the molds *Aspergillus, Fusarium,* and *Scopulariopsis* spp. Proximal subungual onychomycosis caused by molds can result in an inflammatory response, and is often accompanied by a paronychia. A rapidly progressive subtype of proximal subungual onychomycosis is proximal white subungual onychomycosis that has been seen in patients infected with HIV. The clinical presentation is similar to that described, with the distinction that the discoloration at the proximal nail fold is white (leukonychia). In this patient population, the cause is usually *T. rubrum.* Because of this association with HIV, a clinician should consider laboratory testing to investigate a patient's immune status when a diagnosis of superficial white onychomycosis especially proximally is made.

Total dystrophic onychomycosis, or secondary total dystrophic onychomycosis, usually occurs because of extensive fungal infection involving the entire nail plate from distal and lateral subungual onychomycosis or proximal subungual onychomycosis. The entire nail plate is extensively thickened and can easily collapse. Primary total dystrophic onychomycosis is seen in patients with chronic mucocutaneous candidiasis, and is caused by infection of all portions of the nail unit by *Candida.*

Differential Diagnosis

A variety of disease states affecting the nail can mimic onychomycosis and should be considered in the differential diagnosis. These possible simulators of onychomycosis include psoriasis, chronic onycholysis, lichen planus, alopecia areata, chronic paronychia, hemorrhage/trauma, onychogryphosis, aging, median canaliform dystrophy, pincer nail deformity, yellow nail syndrome, subungual malignant melanoma, and subungual squamous cell carcinoma. One must also recognize that any of these disease states can coexist with onychomycosis, and proof of dermatophyte infection in the nail (Fig. 29-3) does not exclude a separate, concurrent disease occurring in the nail unit.

Treatment

Therapy for onychomycosis includes oral and topical medication, as well as periodic clipping and filing of infected portions of the nail plate. Superficial onychomycosis often responds to topical therapy alone. The first-line oral treatment for onychomycosis is terbinafine 250 mg/d (12 weeks for toenails and 6 for fingernails). Terbinafine is an allylamine antifungal medication that is fungicidal. Other options of systemic medications for onychomycosis include the azole antifungal drugs itraconazole and fluconazole. Itraconazole can be given as 100 mg twice daily (12 weeks for toenails or 6 for fingernails). Alternatively, itraconazole can be "pulsed" at 200 mg twice daily for 1 week per month (total of 3 months for toenails and 2 for fingernails).

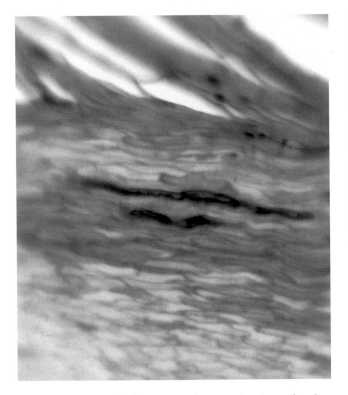

FIGURE 29-3 ■ High power microscopic view of a dermatophyte in nail plate (PAS stain; original magnification400×. *(Courtesy of Dr. George W. Niedt).*

Various pulse therapies have also been advocated for oral terbinafine therapy by some authors. Fluconazole can be dosed from 150 to 300 mg once per week until the nails are clear. Griseofulvin is no longer used frequently for onychomycosis for a variety of reasons, one of which is that it is taken until there is clinical cure, much longer than the therapies mentioned. Ketoconazole has also been used for onychomycosis, but less frequently now than in the past because of possible hepatotoxicity. In a meta-analysis of randomized clinical trials, terbinafine was superior to placebo, itraconazole, and griseofulvin in achieving mycological cure in patients with onychomycosis.

Topical ciclopirox nail lacquer is often used as an adjunctive treatment to improve cure rates. Factors indicating a likely poor response to treatment with oral therapy alone include lateral nail disease, involvement of the entire nail unit, longitudinal streaks of fungal infection in the nail plate, presence of a dermatophytoma (a mass of fungi between the nail plate and nail bed), and extensive onycholysis. If a dermatophytoma is present, removing the portion of nail plate overlying it and removing the concentration of fungi can help to achieve a cure. Ciclopirox has a broad range of antifungal activity against dermatophytes, as well

as *C. albicans*. Additionally, ciclopirox has antibacterial and anti-inflammatory actions. This medication can be particularly useful in patients with onychomycosis who cannot tolerate oral antifungal medication because of the presence of liver or kidney disease, or those taking multiple systemic medications where drug interactions may be a concern.

Onychomycosis is difficult to cure permanently. Many patients have recurrent infections. Factors leading to recurrent disease include persistent predisposing factors such as peripheral vascular disease or diabetes mellitus, trauma, as well as insufficient treatment from early termination of treatment or insufficient dose of medication. A variety of measures have been suggested to avoid recurrence of onychomycosis. These actions include wearing footwear when walking in areas of high concentrations of dermatophytes (*e.g.,* communal areas by pools, spas), avoiding shoes that may have dermatophytes present, drying feet (and interdigital spaces) after a bath or shower, using socks made of absorbent material, treating concurrent tinea pedis, and considering the prophylactic use of topical antifungal agents.

Nail Psoriasis

Nail involvement in psoriasis patients is common, occurring in up to half of all patients with skin psoriasis. Clinical features include

- pitting,
- discoloration,
- onycholysis,
- subungual hyperkeratosis,
- nail plate crumbling and grooving, and
- splinter hemorrhages (Fig. 29-4).

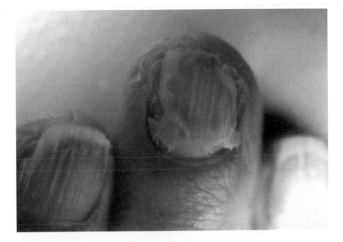

FIGURE 29-4 ■ Nail psoriasis.

Nail pits, the most common sign, are formed by small psoriatic lesions in the proximal nail matrix, which forms the superficial layers of the nail plate. The oil drop sign, a yellow-red discoloration of the nail plate, found in psoriatic nails, is caused by inclusion of neutrophils and exudates between the nail bed and nail plate. Nail changes in psoriasis are variable, ranging from a few pits to total nail dystrophy. Psoriasis can affect all of the components of the nail unit, and biopsy from affected areas including the proximal nail fold, nail plate, nail bed, and matrix may be appropriate to establish the diagnosis.

Diagnosis

Pustular psoriasis of the nails (also known as *acrodermatitis continua of Hallopeau*) is a variant of nail psoriasis in which the characteristic clinical features include periungual or subungual pustules (Fig. 29-5). Pustular psoriasis of the nails can be difficult to distinguish from other nail disorders. In an evaluation of 38 patients with pustular psoriasis of the nails, all of whom had been evaluated by a prior physician, 35 (92%) had not been correctly diagnosed. The diagnosis of pustular psoriasis of the nails should be considered in patients with recurrent subungual and periungual pustules, recurrent painful onycholysis, and patients with painful dystrophic and crusted nails. Nail bed biopsy can be useful in confirming the diagnosis of pustular psoriasis of the nails.

Treatment

Treatment of nail psoriasis requires patience, as correction of abnormal findings can require up to 6 months to show in fingernails and even longer in toenails. The mainstay of psoriatic nail treatment is injected steroid, usually triamcinolone acetonide 2.5% to 10% to the nail matrix. Topical therapies for nail psoriasis include

- corticosteroids,
- vitamin D analogs,
- 5-fluorouracil, and
- topical psoralen plus ultraviolet A (PUVA) therapy.

Other local therapies that have shown efficacy in treating psoriatic nails include

- superficial radiotherapy,
- electron beam therapy, and
- Grenz ray therapy.

Systemic therapies used to treat skin psoriasis, including cyclosporine, acitretin, and methotrexate, have also been effective in treating psoriatic nail disease. For the treatment of pustular psoriasis of the nail, systemic retinoids have been recommended for severe relapses and topical calcipotriol for maintenance therapy in patients with multiple nail involvement. For patients with one or two affected nails, topical calcipotriol alone is suggested.

Subungual Hematoma

A common problem encountered by both dermatologists and primary care physicians is the subungual hematoma, a collection of blood beneath the nail plate. Clinically, it appears as a bluish or violaceous discoloration under the nail plate (Fig. 29-6). The hematoma can produce a significant amount of pressure in the space between the nail bed and nail plate, causing intense pain. The most common cause of subungual hematoma is trauma to the nail: either a sudden, strong, external force, or repeated minor traumatic events occurring over time. Subungual hematomas form easily because the nail bed is a highly vascular structure, prone to bleeding if traumatized.

Diagnosis

The most important distinction a physician must make regarding the evaluation of a discoloration under the nail plate is differentiating a subungual hematoma from a subungual melanoma. Differentiation between these two entities can be partially clarified by the clinical history. A rapidly developing lesion with a history of trauma is more likely to be a subungual hematoma. However, one must remember that some patients with subungual melanoma also report a history of trauma. Only a biopsy can render a final diagnosis.

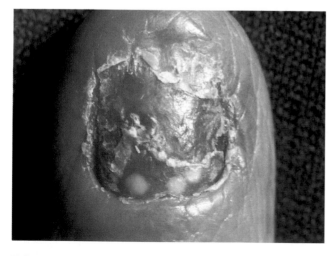

FIGURE 29-5 ■ Pustular nail psoriasis.

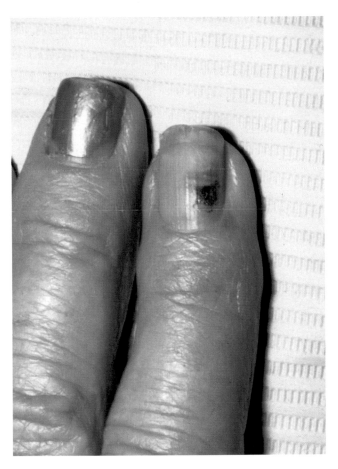

FIGURE 29-6 ■ Subungual hematoma.

Treatment

The classic treatment for a subungual hematoma is nail trephining, which removes the collection of blood under the nail plate. This maneuver relieves the pressure in the confined space created by the hematoma and delivers rapid relief of pain. A number of instruments have been used for this purpose, including a heated paper clip, heated needle, scalpel blade, cautery device, and carbon dioxide laser. The use of an extra-fine insulin syringe needle for the evacuation of subungual hematoma has been reported. To avoid secondary nail dystrophy resulting from the subungual hematoma, it is recommended that evacuation not be delayed past 6 to 12 hours after injury. Nail avulsion is a more drastic measure but also allows for evacuation of the hematoma. A study of 123 patients with 127 subungual hematomas showed that the majority of patients required only simple trephining for symptomatic relief, and that aggressive surgical treatment was unnecessary.

Pincer Nail

The pincer nail deformity is defined as a transverse overcurvature of the nail plate, progressively pinching the nail bed. The lateral edges of the nail plate can break through the skin, resulting in granulation tissue formation (Fig. 29-7). There can be a trumpet-like appearance when the curvature increases from the proximal to distal portion. Involvement of the toenails is more common than the fingernails. A patient's life can be greatly affected by the pain, inflammation, difficulty with ill-fitting footwear, and an undesirable cosmetic appearance. Pincer nails can be both familial and acquired. In the hereditary form, involvement is usually symmetric, whereas acquired pincer nails generally do not show symmetric involvement.

Pincer nails can be divided into three clinical types. The most common form is the trumpet nail deformity described. The second clinical type of pincer nail is the tile-shaped nail, which displays an even, transverse overcurvature with the lateral nail plate edges remaining parallel. The third form of pincer nail is the pilicated nail, which shows a less drastic overcurvature with one or both lateral nail plate edges forming a vertical sheet pressing into the lateral nail groove.

Diagnosis

There are a variety of causes of acquired pincer nails. The most common cause is deviation of the phalanges of the feet secondary to ill-fitting shoes. The most common skin disease causing an acquired pincer nail deformity is psoriasis. When tumors, such as an exostosis, implantation cyst, or myxoid cyst, are responsible for the pincer nail deformity, removal of the tumor may reverse the nail defect.

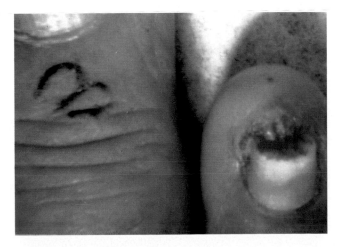

FIGURE 29-7 ■ Pincer nail.

Pincer nails have also been reported in association with metastasis of colon carcinoma. Other causes of acquired pincer nail deformity include nail infection with the dermatophyte *T. rubrum*, placement of an arteriovenous fistula for hemodialysis, and use of β-blocker medications. Finger pincer nail deformity can be seen in association with osteoarthritis.

Treatment

Treatment of the pincer nail can be attempted without surgery by use of a brace placed on the nail plate and fixed on the lateral edges. This brace can be gradually adjusted and results in flattening of the nail plate. Recurrences with this method are common. Nail avulsion has not been shown to be a successful treatment, and in fact can aggravate the problem. Successful surgical treatments have corrected the pincer nail deformity by selective destruction of the lateral matrix horns. Further improvement can be obtained by surgically removing any possible bony defects contributing to the nail deformity. Permanent destruction of the nail matrix by phenol or surgical ablation may be required as a last resort.

Onychocryptosis (Ingrown Nails)

Onychocryptosis occurs most commonly when the distal lateral edge of the nail plate presses on the nail fold resulting in inflammation and soft tissue hypertrophy, which can become secondarily infected. The great toenail is the most often affected site (Fig. 29-8). This condition can be painful for patients and significantly restrict mobility. Heifitz has classified onychocryptosis into stages, depending on the extent of disease. Stage I is pain with mild nail fold erythema and swelling. Stage II is swelling, drainage, and ulceration of the nail fold. Stage III is chronic inflammation with granulation tissue and extensive nail fold hypertrophy.

Diagnosis

Onychocryptosis is often caused by, and is associated with, onychomycosis, resulting in a thickened and dystrophic nail. Incorrect technique in nail trimming can cause onychocryptosis. This occurs when the nail plate corners are cut in a curved manner and not allowed to grow over the toe. Other conditions predisposing patients to onychocryptosis include arthritis, circulatory disorders, hyperhidrosis, and obesity. In younger patients, repetitive trauma, and poor foot hygiene are thought to contribute to this problem.

Treatment

Early disease can be treated with nonsurgical therapy including the placement of a barrier (such as a wedge of fabric treated with an antiseptic solution) between the nail plate and nail fold that stays in place until the nail plate grows beyond the end of the toe. A separate option is excising the portion of the nail plate which is pressing on the nail fold. With the offending area removed, the inflamed nail fold can recover to its normal state while new nail forms. If the area is secondarily infected, antibiotics should be included in the regimen. Ablation of the nail matrix corresponding to the excised segment of the nail plate, known as "angular phenolization," is a useful adjunctive treatment. Phenol is applied to the exposed area of the nail matrix and destroys that area of nail production. Angular phenolization can be complicated by prolonged healing times. Another maneuver, known as the "Zadik procedure," involves avulsing the whole nail plate and then destroying the entire nail matrix. This procedure prevents any nail regrowth, and greatly reduces recurrence rates of onychocryptosis.

Racket Nail

The racket nail is named after its similarity in shape to a tennis racket. The nail is short, broad, and flat. The cause is not because of the nail itself, but occurs rather in response to a deformity in the underlying soft tissue. The most common location is the thumb involved alone, but other digits may be involved as well. It is found more often in women, and affected patients are normal otherwise. Racket nails may be inherited in an autosomal dominant manner. One or both hands can be affected. This finding can be a source of embarrassment to patients, but does not otherwise affect functioning of the affected digit. Most cases of racket nail

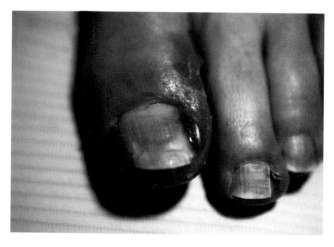

FIGURE 29-8 ■ Onychocryptosis.

are congenital, but an acquired case of racket nails was reported in association with tertiary hyperparathyroidism.

Habit-Tic Deformity

The habit-tic deformity presents as evenly spaced, parallel transverse grooves with central depression in the nail plate (Fig. 29-9). The lunula is enlarged and the cuticle is often disrupted. The most commonly affected site is the thumb nail, but other nails can also be affected. This deformity is caused by repeated trauma to the nail matrix at the proximal nail fold secondary to picking. This can be a conscious or unconscious habit developed by the patient. Body dysmorphic disorder, obsessive–compulsive disorder, and other psychiatric illnesses that involve a loss of impulse control can include ritualistic nail picking as part of the disease spectrum. The picking action can also be a nervous habit, unrelated to a specific psychiatric disorder. A case of the habit-tic deformity responding to treatment with fluoxetine (Prozac) has been reported.

Median Canaliform Dystrophy

Median canaliform dystrophy, also known as *dystrophia unguium mediana canaliformis,* is a nail plate defect in which a median (central) ridge develops, with short transverse ridges running from both sides of the central split. This has been described as an "inverted fir tree configuration." The thumb nails are the site most commonly affected. Median canaliform dystrophy can be hereditary. In most cases, an inciting cause cannot be identified, and the nails normalize in a period of months to years. Although the pathogenesis of this disorder is not known, it is speculated that localized dyskeratinization of the nail matrix may be responsible. Self-inflicted damage to the middle part of the

posterior nail fold has also been speculated to be the cause of median canaliform dystrophy. There are three case reports identifying three patients who developed median canaliform dystrophy after treatment with isotretinoin for acne. In all cases, the nail changes reverted to normal after discontinuation of the drug.

Trachyonychia

Trachyonychia means "rough nails" and can be associated with a variety of dermatoses including

- lichen planus,
- psoriasis,
- alopecia areata,
- atopic dermatitis, and
- ichthyosis vulgaris.

It has also been associated with immunoglobulin A deficiency. The clinical appearance of trachyonychia has been described as having a "sandpapered" appearance, with a rough, lusterless nail plate (Fig. 29-10). The presence of numerous small, superficial pits in the nail plate in less severe cases can cause the nail to appear shiny. One or more nails can be affected. When all 20 nails are affected, this condition is known as "twenty nail dystrophy." The peak incidence is between 3 and 12 years of age. Trachyonychia usually resolves with time when it occurs as a consequence of lichen planus in children. Identification of a specific cause can be accomplished by nail matrix biopsy.

Treatment

Local treatment of trachyonychia can be accomplished with intralesional triamcinolone acetonide into the proximal nail folds, as well as topical PUVA. A case report shows

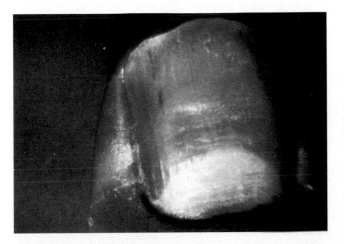

FIGURE 29-9 ■ Habit-tic deformity.

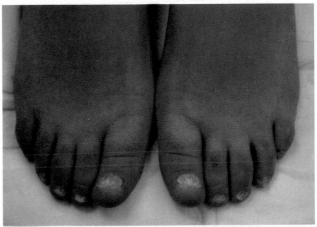

FIGURE 29-10 ■ Trachyonychia.

a beneficial effect of topical 5% 5-flurouracil cream in the treatment of psoriatic trachyonychia.

Brittle nails

Nails can be considered brittle when they are easily damaged (Fig. 29-11). The free end of the nail plate is often affected by longitudinal or horizontal cracking or splitting. Dehydration causes loss of flexibility and elasticity of the nail plate. This can occur commonly in patients who are exposed to solvents. The amino acid cysteine has been found to be decreased in brittle nails. Dermatoses such as psoriasis, lichen planus, and alopecia areata can be associated with brittle nails.

Several systemic diseases are associated with brittle nails, including

- tuberculosis,
- endocrinopathies,
- iron deficiency anemia,
- hemochromatosis,
- glucagonoma, and
- vitamin deficiencies.

Treatment

Treatment should first address any dermatologic or systemic disease that may be contributing to brittle nails. Cases of brittle nails can be divided into nails that are hard and brittle and nails that are soft and brittle. Hard and brittle nails develop as a result of too little moisture, and the treatment goal is nail plate rehydration with the addition of a humidifier to the surrounding environment, daily emolliation, and nighttime nail soaks in water followed by urea or lactic acid creams. The nail plate can also be massaged with mineral oil after soaking to prevent drying. Soft and brittle nails develop as a result of too much moisture. The treatment goal here is to avoid excess moisture by the use of cotton gloves under vinyl gloves for wet work, and avoidance of irritants. Oral biotin, a B-complex vitamin, is considered the systemic treatment of choice for brittle nails. The recommended dose is 2.5 mg/d, taken for 3 to 6 months. The average time before clinical improvement is seen with biotin therapy is 2 months.

Longitudinal Melanonychia (Melanonychia Striata)

Longitudinal melanonychia refers to a tan, brown, or black longitudinal band or streak affecting a nail (Fig. 29-12). One or multiple nails can be involved. When multiple bands are present, the inciting cause is most likely non-neoplastic. Causes of multiple bands of longitudinal melanonychia include

- dermatologic disorders (Laugier-Hunziker syndrome, lichen planus, lichen striatus),
- drugs (antimalarials, ketoconazole, minocycline, zidovudine, many chemotherapeutic agents),
- bacterial and fungal infections,
- racial variation (African American, Hispanic, Indian, Japanese),

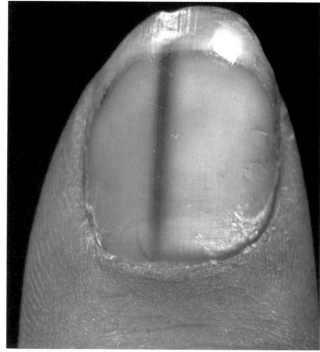

FIGURE 29-12 ■ Longitudinal melanonychia.

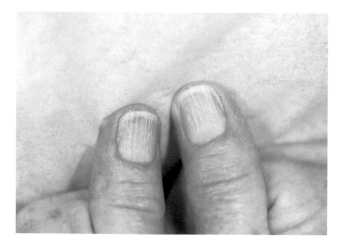

FIGURE 29-11 ■ Brittle nails.

- a variety of systemic diseases (Addison's disease, hyperbilirubinemia, hyperthyroidism, malnutrition, Peutz-Jeghers syndrome, porphyria, and others).

The diagnosis of a nail unit melanoma is always in the differential diagnosis of longitudinal melanonychia, and can only be established or excluded by biopsy.

Presentation and Characteristics

A variety of other causes can be responsible for the clinical presentation of longitudinal melanonychia. Pigment present from exogenous sources, such as dirt, tobacco, or tar, can usually be scratched off the nail plate. These sources usually do not present as a longitudinal streak. Nail plate infection with gram negative bacteria, such as *Klebsiella* and *Proteus* spp. can cause longitudinal melanonychia. When a greenish discoloration is present, infection with *Pseudomonas aeruginosa* is likely. Bacterial infection causing a pigmented streak usually presents at the junction of the lateral and proximal nail folds. The border of this streak is usually variable. Fungal infections of the nail plate can also cause hyperpigmented streaks. These streaks are usually wider distally than proximally. Subungual hematomas caused by repeated minor trauma, usually from shoe friction, can cause an elliptical streak similar to longitudinal melanonychia. Local irradiation has also been reported to cause longitudinal melanonychia. A variety of melanocytic lesions, including acquired and congenital melanocytic nevi, benign and atypical melanocytic hyperplasias, and melanoma, can cause longitudinal melanonychia.

Situations in which ungual melanoma should be suspected in the presence of longitudinal melanonychia include longitudinal melanonychia, which

- begins in a single digit of a person during the fourth to sixth decade of life or later,
- develops abruptly in a previously normal nail plate,
- becomes suddenly darker or wider than 5 mm,
- occurs in the thumb, index finger, or great toe,
- occurs in a person with a history of digital trauma,
- occurs singly in the digit of a dark-skinned patient,
- demonstrates blurred lateral borders,
- occurs in a person with a history or increased risk of melanoma, or
- is accompanied by nail dystrophy.

Longitudinal melanonychia in children must be evaluated on a case-by-case basis, and a biopsy must be seriously considered. Among 85 cases of longitudinal melanonychia in children, which occurred over a period of 35 years, no more than 5 (5.9%) displayed histologic evidence of malignancy. Although detection of a subungual melanoma in a child related to longitudinal melanonychia is a rare event, the risk of nail dystrophy and possible risks of anesthesia are far outweighed by the possibility of identifying a malignant lesion.

Treatment

Treatment of longitudinal melanonychia depends on the underlying cause.

Tumors of the Nail Unit

Subungual Melanoma

Subungual melanoma is an uncommon site for melanoma, with an incidence of between 0.7% and 3.5% of all melanoma cases in the general population. The peak age of incidence of subungual melanoma is in the fifth to seventh decades. The two important signs of subungual melanoma are longitudinal melanonychia (discussed above) and Hutchinson's sign (Fig. 29-13). Hutchinson's sign refers to the spread of pigment from the nail bed, matrix, and nail plate onto the adjacent cuticle and proximal and/or lateral nail folds. Pseudo-Hutchinson's sign refers to periungual pigmentation unrelated to melanoma and can be found in the Laugier-Hunziker syndrome, use of certain medications, with the presence of infectious agents in the nail, secondary to ethnic variation, with a variety of systemic diseases, and other causes.

Diagnosis

It is important for physicians to be aware of the diagnostic criteria for subungual melanoma, because this life-threatening

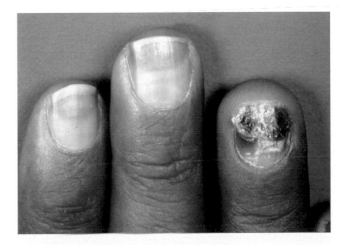

FIGURE 29-13 ■ Subungual melanoma.

disease has been misdiagnosed as onychomycosis, thereby causing delay in adequate treatment. The 5-year survival rate ranging from 16% to 87% for subungual melanoma has a worse prognosis when compared to cutaneous melanoma. There are four histologic subtypes of subungual melanoma, which includes lentigo maligna melanoma, superficial spreading melanoma, acral lentiginous melanoma, and nodular melanoma. It is also possible to develop a subungual melanoma without pigment, termed an *amelanotic melanoma*. The most important factors contributing to prognosis include the Breslow depth of invasion of the melanoma, presence of tumor ulceration, and presence of bone invasion.

The ABCDEF rule for clinical detection of subungual melanoma, which was developed after a review of the world literature on the subject. The ABCDEF is an acronym by which a physician can recall the important points regarding the diagnosis of subungual melanoma.

- *A* stands for *African Americans, Asians,* and Native *Americans,* the races most commonly affected by subungual melanoma.
- *B* stands for the diagnostic sign of a *b*rown to *b*lack pigmented nail *b*and with *b*lurred *b*orders and a *b*readth of 3 mm or more.
- *C* stands for a recent, sudden, or rapid *c*hange in the size of the nail band or lack of change despite treatment.
- *D* stands for the *d*igit most commonly affected by subungual melanoma, the thumb, followed by the hallux or index finger. A single digit affected by a pigmented band should raise the suspicion of subungual melanoma more than a situation where multiple digits are affected by pigmented bands.
- *E* stands for *e*xtension of pigment onto the proximal and/or lateral nail fold (Hutchinson's sign).
- *F* stands for *f*amily or personal history of the dysplastic nevus syndrome or previous melanoma, which would indicate an increased overall risk for subungual melanoma.

Final diagnosis of subungual melanoma requires a biopsy.

Treatment

Treatment of subungual melanoma depends on the extent of disease and the presence or absence of systemic metastasis. Evaluation of tumor burden can be accomplished with elective lymph node dissection or sentinel lymph node mapping and biopsy. However, such evaluation must be decided on a case-by-case basis, as lymph node dissection itself carries morbidity. Therapy includes surgical removal of the tumor with clear margins with local excision or amputation of the affected digit and, depending on the tumor burden, can include systemic chemotherapy and the use of interferon.

Nail Unit Squamous Cell Carcinoma

Subungual squamous cell carcinoma is rare. It is often associated with inciting factors including prior radiation therapy (especially in physicians and dentists), nail unit infections with human papillomavirus, tar exposure, and trauma. The incidence of subungual squamous cell carcinoma is highest during 50 to 69 years of age. Most reported cases of subungual squamous cell carcinoma occur on the fingers, but cases have been described occurring on the toes as well. Usually only one digit is affected, the most common site being the thumb (Fig. 29-14).

Diagnosis

Definitive diagnosis requires a biopsy. Delay in diagnosis is common as the presentation can resemble other common diseases of the nail unit including onychomycosis, verruca vulgaris, or a paronychia. Subungual squamous cell carcinoma involves the bone in between 20% and 55% of cases. Squamous cell carcinoma of the nail unit is considered to have a good prognosis when compared with the prognosis of squamous cell carcinomas of other cutaneous sites. Metastasis is an unusual progression of the disease.

Treatment

The treatment of choice for the distal digital segment is Mohs micrographic surgery when there is no involvement of the underlying bone. Amputation of the affected digit may

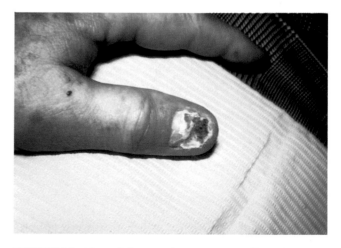

FIGURE 29-14 ■ Subungual squamous cell carcinoma.

be recommended depending on the extent of disease. Radiation therapy has been employed successfully in the treatment of unresectable subungual squamous cell carcinoma.

Subungual Metastases

A comprehensive review of 133 patients diagnosed with subungual metastases shows that the three most common primary malignancy sites are the lung (41% of cases), kidney (11% of cases), and breast (9% of cases). The appearance of these lesions took a variety of forms, with some cases masquerading as other dermatoses such as a pyogenic granuloma, or infections such as acute paronychia, erysipelas, and herpes zoster. Subungual metastases are usually painful. Anatomic sites of presentation include both the hands and feet. One or multiple digits can be affected. An x-ray of the affected digit should be performed to evaluate bone involvement, a common complication of subungual metastases. A review of 39 patients with subungual metastases showed that in 44% of these cases the metastatic lesion was the initial expression of an undiagnosed malignancy or presented in the same month that the tumor was discovered.

Digital Myxoid Cyst

The digital myxoid cyst is also known as a digital mucoid cyst, digital mucous cyst, myxoid pseudocyst, and synovial cyst. The variety of terms for this disorder reflects the controversial origin of the cyst development. It usually presents as an asymptomatic, single, soft to rubbery nodule on the dorsal surface of a finger, located between the proximal nail fold and distal interphalangeal joint, lateral to the midline. The material encased in the cyst has been described as viscous or gelatinous. The surface of the cyst is usually smooth, but verrucous variants have also been reported. Most cases occur in patients between ages 40 and 70. Women are more commonly affected than men. The most commonly affected anatomic sites are the middle and index fingers, but are also sometimes found on the toes. Because of its location, the cyst can exert pressure on the nail matrix, resulting in a linear nail plate dystrophy and a groove in the nail. Occasionally, these cysts can have a connection with the nearby distal interphalangeal joint.

Treatment

When surgically excised, care must be taken to remove any communicating tracts between the cyst and joint, if present, to prevent recurrence. Other treatment options include cryotherapy, carbon dioxide laser vaporization, and injection of sclerosing solutions. Treatment with aspiration of the cyst contents and injection of intralesional steroids can have high recurrence rates.

Suggested Reading

Baran R, Hay RJ, Tosti A, et al. A new classification of onychomycosis. Br J Dermatol 1998;139:567–571.

Baran R, Dawber RPR. Baran and Dawber's diseases of the nails and their management, ed 3. Malden, MA, Blackwell Science, 2001.

Cohen PR. Metastatic tumors to the nail unit: Subungual metastases. Dermatol Surg 2001;27:280–293.

de Berker D. Management of nail psoriasis. Clin Exp Dermatol 2000;25:357–362.

Faergemann J, Baran R. Epidemiology, clinical presentation and diagnosis of onychomycosis. Br J Dermatol 2003;149(Suppl 65):1–4.

Farber EM, Nall L. Nail psoriasis. Cutis 1992;50:174–178.

Gupta AK. Types of onychomycosis. Cutis 2001;68 (2 Suppl):4–7.

Gupta AK. Ciclopirox nail lacquer: A brush with onychomycosis. Cutis 2001;68:13–16.

Gupta AK, Baran R, Summerbell R. Onychomycosis: Strategies to improve efficacy and reduce recurrence. J Eur Acad Dermatol Venereol 2002;16:579–586.

Haneke E, Baran R. Longitudinal melanonychia. Dermatol Surg 2001;27:580–584.

Helms A, Brodell RT. Surgical pearl: Prompt treatment of subungual hematoma by decompression. J Am Acad Dermatol 2000;42:508–509.

Hordinsky MK, Sawaya ME, Scher RK. Atlas of hair and nails, ed 1. Philadelphia, Churchill Livingstone, 2000.

Levit EK, Kagen MH, Scher RK, et al. The ABC rule for clinical detection of subungual melanoma. J Am Acad Dermatol 2000;42:269–274.

Peterson SR, Layton EG, Joseph AK. Squamous cell carcinoma of the nail unit with evidence of bony involvement: A multidisciplinary approach to resection and reconstruction. Dermatol Surg 2004;30:218–221.

Rich P, Scher RK. An atlas of diseases of the nail, ed 1. New York, Parthenon Publishing Group, 2003.

Sonnex TS. Digital myxoid cysts: A review. Cutis 1986;37:89–94.

Thai KE, Young R, Sinclair RD. Nail apparatus melanoma. Australas J Dermatol 2001;42:71–81; quiz 2–3.

Usman A, Silvers DN, Scher RK. Longitudinal melanonychia in children. J Am Acad Dermatol 2001;44:547–548.

Uyttendaele H, Geyer A, Scher RK. Brittle nails: Pathogenesis and treatment. J Drugs Dermatol 2003;2:48–49.

CHAPTER 30

Diseases of the Mucous Membranes

John C. Hall

The mucous membranes of the body adjoin the skin at the oral cavity, nose, conjunctiva, penis, vulva, and anus. Histologically, these membranes differ from the skin in that the horny layer and the hair follicles are absent. Disorders of the mucous membranes are usually associated with existing skin diseases or internal diseases. Only the most common diseases of the mucous membranes are discussed herein. At the end of the chapter is a listing of the uncommon conditions of these areas.

Geographic Tongue

Geographic tongue is an extremely common condition of the tongue that usually occurs without symptoms. When these lesions are noticed for the first time by the individual, they may initiate fears of cancer.

Presentation and Characteristics

Clinical Appearance

Irregularly shaped (map-like or geographic) pale red patches are seen on the tongue (Fig. 30-1). Close examination reveals that the filiform papillae are flatter or denuded in these areas. The patches slowly migrate over the tongue surface and heal without scarring.

Course

The disorder may come and go but may be constantly present in some persons.

Cause

The cause is unknown, but the lesions seem to be more extensive during a systemic illness. It has been suggested the geographic tongue is a form of psoriasis by some authors.

Subjective Symptoms

Some patients complain of burning and tenderness, especially on eating sour or salty foods.

Differential Diagnosis

- *Syphilis,* secondary mucous membrane lesions: Similar clinically, but acute in onset, usually more inflammatory; other cutaneous signs of syphilis; darkfield examination and serology positive (see Chap. 22); does not come and go as rapidly

Treatment

1. Reassure patient that these are not cancerous lesions.
2. There is no effective or necessary therapy. However, if patient complains of burning and tenderness, prescribe

   Triamcinolone (Kenalog) in Orabase 15.0
   Sig: Apply locally q.i.d. 1/2 hour p.c. and h.s.

Aphthous Stomatitis

Canker sores are extremely common, painful, superficial ulcerations of the mucous membranes of the mouth (Fig. 30-2).

Presentation and Characteristics

Course

One or more lesions develop at the same time and heal without scarring in 5 to 10 days. They can recur at irregular intervals.

Cause

The cause is unknown, but certain foods, especially chocolate, nuts, and fruits, can precipitate the lesions or may even be causative. Trauma from biting or dental procedures can

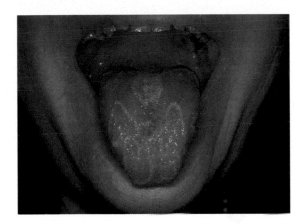

FIGURE 30-1 ■ Geographic tongue. *(Courtesy of Neutrogena Corp.)*

initiate lesions (pathergy). Some cases in women recur in relation to menstruation. A viral cause has not been proved. A pleomorphic, transitional L-form of an α-hemolytic *Streptococcus* species (*S. sanguis*) has also been implicated as causative.

Differential Diagnosis

■ *Syphilis*, secondary lesions: Clinically similar; less painful; other signs of syphilis; darkfield examination and serology positive (see Chap. 22)

Treatment

Most persons who get these lesions learn that very little can be done for them and that the ulcers heal in a few days.

1. Toothpaste swish therapy: Brush the teeth and swish the toothpaste around in the mouth after each meal and at bedtime. If done soon after the onset of ulcers, extension of the lesions can be prevented and early healing can be helpful in many cases.
2. Triamcinolone in Orabase (prescription needed) applied locally after meals relieves some of the pain.
3. Tetracycline therapy: An oral suspension in a dosage of 250 mg per teaspoonful (or the powdery contents of a 250-mg capsule in a teaspoon of water) kept in the mouth for 2 minutes and then swallowed, four times a day, is beneficial. This mixture can be applied with a piece of cotton soaked in this solution.
4. Systemic corticosteroids may occasionally be used for severe ulcers.

Herpes Simplex

Herpes simplex virus infection can occur as a group of umbilicated vesicles on the mucous membranes of the lips, the conjunctiva, the penis, and the labia. Frequently recurring episodes of this disease can be quite disabling (see Chap. 17). Recurrent intraoral herpes simplex is uncommon but the primary outbreak can have extensive intraoral mucous membrane involvement.

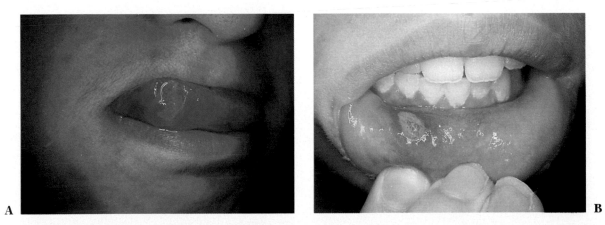

A   B

FIGURE 30-2 ■ **(A)** Recurrent aphthous ulcer of tongue. **(B)** Aphthous ulcer in patient with cyclic neutropenia. *(Courtesy of Neutrogena Corp.)*

Fordyce's Disease

This is a physiologic variant of oral sebaceous glands in which more than the normal number exist. When they are suddenly noticed, the person becomes concerned as to the diagnosis. The lesions are asymptomatic, yellowish-orange, 1- to 2-mm papules on the lips and labia minora. No treatment is necessary; they are benign.

Other Mucosal Lesions and Conditions

Mucosal lesions can also be caused by the following:

- *Physical causes:* Sucking of lips, pressure sores, burns, actinic or sunlight cheilitis, factitial disorders, tobacco, and other chemicals. Allergens are not commonly caused.
- *Infectious diseases* (from viruses, bacteria, spirochetes, fungi, and animal parasites): Gangrenous bacterial infections are called *noma. Ludwig's angina* is an acute cellulitis of the floor of the mouth caused by bacteria, abscesses, and sinuses and may be due to dental infection. *Trench mouth,* or *Plaut-Vincent's disease,* is an acute ulcerative infection of the mucous membranes caused by a combination of a spirochete and a fusiform bacillus.
- *Systemic diseases* (Fig. 30-3): These include lesions seen with hematologic diseases (e.g., leukemia, agranulocytosis from drugs or other causes, thrombocytopenia, pernicious anemia, cyclic or periodic neutropenia), immunocompromised conditions (such as the acquired immunodeficiency syndrome, organ transplants, lymphomas), collagen diseases (lupus erythematosus and scleroderma), pigmentary diseases (e.g., Addison's disease, Peutz-Jeghers

syndrome), and autoimmune diseases, which crossover in several categories but include pemphigus and benign mucosal pemphigoid.
- *Drugs:* Phenytoin sodium causes a hyperplastic gingivitis; bismuth orally and intramuscularly causes a bluish-black line at the edge of the dental gum (see Fig. 9-12); certain drugs cause hemorrhage and secondary infection of the mucous membranes.
- *Metabolic diseases:* Mucosal lesions are seen in primary systemic amyloidosis, lipoidosis, reticuloendothelioses, diabetes, and other disorders.
- *Tumors, local or systemic:* These include leukoplakia, squamous cell carcinoma, epulis, and cysts.

Rarer Conditions of Oral Mucous Membranes

- *Halitosis:* Halitosis, or fetor oris, is a disagreeable odor of the breath.
- *Periadenitis mucosa necrotica recurrens* (Fig. 30-4): Also known as Sutton's disease, this is a painful, recurrent, ulcerating disease of the mucous membranes of the oral cavity. The single or multiple deep ulcers exceed 10 mm and heal with scarring. Systemic corticosteroids may be indicated. It is considered by some to be a very severe type of aphthous ulcer.
- *Hand–foot–mouth disease:* A common vesicular eruption of the hands, feet, and mouth. Usually affecting children, it lasts up to 2 weeks. Most cases are caused by coxsackievirus A16.

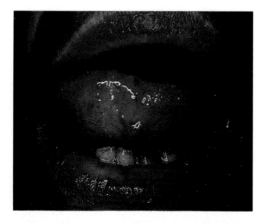

FIGURE 30-3 ■ Rendu-Osler-Weber disease of lips and tongue. *(Courtesy of Neutrogena Corp.)*

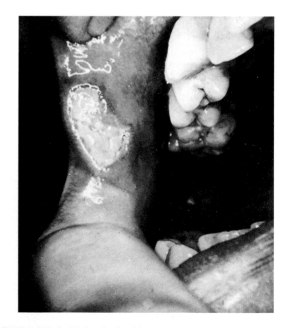

FIGURE 30-4 ■ Periadenitis mucosa necrotica recurrens.

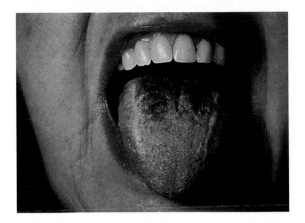

FIGURE 30-5 ■ Black tongue. *(Courtesy of Neutrogena Corp.)*

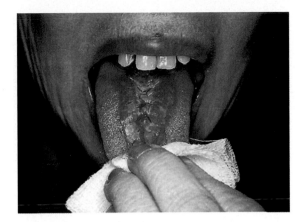

FIGURE 30-6 ■ Glossitis rhomboidea mediana. *(Courtesy of Neutrogena Corp.)*

- *Koplik's spots:* Bright red, pinpoint-sized lesions on the mucous membranes of the cheek are seen in patients before the appearance of the rash of measles.
- *Erythema multiforme* (Fig. 30-8): Causes "bulls eye" lesions on the skin and erosions of the mucus membranes that may be severe. The commonest causes are herpes simplex and drug allergies.
- *Burning tongue* (glossodynia): This rather common complaint, particularly among middle-aged women, is usually accompanied by no visible pathology. The cause is unknown, and therapy is of little value, but the many diseases and local factors that cause painful tongue must be ruled out from a diagnostic viewpoint. The entire mouth can also burn. Tricyclic antidepressants have been used with some success.
- *Black tongue* (hairy tongue, lingua nigra; Fig. 30-5): Overgrowth of the papillae of the tongue, apparently caused by an imbalance of bacterial flora, is due to the use of antibiotics and other agents. Black tongue without papillae hypertrophy can be seen with tobacco abuse, crack cocaine smoking, lansoprazole, chewing bismuth, methyldopa, minocycline, and hydroxychloroquin.
- *Hairy leukoplakia of the tongue:* A slightly raised, poorly demarcated lesion with a corrugated or "hairy" surface appears on the sides of the tongue. It is seen mainly in immunosuppressed homosexual men infected with human immunodeficiency virus. Human papillomavirus and Epstein-Barr virus have been identified in biopsy specimens (see Chap. 24). It is benign and no therapy is necessary.
- *Moeller's glossitis:* This painful, persistent, red eruption on the sides and the tip of the tongue

persists for weeks or months, subsides, and then recurs. The cause is unknown.

- *Furrowed tongue* (grooved tongue, scrotal tongue): The tongue is usually larger than normal, containing deep longitudinal and lateral grooves of congenital origin, due to syphilis, or as part of Melkersson-Rosenthal syndrome (see Dictionary–Index).
- *Glossitis rhomboidea mediana* (Fig. 30-6): This rare disorder, characterized by a smooth reddish lesion, usually occurs in the center of the tongue. This term is poor because there is no inflammation and the reddish plaque may not always be in the center.
- *Sjögren's syndrome:* This rare entity is characterized by dryness of all of the mucous membranes and of the skin in middle-aged women. *Keratoconjuntivitis*

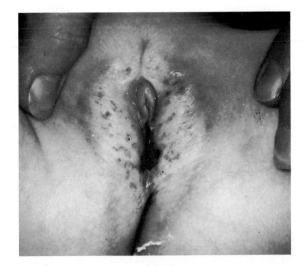

FIGURE 30-7 ■ Lichen sclerosis et atrophicus of labia, age 3 years.

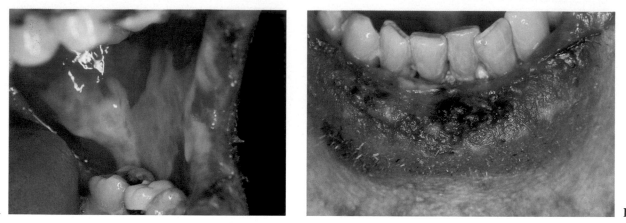

FIGURE 30-8 ■ Erythema multiforme of left buccal mucosa (**A**) and on lower lip (**B**).

sicca is used to describe the severe dryness of the eyes seen in this syndrome. The primary form of this syndrome is in many cases associated with a cutaneous vasculitis. The secondary type of Sjögren's syndrome is associated with rheumatic and collagen diseases. Evoxac is an oral medication which may help with the dry mouth. Sucking on hard lemon candy and artificial saliva can be tried. Evoxac is an oral medication that can be tried.

■ *Cheilitis glandularis:* This chronic disorder of the lips is manifested by swelling and secondary inflammation, caused by hypertrophy of the mucous glands and their ducts.

Rarer Conditions of Genital Mucous Membranes

■ *Fusospirochetal balanitis:* This uncommon infection of the penis is characterized by superficial erosions. It must be differentiated from syphilis by a darkfield examination and blood serology.

■ *Balanitis xerotica obliterans* (see *Atrophies of the Skin* in the Dictionary–Index): This whitish atrophic lesion on the penis is to be differentiated from leukoplakia. The female counterpart is lichen sclerosus et atrophicus.

■ *Lichen sclerosus et atrophicus:* This is a rare atrophy of the skin usually of the genital and perirectal mucous membranes. In children (Fig. 30-7), it is the most common chronic genital dermatitis. The prognosis is better in younger patients. In older patients there is a slight increase in the incidence of squamous cell cancer (approximately 5%). (See *Atrophies of the Skin* in the Dictionary–Index.)

Suggested Reading

Axell T. The oral mucosa as a mirror of general health or disease. Scand J Dent Res 1992;100:9.

Daley TD. Common acanthotic and keratotic lesions of the oral mucosa: A review. Can Dent Assoc J 1990; 56:407.

Eisen D, Lynch DP. The mouth: Diagnosis and treatment. St Louis, Mosby, 1998.

Eversole LR. Immunopathology of oral mucosal ulcerative, desquamative and bullous disease: selected review of the literature. Oral Surg Oral Med Oral Pathol 1994; 77:555.

Novick NL. Diseases of the mucous membrane. Clin Dermatol 1987;5.

Van der Waal I. Diseases of the salivary glands and Sjögren's syndrome. 1997.

SPECIALIZED DISEASE CATEGORIES

Pigmentary Dermatoses

John C. Hall

There are two variants of pigmentation of the skin: hyperpigmentation and hypopigmentation. The predominant skin pigment discussed in this chapter is melanin, but other pigments can be present in the skin. A complete classification of pigmentary disorders appears at the end of this chapter.

The melanin-forming cells and their relationship to the tyrosine–tyrosinase enzyme system are discussed in Chapter 1. The common clinical example of abnormal hyperpigmentation is *chloasma*, but secondary melanoderma can result from many causes. The most common form of

hypopigmentation is *vitiligo*, but secondary leukoderma does occur.

Chloasma (Melasma)

Presentation and Characteristics

Clinical Lesions

An irregular hyperpigmentation of the skin that varies in shades of brown is seen. It is well demarcated and

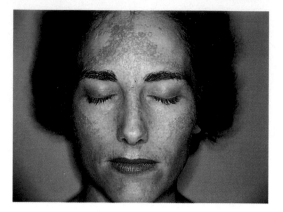

FIGURE 31-1 ■ Chloasma of face. *(Neutrogena Skin Care Institute.)*

located most often on the face in sun-exposed areas (Fig. 31-1).

Distribution

The lesions usually occur on the sides of the face, forehead, and sides of the neck.

Course

The disorder is slowly progressive, but remissions do occur. It is more obvious in the summer.

Cause

The cause is unknown, but some cases appear during pregnancy (called "mask of pregnancy") or with chronic illness. There is an increased incidence of chloasma in women taking contraceptives, postmenopausal hormone replacement, or fertility hormones. The melanocyte-stimulating hormone of the pituitary may be excessive and affect the tyrosine–tyrosinase enzyme system.

Differential Diagnosis

The causes of *secondary melanoderma* should be ruled out (see end of this chapter).

Treatment

1. The patient should not be promised great therapeutic results. Most cases associated with pregnancy slowly fade or disappear completely after delivery. The pigmentation may be prolonged if the patient elects to breastfeed.

2. For a mild case in an unconcerned patient, cosmetic coverage can be adequate. Dermablend or Lydia O'Leary Covermark are two useful products.

3. Sunlight intensifies the pigmentation, so a sunscreen should be added to the routine.

4. Hydroquinone preparations (any of the following):

Melanex solution 3%	30.0
Lustra Cream 4%	
Eldopaque Forte cream (tinted)	30.0
Solaquin Forte cream (nontinted)	30.0
Eldoquin Forte	30.0
Lustra AF (sunscreen)	
Lustra-Ultra (sunscreen, retinol)	
Tri-Luma (Fluocinolone, tretinoin)	
EpiQuin (microsponge)	
Glyquin (glycolic acid)	

   Comment: Tri-Luma contains a retinoid, a class VI corticosteroid, and hydroquinone. This product should show a response within 8 weeks and some authors restrict its use to this time period and then have a rest period because it contains a corticosteroid. They then switch to a sunscreen and hydroquinone combination. There are many variants of these topicals, all with hydroquinone and some with sunscreens, glycolic acid, and retinoids.

   Sig: Apply locally b.i.d. Stop if irritation develops.

   Comment: The treatment with any of these hydroquinone preparations should be continued for at least 3 months. Response to therapy is slow. When they are stopped the disease tends to recur. Prolonged use over many months to years can cause increased pigmentation owing to an acquired ochronosis. This resolves on discontinuing the hydroquinone.

5. Retinoic acid (Retin-A cream or gel Renova [0.02%, 0.05%]) applied at night can slowly decrease the pigmentation, if tolerated.

Vitiligo

Presentation and Characteristics

Clinical Lesions

Irregular areas of depigmented skin are occasionally seen with a hyperpigmented border (Fig. 31-2). There is a segmental variety that has pigment loss in a dermatomal (especially trigeminal) distribution.

Distribution

Most commonly, the lesions occur on the face and the dorsum of hands and feet, but they can occur on all body areas.

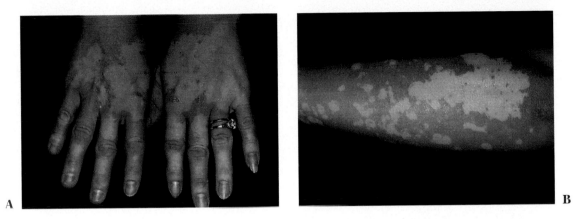

FIGURE 31-2 ■ **(A)** Vitiligo of hands in a white patient. **(B)** Vitiligo of forearm in a black patient. *(Neutrogena Skin Care Institute.)*

Course

The disease is slowly progressive, but remissions and changes are frequent. It is more obvious during the summer because of the tanning of adjacent normal skin.

Cause

The cause is unknown, but believed by some to be an autoimmune disease. Heredity is a factor in some cases. Autoimmune diseases, especially thyroiditis, can be associated with vitiligo.

Differential Diagnosis

Causes of *secondary hypopigmentation* need to be ruled out (see end of this chapter and Fig. 31-3).

Treatment

Case Example. A young woman with large depigmented patches on her face and dorsum of hands asks if something can be done for her "white spots." Her sister has a few lesions.

- *Cosmetics:* The use of the following covering or staining preparations is recommended: pancake-type cosmetics, such as Covermark, by Lydia O'Leary; Vitadye (Elder); dihydroxyacetone containing self-tanning creams, gels, and foams; walnut-juice stain; or potassium permanganate solution in appropriate dilution. Many patients with vitiligo become quite proficient in the application of these agents. A sunscreen used on the surrounding skin makes the contrast of light and dark skin less apparent.
- *Corticosteroid cream therapy:* This is effective for early mild cases of vitiligo, especially when one is mainly concerned with face and hand lesions. Betamethasone valerate (Valisone) cream 0.1% can be prescribed for use on the hands for 4 months or so and for use on the face for only 3 months. It should not be used on the eyelids or as full-body therapy. Even class I topical corticosteroids can be used for a while if appropriate precautions are observed.
- *Protopic 0.1% ointment* used twice a day avoids topical corticosteroid side effects and may be quite beneficial. Concern over induction of cutaneous lymphoma has been hypothesized but not proven.
- *Sun avoidance:* Sun tanning should be avoided because this accentuates the normal pigmentation and makes the nonpigmented vitiligo more noticeable. The white areas of vitiligo are more susceptible to sunburn. If the patient desires a more specific treatment, the following can be suggested with certain reservations:
- *Psoralen derivatives:* For many years, Egyptians along the Nile River chewed certain plants to cause the disappearance of the white spots of vitiligo. Extraction of the chemicals from these plants revealed the psoralen derivatives to be the active agents, and one of these, 8-methoxypsoralen, was found to be the most effective. This chemical is available as Oxsoralen in 10-mg capsules and also as a topical liquid form. The oral form is to be ingested 2 hours before exposure to measured sun radiation. The package insert should be consulted. Our results with this long-term therapy have been disappointing.
- Trisoralen is a synthetic psoralen in 5-mg tablets. The recommended dosage is 2 tablets taken 2 hours before measured sun exposure for a long-term course. Detailed instructions accompany the

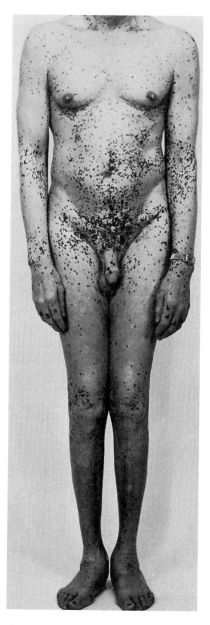

FIGURE 31-3 ■ Secondary hypopigmentation. A marked example of loss of pigment that occurred in an African-American man following healing of an exfoliative dermatitis. Corticosteroids were used in the therapy.

package. Some dermatologists believe this therapy to be more effective than Oxsoralen.

■ A short 2-week course of Oxsoralen capsules (20 mg/d) has been advocated for the purpose of acquiring a better and quicker suntan. The value of such a course has been questioned. The sun exposure must be gradual. Oral psoralens plus self-administered UVA or UVB in "tanning booths" can produce severe burns, which may be fatal.

■ *Psoralens and ultraviolet light (PUVA) therapy:* The combination of topical or oral psoralen therapy with UVA radiation has been somewhat successful in repigmenting vitiligo. The psoralen can be given orally, topically, or as a bath. Precautions concerning photoaging and skin cancer apply.

■ *Depigmentation therapy:* In the hands of experts, monobenzyl ether of hydroquinone (Benoquin) can be used to remove skin pigment to even out the patient's skin color.

■ *Skin grafting:* Autologous minigrafting and other similar surgical procedures have been used with success by some.

■ *Surgical therapy:* Various grafting procedures are valuable in recalcitrant disease. Epidermal or full-thickness autographs have been advocated by some authors.

Classification of Pigmentary Disorders

Melanin Hyperpigmentation or Melanoderma

1. Chloasma (melasma) (see Fig. 31-1)
2. Incontinentia pigmenti
3. Secondary to skin diseases
   a. Chronic discoid lupus erythematosus
   b. Tinea versicolor
   c. Stasis dermatitis
   d. Lichen planus
   e. Fixed drug eruption
   f. Many cases of dermatitis in African Americans and other dark-skinned individuals (see Fig. 31-3)
   g. Scleroderma
   h. Porphyria cutanea tarda (Fig. 31-4)
   i. Dermatitis herpetiformis

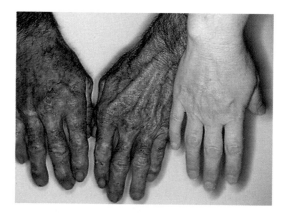

FIGURE 31-4 ■ Porphyria cutanea tarda hyperpigmentation. *(Neutrogena Skin Care Institute).*

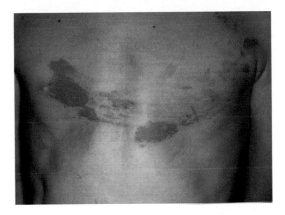

FIGURE 31-5 ■ Berlock dermatitis: photosensitivity reaction from mother's perfume, age 7 years. *(Neutrogena Skin Care Institute.)*

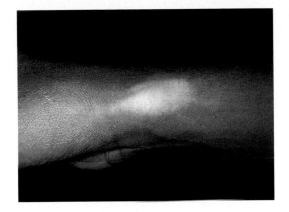

FIGURE 31-6 ■ Leukoderma on wrist from corticosteroid intralesionally in a black patient. *(Neutrogena Skin Care Institute.)*

4. Secondary to external agents
   a. X-radiation
   b. Ultraviolet light
   c. Sunlight
   d. Tars
   e. Photosensitizing chemicals, as in cosmetics, causing development of clinical entities labeled as Riehl's melanosis, poikiloderma of Civatte on the sides of the neck due to chronic sun exposure, berlock dermatitis (Fig. 31-5), and others

5. Secondary to internal disorders
   a. Addison's disease (see Fig. 33-1)
   b. Chronic liver disease
   c. Pregnancy
   d. Hyperthyroidism
   e. Internal carcinoma causing malignant form of acanthosis nigricans
   f. Hormonal influence on benign acanthosis nigricans
   g. Intestinal polyposis causing mucous membrane pigmentation (Peutz-Jeghers syndrome)
   h. Albright's syndrome
   i. Schilder's disease
   j. Fanconi's syndrome (in HIV-positive patients)

6. Secondary to drugs such as adrenocorticotropic hormone, estrogens, progesterone, melanocyte-stimulating hormone

Nonmelanin Pigmentations

1. Argyria owing to silver salt deposits
2. Arsenical pigmentation caused by ingestion of inorganic arsenic, as in Fowler's solution and Asiatic pills
3. Pigmentation from heavy metals such as bismuth, gold, and mercury

4. Tattoos
5. Black dermographism, the common bluish black or green stain seen under watches and rings in certain persons from the deposit of the metallic particles reacting with chemicals already on the skin
6. Hemosiderin granules in hemochromatosis or pigmented purpuric eruptions (see Chap. 12)
7. Bile pigments from jaundice
8. Yellow pigments following atabrine and chlorpromazine ingestion
9. Carotene coloring in carotenemia
10. Homogentisic acid polymer deposit in ochronosis
11. Minocycline hyperpigmentation (characteristic histopathology) diffuse and also localized at scar sites (and rarely teeth).

Hypopigmentation

1. Albinism
2. Vitiligo
3. Leukoderma or acquired hypopigmentation (Fig. 31-6)
   a. Secondary to skin diseases such as tinea versicolor, chronic discoid lupus erythematosus, localized scleroderma, psoriasis, secondary syphilis, or pinta (see Fig. 31-3)
   b. Secondary to chemicals such as mercury compounds, monobenzyl ether of hydroquinone, and cortisone-type drugs given intralesionally, especially in people of color (see Fig. 31-6)
   c. Secondary to internal diseases, such as hormonal diseases, and in Vogt-Koyanagi syndrome
   d. Associated with pigmented nevi (halo nevus or leukoderma acquisitum centrifugum)

Suggested Reading

Boersma BR, Westerhof W, Bos JD. J Am Acad Dermatol 1995;33:6.

Drake LA, Dinehart SM, Farmer ER, et al. Guidelines of care for vitiligo. J Am Acad Dermatol 1996;35: 620.

Fulk CS. Primary disorders of hyperpigmentation. J Am Acad Dermatol 1984;10:1.

Grimes PE. New insights and new therapies in vitiligo. JAMA 2005;293:730–735.

Kovacs SO. Vitiligo. J Am Acad Dermatol 1998;38:5.

Levine N. Pigmentation and pigmentary disorders. Boca Raton, FL, CRC Press, 1994.

Nordlund JJ, Boissy R, et al. The pigmentary system: Physiology and pathophysiology. 1998.

Victor FC, Gelber J, Rao B. Melasma: A review. J Cutan Med Surg 2004;8:97–102. Epub 2004 May 4.

CHAPTER 32

Collagen Vascular Diseases

Gary Goldenberg, MD, and Joseph L. Jorizzo, MD

The collagen vascular diseases are a group of autoimmune diseases including lupus erythematosus (LE), scleroderma, dermatomyositis (DM), rheumatoid arthritis, Sjögren's syndrome, and many others. LE, scleroderma, and DM are discussed in detail herein. These diseases are characterized by autoimmune phenomena, including circulating autoantibodies (aAb). There is a great deal of overlap, including clinical features and laboratory findings. Cutaneous manifestations of these diseases may be the presenting or dominant feature. However, systemic, multiorgan disease needs to be excluded in each case.

A thorough laboratory evaluation is required. Much has been written about antinuclear antibody (ANA) testing. This assay identifies aAbs present in serum to autoantigens present in nuclei of mammalian cells. ANA testing is reported as a titer and most commercial kits reports ANA titer of 1:40 or 1:80 as abnormal. However, titers less than 1:160 are not diagnostic; approximately 5% of otherwise healthy young individuals have an ANA titer of 1:160 or higher. The prevalence of "positive" ANA increases with age. Therefore, it is important not to label patients with LE or another autoimmune disease simply based on one laboratory test.

Lupus Erythematosus

Chronic cutaneous lupus erythematosus (CCLE) characterized by discoid lesions, subacute cutaneous lupus erythematosus (SCLE) (Figs. 32-1 and 32-2), and acute cutaneous lupus erythematosus (ACLE) are the most common variants encountered by dermatologists.

It has been estimated that cutaneous variants of LE are two to three times more common than systemic disease. LE is much more common in women than in men; the female to male ratio is at least 6:1. The average age of onset is 30 years old in women and 40 years old in men. LE is more common in blacks than in whites, and blacks have a higher frequency of systemic disease.

Drug-induced lupus has been reported with multiple medications, including hydrochlorothiazide, calcium channel blockers, isoniazid, phenytoin, angiotensin-converting enzyme inhibitors (captopril), tetracyclines (minocycline), and many others including over-the-counter nonsteroidal anti-inflammatory drugs. Anti-histone aAb is a serologic marker that occurs in patients with drug-induced LE.

Neonatal LE (NLE) is seen in newborns whose mothers have anti-Ro aAb. Nearly 100% of patients with NLE also have anti-Ro aAbs. SCLE-like lesions are usually seen on the face of newborns. Congenital heart block is an important complication and is usually present at birth. Therefore, screening for heart disease should be performed in all patients with NLE. Children with this complication have a 20% mortality rate and two-thirds require pacemakers.

Diagnosis of LE and its subtypes depends on a constellation of findings that include history, physical examination, histopathologic correlation, and laboratory evaluation, which focuses on published American College of Rheumatology criteria. See Table 32-1 for a comparison of CCLE, SCLE, and ACLE. The treatment approach is outlined in Table 32-2.

Scleroderma

Localized scleroderma (morphea), systemic (diffuse) sclerosis (Fig. 32-3), and CREST syndrome (*C*alcinosis cutis, *R*aynaud's phenomenon, *E*sophageal dysfunction, *S*clerodactyly, *T*elangiectasias) are variants included under the general heading of scleroderma.

Systemic sclerosis is a systemic disease that affects the skin, lungs, heart, GI tract, and other organ systems. It is up to 15 times more common in women and the age of onset is between 30 and 50 years old. Ten-year survival of patients with systemic sclerosis is under 70%. Pathogenesis of systemic sclerosis is unknown, but endothelial

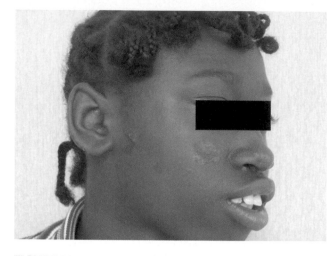

FIGURE 32-1 ■ CCLE with discoid lesions—erythematous, hyperpigmented plaques with scarring characteristic of CCLE with discoid lesions.

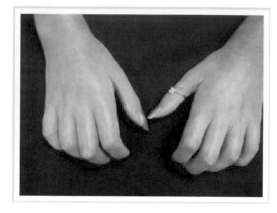

FIGURE 32-3 ■ Systemic sclerosis. This patient demonstrates typical loss of wrinkles on the hands with waxy, shiny, bound down skin.

cell damage is suspected as the key pathogenic abnormality. Cutaneous and systemic findings of systemic sclerosis and other variants of scleroderma are summarized in Table 32-3.

Dermatomyositis

DM is an autoimmune proximal extensor inflammatory myopathy with specific cutaneous manifestations (Fig. 32-4). Polymyositis is an inflammatory myopathy without any skin involvement. DM sine myositis presents with the characteristic eruption of DM without muscle involvement.

Cutaneous disease is characteristic (Table 32-4) and can either precede or follow muscle disease. Adult and juvenile variants exist. Differential diagnosis of skin disease includes SLE, psoriasis, allergic contact dermatitis, phototoxic drug eruption, cutaneous T-cell lymphoma, atopic dermatitis, and scleroderma.

The pathogenesis of DM is unclear, but it is believed to be an autoimmune disease triggered by outside factors in genetically predisposed individuals. Photosensitivity plays an important role in inducing cutaneous DM. Average age

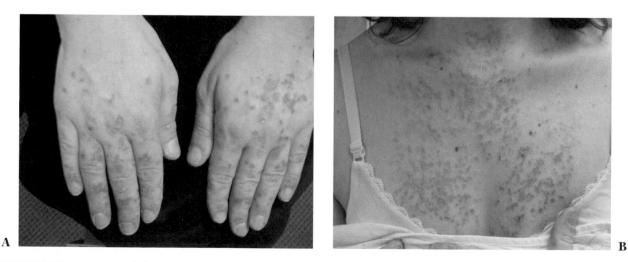

FIGURE 32-2 ■ SCLE. (**A**) Erythematous papules and plaques on dorsal hands, typical distribution spares the knuckles. (**B**) Erythematous papules and plaques in a typical sun-exposed distribution of the V of the chest.

TABLE 32-1 ■ Comparison of Three Most Common Types of LE Encountered by Dermatologists

LE Subtype	CCLE	SCLE	ACLE
Distribution	Face, scalp, ears, extensor arms	V of the neck, upper back, shoulders, extensor arms, less commonly face	"Butterfly" malar distribution on face, V of neck, arms, hands (sparing knuckles)
Clinical features	*Early lesions:* sharply demarcated erythematous papules and plaques with prominent scale, follicular plugging and early scarring; *Late lesions:* atrophic plaques with central scarring, telangiectasia and hypopigmentation; photosensitivity	Erythematous papules and scaly, hyperkeratotic, annular/polycyclic plaques; photosensitivity; nonscarring	Poorly marginated erythematous macules, fine scaling, poikiloderma, edema; photosensitivity; nonscarring
Course	Chronic with disease progression without treatment; 5–10% eventually meet ACR criteria for SLE	50% meet ACR criteria for SLE	Acute onset, usually with systemic signs and symptoms
Histopathology	Vacuolar change, dyskeratotic keratinocytes, follicular plugging, basement membrane thickening, superficial and deep perivascular and perifollicular lymphohistiocytic infiltrate, increased dermal mucin	Vacuolar change, dyskeratotic keratinocytes, epidermal atrophy, superficial and mid perivascular lymphohistiocytic infiltrate, increased dermal mucin	Vacuolar change, dyskeratotic keratinocytes, superficial perivascular lymphohistiocytic infiltrate, dermal edema
Laboratory findings	Positive ANA (5%)	Positive ANA, anti-Ro aAb (>90%);	Positive ANA (99%), double-stranded DNA (60%); anemia (normocytic), leukopenia, thrombocytopenia, elevated ESR, proteinuria, cellular casts
Differential diagnosis	Polymorphous light eruption, psoriasis, sarcoidosis, lichen planus, granuloma faciale	Annular erythemas, atopic dermatitis, psoriasis, dermatophyte infection, secondary syphilis	Sunburn, rosacea, DM, phototoxic drug eruption, seborrheic dermatitis

Abbreviations: ACLE, acute cutaneous lupus erythematosus; ANA, antinuclear antibody; ACR, American College of Radiology; CCLE, chronic cutaneous lupus erythematosus; DM, dermatomyositis; ESR, erythrocyte sedimentation rate; SCLE, subacute cutaneous lupus erythematosus.

TABLE 32-2 ■ Therapeutic Options for LE

Mild local disease	Sunscreens (high SPF with UVA blocker) Topical or intralesional corticosteroids Topical immunomodulators (e.g., tacrolimus) Hydroxychloroquine (may add quinacrine)	Systemic disease	Prednisone Azothioprine Mycophenolate mofetil Cyclophosphamide
Extensive cutaneous disease	Oral retinoids Dapsone/sulfapyridine Clofazimine Methotrexate Thalidomide Azothioprine		Cyclosporine Interferon IVIG Newer biological therapies Extracorporeal immunomodulation Stem cell transplantation

Abbreviations: IVIG, intravenous immunoglobulin; LE, lupus erythematosus; SPF, sun protective factor; UVA, ultraviolet A.

TABLE 32-3 ■ Clinical Features of Scleroderma Variants

Scleroderma Subtype	Systemic Sclerosis	CREST Syndrome	Morphea
Cutaneous findings	Sclerodactyly (induration of fingers, waxy, shiny, hardened, bound down skin, loss of wrinkling), Raynaud's phenomenon (coldness, triphasic color changes, i.e., pallor, cyanosis, rubor), diffuse and salt-and-pepper hyperpigmentation, cutaneous ulcers ("rat bite necrosis"), trunk involvement	Telangiectasias, Raynaud's phenomenon, calcinosis cutis (especially over bony prominences), cutaneous ulcers ("rat bite" necrosis), sclerodactyly	*Plaque type:* erythematous, edematous plaque that becomes sclerotic and scar-like with hypopigmentation and hyperpigmentation; *Deep (profunda) morphea:* deep tissue sclerosis; *En coupe de saber:* linear morphea affecting the forehead and scalp; *Parry-Romberg syndrome:* hyperpigmentation and soft tissue atrophy affecting the entire distribution of the trigeminal nerve leading to facial asymmetry
Systemic findings	*Esophagus:* reflux disease, dysmotility, dysphagia; *GI tract:* decreased peristalsis leading to constipation, diarrhea, bloating, malabsorption; *Heart:* constrictive pericarditis, conduction abnormalities; *Lungs:* diffuse pulmonary fibrosis; *Kidneys:* uremia, renal hypertension	*Esophagus:* reflux disease, dysmotility, dysphagia; *GI tract:* telangiectasias	None
Histopathology	Diffuse dermal sclerosis, mild vacuolar change, excessive collagen deposition, decreased adnexal structures, mild perivascular infiltrate with plasma cells	Same (for sclerodactyly)	Same
Laboratory findings	Positive ANA (90–95%), anti–Scl-70 aAb (DNA topoisomerase I; 60%)	Positive ANA, anti-centromere aAb (80%)	Possibly a positive ANA (especially linear morphea), anti-fibrillin 1 aAb
Differential diagnosis	Eosinophilic fasciitis, scleromyxedema, scleredema, L-tryptophan syndrome, nephrogenic fibrosing dermopathy, toxic oil syndrome, graft-versus-host disease, drug reaction (bleomycin)	Pathognomonic if all features are present	Toxic oil syndrome, drug reaction (bleomycin), silicosis; chemical exposure (vinyl chloride, organic solvents, pesticides and epoxy resin), graft-versus-host disease
Treatment	*Skin sclerosis:* physical therapy, prednisone (controversial), methotrexate, D-penicillamine; *Raynaud's phenomenon:* calcium channel blockers, Viagra; *Calcinosis cutis:* excision; *Renal disease:* ACE inhibitors; *Esophageal disease:* proton pump inhibitors; *Pulmonary disease:* cyclophosphamide	*Calcinosis cutis:* excision; *Raynaud's phenomenon:* calcium channel blockers, Viagra; *Esophageal disease:* proton pump inhibitors; *Skin sclerosis:* physical therapy, methotrexate, D-penicillamine	*Mild disease:* Topical/intralesional corticosteroids, topical immunomodulators (e.g., tacrolimus); with keratolytics; *Severe disease:* hydroxychloroquine, methotrexate, D-penicillamine, cyclosporine, phototherapy, physical therapy

Abbreviations: ACE, angiotensin-converting enzyme; ANA, antinuclear antibody.

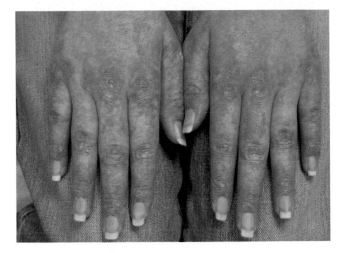

FIGURE 32-4 ■ GOTTRON'S papules on dorsal hands of a patient with juvenile DM.

TABLE 32-5 ■ Therapeutic Options for Treatment of Dermatomyositis

Cutaneous lesions	Sunscreens (high SPF with UVA blocker) Topical corticosteroids Topical immunomodulators (e.g., tacrolimus) Hydroxychloroquine Low-dose methotrexate Mycophenolate mofetil Retinoids
Systemic disease	Oral prednisone Low-dose methotrexate Cyclosporine Cyclophosphamide Chlorambucil Newer biological therapies IVIG

Abbreviations: DM, dermatomyositis; IVIG; intravenous immunoglobulin; SPF; sun protective factor; UVA, ultraviolet A.

of onset of adult disease is 52 years old and juvenile disease is 8 years old. Adult DM is more common in women; the male to female ratio is 1:6. Juvenile DM is slightly more common in boys.

The inflammatory myopathy affects proximal muscle groups, especially the triceps and quadriceps. Patients present with proximal muscle weakness, muscle tenderness, and fatigue. Muscle disease workup should include creatine phosphokinase and aldolase, magnetic resonance imaging, electromyography, and triceps muscle biopsy. Pulmonary fibrosis can be seen in 15% to 30% of patients and is more common in patients with anti–transfer-RNA syndrome.

Internal malignancy is estimated to occur in 10% to 50% of patients with adult DM. Genitourinary malignancies (especially ovarian), breast, lung, and gastric cancers have been described. The risk of malignancy may return to normal after 2 years. Juvenile DM is not associated with increased malignancy risk.

Histopathology reveals vacuolar change, sparse lymphocytic infiltrate, epidermal atrophy, and basement membrane degeneration. Autoantibodies to Jo-1 and Mi-2 are found in 30% of patients with polymyositis and 10% of patients with DM, respectively. Treatment is outlined in Table 32-5.

TABLE 32-4 ■ Cutaneous Manifestations of Dermatomyositis

Gottron's papules (see Fig. 32-4)	Violaceous papules overlying dorsal interphalangeal and metacarpophalangeal joints
Gottron's sign	Confluent violaceous erythema overlying dorsal interphalangeal and metacarpophalangeal joints
Periorbital heliotrope rash	Confluent violaceous erythema and edema of the eyelids and periorbital tissue
Poikiloderma	Violaceous erythema with hypopigmentation, hyperpigmentation, and atrophy in sun exposed distribution and over extensor surfaces

Suggested Reading

Buyon JP, Hiebert R, et al. Autoimmune-associated congenital heart block: Demographics, mortality, morbidity and recurrence rates obtained from a national neonatal lupus registry. J Am Coll Cardiol 1998 Jun;31:1658–1666.

Falanga V. Systemic sclerosis (scleroderma). In Bolognia JL, Jorizzo JL, Rapini RP, eds. Dermatology. St. Louis, Mosby, 2003, pp. 625–632.

Hachberg MC, Boyd RE, Ahearn JM, et al. Systemic lupus erythematosus: A review of clinico-laboratory features and immunogenetic markers in 150 patients with emphasis on demographic subsets. Medicine 1985;64:285–295.

Hochberg MC. The epidemiology of systemic lupus erythematosus. In: Wallace DJ, Hahn BH, eds. Dubois' lupus erythematosus, ed 4. Philadelphia, Lea & Febiger, 1993, pp. 49–57.

Jacobe H, Sontheimer RD. Autoantibodies encountered in patients with autoimmune connective tissue diseases. In Bolognia JL, Jorizzo JL, Rapini RP, eds. Dermatology. St. Louis, Mosby, 2003, pp. 601–613.

Jorizzo JL. Dermatomyositis. In Bolognia JL, Jorizzo JL, Rapini RP, eds. Dermatology. St. Louis, Mosby, 2003, pp. 615–623.

Sontheimer R. Skin manifestations of systemic autoimmune connective tissue disease: Diagnostics and therapeutics. Best Pract Res Clin Rheumatol 2004;18:429–462.

Tebbe B, Orfanos CE. Epidemiology and socioeconomic impact of skin disease in lupus erythematosus. Lupus 1997;6:96–104.

Uitto J, Jimenez S. Fibrotic skin diseases. Clinical presentations, etiologic considerations, and treatment options. Arch Dermatol 1990;126:661–664.

CHAPTER 33

The Skin and Internal Disease

Warren R. Heymann, MD, and Larisa Ravitskiy, MD

A practicing dermatologist must be cognizant of the potential cutaneous manifestations of systemic diseases. Although certain skin findings are pathognomic for a particular malady, more often than not cutaneous eruptions must be interpreted in the context of the complete clinical picture. On occasion, a cutaneous finding may guide the clinician toward a previously undiagnosed systemic disease. It is the interplay between the skin and the internal organs that requires the physician to be aware of such relationships.

Cutaneous findings can be classified as specific and nonspecific. *Specific changes* demonstrate the same pathologic process as internal disease and can, therefore, be diagnostic of disease. *Nonspecific changes* do not demonstrate the primary disease process (Figs. 33-1 and 33-2). These changes can be helpful in establishing the diagnosis only if interpreted within the context of the clinical data. The following cases are a few selected examples of the many systemic diseases with skin involvement. Table 33-1 lists some internal diseases and their dermatologic manifestations.

Cardiology

Kawasaki's Syndrome

Kawasaki's syndrome, also known as *mucocutaneous lymph node syndrome,* is a self-limited acute vasculitis of childhood. It has a propensity for coronary artery involvement with aneurysms, angina pectoris, or myocardial infarction in up to 18% to 23% of untreated cases. With proper treatment, the percentage of coronary artery aneurysms decreases to 4% to 8%. Usually young children under the age of 5 are affected, with cases reported in infants and teenagers as well. There is a slight female preponderance. The diagnosis of Kawasaki's syndrome is based on a constellation of clinical findings including fever lasting at least 5 days, nonsuppurative cervical adenopathy, bilateral nonpurulent conjunctival injection, reddening and fissuring of the lips, "strawberry tongue", and several cutaneous findings. The skin changes begin with erythema of palms and soles, which may spread to the trunk. Indurative edema and desquamation starting on the tips of the fingers and toes and around nails is then noted. A polymorphous rash that can vary from morbilliform to scarlatiniform may also be present.

LEOPARD Syndrome

Multiple lentigines syndrome is an autosomal dominant disorder with abnormalities of various clinical expression. LEOPARD is an acronym for the following abnormalities that may be present in an individual patient with this syndrome:

- *L*entigines: multiple lentigines are present at birth and may cover the entire body, including the palms and soles, sparing the lips and oral mucosa. The pigment can be seen in the iris and retina as well.
- *E*lectrocardiogram conduction defects
- *O*cular hypertelorism
- *P*ulmonary stenosis
- *A*bnormalities of genitalia
- *R*etardation of growth
- *D*eafness (sensorineural)

Pseudoxanthoma Elasticum

Pseudoxanthoma elasticum is a genetic disorder of connective tissue disease characterized by progressive mineralization of elastic fibers with cutaneous, cardiovascular, and ophthalmologic complications. The disease manifests as angioid streaks of the retina, retinal and gastrointestinal hemorrhages, hypertension, and occlusive vascular disease secondary to progressive calcification and fragmentation of the elastic fibers in the eye and blood vessels. Characteristic yellowish papules that appear like a "plucked chicken" are seen in flexural areas of the neck and periumbilical areas. These lesions can also be seen in the oral, vaginal, and rectal mucosa.

FIGURE 33-1 ■ Nonspecific skin changes indicating an underlying psychological disease state. **(A)** Delusional excoriation on the arm ("have to get the hairs out"). **(B)** Neurotic excoriations on the arm.

Endocrinology

Diabetes Mellitus

Cutaneous manifestations associated with diabetes mellitus may correlate with metabolic derangements, present as chronic degenerative changes with no apparent correlation to the degree of hyperglycemia. Metabolic changes in patients with poorly controlled diabetes tend to cause a higher risk for the development of cutaneous infections by bacterial, fungal, and yeast pathogens. Diabetic dermopathy (atrophic, circumscribed, brownish plaques on the pretibial surfaces; Fig. 33-3) or bullous diabeticorum (spontaneous development of bullae on the extremities) can be seen as a result of chronic degenerative changes. The latter, further compounded by vascular compromise, may eventuate in neuropathic foot ulcers (Fig. 33-4).

Necrobiosis lipoidica (NL) is seen in less than 1% of diabetics, but many of the patients with NL have diabetes mellitus (Fig. 33-5). NL begins as sharply circumscribed dusky-red nodules or papules located most commonly on anterior and lateral surfaces of lower extremities. The lesions expand to form atrophic, waxy, yellowish, telangiectatic plaques with active brawny borders. The plaques occasionally ulcerate. New NL lesions may appear at the site of surgery or trauma (Koebner phenomenon).

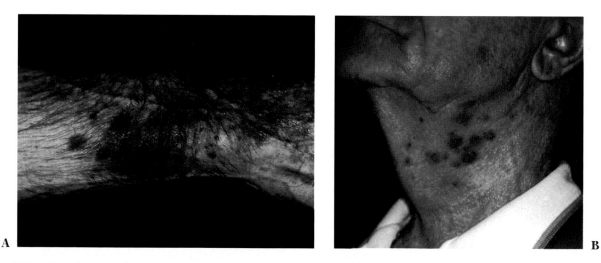

FIGURE 33-2 ■ Nonspecific skin changes resulting from an internal disease. Purpura of the arm **(A)** and folliculitis of the neck **(B)** in a patient with myelogenous leukemia. *(Courtesy of Syntext Laboratories Inc.)*

TABLE 33-1 ■ **Internal Diseases with Cutaneous Manifestations**

Disorder	Cutaneous Findings	Associated Malignancies
Acanthosis nigricans	Velvety hyperpigmentation of flexures and, less commonly, mucosal surfaces, and palms (tripe palms)	Adenocarcinoma of GU or GI tract. Most commonly associated with adenocarcinoma of stomach (55.5%)[1]
Acquired ichthyosis	Adult onset hyperkeratosis indistinguishable from ichthyosis vulgaris	Hodgkin's lymphoma, mycosis fungoides, multiple myeloma, leiomyosarcoma
Acrokeratosis paraneoplastica (Bazex syndrome)	Acromelic psoriasiform plaques with nail dystrophy	Carcinomas of upper digestive and respiratory tracts. Also was described in association with transitional cell bladder carcinoma[2]
Carcinoid syndrome	Deeply erythematous or violaceous flushing of upper body associated with pruritus, diaphoresis, lacrimation, and facial edema	Foregut, midgut, and bronchial neuroendocrine tumors
Cushing's syndrome	Generalized hyperpigmentation, including areolae, palmar creases, and scars hirsuitism, central obesity, moon facies, striae	Ectopic ACTH production by small cell lung cancer, bronchial carcinoid tumors, cancers of thyroid, pancreas, and adrenals
Dermatomyositis	Heliotrope dermatitis, proximal nailfold telangiectasias, Gottron's papules, cutaneous necrosis	Ovarian, digestive, amd nasopharyngeal carcinomas; adenocarcinomas of lung and prostate; hematologic malignancies
Erythema gyratum repens	Migratory figurate erythema with "wood grain" pattern	Malignancies of lung, breast, female reproductive tract, GI tract, prostate
Hypertrichosis lanuginosa acquisita	Excessive growth of vellus hairs on neck and face, but can involve any body surface	Most commonly observed with colorectal, breast, and lung cancers
Necrolytic migratory erythema (NME)	Acral and intertriginous papulosquamous dermatitis with occasional vesiculation	Pancreatic α-cell tumor presents with glucagonoma syndrome (see text)
Paget's disease	1) Unilateral eczematous nipple plaque 2) Eczematous plaque of anorectal, genital, and axillary regions	1) Associated with ductal adenocarcinoma 2) Regional associations are: a) anorectal—adenocarcinoma of anus and colorectum, b) vulvar—epithelial, eccrine and apocrine neoplasms, c) male genitalia—GU and male reproductive tract malignancies
Paraneoplastic pemphigus	Diffuse mucocutaneous involvement with blisters, erosions, lichenoid, and erythema multiforme-like lesions. Head and neck skin is usually spared. Extensive oral erosions are notable.	Hematologic malignancies

(continued)

TABLE 33-1 ■ (*Continued*)

Porphyria cutanea tarda	Vesicles and bullae with subsequent scarring, skin fragily on dorsal hands, milia formation, and hypertrichosis on sun-exposed surfaces	Hepatocellular carcinoma, hematologic malignancies, myelodysplastic syndromes
Sweet's syndrome–atypical bullous pyoderma gangrenosum overlap	Indurated erythematous to violaceous plaques with or without bulla formation and ulceration	Hematologic malignancies, myeloproliferative disorders
Sign of Leser-Trélat	Eruptive multiple seborrheic keratoses	Adenocarcinomas of the lung and GI tract

[1.] Rigel DS, Jacobs MI. Malignant acanthosis nigricans: a review. *J Dermatol Surg Oncol.* Nov 1980;6(11):923–927.

[2.] Arregui MA, Raton JA, Landa N, Izu R, Eizaquirre X, Diaz-Perez JL. Bazex's syndrome (acrokeratosis paraneoplastica)–first case report of association with a bladder carcinoma. *Clin Exp Dermatol.* Sep 1993;18(5):445–448.

Disorders of the Hypothalamic–Pituitary–Adrenal Axis

Cushing's syndrome of glucocorticoid excess is caused by either endogenous overproduction of the adrenal glands or by iatrogenic steroids, whereas Cushing's disease is caused by an adrenocorticotrophic hormone–secreting anterior pituitary or nonpituitary neoplasm. The most profound cutaneous manifestations of Cushing's syndrome (and disease) including epidermal atrophy, striae, plethoric moon facies, buffalo hump, supraclavicular fat pads, and central obesity. There is a marked susceptibility to cutaneous fungal infections. The following findings are limited to Cushing's syndrome:

■ Addisonian hyperpigmentation,
■ Precocious puberty,
■ Virilization, and
■ Pattern alopecia in females.

Patients with Addison's disease, or primary adrenocortical insufficiency, suffer from deficiency of glucocorticoids as well as mineralocorticoids. There is hyperpigmentation

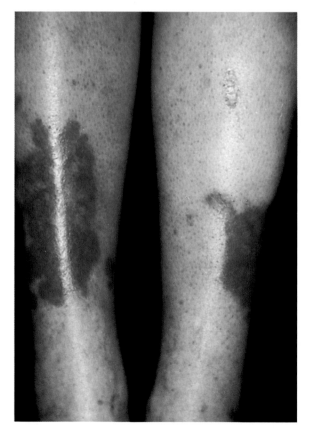

FIGURE 33-3 ■ Diabetic dermopathy. Necrobiosis lipoidica diabeticorum on the anterior tibial area of the legs. (*Courtesy of Smith Kline & French Laboratories.*)

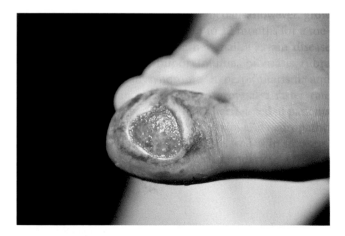

FIGURE 33-4 ■ Mal perforans ulcer on the great toe of a diabetic man.

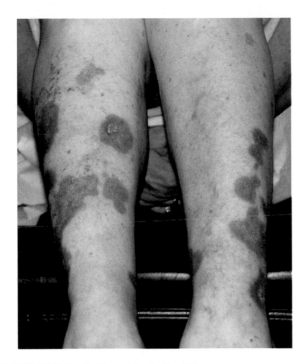

FIGURE 33-5 ■ Necrobiosis lipoidica.

of sun-exposed surfaces, flexural areas, pressure points, scars and palmar creases (Fig. 33-6). Women may experience loss of axillary and pubic hair.

Multiple Mucosal Neuroma Syndrome

Multiple mucosal neuroma syndrome is also known as *multiple endocrine neoplasia IIB*. In this autosomal dominant disorder, medullary thyroid carcinoma (MTC) and pheochromocytoma are associated with oral, nasal, upper gastrointestinal tract, and conjunctival neuromas. The skin lesions typically range from soft to firm intradermal nodules, which tend to precede the MTC. However, the MTC can occur in early childhood prior to the development of the neuromas. Additional skin findings include "blubbery" lips, lentigines, café-au-lait macules, and localized intense unilateral pruritus on the back (nostalgia paresthetica).

Thyroid Disease

The activity of the thyroid gland is intimately reflected by changes in the skin and its appendages. In hyperthyroidism, the skin is thin, warm, moist, and flushed secondary to vasodilation of dermal vasculature. Erythema and hyperhidrosis of palms and soles may be present. Adnexal changes include rapidly growing fine soft hair with attendant nonscarring alopecia, and soft nails with distal onycholysis. Graves' disease is associated with ophthalmopathy (proptosis, exophthalmos, and lid lag) and acropachy.

In hypothyroidism, the skin is cold dry, and pale secondary to vasoconstriction of the cutaneous vessels (Fig. 33-7). There is generalized thinning and hyperkeratosis of the epidermis. Fine wrinkling and a yellow discoloration are sometimes present. The hair is coarse, dry, brittle, and slow growing. Patchy or diffuse alopecia can be seen. Loss of the outer third of the eyebrow (madarosis) is a characteristic finding. Myxedema is also found but in a more diffuse distribution than seen in hyperthyroidism. Hypothyroid facies typically is expressionless, with thickening of the lips, broadening of the nose, drooping of the upper eyelids, and overall puffiness.

Gastroenterology

Dermatitis Herpetiformis

Also known as Duhring disease, dermatitis herpetiformis causes vesicles on the buttocks, elbows, and knees. Dermatitis

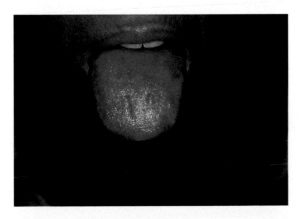

FIGURE 33-6 ■ Hyperpigmentation of skin and tongue in a white woman with Addison's disease.

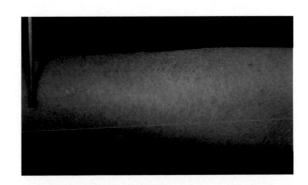

FIGURE 33-7 ■ Year-round dry skin associated with hypothyroidism. *(Courtesy of Reed and Carnick.)*

herpetiformis is associated with celiac sprue (gluten-sensitive enteropathy). Celiac sprue is often subclinical but can be confirmed by jejunal biopsy.

Inflammatory Bowel Disease

Ulcerative colitis is most commonly associated with pyoderma gangrenosum, a destructive neutrophilic dermatosis (Fig. 33-8). In pyoderma gangrenosum, a painful violaceous nodule or pustule breaks down to form an enlarging ulcer with a raised, undetermined border and a boggy, necrotic base. Pyoderma gangrenosum has also been observed with Crohn's disease as well as hematologic malignancies, monoclonal gammopathies, and various arthritides.

Peutz-Jeghers Syndrome

Peutz-Jeghers syndrome is an autosomal dominant disorder characterized by hamartomatous gastrointestinal polyposis and mucocutaneous pigmentation. Patients may present with abdominal pain, rectal bleeding, rectal prolapse, or intussusception. There is an increased risk of gastrointestinal tumors, ovarian and breast malignancies in females, and Sertoli cell tumors in males. Lentigines may be present at birth or develop in early childhood. Discrete brown, blue, or blue-brown macules are almost always located on the lips and oral mucosa, most commonly on buccal surfaces. Lentigines may also appear on the vac, nail beds, hands, and feet, especially on palmar and plantar areas. With age, the cutaneous lesions may fade and even disappear, but the buccal mucosal lesions tend to persist into adulthood.

Hematology-Oncology

Although cutaneous manifestations of systemic neoplastic disorders are diverse and often nonspecific, a practitioner

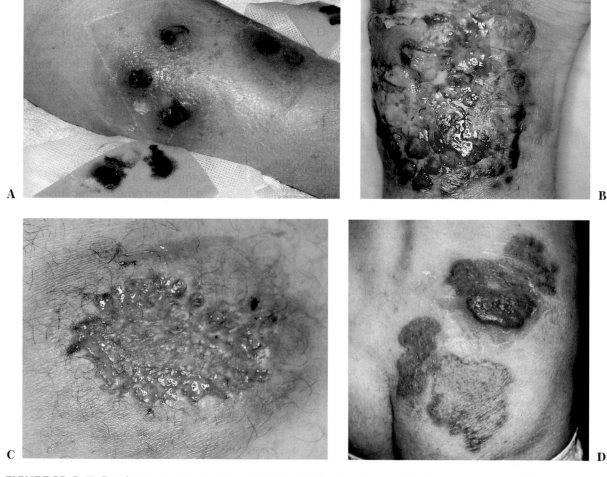

FIGURE 33-8 ■ Pyoderma gangrenosum associated with ulcerative colitis. *(Part D courtesy of Schering Corp.)*

in the course of his or her career is likely to encounter a warning sign that may warrant further investigation. Pioneered by Curth and later expanded by Hill, criteria of association are applied to determine whether any given malignancy and a dermatologic condition are indeed correlated. These criteria are invaluable prognostically in both managing patients concerned with the outcome and determining cause and outcome in suspect dermatoses and underlying conditions. Application of these epidemiologic principles allows identification of specific dermatoses/syndromes and associated malignancies.

Acquired ichthyosis (Fig. 33-9), which clinically appears as severely dry skin, is most often associated with lymphoproliferative disorders and other malignancies, including

- Hodgkin's disease,
- mycosis fungoides,
- multiple myeloma,
- Kaposi's sarcoma,
- leiomyosarcomas, and
- breast, cervical, and lung cancers.

It is most often a later manifestation of lymphoma but may precede the diagnosis by many years. Erythroderma is diffuse erythema of the skin, usually with induration and scaling. When scaling is diffuse, the condition is defined as exfoliative erythroderma. When associated with internal malignancy, erythroderma is seen more commonly with hematologic malignancies, especially leukemia, lymphoma, and Sézary syndrome.

Acanthosis nigricans (AN) can be benign or malignant (Fig. 33-10). "Benign" forms are generally seen in obese patients or associated with endocrinopathies such as hyper-

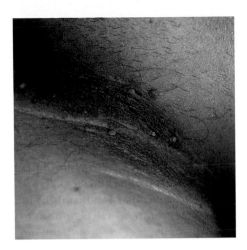

FIGURE 33-10 ■ AN of the base of the neck.

androgenism and insulin resistance, as well as diabetes mellitus and the polycystic ovarian syndrome. AN is also observed in a number of genetic disorders. Occasionally, AN is induced by systemically administered corticosteroids, somatotropin, nicotinic acid, and insulin. The pathophysiology of AN in metabolic disturbances is purportedly related to insulin and insulin-like growth factor (IGF) and their interaction with corresponding keratinocytic receptors (IGFR-1), and is likely to be a reflection of insulin resistance.

"Malignant" AN is suspected in thin, older individuals with extensive involvement of the mucocutaneous integument. These gray-brown, symmetric, velvety, papillomatous plaques involve axillae, neck, groin, antecubital fossae, vermilion border of the lip, and eyelids. Mucosal AN presents with verrucous pigmented plaques on oral mucosa and conjunctivae and is especially suggestive of a neoplastic process. Association with rugated velvety plaques of palmar surfaces (tripe palms) is observed. Malignant AN is most often associated with lung, ovarian, breast, gastric, bladder, and endometrial carcinomas.

Necrolytic migratory erythema (NME) is an integral part of a paraneoplastic syndrome observed in the context of glucagonoma, a neuroendocrine pancreatic tumor. Although no longer considered pathognomic of glucagonoma, NME accompanied by the new onset of diabetes, weight loss, glossitis, and angular cheilitis may be observed in a majority of patients with a glucagonoma at some point of their illness. NME frequently presents as an annular psoriasiform eruption in acral distribution affecting the central face, extremities, and groin. Disseminated lesions are not uncommon. The lesions tend to have a waxing and waning course, healing without scarring. The NME course does not reflect the activity of the underlying tumor.

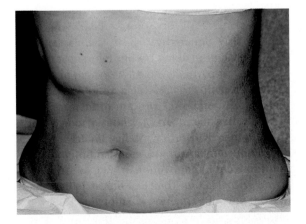

FIGURE 33-9 ■ Acquired ichthyosis, which can be a sign of lymphoproliferative disorders.

Paraneoplastic rheumatologic syndromes include rheumatoid arthritis, systemic lupus erythematosus (SLE), vasculitides, Sjögren's syndrome, and dermatomyositis. Although presentation of malignancy-associated rheumatologic disturbances is very similar to non-paraneoplastic rheumatologic diseases, there are certain laboratory and clinical findings that may suggest malignancy in otherwise typical cases. Rapid onset, cutaneous necrosis, extensive vasculitis, and a history of malignancy are all likely predictors of a concurrent neoplasm. Rheumatic symptoms and primary tumors follow parallel clinical courses. Dermatologic manifestations of some lymphoproliferative disorders are shown in Fig. 33-11.

Infectious Diseases

Lyme Disease

Lyme borreliosis, a spirochetal multisystem illness borne by *Ixodes* spp. ticks, is prevalent in Northeastern, North Central, and Pacific coastal regions. In the United States, *Borrelia burgdorferi* is the most commonly isolated causative organism, whereas in the European countries *B. afzelii* and *B. garinii* predominate. Erythema chronicum migrans (ECM) is the principal cutaneous hallmark of new-onset Lyme disease (Fig. 33-12). An early lesion displays homogenous erythema at the site of the tick bite that subsequently spreads centrifugally. The center may fade or clear completely, leaving an annular expanding erythema. ECM may present with

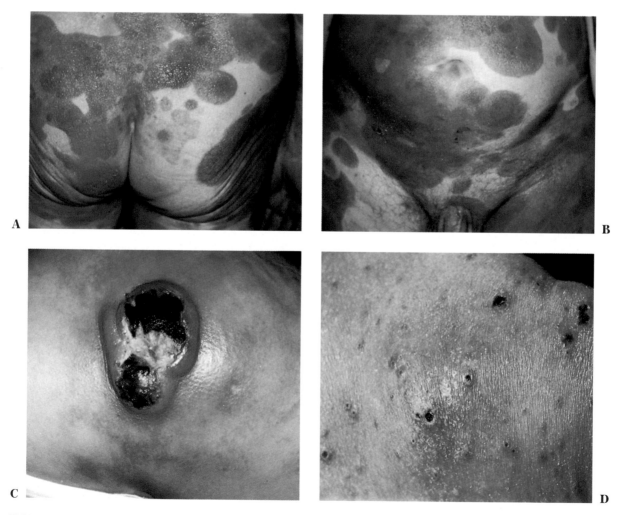

FIGURE 33-11 ■ Dermatoses associated with lymphomas. (**A, B**) Mycosis fungoides in plaque stage of the buttocks (**A**) and abdomen (**B**) of a 79-year-old man. (**C**) Mycosis fungoides in tumor stage on the thigh. (**D**) Non-specific pyoderma with lymphocytic leukemia.

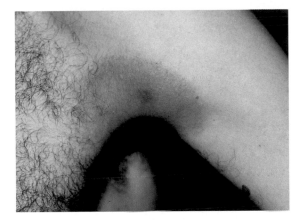

FIGURE 33-12 ■ ECM of the axilla.

a single or, less often, multiple lesions. Although ECM is by far the most common Lyme-associated dermatosis in the United States and Europe, other cutaneous disorders, borrelial lymphocytoma (BL), and acrodermatitis chronica atrophicans (ACA), are observed more frequently in Europe. BL, also known as *lymphadenosis benigna cutis,* is usually noted at or near the tick bite site. Typically, BL presents as a solitary bluish-red nodule with regional lymphadenopathy. Sites of predilection include the earlobe, nipple and areola, scrotum, and nose. Patients with BL may present with or without proceeding or concomitant ECM. Late Lyme disease may be associated with ACA, a chronic acral dermatitis that develops 6 months to 10 years after the initial arthropod assault. The onset is insidious with waxing and waning edema and a reddish-blue discoloration of distal extremities, reminiscent of venous insufficiency. With time, the epidermis and dermis become atrophic and translucent. Late findings include fibrotic bands and nodule formation.

Syphilis

With its incidence on the rise, syphilis has reemerged as an important treponemal disease. Syphilis (lues) is caused by the spirochete *Treponema pallidum.* The mode of acquisition (sexual versus vertical) and stage determine cutaneous and systemic manifestations. Lesions of primary syphilis present as a syphilitic chancre—a firm, painless, eroded plaque at the site of treponemal entry. These are commonly seen on the glans penis and prepuce in males and external genitalia and fourchette in females. Often syphilitic chancres are unrecognized as such because of their perianal, anal, intravaginal, or oral locations. Untreated, the classic Hunterian chancre heals spontaneously. If the chancre is coinfected with other sexually transmitted agents, the presentation may be atypical.

Roughly one third of patients with untreated primary syphilis progress to secondary syphilis. More than 80% of these patients develop generalized cutaneous eruptions—syphilids that vary widely in their presentations including macular, maculopapular, papular, annular, and less frequently, nodular and pustular lesions (Fig. 33-13). Patchy alopecia of the scalp, eyebrows, beard, and, rarely, body, is infrequently observed. Mucous membrane lesions are not uncommonly seen. Condyloma lata are moist, macerated, cauliflower-like vegetations seen in the anogenital areas. Mucous patches are macerated—gray papules and plaques with denuded areas over oral mucosa—especially common on the tongue and lips. These lesions are highly infectious.

Nearly one third of untreated patients develop tertiary syphilis, which also presents with polymorphous lesions. Gummas are painless, pink to dusky-red nodules that can affect any organ system. These lesions may ulcerate and cause local tissue destruction. Whereas gummas involving visceral organs, skeletal structures, and skin are seen in the majority of cases, neurosyphilis and cardiovascular syphilis each affect 25% of patients with tertiary syphilis.

Presenting signs and symptoms of cerebrovascular syphilis range from the Argyll Robertson pupil that accommodates and converges but does not react to light, to blindness, deafness, and dementia. Tabes dorsalis is the degeneration of posterior columns of the spinal cord leading to lancinating pain, ataxia, urinary incontinence, and loss of proprioception with resultant joint deterioration (Charcot's

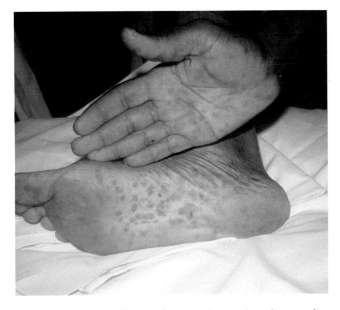

FIGURE 33-13 ■ Ham-colored palm and scale papules of secondary syphilis.

joints). Cardiovascular syphilis leads to a spectrum of manifestations: uncomplicated aortitis, aortic aneurysm (usually affecting the ascending aorta), aortic valvulitis with aortic insufficiency, coronary ostial stenosis, and myocarditis. Interestingly, early atherosclerosis in individuals with no known risk factors has been associated with tertiary syphilis.

Congenital syphilis tends to present soon after birth. However, a delay in presentation of up to 2 years may occur. Early manifestations are remarkably similar to syphilids in adults. In neonates, pemphigus syphiliticus with vesiculobullous lesions of palms and soles, as well as other areas, have been described. Classically, syphilitic rhinitis (snuffles) is one of the more frequent specific signs of congenital syphilis. Mucosanguineous discharge with attendant nasal obstruction is present early in the disease; saddle nose deformity with septal perforation and perioral rhagades are stigmata of late congenital syphilis. Hutchinson's triad of congenital syphilis consists of Hutchinson's teeth (notched incisors), interstitial keratitis, and sensorineural deafness. Among other important presenting signs are bone lesions (saddle nose deformity, epiphysitis with resultant pain on motion—Parrot's pseudoparalysis) and Higoumenakia's sign (unilateral clavicular thickening lateral to the patient's dexterity), neurosyphilis (seizures, hydrocephalus, cranial nerve palsies, tabes dorsalis), lymphadenopathy, and hepatosplenomegaly.

Nephrology

Acquired Perforating Disease

Acquired perforating disease (APD) of end-stage renal disease (ESRD) presents as a clinical aggregate of three primary perforating disorders:

- Kyrle's disease,
- reactive perforating collagenosis, and
- perforating folliculitis.

APD has also been associated with patients on dialysis. As with primary perforating disorders, an alteration in connective tissue (collagen or elastin) and transepithelial elimination have been implicated in the pathophysiology of APD. The lesions appear clinically as dome-shaped papules with keratotic plugs on the trunk and extensor extremities. Severe pruritus may accompany cutaneous eruption of APD. Koebnerization is frequently observed.

Calcinosis Cutis and Calciphylaxis

Abnormal calcium and phosphate metabolism with subsequent secondary hyperparathyroidism predispose patients with renal disease to metastatic calcifications. Calcinosis cutis frequently affects periarticular soft tissues. Discrete,

mobile, skin-colored subcutaneous nodules are tender when present on the digits. Pasty or chalky contents occasionally extrude from these lesions. Calciphylaxis is a systemic vascular disease with mural calcification of small and medium-sized arteries. Typical lesions are exquisitely tender, poorly defined, deep subcutaneous nodules and plaques with overlying livedoid purpura of proximal thighs and buttocks. Stellate ulcerations are not uncommon. Cutaneous necrosis occurs and not uncommonly fatal.

Chronic Renal Failure and Dialysis

As the number of ESRD patients and those on dialysis continues to increase, previously known diseases affecting this population become better characterized and new entities continue to emerge. Several cutaneous changes are particularly prevalent in patients on dialysis. Generalized pruritus without a primary cutaneous eruption could be a sign of various underlying disorders, including uremia or chronic renal failure. Dialysis seems to be an important trigger of pruritus. Uremic frost is exceedingly rare in the present day but can be seen as white crystalline precipitation on the skin. Pallor of the proximal nail bed, known as Lindsay's nail (half-and-half nail), may be observed in azotemic patients.

Henoch-Schönlein Purpura

Henoch-Schönlein purpura is an IgA-mediated systemic leukocytoclastic vasculitis of small vessels that typically affects the skin, joints, gastrointestinal tract, and kidneys (see Chap. 12). Clinically, pediatric patients present with the classic tetrad of abdominal pain, polyarthritis, nephritis, and a purpuric eruption. Palpable purpura, typically of the lower legs and buttocks, occurs in almost every case and is the presenting sign in more than 50% of cases. Petechiae and ecchymoses may also be present. Urticarial and erythematous maculopapular lesions preceding the purpura have been described. Nail fold capillaroscopy reveals tortuous capillaries with granular capillary wall appearance and edema during the acute episode and on follow-up. A characteristic finding in children is painful edema of the face, scalp, ears, periorbital region, extremities, and genitalia. Scrotal edema and bruising is observed in up to one third of male patients. Rare cases of penile edema and purpura involving the glans penis have been reported.

Fabry's Disease

Fabry's disease is an X-linked recessive defect in the activity of a lysosomal enzyme, α-galactosidase A, with ensuant accumulation of glycosphingolipids in tissues. The glycosphingolipid deposits primarily affect the vascular endothelium, which leads to cardiovascular, cerebral, and renal manifestations. Cutaneous findings give rise to the alternative name for this disease: angiokeratoma corporis diffusum universale. Angiokeratomas are of the utmost diagnostic importance as they appear in childhood and may be one of the earliest signs of the disease. These are nonblanchable, punctuate, red to blue-black keratotic papules with slight hyperkeratosis in the larger lesions. Angiokeratomas, with time, increase in size and number. Lesions are mostly located between the umbilicus and the knees and are usually symmetrically distributed. Acroparesthesias and hypohidrosis with resultant heat intolerance have been described.

Nephrogenic Sclerosing Dermopathy

First described in 1997, nephrogenic sclerosing dermopathy (NFD) has been recognized in patients with renal insufficiency with nearly 150 cases identified between 1997 and 2004. Patients may or may not require hemodialysis. NFD has been described equally in males and females without ethnic predilection. Clinically, patients initially present with erythematous papules as well as a peau d'orange appearance of distal extremities. These primary lesions coalesce into woody, sclerodermoid red-brawny plaques with an edge that advances proximally. Dependent areas are more severely involved. There is accompanying pruritus, burning, and lancinating pain. A marked decrease in the affected joints' range of motion progresses to full joint contractures, incapacitating a patient in a short period of time. Systemic involvement with extensive calcifications and fibrosis of vital structures had been reported. The disease course closely parallels that of renal function.

Porphyria Cutanea Tarda

Porphyria cutanea tarda (PCT) in renal disease patients is most often of the sporadic type. Clinical and laboratory findings are analogous to those of the inherited form of PCT, with photodistributed tense bullae that tend to rupture and heal with scars and milia. Hypertrichosis and hyperpigmentation are common. Pseudoporphyria, a bullous dermatosis clinically similar to PCT, has been described in patients on chronic hemodialysis. However, patients with pseudoporphyria lack abnormal porphyrin levels and do not exhibit either hypertrichosis or sclerodermoid changes.

Neurology

Atopic Dermatitis

Asthma penicillin allergy, urticaria, marked reaction to insect bites, multiple food allergies, allergic rhinitis, and conjunctivitis have all been associated with atopic dermatitis (see

Chap. 9). These disorders may occur concomitantly or independently, and most patients develop only one or two components of an atopic diathesis. Several genetically inherited cutaneous disorders include atopic dermatitis as an integral part of the syndrome. Netherton's syndrome is an autosomal recessive genodermatosis characterized by pathognomic erythematous patches with a double-edge scale termed *ichthyosis linearis circumflexa*, a "ball-and-socket" hair deformity (trichorrhexis invaginata), and atopic dermatitis. Other diseases associated with atopic dermatitis include ichthyosis vulgaris and the Wiskott-Aldrich syndrome. Recently, chronic atopic dermatitis has been implicated in increased susceptibility to CD30[+] cutaneous lymphoma. However, the causal relationship between the two entities remains under scrutiny.

Neurofibromatosis

Neurofibromatosis (NF) is an autosomal dominant genodermatosis (see Chap. 35). There are two subtypes of NF: Recklinghausen's disease (NF-1) and bilateral acoustic neurofibromatosis (NF-2). Both types involve congenital and acquired hamartomatous tumors of the central nervous system (CNS), skin, bone, endocrine glands, and eyes. Café-au-lait macules develop shortly after birth and may be found anywhere on the body. These hyperpigmented lesions can be found in normal individuals, but the presence of six or more macules 1.5 cm or greater in adults ($\geq$0.5 cm in children) have nearly always been found to indicate NF. Intertriginous freckling (Crowe's sign) as well as pigmented hamartomas of the iris (Lisch nodules) are almost always diagnostic of NF. The principal dermatologic manifestations of this disease are cutaneous, subcutaneous, or plexiform neurofibromas (Fig. 33-14). These vary in size and shape and range from a few to as many as 9,000. Less common features include total or partial limb enlargement (elephantiasis neuromatosa), multiple lipomas, or a cutaneous sclerosing perineuroma. Segmental involvement with either NF subtype may represent postzygotic mutation.

Sarcoidosis

Sarcoidosis is a granulomatous process affecting various organ systems (see Chap. 16). The most characteristic cutaneous sarcoidal lesion is lupus pernio. Lesions of lupus pernio consist of chronic reddish-brown to violaceous, indurated papules and plaques with a predilection for the nose, ears, and lips (Fig. 33-15). Sarcoidal skin plaques are also located on the limbs, back, and buttocks. These plaques may have central atrophy or a hypopigmented appearance. Erythema nodosum is the most common nonspecific cutaneous manifestation of sarcoidosis. Erythema nodosum is a hypersensitivity reaction to various agents

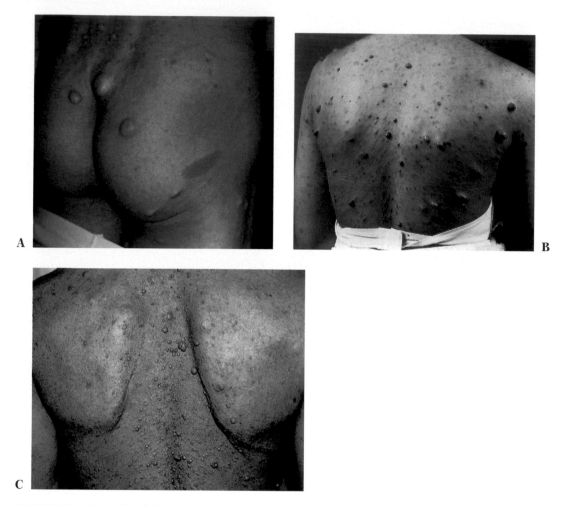

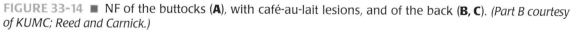

FIGURE 33-14 ■ NF of the buttocks (**A**), with café-au-lait lesions, and of the back (**B, C**). *(Part B courtesy of KUMC; Reed and Carnick.)*

and appears clinically as tender erythematous, subcutaneous nodules predominantly on the anterior shins. Lofgren's syndrome is a triad of erythema nodosum, fever, and polyarthralgia. Lupus pernio is more frequent in African American patients; erythema nodosum is commonly found in European and Latin American patients. Heerfordt's syndrome is a manifestation of acute sarcoidosis and presents with fever, uveitis, parotitis, and Bell's palsy. Although rare in the general population, this syndrome has been most often reported in young Japanese patients, with females outnumbering males. Koebnerization of sarcoidal lesions is observed. Uncommon manifestations such as leonine facies, psoriasiform or lichenoid plaques, and pyoderma gangrenosum have been reported. Other nonspecific skin findings include scarring and nonscarring alopecia, hypopigmented patches, erythroderma, erythema multiforme, acquired ichthyosis, and dystrophic calcifications.

Sturge-Weber Syndrome

In this neurocutaneous syndrome, a port-wine stain (nevus flammeus) involves the unilateral or, less commonly, the bilateral distribution of the ophthalmic division of the trigeminal nerve. Typically, the cutaneous involvement precedes the cerebral involvement, which appears later in childhood as a contralateral spastic hemiparesis, unilateral seizures, hemisensory defects, mental retardation, glaucoma, and homonymous hemianopia. Although plain skull x-rays reveal the classic "tram-track" calcifications, these do not appear until later in life. Therefore, either MRI/MRA or PET scans are

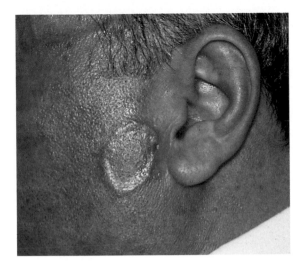

FIGURE 33-15 ■ A granulomatous skin plaque in a man with sarcoidosis.

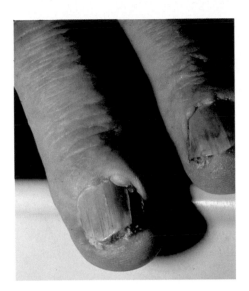

FIGURE 33-17 ■ Periungual fibromas (Koenen tumor) associated with tuberous sclerosis.

better modalities to screen for leptomeningeal angiomatosis and brain involvement.

Tuberous Sclerosis

Tuberous sclerosis is a highly penetrant, genetically heterogeneous autosomal dominant genodermatosis characterized by the triad of multiple hamartomas, seizures, and developmental difficulties. Hamartomas can involve any organ system, especially the skin, CNS, renal system, and cardiovascular system. Adenoma sebaceum (Fig. 33-16), Koenen tumors (Fig. 33-17), and fibrous plaques are the major cutaneous findings.

Adenoma sebaceum is actually a misnomer. These red-to-pink papules and nodules are in fact angiofibromas.

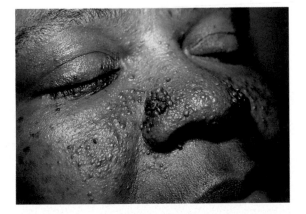

FIGURE 33-16 ■ Adenoma sebaceum (angiofibromas) on the face of a patient with tuberous sclerosis.

They tend to appear after 4 years of age and localize to the nasolabial folds, cheeks, and chin. Fibrous forehead plaques may present as early as the first weeks of life. The Koenen tumor is an ungual angiofibroma. A later finding appearing during childhood or adolescence is the shagreen patch, a connective tissue hamartoma. It is characteristically found in the lumbosacral region and appears as a skin-colored, slightly elevated plaque with the texture and appearance of an orange peel. When fewer than three in number, hypomelanotic macules may be observed in normal individuals; congential hypomelanotic macules have been found in up to 90% of patients with tuberous sclerosis. These lesions, typically located on the trunk and limbs, appear before any other skin findings. Their configurations vary from guttate leukodermatous "confetti" macules to lance ovate ash-leaf macules. Fibroepithelial polyps (molluscum fibrosum pendulum), café-au-lait macules, and port-wine hemangiomas may be observed but are not diagnostic of tuberous sclerosis.

Rheumatology
(see Chap. 32)

Dermatomyositis

Dermatomyositis is a complex autoimmune disease of adults and children that causes progressive muscular inflammation and weakness. Myositis preferentially involves the shoulder and hip girdles, resulting in difficulties with such activities as combing hair and getting up from a chair. Interstitial lung disease is an uncommon presenting sign of dermatomyositis, with 65% of newly diagnosed patients affected. Rarely, dermatomyositis may be complicated by associated malignancies, including cancers of lung, ovary, and hematopoietic systems.

The cutaneous manifestations are pathognomic. The most specific skin finding are the Gottron's papules, erythematous papules of distant interphalangeal joints. The heliotrope rash, a subtle, erythematous or violaceous blush on the eyelids and periorbital region, is seen in approximately 60% of cases. Erythema may develop on sun-exposed areas, and chronic changes may include poikilodermatous lesions on the trunk and proximal extremities. Periungual telangiectasias and cuticular thromboses may also be noted. Of note, myositis and cutaneous manifestations often have divergent courses in terms of onset, progress, and severity. "Amyopathic" dermatomyositis displays classic cutaneous findings without an associated myopathy. These patients may also be at risk for associated malignancies.

Lupus Erythematosus

SLE is an autoimmune connective tissue disease characterized by multiorgan involvement and the presence of autoantibodies to nuclear antigens (see Chap. 32). The stringent diagnostic criteria for SLE were originally set forth by the American College of Rheumatology in 1982 and revised in 1997. The butterfly rash is the *sine qua non* of an acute SLE eruption (Fig. 33-18). The shape of the eruption indeed resembles a butterfly with open wings, with erythematous to violaceous edematous plaques over the malar cheeks and

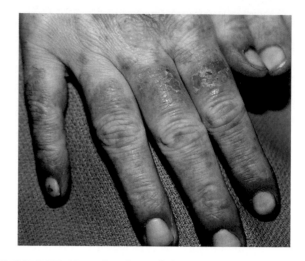

FIGURE 33-19 ■ Sporing of the knuckles in systemic lupus erythematosus (the opposite of dermatomyositis).

dorsal nose. The nasolabial folds are typically spared. As with all SLE cutaneous manifestations, the malar rash appears typically after sun exposure. Other sites of predilection are the V of the chest, extensor extremities, mid-upper back, and shoulders (Fig. 33-19). On rare occasions, the atrophic, hyperpigmented scarring lesions of chronic cutaneous lupus erythematosus (discoid lupus erythematosus) may develop; the annular or papulosquamous lesions of subacute cutaneous lupus erythematosus have a more frequent association with systemic disease than discoird lupus erythematosus.

Mucous membranes may also be affected, with lesions on either palatal or buccal mucosa. The former is involved with honeycomb plaques, hyperemia, and punched-out ulcerations, whereas lichen planus–like leukoplakia appears on the latter. Discoid lesions may be observed on the palatal and buccal mucosae. Panniculitis (lupus profundus), alopecia, livedo reticularis, and periungual telangiectasias are other cutaneous features that can be seen in SLE.

Scleroderma

Systemic scleroderma is a chronic disease of unknown origin that affects the connective tissue and the vasculature. The disease is characterized by fibrosis and obliteration of the vessels in the skin, lungs, heart, gastrointestinal tract, and kidneys (Fig. 33-20). Whereas the localized form of scleroderma, morphea is confined to the skin, systemic scleroderma manifests based on the systems involved.

There are two forms of systemic scleroderma: progressive and limited. Limited systemic scleroderma or

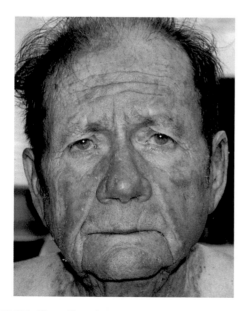

FIGURE 33-18 ■ Papulosquamous eruption of subacute cutaneous lupus.

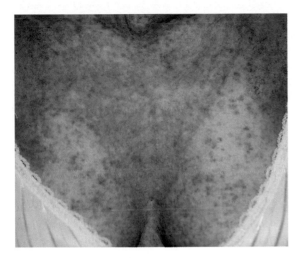

FIGURE 33-20 ■ Hypopigmentation with perifollicular pigment retention and skin tightening of scleroderma.

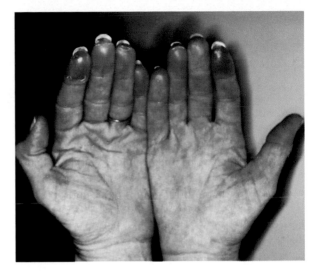

FIGURE 33-21 ■ Raynaud's disease with gangrene.

CREST syndrome (*c*alcinosis, *R*aynaud's phenomenon, *e*sophageal dysmotility, *s*clerodactyly, *t*elangiectasias) predominantly affects the hands and may start as Raynaud's phenomenon or nonpitting edema of the hands and fingers (Fig. 33-21). Flexion contractures and sclerodactyly may eventually supervene. Progressive systemic scleroderma may also present with Raynaud's phenomenon and, as the name implies, evolve to affect viscera and the skin. The disease slowly extends to involve upper extremities, face, trunk, and possibly the lower extremities. It begins as a painless edema, which leads to tightening of the skin. In the final or atrophic stage, the skin becomes taut, smooth, and discolored, being tightly bound to underlying bony structures with a resultant decrease in range of motion. The face takes on a mask-like quality with microstomia with radial furrowing around the mouth, a beaked nose, and an unnaturally youthful countenance. Mat-like telangiectasias of the face and upper trunk, alopecia, and anhidrosis are also seen.

Suggested Reading

Callin J. Dermatological signs of internal disease, ed 2. Philadelphia, WB Saunders, 1995.

Christova I, Komitova R. Clinical and epidemiological features of Lyme borreliosis in Bulgaria. Wien Klin Wochenschr 2004;116:42–46.

Coens JL, Janninger CK, DeWolf K. Dermatologic and systemic manifestations of syphilis. Am Fam Physician 1994;50:1013.

Cohen PR. Cutaneous paraneoplastic syndromes. Am Fam Physician 1994;50:1273.

Kirsner RS, Federman DG. Cutaneous clues to systemic disease. Postgrad Med 1997;101:137, 144–147.

Lebwohl M. Atlas of the skin and systemic disease. New York, Churchill Livingstone, 1995.

Loucas E, Russo G, Millikan LE. Genetic and acquired cutaneous disorders associated with internal malignancy. Int J Dermatol 1995;34:749.

Lucky AW. Pigmentary abnormalities in genetic disorders. Dermatol Clin 1988;6:193.

Lyme disease—United States, 2001–2002. MMWR Morb Mortal Wkly Rep 2004;53:365–369.

Mana J, Marcoval J, Graells J, et al. Cutaneous involvement in sarcoidosis: Relations to systemic disease. Arch Dermatol 1997;133:882.

Mannis MJ, Mascal MS, Huntley AC. Eye and Skin Disease. Philadelphia, Lippincott-Raven, 1996.

Ostezan LB, Callen JP. Cutaneous manifestations of selected rheumatologic diseases. Am Fam Physician 1996;53:1625.

Perez MI, Kohn SR. Cutaneous manifestations of diabetes mellitus. J Am Acad Dermatol 1994;30:519.

Weschesler HL. Cutaneous disease in systemic lupus erythematosus. Clin Dermatol 1985;3:79.

CHAPTER 34

Dermatologic Reactions to Ultraviolet Radiation and Visible Light

Laurie Linden, MD and Henry W. Lim, MD

The UV Spectrum

By convention, ultraviolet (UV) radiation is divided into UVA, UVB, and UVC. UVA ranges from 320 to 400 nm. UVB spans from 290 to 320 nm, and UVC includes wavelengths measuring from 200 to 290 nm. UVC radiation emitted by the sun is absorbed by the atmosphere; therefore, it does not reach the earth's surface and has no medical relevance. Sixty-five percent of UV radiation reaches the earth's surface between 10 AM and 2 PM, when the sun is most directly overhead. UV radiation in noonday sun consists of 95% UVA and 5% UVB. This is the reason that for optimal photoprotection, broad-spectrum sunscreens that absorb in both the UVA and UVB range are recommended. The type of UV and chromophores in the skin, such as nucleic acids, melanin, and aromatic amino acids, determine the depth of penetration of UV radiation. UVA, being of a longer wavelength, penetrates deeper than UVB. Twenty to thirty percent of UVA radiation reaches the deep dermis, whereas only 10% of UVB reaches the superficial dermis. UVA, but not UVB radiation, can penetrate window glass.

Sunburn and Tanning: Acute Effects of UV Light

Skin type plays an important role in the clinical outcome of sun exposure. Fitzpatrick's classification of skin types is widely used (Table 34-1). Sensitivity to UV is best assessed by the determination of minimal erythema dose (MED), which is defined as the smallest dose of radiation causing perceptible erythema covering the entire irradiated area. For individuals with skin type I, the MED for broadband UVB is between 20 and 40 mJ/cm^2, and for broadband

UVA, 20-40 J/cm^2, illustrating the 1000-fold less efficiency of UVA radiation in causing erythema.

Presentation and Characteristics

UVA-induced erythema has two phases: immediate and delayed. In skin type I individuals with sufficient exposure, erythema is typically apparent by the end of the irradiation period and may quickly fade. The delayed phase constitutes peak reappearance of erythema anywhere from 6 to 24 hours after exposure. For darker skinned individuals, all that may be observed is the delayed-phase reaction.

UVA is much more effective at inducing a tan than causing erythema. Exposure to UVA radiation results in two types of pigmentation changes: immediate pigment darkening (IPD) and persistent pigment darkening (PPD). IPD occurs immediately after exposure and fades within 10 to 20 minutes; it presents as a bluish-gray discoloration of the skin. The mechanism of IPD is oxidation of preexisting melanin in the epidermis; there is no neomelanogenesis. PPD occurs by the same mechanism and follows IPD if the UVA dose is sufficiently high. PPD lasts from 2 to 24 hours.

UVB-induced erythema also consists of an immediate and delayed phase; the latter peaks at 12 to 24 hours. Erythema is a necessary prerequisite for pigmentation changes secondary to UVB exposure. There is no IPD/PPD seen with UVB—just a delayed tanning reaction that is also observed with UVA exposure. For both UVA and UVB, delayed tanning occurs within 3 days; neomelanogenesis takes place in delayed tanning reaction. Delayed tanning after UVA radiation can last for weeks to months; in contrast, delayed tanning after UVB exposure fades much more quickly.

Sunburn reactions present as erythema, edema, vesiculation, and pain, followed by scaling and desquamation.

TABLE 34-1 ■ Fitzpatrick Skin Types

Skin Type	Characteristics
I	Never tan, always burn
II	Occasionally tan, usually burn
III	Usually tan, occasionally burn
IV	Easily tan, rarely burn
V	Brown skin
VI	Black skin

SAUER'S NOTES

1. UVB is most efficient in inducing sunburn; UVA delays tanning.
2. Photoprotection includes minimizing sun exposure between 10 AM and 2 PM, the use of photoprotective clothing, wide-brimmed hats, sun protective glasses, and the application of sunscreen.
3. Broad-spectrum sunscreen with SPF >15 should be applied generously, and reapply every 1 to 2 hours when outdoors.

Acute reactions, when severe, may be accompanied by weakness, fatigue, and pruritus.

Treatment

- *Photoprotection:* Photoprotection consists of minimizing sun exposure between 10 AM and 2 PM, the use of photoprotective clothing, wide-brimmed hats, sunglasses, and the application of sunscreen. Sunscreens with a sun protection factor (SPF) of 15 or greater should be applied 30 minutes before sun exposure, and reapplied every 1 to 2 hours, especially after sweating or swimming. Sunscreens should be applied generously: 1 ounce (30 mL) is needed to cover the entire body surface. Broad-spectrum sunscreens, which protect against both UVB and UVA radiation, should be recommended. Commonly used sunscreen ingredients in the United States are listed in Table 34-2.
- *Nonsteroidal anti-inflammatory agents and corticosteroids:* These should be taken within 4 to 6 hours after sun exposure. Topical corticosteroids and cool compresses are helpful in reducing the inflammation. Oral prednisone (1 mg/kg) may be used for 5 to 7 days in severe cases.

TABLE 34-2 ■ Commonly Used Sunscreen Ingredients in the United States

UVB Filters	UVA Filters
PABA derivatives	Benzophenones
Cinnamates	Avobenzone (Parsol 1789)
Salicylates	Anthranilate
Octocrylene	Titanium dioxide
	Zinc oxide

Abbreviation: PABA, para-aminobenzoic acid

Photoaging: Chronic Effects of UV Radiation

Presentation and Characteristics

Photoaging accounts for 90% of age-associated cosmetic problems. The effects of photoaging can be broken down into the following categories:

- pigmentation changes,
- texture changes,
- vascular changes, and
- papillary changes.

Pigmentation changes result from UV damage to the epidermis; the other changes result from dermal pathology. Both UVA and UVB radiation contribute to the process of photoaging.

The prototypical pigmentary change seen in older adults is the solar or senile lentigo. Solar lentigines, or "age spots," appear in chronically sun-exposed areas during the 40s through 60s. They usually present with multiple macular lesions, have well-demarcated borders, and vary in color from yellowish brown to dark brown. The mechanism of occurrence is thought to be an increase in melanin content within the keratinocytes and possibly reactive hyperplasia of melanocytes. Areas near the lentigines may be hypopigmented, giving the skin an overall mottled appearance.

The leathery texture and deep wrinkling of the skin from photoaging is called *solar elastosis* and is very characteristic of severe sun damage. This typically occurs on the face and neck and gives the skin a yellowish hue. The pathologic hallmark is deposition in the papillary dermis of amorphous elastotic material that does not form functional elastic fibers. This altered connective tissue does not demonstrate the resilient properties of normal elastic tissue. There is also epidermal acanthosis seen on histology. Furthermore, collagen destruction, induced by downstream effects of oxidative and direct DNA damage from UV radiation, plays a role in the loss of the skin's tensile strength.

Blood vessel damage occurs with photoaging, as well. Thinning of vessel walls and a decrease in vessel number are observed. Connective tissue support of the vasculature is diminished. Thus, fragility of vessels is demonstrated by the development of ecchymosis after minimal trauma. Telangectasias are also seen in chronically sun-exposed regions.

A common example of a papillary change seen in photoaging is the seborrheic keratosis. This "wisdom spot" results from disrupted keratinocyte maturation imposed by accumulated UV radiation. Seborrheic kerastoses appear "stuck on" to the skin and are more frequent on exposed skin of the trunk and extremities. They are completely benign growths and pose no risk of malignant transformation.

Treatment

- *Topical retinoids:* These can cause slight reversal of photoaged skin. They increase collagen levels, which effaces wrinkles. Retinoids also stimulate epidermal hyperplasia, which manifests clinically as smoother skin with fewer fine lines. Deeper wrinkles causes by chronologic aging persist. Retinoids also lighten pigmentary changes associated with photodamage. Side effects include peeling, erythema, and dryness. Topical retinoids are not recommended during pregnancy.
- *Photorejuvenation:* It entails stimulation of dermal collagen synthesis by exposure to laser, intense pulse (visible) light, radiofrequency, or photodynamic therapy. This is a rapidly evolving area with numerous methods and equipments on the market. More studies are needed for many of the methods used.
- *Resurfacing:* This can occur at a superficial, medium, or deep level. Techniques employed include microdermabrasion, chemical peels, and laser resurfacing; efficacy depends on the depth of wound infliction. The mechanism of wrinkle

reduction is stimulation of wound healing with new collagen formation. Reepithelialization occurs from stem cells located in adnexal appendages. Side effects of resurfacing include permanent pigmentary changes and scarring.

Photocarcinogenesis

Actinic Keratoses

Presentation and Characteristics

Actinic keratoses (AK) are premalignant lesions that predominately form on the chronically sun-exposed areas of skin type I and II patients. They occasionally appear in type III and IV individuals as well. Clinically, they present as discrete rough hyperkeratotic areas with a scale; they may be brown, yellowish-brown, flesh-colored, or red. When the lower lip is involved, *actinic cheilitis* is used (Fig. 34-1). Texture is the key to diagnosis. Histologically, an AK is an abnormal proliferation of cells confined to the epidermis with some evidence of cellular atypia. It has been estimated that over 10 years, 10.2% of AK would evolve into invasive squamous cell carcinoma, thus necessitating treatment for lesions that do not spontaneously remit.

Treatment

- *Cryotherapy:* It is the treatment of choice for most superficial lesions. For AK lesions that appear indurated, painful, or with a thick crust, surgical removal may be required, and a specimen should be sent for pathologic examination to rule out squamous cell carcinoma.

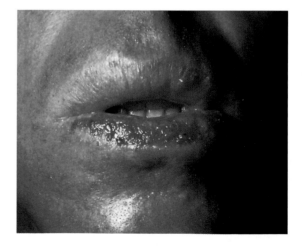

FIGURE 34-1 ■ Actinic cheilitis, presenting as rough, keratotic patches on the lower lip.

SAUER'S NOTES

1. Photoaging changes include solar lentigines, solar elastosis, loss of elasticity of skin, and telangiectasias.
2. Treatment includes topical retinoids, photorejuvenation, and resurfacing.

■ *Topical agents:* 5-Fluorouracil, imiquimod cream, and diclofenac sodium gel are useful for patients with multiple or recurrent lesions.

■ *Photodynamic therapy:* Photodynamic therapy, which utilizes 5-aminolevulinic acid (which gets converted to protoporphyrin) and blue light, or methyl aminolevulinate and red light, have been shown to successfully eliminate AK.

Nonmelanoma Skin Cancer

Basal cell carcinomas (BCCs) comprise 80% of non-melanoma skin cancers (NMSCs) diagnosed; squamous cell carcinomas (SCCs) comprise 20%. SCCs demonstrate a more linear correlation to the amount of UV exposure than do BCCs. Among white people, the incidence of NMSCs and melanomas has been increasing annually for several decades.

Squamous Cell Carcinoma

Presentation and Characteristics. The in situ form of SCC is known as Bowen's disease. Clinically, it appears as a well-demarcated, red, scaly patch, usually in sun-exposed areas. It is more likely to be found on the lower extremity of women and the scalp and ears of men. Treatment options include electrodessication and curettage, cryosurgery, and surgical excision.

Risk factors for development of SCCs include fair skin, light eyes, intermittent burns during childhood, ionizing radiation, immunosuppression, chronic inflammation, environmental carcinogens, certain genodermatoses, proximity to the equator, and cumulative exposure to UVR—specifically UVB radiation. UVB induces DNA damage and mutates tumor suppressor genes, such as *p53*. UVA also damages DNA and is thought to enhance the carcinogenic potential of UVB radiation.

SCCs are typically distributed on the scalp, dorsal hands, and pinna. SCCs have a greater potential for metastasis than BCC's. The risk of metastasis depends on a multitude of factors including location of the primary lesion, immune status, size of tumor, degree of differentiation on histopathology examination, and depth of invasion.

Treatment. Treatment entails electrodessication and curettage, surgical excision, or Mohs micrographic surgery.

Basal Cell Carcinoma

Presentation and Characteristics. BCCs are the single most common malignant neoplasms of the skin. They occur most often after the age of 40. Although sun exposure is an important cause of BCC's, other factors, such as ethnicity and skin type, play a role in its etiology. It seems that intermittent, as opposed to cumulative, sun exposure is the more prominent factor in the development of BCCs. BCCs often appear in areas protected from the sun, like behind the ears. However, 25% to 30% of BCCs occur on the nose.

Clinically, BCCs appear as pink or white pearly papules with areas of telangiectasia. As lesions progress, they may ulcerate and look as if they have been gnawed upon: the classic "rat bite" description. There are five histologic patterns of BCCs: nodular, superficial, micronodular, infiltrative, and morpheaform. Microscopically, BCCs are nests of basophilic cells originating from basal keratinocytes and hair follicles. Peripheral palisading is a hallmark histologic feature.

Risk factors include poor ability to tan, fair skin, immunosuppression, old age, and exposure to UV radiation. There are also genodermatoses associated with the development of BCCs, such as Gorlin's syndrome. Just as with SCCs, UVB radiation is thought to be more effective in photocarcinogenesis than UVA radiation. DNA mutations involving the Sonic hedgehog pathway are thought to play a role. Whether or not these are caused by UV radiation has not yet been elucidated.

BCCs grow by direct extension; therefore, the incidence of metastasis is low. Diagnosis is made only from biopsy.

Treatment. Treatment options include electrodessication and curettage, surgical excision, Mohs micrographic surgery, or radiation therapy for elderly patients who cannot tolerate surgical procedures.

Melanoma

Presentation and Characteristics. Melanoma demonstrates a less clear-cut relationship with sun exposure. Unlike BCCs, melanoma does not typically appear on skin that has received the most cumulative UVR. Furthermore, melanoma has a peak incidence in younger patients, who have acquired less lifetime sun exposure than their elderly counterparts. Melanoma occurs more frequently in people who work indoors, as opposed to outdoors. One proposed explanation for why indoor workers have a higher incidence of melanoma is that melanoma may be related to intense, intermittent sun exposure of untanned skin. This also supports the distribution pattern of melanoma seen on the trunk in men and lower extremities in women.

A helpful guideline to distinguish melanomas from benign nevi (moles) is the ABCD rule. Melanoma tends to be *a*symmetrical, with *b*order irregularity, *c*olor variegation, and a *d*iameter greater than 6 mm. This is, of course, just a clinical tool and does not help in the diagnosis of all melanomas. Changing moles, or moles that look different from the other moles on the patient, are two other clinical clues that should be considered.

There are four major clinicohistopathologic subtypes:

- superficial spreading,
- lentigo maligna,
- nodular, and
- acral lentigines.

They differ with respect to the pattern of sun exposure and location. A more detailed discussion of these subtypes is beyond the scope of this chapter. Other risk factors for melanoma include

- a first-degree relative with melanoma,
- the presence of atypical or dysplastic nevi,
- fair skin and light eyes,
- a history of severe childhood sunburns,
- a history of NMSC and
- immunosuppression.

One gene that has been linked to melanoma in certain families is *p16;* its protein products code for cell cycle arrest. Mutation of *p16* would theoretically allow damaged DNA to replicate, leading to oncogenesis.

Diagnosis. The diagnosis of melanoma is also made from biopsy. Under the microscope, melanomas appear as clusters of large and atypical melanocytes with visible mitotic figures proliferating above the epidermis. The pathology report includes the Breslow's depth (full tumor thickness) and the presence or absence of ulceration. The depth of the lesion is the strongest histologic factor influencing prognosis. Thus, superficial shave biopsies are not appropriate in

cases of suspected melanoma, because they have the potential to obscure an accurate report of tumor depth. Wide local excision is the only acceptable treatment and surgical margins are determined by Breslow's depth and the diameter of the lesion. α-Interferon is considered for adjuvant therapy in certain cases. Melanomas, especially the deeper ones, are frequently lethal; they are responsible for 75% of skin cancer deaths.

Photodermatoses

Although the aforementioned acute and chronic effects of UV radiation occur in exposed skin of all individuals, there are some abnormal reactions to sunlight that only manifest in the predisposed. These reactions are known as the *photodermatoses;* the more commonly encountered ones (Table 34-3) are discussed below. Photoprotection is an integral part of the management of photodermatoses.

Idiopathic, or Immunologically Mediated Dermatoses

Polymorphous Light Eruption

Presentation and Characteristics. Polymorphous light eruption (PMLE) is the most common photodermatosis in humans. It effects patients of all backgrounds and races and occurs more often in women than men. Its peak onset is during a person's 20s and 30s. It flares during the spring

---

TABLE 34-3 ■ Commonly Encountered Photodermatoses
Idiopathic, or immunologically mediated photodermatoses
Polymorphous light eruption
Chronic actinic dermatitis
Solar urticaria
Endogenous photodermatoses
Porphyria cutanea tarda
Erythropoietic protoporphyria
Exogenous photodermatoses
Phototoxicity
Photoallergy
Photoaggrevated dermatoses
Lupus erythematosus
Dermatomyositis
Atopic dermatitis
Seborrheic dermatitis

SAUER'S NOTES

1. Chronic sun exposure, or repeated sunburn, is associated with the development of AK, basal cell carcinomas, squamous cell carcinomas, and melanomas.
2. Treatment

    i. *Actinic keratoses:* cryotherapy, topical 5-fluorouracil, imiquimod cream, and diclofenac sodium gel.

    ii. *Basal cell carcinomas, squamous cell carcinomas:* electrodessication and curettage, surgical excision, Mohs micrographic surgery.

    iii. *Melanomas:* wide local excision, α-interferon.

and summer, after exposure to a certain threshold of UV radiation. Association with lupus erythematous and thyroid disease has been reported.

Patients are usually susceptible to broadband UVA and UVB radiation, with either able to elicit the symptoms. Doses less than the MED have been sufficient to induce the reaction. There is recent evidence to suggest that pathogenesis of PMLE stems from a delayed-type hypersensitivity response to a photo-induced antigen. Clinically, PMLE presents minutes to hours after exposure to UVR and can persist from 1 day to weeks. Initial symptoms include burning and pruritus. Grouped erythematous papules and rarely vesicles appear in a symmetrical distribution on sun exposed skin—notably, forehead, the upper chest, dorsum of hands, and forearms (Fig. 34-2). There are several different clinical manifestations, such as papules, plaques, nodules, and rarely, vesicles. General malaise, headache, fever, and nausea may infrequently accompany the cutaneous findings. Histologically, PMLE appears as a nonspecific dermal lymphocytic perivascular infiltrate. Diagnosis is made by history and clinical findings in the context of a negative rheumatologic (lupus erythematosus, dermatomyositis) serology workup. Biopsy is not typically helpful and phototesting is often unnecessary.

Treatment

- *Desensitization:* This is attained by narrowband UVB phototherapy, two to three times per week for 15 treatments, usually done in the spring. 8-Methoxypsoralen and UVA (PUVA) therapy is also effective.
- *Antimalarials:* They have been shown to provide moderate protection during the spring and summer, but patients must be warned of their ocular

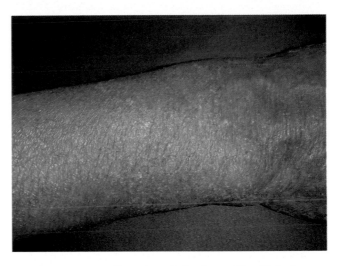

FIGURE 34-3 ■ Chronic actinic dermatitis. Note hyperpigmentation and lichenification on dorsum of the hand with sparring of photoprotective area above the wrist.

side effects. Once the outbreak has occurred, the symptoms are best treated with topical or oral corticosteroids.

Chronic Actinic Dermatitis

Description. Chronic actinic dermatitis is a chronic photodermatosis that occurs more commonly among older men; it is most severe during the summer months. Clinically, it presents with lichenified papules or plaques on sun-exposed areas (Fig. 34-3); the lesions are usually pruritic. Histologically, there is mild epidermal spongiosis, perivascular lymphocytic infiltrate, and not infrequently, there are atypical mononuclear cells in the dermis and epidermis. Therefore, histologic changes of chronic actinic dermatitis may resemble those of cutaneous T-cell lymphoma. Diagnosis is confirmed by phototesting: there is an abnormal response to UVB, and/or UVA, and/or visible radiation.

Treatment

- *Corticosteroids and tacrolimus:* Symptom relief is accomplished with the use of topical and oral corticosteroids. Topical tacrolimus has been used with success in some patients.
- *Others:* Management of refractory cases includes low-dose PUVA, mycophenolate mofetil, cyclosporine, and azathioprine.

Solar Urticaria

Presentation and Characteristics. Solar urticaria occurs slightly more often in females and is associated with

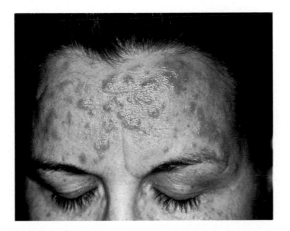

FIGURE 34-2 ■ Polymorphous light eruption. Note erythematous papules on the forehead.

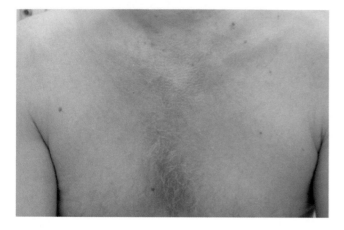

FIGURE 34-4 ■ Solar urticaria. Patient developed urticaria on chest within minutes of exposure to sunlight.

atopic dermatitis in 21% to 48% of patients. Patients typically present in their 20s and 30s. The pathogenic mechanism is thought to involve IgE formation with mast cell degranulation in response to a yet-unidentified photosensitized allergen.

Patients present with urticaria minutes after exposure to the instigating wavelength (Fig. 34-4). Like all urticarias, lesions disappear within hours. The wheals may be pruritic and occasionally burn. In rare instances, patients may also experience a systemic anaphylactic reaction. Biopsy of the lesion shows mild dermal edema with a perivascular infiltrate consisting of neutrophils and eosinophils. Phototesting reveals the wavelength range responsible and reliably recreates the symptoms.

Treatment

- *Antihistamines*
- *Desensitization:* This is done with incrementally increasing doses of UVA or PUVA.
- *Plasmapheresis:* For refractory cases.

Endogenous Photodermatoses: The Cutaneous Porphyrias

The porphyrias are a group of disorders caused by congenital defects of enzymes in the heme biosynthesis pathway. This section discusses the two most common porphyrias that exhibit skin involvement most prominently.

Porphyria Cutanea Tarda

Presentation and Characteristics. Porphyria cutanea tarda (PCT) is the most common cutaneous porphyria. There a two forms: an inherited autosomal dominant form and an acquired form. Men present with PCT slightly more commonly than women. Men with PCT are more likely to use alcohol, and women are more likely to be exposed to estrogen replacement. Most patients present after their 40s, although childhood onset has been infrequently reported. There is a strong association of PCT with hepatitis C as well as with hemochromatosis. Association of PCT with HIV infection has been well reported; therefore, HIV testing should be offered to all newly diagnosed patients with acquired PCT.

PCT is caused by a defect in hepatic uroporphyrinogen decarboxylase activity, which creates an excess of uroporphyrinogen, 7-, 6-, 5-, and 4-carboxyl porphyrinogens; all porphyrinogens are spontaneously oxidized to the corresponding porphyrins. These porphryins are phototoxic when exposed to visible light (Soret band, 400 to 410 nm).

Clinically, PCT manifests with skin fragility, blisters, erosions, crusting, and milia on sun-exposed areas (Fig. 34-5). Mottled hyper- and hypopigmentation and hypertrichosis on periorbital area are frequently observed; scarring alopecia and sclerodermoid lesions are uncommon presentations.

Histologically, subepidermal blister with cell-poor dermal infiltrate is seen. Diagnosis is confirmed by the characteristic porphyrin profile: there are elevated levels of uroporphyrin, 7-, 6-, 5-, and 4-carboxyl porphyrins in urine and plasma, and elevated isocoproporphyrin in the stool.

Treatment

- *Photoprotection:* Because the action spectrum is in the visible light range, photoprotection with

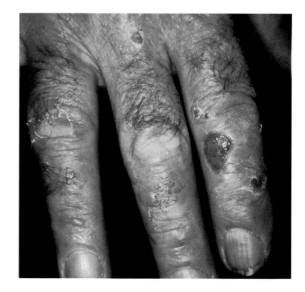

FIGURE 34-5 ■ PCT, presenting with vesicles and postinflammatory hyperpigmentation on dorsum of hand.

physical agent (nonmicronized titanium dioxide or zinc oxide, clothing, etc.) is required.

- *Phlebotomy:* This is done to decrease the iron load; it is the most effective treatment for patients. One unit of blood is usually removed weekly for 10 to 15 treatments. Alcohol, other hepatic toxins, and iron should be avoided. Interferon-α may be beneficial in the treatment of PCT in those patients with concomitant hepatitis C virus infection.
- *Antimalarials:* Low-dose chloroquine or hydroxychloroquine also produces a therapeutic response; its mechanism of action is to cause release of tissue-bound hepatic porphyrins for elimination.

Erythropoietic Protoporphyria

Presentation and Characteristics. Unlike PCT, erythropoietic protoporphyria (EPP) presents in children, usually by age 2. It is inherited in an autosomal dominant fashion with variable penetrance. The enzyme deficiency in EPP is ferrochelatase, which converts protoporphyrin to heme by insertion of iron. Elevated levels of phototoxic protoporphyrin in erythrocytes, plasma, and stool are seen in EPP; because protoporphyin is lipophilic, urine porphyrin level is normal in EPP.

Clinically, children with EPP usually cry or scream in pain minutes after exposure to sunlight. Sometimes this is misdiagnosed as psychoneurosis. The burning sensation lasts for hours and is followed by erythema, induration, and purpura; vesicles are rarely seen. With repeated attacks, shallow erosions on forehead and nose bridge, and waxy thickening of the skin of knuckles may be apparent. In rare instances, hepatic failure may occur. Histologically, thickening of dermal epidermal junction and blood vessel wall of superficial capillaries is observed.

Treatment

- *Oral β-carotene:* This is used to quench the reactive oxygen species. Lumitene, an over-the-counter preparation, at 30 to 300 mg/d, is usually recommended.
- *PUVA or narrowband UVB:* These are utilized to induce tolerance.

Exogenous Photodermatoses

Phototoxicity and Photoallergy

Presentation and Characteristics. Exogenous agents can be categorized by whether they cause a phototoxic or photoallergic cutaneous reaction. *Phototoxic responses* occur when UV radiation activates a drug or chemical which sub-

TABLE 34-4 ■ Common Exogenous Photosensitizers

Common Phototoxic Agents	Common Photoallergic Agents
Antiarrhythmics	Sunscreen filters
Diuretics	Fragrances
NSAIDs	Antibacterials
Phenothiazines	
Psoralens	
Quinolones	
Tetracyclines	
Thiazides	
Sulfonamides	
Sulfonylureas	

Abbreviation: NSAID, nonsteroidal anti-inflammatory drug.

sequently produces tissue injury; it occurs in 100% of individuals provided they are exposed to sufficient doses of phototoxic agent and the radiation. *Photoallergy* is a delayed-type hypersensitivity reaction, consisting of a sensitization phase on first exposure; subsequent exposures precipitate a photoallergic response. Commonly encountered Photosensitizers are listed in Table 34-4.

Clinically, phototoxic eruptions consist of erythema, edema, stinging, and burning in sun-exposed areas (Fig. 34-6). Relatively sun-protected areas such as the

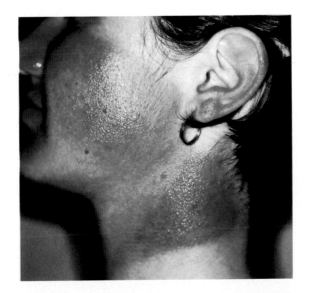

FIGURE 34-6 ■ Phototoxicity secondary to demeclocycline.

submental, retroauricular areas and eyelids are usually spared. Occasionally, vesicles, bullae, and onycholysis may be observed. Symptoms resolve with hyperpigmentation over the course of days to weeks. Histologically, phototoxic reactions present with lymphocytic and neutrophilic dermal infiltrates and occasional necrotic keratinocytes.

UVA is the most common action spectrum for systemic drug-induced phototoxicity. Exposure to furocumarin producing plants causes a topical phototoxic reaction called *phytophotodermatitis.* Common plants evoking this condition include celery, parsnip, lime, and parsley.

Photoallergic reactions present with pruritus and eczematous dermatitis. Bullae and vesicles are rarely seen. The histologic changes are similar to those of contact dermatitis, namely, lymphohisticocytic dermal infiltrates and spongiosis. Currently, the most common cause of photoallergic reactions is sunscreen filters. However, it should be noted that considering the large number of individuals exposed to sunscreens, the incidence of photoallergy to sunscreen agents is very low.

Careful history taking, paying special attention to medication and recent chemical exposures, is crucial for diagnosis. Photoallergy can be confirmed by photopatch testing.

Treatment. Avoidance of the offending agents along with appropriate photoprotection; symptomatic treatment, including topical or systemic corticosteroids, may be necessary in severe cases.

Photoaggravated Dermatoses

Exacerbation of cutaneous lesions in lupus erythematosus following sun exposure is frequently seen, especially in subacute lupus erythematous and in tumid lupus erythematous. Patients with dermatomyositis also frequently complain of photosensitivity. Photoexacerbation of atopic dermatitis and less commonly, seborrheic dermatitis, has been well reported.

Treatment

In addition to treatment of the primary disease, photoprotection is the appropriate management for these conditions.

Suggested Reading

Hawk JLM, Lim HW. Photodermatoses. In Bolognia JL, Jorizzo JL, Rapini RP, eds. Dermatology. London, Mosby, 2003, pp. 1365–1384.

Lim HW, ed. The diagnosis and treatment of photodermatitis. Dermatol Ther 2003;16:1–72.

Lim HW, Khoo SW. Carcinogenesis and ultraviolet radiation. In Taylor S, Kelly P, eds. Dermatology for Skin of Color. New York, McGraw-Hill, 2004.

Moyal D, Fourtanier A. Acute and chronic effects of UV on skin: What are they and how to study them? In Rigel DS, Weiss RA, Lim HW, et al, eds. Photoaging. New York, Marcel Dekker, 2004; pp. 15–33.

Murphy GM. Porphyria. In Bolognia JL, Jorizzo JL, Rapini RP, eds. Dermatology. London, Mosby, 2003, pp. 679–688.

CHAPTER 35

Genodermatoses

Amy Y. Jan, MD, PHD, and Virginia P. Sybert, MD

The inherited skin disorders are individually rare, but in the aggregate comprise a significant proportion of dermatologic practice. Some are of minimal medical significance; others are life threatening, life shortening, or debilitating. For some, treatment is available. For others, there is no management beyond diagnosis. For a growing number of conditions, both the causal mutations and the specific perturbations in cellular function are known.

Genetic skin disorders are unique in that the diagnosis automatically invokes the issues of recurrence risk to relatives and prenatal diagnosis (Table 35-1). These are topics not usually in the domain of the dermatologist. Identification of a genodermatosis may require referral for medical genetics evaluation and counseling. The availability and applicability of molecular (DNA) testing changes daily. Medical genetics centers are most likely to be aware of these resources. On-line resources include:

- GENECLINICS
- www.geneclinics.org
  Includes a listing of laboratories offering molecular testing for research and/or clinical purposes and for many disorders, a review that is clinically focused with molecular information as well, along with support group information.
- OMIM
- www3.ncbi.nlm.nih.gov/omim/
  A catalog of Mendelian disorders in humans with references, clinical synopses, and hyperlinks to other databases.

Many common skin disorders also have a significant genetic component. The risk for psoriasis, atopic dermatitis, vitiligo, alopecia areata, or systemic lupus erythematosus is much higher among close relatives of affected individuals than for the general population. Even acne and onychomycosis enjoy genetic contribution. These disorders are discussed elsewhere and are not further addressed here. This chapter deals with only a handful of the many inherited skin disorders.

Disorders of Keratinization

Ichthyoses

Presentation and Characteristics

The ichthyoses (Table 35-2; Fig. 35-1) have in common a thickened stratum corneum, which results in scaly skin. The distribution and severity of scaling, the presence of erythroderma, the mode of inheritance, and the associated abnormalities differ among them. The degree to which life is impaired ranges from minimal to lethal. The genetic alterations responsible for some of these conditions are known.

Treatment

Treatment remains general and nonspecific. Use of keratolytics (α-hydroxy acids such as lactic acid, glycolic acid, and urea-based emollients) can be helpful. The oral retinoids are effective and should be considered in the more severe forms of ichthyoses. Their long-term use is limited by significant side effects including dryness of the mucous membranes, alterations in serum lipids, musculoskeletal pain, bony alterations, and teratogenicity.

Palmar–Plantar Keratodermas

Palmar–plantar keratodermas (PPK) (Fig. 35-2) are conditions in which thickening of the stratum corneum and scaling, with or without erythroderma, are limited primarily to the palms and soles. They are distinguished, as are the more generalized ichthyoses, by mode of inheritance and associated findings. One autosomal dominant form (Howell–Evans) is associated with esophageal carcinoma. Papillon–Lefévre is an autosomal recessive PPK caused by mutations in the cathepsin C gene, and is associated with gingivitis and premature tooth loss. Unna–Thost/Voerner disease or PPK with epidermolytic hyperkeratosis results from mutations in either K9 or K1, type I acidic keratins. PPK without epidermolytic hyperkeratosis can be caused by mutations in K1 as well, and by mutations in K16.

373

TABLE 35-1 ■ **Patterns of Inheritance**

Mode of Inheritance	Risk to Relatives	Key Features
Autosomal dominant	50% to offspring born to affected parents	May be sporadic (new mutation) or inherited from affected parent
		Males and females equally affected
Autosomal recessive	25% to offspring born to carrier parents	Parents are heterozygote carriers
		Males and females equally affected
X-linked dominant	50% to inherit gene from affected mother	Usually lethal in males
X-linked recessive	50% to inherit gene from carrier mother	Males express condition
	Daughters of affected fathers = 100% risk to inherit gene	Females show condition to varying degrees, depending on X inactivation.
	Sons of affected fathers = 0% risk to inherit gene	Ranges from no obvious features to full-blown expression.

TABLE 35-2 ■ **Ichthyoses**

Disorder	Inheritance	Basic Defect	Major Dermatologic Findings	Associated Features	Miscellaneous
Ichthyosis vulgaris	AD	Unknown	Mild-to-moderate white scales	None	Improves with age and warm weather
			Spares flexures and neck; involves face		
			Keratosis pilaris		
			Atopic dermatitis (50%)		
X-linked ichthyosis (sterol sulfatase deficiency)	XLR	Mutation/deletion of steroid sulfatase gene	Moderate-to-severe white-brown scale	Corneal opacities	Pregnancies with affected males have low to absent estriol levels; failure of spontaneous initiation of labor is common
			Spares face; involves neck	Possible increased risk of testicular malignancy	
Bullous congenital ichthyosiform erythroderma (epidermolytic hyperkeratosis)	AD	Mutations in K1 or K10 (suprabasal keratins)	Red skin with blisters and scale evident at birth	Secondary skin infection, bacterial and fungal common	Skin is tender; skin fragility improves with age
			Marked hyperkeratosis		
			Face usually least affected		
			Inter- and intrafamilial variability		
Lamellar ichthyosis/ nonbullous congenital ichthyosiform erythroderma/ congenital autosomal recessive ichthyosis	AR	Heterogenous. Some caused by mutations in transglutaminase 1 (*TGM1*), 12-R lipoxygenase (*ALOX12B*), lipoxygenase-3 (*ALOXE3*), ATP	LI: mild erythroderma; brown, adherent plate-like scale	Secondary tinea infection common.	Collodion membrane common at birth
			NCIE: Erythroderma; fine, white scale		Ectropion/eclabium common
			Many cases with overlap in phenotype		

(*continued*)

TABLE 35-2 ▪ *(Continued)*

Disorder	Inheritance	Basic Defect	Major Dermatologic Findings	Associated Features	Miscellaneous
		binding cassette transporter 2 (*ABCA2*)			
Harlequin fetus	AR	Unknown; probably heterogenous	Severe, armor plate-like hyperkeratosis In survivors, phenotype becomes similar to BCIE	Among survivors, mental retardation has been noted in a few	Rare spontaneous survival; handful of survivors treated with oral retinoids
Conradi Hunermann	XLD AR	XLD: mutation in gene encoding delta(8)-delta(7) sterol isomerase emopamil-binding protein AR: mutations in *PEX7* gene	Feathery scale on erythrodermic base Follicular atrophoderma	Seizures; MR Chondrodysplasia punctata Cataracts	Asymmetry typical in XLD form
Sjogren-Larsson syndrome	AR	Fatty aldehyde dehydrogenase deficiency	Mild to moderate fine, adherent scale Pruritus	Progressive spastic paraparesis Mild retardation Glistening white dots on retina	
Netherton syndrome	AR	Mutations in *SPINK5* gene	Variable erythroderma and scale Classic pattern of ichthyosis linearis circumflexa	Trichorrhexis invaginata (bamboo hair)	Failure to thrive Food allergies
Collodion baby	AR if isolated Otherwise, depends on underlying disorder	Heterogenous	Plastic wrap-like membrane peels within few weeks after birth, revealing underlying skin which may range from minimally xerotic to lamellar ichthyosis	This is a feature of many disorders including lamellar ichthyosis, hypohidrotic ectodermal dysplasia, Gaucher disease and lamellar exfoliation of the newborn	

Abbreviations: AD, autosomal dominant; AR, autosomal recessive; BCIE, bullous congenital ichthyosiform erythroderma; XLR, X-linked recessive; K, keratin; MR, mental retardation.

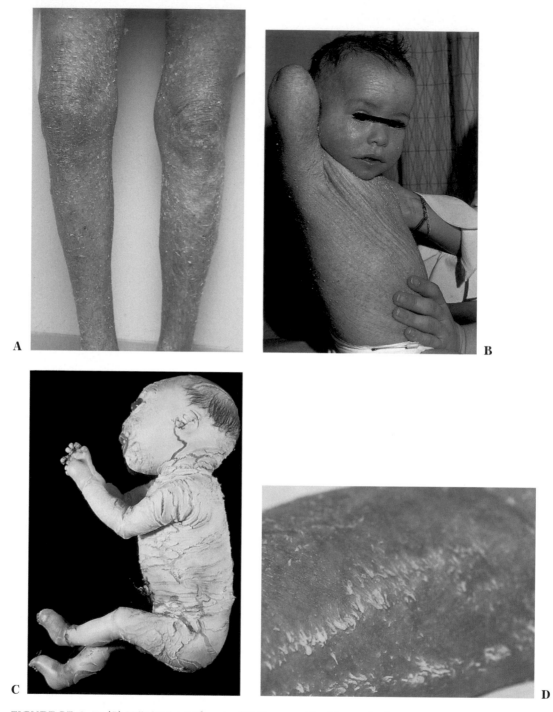

FIGURE 35-1 ■ (**A**) X-linked ichthyosis. (**B**) Young girl with nonbullous congenital ichthyosiform erythroderma. (**C**) Newborn with Harlequin ichthyosis. (**D**) Feathery scale of X-LD Conradi Hunermann disease. *(From Sybert VP. Genetic Skin Disorders. New York, Oxford University Press, 1997.)*

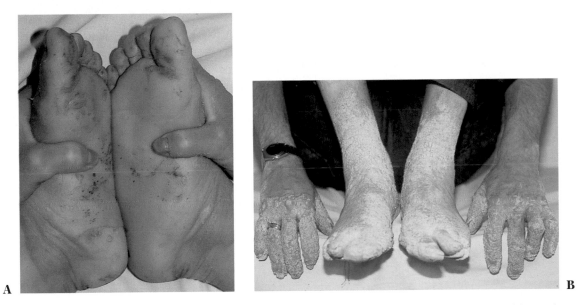

FIGURE 35-2 ■ **(A)** Palmar–plantar hyperkeratosis. The hands and soles are thickened, with erythroderma evident at margins. Young girl shares same condition as her father. **(B)** Palmar–plantar hyperkeratosis with severe palm/sole involvement and extension onto wrists and shins. In this family, elbows, knees, and the gluteal cleft are involved in some affected individuals. *(From Sybert VP. Genetic Skin Disorders. New York, Oxford University Press, 1997.)*

Disorders of Adhesion

The *epidermolysis bullosa syndromes* are mechanobullous disorders that share fragility of the skin (Table 35-3; Fig. 35-3). They are distinguished by the histologic level of blister formation, mode of inheritance, and associated cutaneous features. Most present at birth or soon thereafter. Scarring is primarily limited to the dystrophic forms, where the separation of the skin occurs below the basement membrane of the dermis. Extensive involvement in the newborn period can occur in epidermolysis bullosa simplex–Dowling–Meara, recessive epidermolysis bullosa dystrophica, and in junctional epidermolysis bullosa (JEB). Neonatal or infant death due to sepsis or intestinal protein loss and inanition is common in the most severe forms. Respiratory mucosa is often involved in the Herlitz form of JEB. Accurate diagnosis requires electron microscopy and/or immunofluorescence studies.

Treatment

Treatment consists of protection of skin surfaces and avoidance of trauma, lancing of small blisters to prevent lateral spread by the pressure of blister fluid, topical antibiotics, and nonadherent dressings. More severe forms may require a team approach to management of complications.

Disorders of Pigmentation

There are many molecules that contribute to skin color. This discussion is limited to alterations in melanin, the major contributor. Perturbations in pigment production are due to alterations or defects anywhere along the pathway from the differentiation and migration of neural crest derivatives, through the enzymatic production of melanin, to the packaging and transport of melanosomes.

Hypopigmentation

Presentation and Characteristics

Waardenburg syndromes I and II and *piebaldism* (Fig. 35-4) have in common white patches of skin, a white forelock, premature graying of the hair, and autosomal dominant inheritance. All are caused by a failure of migration and invasion of melanocytes into the epidermis. Individuals with Waardenburg syndrome also have dystophia canthorum and heterochromia irides. Those with Waardenburg I or II may be deaf. *Hirschsprung disease* occurs in approximately 10%. Waardenburg I and some instances of

TABLE 35-3 ■ **Epidermolysis Bullosa**

Disorder	Mode of Inheritance	Basic Defect Mutations In	Major Dermatologic Findings	Associated Features	Electron Microscopy
EBS-WC (Weber-Cockayne) (localized)	AD	Basal keratins (*KRT* 5) (*KRT* 14)	Blisters primarily limited to hands and feet. Onset can be at birth but usually thereafter. Occasionally delayed until adolescence. Palmar/plantar hyperkeratosis may occur.	None	Level of split within basal keratinocyte
EBS-K (Koebner) (generalized)	AD	Basal keratins (*KRT* 5) (*KRT* 14)	Blisters soon after birth, generalized. May have oral involvement/nail involvement.	None	Level of split within basal keratinocyte
EBS-DM (Dowling-Meara) (herpetiform)	AD	Basal keratins (*KRT* 5) (*KRT* 14)	Marked blistering at birth. With time clustering of small blisters in rosettes may occur. Oral involvement common. Nails often dystrophic. Progressive palmar/plantar hyperkeratosis common. Dyspigmentation common.	Can result in neonatal/infant death. Blistering tends to diminish with age.	Clumping of tonofilaments within basal cells with cytolysis
EBS with muscular dystrophy	AR/AD	Plectin (*PLEC1*)	Relatively severe simplex disease, may be mistaken for junctional EB.	Muscular dystrophy of various types has been described.	Split at hemidesmosomal attachment plate
EBS with mottled hyperpigmentation	AD	Basal keratin (*KRT* 5)	Blisters similar to EBS-K. Development of hyper/hypopigmented spots.	None	Level of split within basal keratinocyte
JEB-Herlitz (gravis) (letalis)	AR	Various components of laminin (*LAMA3*) (*LAMC2*) (*LAMB3*)	Widespread severe. GI, respiratory, and GU mucosa often involved. Usually lethal.		Level of split within lamina lucida, decrease/absence of hemidesmosomes.
JEB-mitis (GABEB)	AR	Type 17 collagen; Laminin (*BPAG2/ COL17A1*) (*LAMB3*)	More mild, gradual atopic appearance of healed skin	None	Similar to JEB-H. May have relatively more hemidesmosomes.
JEB with PA	AR	Integrins (*ITGB4*) (*ITGB6*)	Similar to JEB-L, usually lethal.	Pyloric atresia, intestinal malabsorption	Same as JEB-H
EBD-C-T (Cockayne-Touraine)	AD	Type 7 collagen (*COL7A1*)	Blistering and scarring limited and localized to areas of greatest trauma. Mild oral involvement. Milia.	None	Split below basement membrane Decrease in anchoring fibrils.
EBD-H-S (Hallopeau-Siemens)	AR	Type 7 collagen (*COL7A1*)	Widespread, severe blistering, progressive scarring. Pseudamputation of digits. Development of cutaneous malignancy common in adult life. Oral mucosa involved. Milia.	FTT. Anemia, GI involvement is progressive	Same as EBD C-T. Absence of anchoring fibrils.

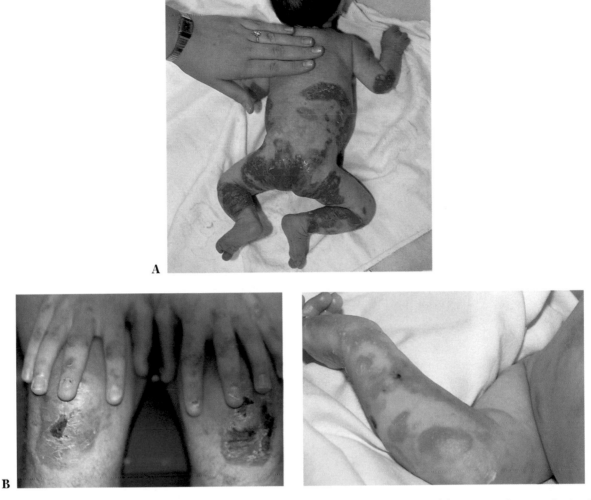

FIGURE 35-3 ■ **(A)** Newborn with junctional epidermolysis bullosa–Herlitz. **(B)** Scarring in a patient with DEBD. **(C)** Extensive superficial blistering in a patient with EBS–Dowling–Meara.

Waardenburg II are due to mutations in *PAX3*. Mutations in *MITF* have been found in some cases of Waardenburg II, confirming genetic heterogeneity within this group. *Piebaldism,* which is caused by mutations in the C-*kit* protooncogene, is usually characterized only by skin changes, although deafness has been reported in some patients. In all three of the disorders there are no melanocytes in the depigmented areas.

The oculocutaneous albinisms are a group of autosomal recessive disorders distinguished by the degree of pigment production and whether they are "tyrosinase positive" or "tyrosinase negative." Affected individuals have

- pink skin,
- transillumination of the irises,
- white to light yellow hair,
- often visual disturbances,
- foveal hypoplasia, and
- nystagmus.

Many mutations in the tyrosinase gene have been identified in both tyrosinase positive and tyrosinase negative forms of oculocutaneous albinism and many affected individuals are compound heterozygotes for mutations at this locus. In addition, mutations in the P gene, located on

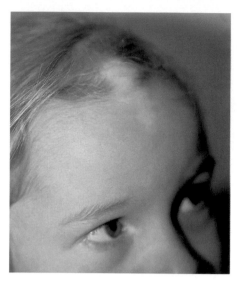

FIGURE 35-4 ■ White forelock and patch of unpigmented skin in young girl with piebaldism.

chromosome 15, have been identified in some tyrosinase-positive albino individuals. There is also an X-linked recessive form of oculocutaneous albinism, which is very rare.

Tuberous sclerosis (Fig. 35-5) is an autosomal dominant disorder which results from mutations in genes at one of at least two loci; one on chromosome 9 (*TSC1*-hamartin), the other at chromosome 16 (*TSC2*-tuberin). It is characterized by a number of cutaneous changes including angiofibromas, connective tissue nevi (shagreen patches), periungal fibromas, and hypopigmented macules (ashleaf spots). Melanocytes and keratinocytes in these light-colored areas contain "effete" or poorly melanized small melanosomes. Mental retardation, seizures, and renal involvement are the other major features of this condition that has very variable expression.

Hypomelanosis of Ito is the term given to the presence of hypopigmentation or hyperpigmentation distributed along the lines of Blaschko (Fig. 35-6). The biologic basis for this phenomenon is not understood. Individuals with these skin changes often have structural malformations and mental retardation. Almost two thirds of patients are mosaic for detectable chromosomal aneuploidy. Mosaicism for X chromosome alterations, tetrasomy 12p, triploidy, trisomy 18, and chimerism are the more common abnormalities reported. It appears that it is the presence of two chromosomally distinct lines, rather than specific cytogenetic alterations that confers this striking pigment anomaly.

Individuals with hypopigmentation due to any cause need to be protected from excessive sun exposure.

Hyperpigmentation

Neurofibromatosis is a relatively common (1/3,000) autosomal dominant disorder caused by mutations in the *NF1* gene, which resides on chromosome 17.

Neurofibromatosis is a disorder of neural crest cells, including the melanocyte. Affected individuals manifest pigment abnormalities, including

- café-au-lait spots (brown macules and patches) (Fig. 35-7), usually numbering more than five and larger than 5 mm in children, 1.5 cm in adults;
- axillary, inguinal, and inframammary freckling (Crowe's sign); and
- a general increase in skin color (hypermelanosis).

Pigment in these areas is packaged in giant melanosomes—a feature also common in café-au-lait spots not associated with neurofibromatosis. Over time, affected persons develop benign tumors, neurofibromas, which arise from Schwann cells and can occur along any myelinated nerve. These may be few or number in the thousands. Severe complications include:

- plexiform neurofibromas—large disfiguring growths, pseudoarthrosis, mental deficiency (5% to 10%),
- sarcomatous degeneration of benign growths,
- optic glioma, and
- leukemia (less than 1%).

This is a progressive condition that is extremely variable in its expression both within and among families.

The clinical features of *McCune–Albright syndrome* (Fig. 35-8) are giant café-au-lait spots, polyostotic fibrous dysplasia, and endocrine abnormalities, primarily precocious puberty. It results from a postzygotic mutation in the *GNAS1* gene. Affected individuals are mosaic for this otherwise lethal dominant mutation. The severity and location of clinical features depends on the proportion of normal to abnormal cells present. It is believed to be lethal in the fully heterozygous state; it is only tolerated by the organism if it is not present in all cells. Almost all cases are sporadic, caused by postzygotic mutations. Affected individuals who reproduce have no risk for affected offspring; embryos with the abnormal gene present in all cells cannot develop.

Incontinentia pigmenti (Fig. 35-9) is an X-linked dominant condition affecting girls almost exclusively. It is usually lethal prenatally in affected boys. Newborns present with blistering distributed along the lines of Blaschko. Over weeks to months, these areas become

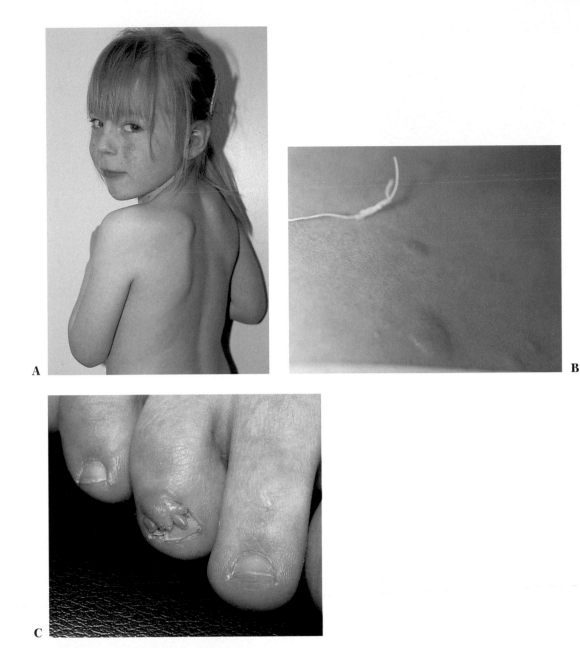

A

B

C

FIGURE 35-5 ■ (**A**) Young girl with tuberous sclerosis; hypopigmented macules; angiofibromas on cheeks. (**B**) Shagreen patches (collagenoma). (**C**) Periungal fibroma. *(B, C, From Sybert VP. Genetic Skin Disorders. New York, Oxford University Press, 1997.)*

hyperkeratotic and warty in appearance. This gradually subsides and hyperpigmentation develops, also along the lines of Blaschko, but not necessarily in or limited to the areas of blistering. This hyperpigmentation persists throughout childhood, but may fade to hypopigmented hairless skin in adult life. The severity of associated problems varies. These include:

- central nervous system abnormalities, including seizures and mental retardation;
- retinal vascular dysplasia and visual defects;
- alopecia;
- hypodontia and peg-shaped teeth;
- nail dysplasia; and
- skeletal abnormalities.

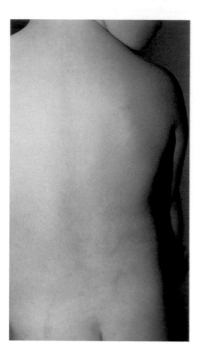

FIGURE 35-6 ■ Streaky pigment variegation, along the lines of Blaschko in patient with mosaicism for 46,XX/47,XX + rea (12).

Disorders of Elasticity

Ehlers–Danlos Syndrome

Ehlers–Danlos syndrome (EDS) is the eponym given to a group of conditions, some of which share little in common. Recent efforts have been made to limit application of this eponym to those conditions in which fragility, thinness, and/or hyperelasticity of the skin is a primary finding.

The classic type of EDS is characterized by soft, velvety hyperextensible skin that is fragile, tears easily, and heals poorly with thin cigarette paper scars. There is easy bruisability. Over time, elastosis perforans serpiginosa can become a significant management problem. Patients have marked ligament laxity. In some families, mutations in type five collagen (*COL5A1* or *COL5A2*) have been identified. Individuals with the hypermobility type of EDS have essentially normal skin, but marked hyperextensibility of large and small joints. Electromicroscopy of skin shows abnormal collagen bundles in these conditions. The vascular type of EDS is autosomal dominant, as are the classical and hypermobility types. The skin in the vascular type of EDS is thin and taut, rather than velvety and soft. This is a disorder of Type III collagen (*COL3A1*) and affects the lining of vessels and viscera. Rupture of these is

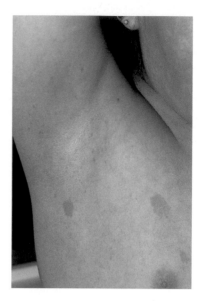

FIGURE 35-7 ■ Café-au-lait spots and axillary freckling in neurofibromatosis. *(From Sybert VP. Genetic Skin Disorders. New York, Oxford University Press, 1997.)*

the major medical complication and death is common before age 50.

Cutis Laxus

Cutis laxa is heterogeneous group of autosomal recessive and X-linked recessive conditions that share laxity, not

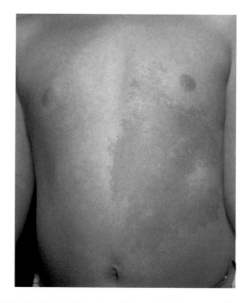

FIGURE 35-8 ■ Giant café-au-lait in a patient with McCune–Albright syndrome. *(From Sybert VP. Genetic Skin Disorders. New York, Oxford University Press, 1997.)*

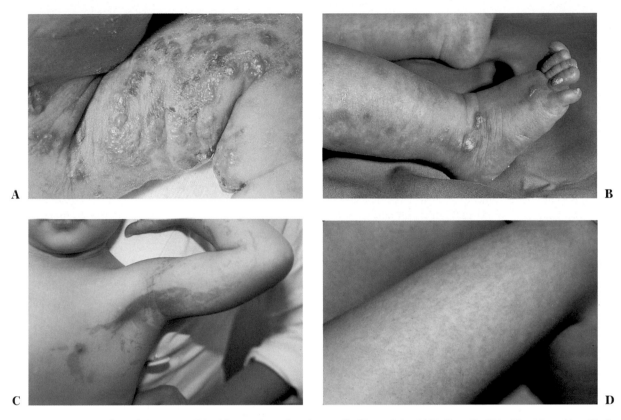

FIGURE 35-9 ■ **(A–D)** Stages I–IV of incontinentia pigmenti. *(From Sybert VP. Genetic Skin Disorders. New York, Oxford University Press, 1997.)*

elasticity, of the skin. The skin is soft and progressively loses tone. Affected individuals have a prematurely aged "hound dog" appearance to the face. X-linked cutis laxa, also referred to as *Occipital Horn Syndrome,* is caused by a defect in the *ATP7A* gene, whose product transports copper. Thus, mutations in *ATP7A* result in secondary deficiency of copper-dependent enzymes. Internal involvement includes progressive hydronephrosis and bladder diverticuli, emphysema and pulmonary blebs, and hernias. Intellect ranges from mild mental retardation to normal. The *ATP7A* gene is also involved in Menkes syndrome, a much more severe disorder. Skin of affected males is thin, pale, with a prominent venus pattern. The hairs are fine, sparse, fragile, and demonstrate pili torti (twisting). Neurologic involvement is usually severe and progressive. Prenatal diagnosis is available for both X-linked cutis laxa and Menkes syndrome. Daily use of a dietary copper histamine supplementation when instituted shortly after birth may have some benefit in slowing progression of neurologic symptoms.

Pseudoanthoma Elasticum

In pseudoxanthoma elasticum, there is progressive deterioration of elastic fibers in the dermis, choroid of the eye and blood vessels. The skin becomes progressively involved by cobblestoned, yellowish plaques, especially at the nape and in the folds. These are clinically similar to solar elastosis. Progressive atherosclerotic disease, presumably owing to calcified plaques developing on abnormal vessel walls, results in claudication, gastrointestinal bleeding, and stroke. Breaks in Brusch's membrane of the eye are seen as angioid streaks on eye examination. This is a feature typical of the disorder. The changes in pseudoxanthoma elasticum are progressive. Making the diagnosis is unusual in childhood unless there is a positive family history and a high index of suspicion. Homozygosity or compound heterozygosity for mutations in the *ABCC6* gene underlies this autosomal recessive condition. Pedigrees with apparent autosomal dominant inheritance of pseudoxanthoma elasticum appear to be the result of pseudodominance.

Disorders of Appendages

Hair

Inherited defects in hair can affect the development of follicles, hair growth, and hair structure. Congenital alopecias are rare. They may be isolated or associated with other organ involvement. Most are autosomal recessive. A disorder of hair growth in childhood is the loose anagen syndrome, in which the anagen roots are structurally abnormal, the hairs are poorly anchored and easily plucked, and the growth period is reduced. Affected children have thin, short hair that "never needs to be cut." It tends to improve with time and by adult life hair may appear normal, although still relatively loosely anchored. Inheritance is uncertain. Structural hair shaft abnormalities are listed in Table 35-4.

Nails

Isolated inherited disorders of nails are rare and most abnormalities are usually part of syndromes. *Pachonychia congenita* (P-C) (Fig. 35-10) is a term used for two autosomal dominant conditions: Type 1, Jadassohn-Lewandowsky and Type 2, Jackson-Lawler. In P-C, the nail plates are thickened or may be small or absent. Nail changes may appear within the first few years of life or not until later. Not all nails are necessarily involved. Other physical findings include palmar

TABLE 35-4 ■ **Hair Disorders**

Name	Inheritance	Basic Defect	Microscopic Features	Associated Abnormalities
Monilethrix	AD	Mutations in Type II hair keratins: *hHb6* *hHb1*	Beaded hairs; regular or irregular narrowing and widening of hair shaft.	None
Pili annulati	AD	Unknown. Bands are due to air-filled cavities in cortex.	Ringed hair; alternating bands of light and dark.	None
Pili torti	XLR	Mutations in *MNK1* (*ATP7A*)	Twisting along longitudinal axis of hair shaft.	Menkes syndrome
	AD	Unknown		None
Pili trianguli et canaliculi (uncombable; spangled hair)	AD	Unknown	Grooved, triangular hair	None
Trichorrhexis invaginata	AR	Unknown	Nodal swelling of hair shaft; similar to bamboo	Netherton syndrome
Trichorrhexis nodosa	AD	Unknown	Fraying of medulla due to abnormal cuticle. Appearance of opposing broom heads.	Argininosuccinic aciduria
	AR	Unknown		
	Acquired	Argininosuccinate lycose deficiency		Trauma
				Can be seen in any fragile hair
Trichothiodystrophy	AR	Decrease in disulfide bonds. Decrease in cysteine in hair. Mutations in *ERCC2/XPD* and *ERCC3/XPB* in some with *PIBIDS*	Thin fragile hairs with birefrigent regions in polarized microscopy	Heterogeneous — may be associated with any of: Ichthyosis Mental retardation Failure to thrive Short stature Infertility or maybe isolated

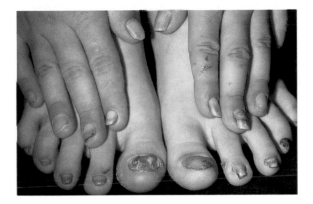

FIGURE 35-10 ■ Nails in pachyonychia–congenita. *(From Sybert VP. Genetic Skin Disorders. New York, Oxford University Press, 1997.)*

plantar hyperkeratosis, leukokeratosis of the oral mucosa, and follicular keratosis at the elbows and knees. Epidermal cysts, steatocystoma multiplex, and natal teeth were typical of P-C 2. Mutations in keratins—keratins 6A and 16 in P-C 1 and keratins 6B and 17 in P-C 2—have been found.

Nail–patella syndrome (Fig. 35-11) is an autosomal dominant disorder marked by variable nail dystrophy with usually symmetric involvement. Skeletal abnormalities are also a feature and include hypoplasia to absence of the patellae, malformations of the elbows and scapulae, and iliac horns. Renal involvement ranges from glomerulonephritis to severe renal failure and occurs in up to a third of affected individuals. The causal gene, *LMX1B* (LIM-homeodomain protein), is linked to the ABO blood group on the long arm of chromosome 9.

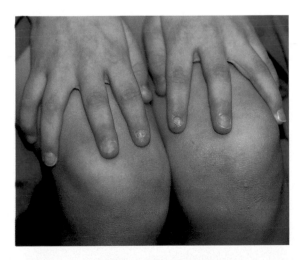

FIGURE 35-11 ■ Nails in nail–patella syndrome. *(From Sybert VP. Genetic Skin Disorders. New York, Oxford University Press, 1997.)*

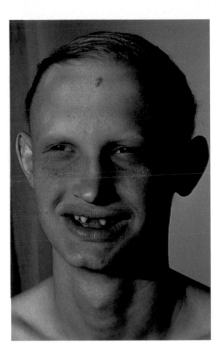

FIGURE 35-12 ■ Male with sparse hair; peg-shaped teeth and hypodontia, and typical facies of hypohidrotic ectodermal dysplasia. *(From Sybert VP. Genetic Skin Disorders. New York, Oxford University Press, 1997.)*

Ectodermal Dysplasias

There are over 100 genetic conditions whose major findings involve alterations in two or more of the primary ectodermal derivatives—hair, teeth, sweat glands, and nails. Historically, the ectodermal dysplasias have been divided into those with relatively normal sweating (hidrotic) and those with heat intolerance (hypohidrotic or anhidrotic). The most common of the ectodermal dysplasias is X-linked recessive hypohidrotic ectodermal dysplasia (Christ–Siemens–Touraine syndrome), which is caused by mutation in the gene encoding ectodysplasin A (Fig. 35-12). Affected boys may present with a collodion membrane at birth, have heat intolerance because of inability to sweat, hypodontia, peg-shaped teeth, and sparse hair. Female carriers may have patchy hair loss and patchy distribution of sweat glands, with minimal to significant tooth involvement.

Hamartomas/Malignancies

A number of genetic skin conditions are marked by development of cutaneous and extracutaneous malignancy. Table 35-5 lists some of these.

TABLE 35-5 ■ Disorders Associated With Malignancy

Disorder	Mode of Inheritance	Gene	Major Dermatologic Findings	Associated Features	Typical Malignancy
Ataxia telangiectasia	AR	ATM	Progressive telangiectases on skin conjunctiva. Premature graying of the hair.	Ataxia CNS degeneration Immunodeficiency	Lymphoreticular
Basal cell nevus syndrome	AD	PTCH	Basal cell nevi Palmar/plantar pits Epidermal cysts	Many, including odontogenic keratocysts and skeletal abnormalities	Basal cell carcinoma Medulloblastoma Ovary
Bloom syndrome	AR	BLM	Malar telangiectases	Immunodeficiency Growth failure Infertility in males	Many different organs
Cowden syndrome	AD	PTEN	Tricholemmomas Acral keratoses Palmar/plantar keratoses Oral papillomas	Thyroid abnormalities Fibrocystic breast disease GI polyps	Breast Ovary Thyroid
Dyskeratosis congenita	XLR AD ?AR	DKC1 TERC unknown	Progressive reticular hyperpigmentation Nail dystrophy Oral leukoplakia.	Bone marrow failure	Squamous cell cancer
Fanconi syndrome	AR	FACA FACC	Café-au-lait spots Patchy hyperpigmentation Sweet's syndrome	Bone marrow failure Radial ray defects Short stature	Hematopoietic Hepatocellular
Gardner syndrome	AD	APC	Epidermal inclusion cysts Fibromas Desmoid tumors	Intestinal polyps Mandibular osteomas	GI malignancies
MEN 2A/2B	AD	RET	Mucosal neuromas	Marfanoid habitus Ganglioneuromas of GI tract Pheochromocytoma	Thyroid
Peutz-Jeghers	AD	STK11	Lentigines on lips, mucosa palms, soles, fingertips	GI polyposis	GI malignancy Ovary Testicle Uterus Pancreas
Rothmund-Thomson syndrome	AR	RECQL4 in some cases	Facial telangiectases Poikiloderma Alopecia	Short stature Radial ray defects Hypogonadism Cataracts	Squamous cell cancer
Xeroderma pigmentosa (many complementation groups)	AR	ERCC 2 ERCC3 ERCC5 XPCC XPAC	Progressive dyspigmentation Telangiectases Atrophy Progressive acinic changes	Neurologic involvement in XPA, XPC, XPD	Squamous cell cancer Basal cell cancer Malignant melanoma

Suggested Reading

Beighton P, Paepe AD, Steinmann B, et al. Ehlers-Danlos Syndromes: Revised Nosology, Villefranche, 1997. Am J Med Genet 1998;77:31–37.

Birnbaum PS, Baden IH. Heritable disorders of hair. Dermatol Clin 1987;5:137–153.

Byers PH. Disorders of collagen biosynthesis and structure. Chapter 25 in Scriver CR, Beaudet AL, Sly WS, Valle D, eds. The Metabolic and Molecular Bases of Inherited Disease, ed 8. New York: McGraw-Hill, 2001.

Freire-Maia N, Pinheiro M. Ectodermal Dysplasias: A Clinical and Genetic Study. New York, Alan R. Liss, 1984.

Hu X, Plomp AS, van Soest S, et al. Pseudoxanthoma elasticum: a clinical, histopathological, and molecular update. Surv Ophthalmol 2003;48:424–438.

Juhlin L, Baran R. Hereditary and congenital nail disorders. In Baran R, Dawber RPR, eds. Diseases of the Nails and their Management, ed 2. Oxford, Blackwell 1994.

King RA, Hearing VJ, Creel DJ, et al. Albinism. Chapter 220 in Scriver CR, Beaudet AL, Valle ED, Sly WS, et al., eds. The Metabolic and Molecular Bases of Inherited Disease, ed 8. New York, McGraw-Hill, 2001.

Lamartine J. Towards a new classification of ectodermal dysplasias. Clin Exp Dermatol 2003;28(4):351–355.

Lin A, Carter DM, eds: Epidermolysis Bullosa. Basic and Clinical Aspects. New York, Springer-Verlag, 1992.

Neldner KH. Pseudoxanthoma elasticum. Clin Dermatol 1988;6:1–159.

Steinmann B, Royce PM, Superti-Furga A. The Ehlers-Danlos syndrome. In Royce PM, Steinmann B eds. Connective Tissue and Its Heritable Disorders. New York, Wiley-Liss, 1992, pp. 351–407.

Stratigos AJ, Baden HP. Unraveling the molecular mechanisms of hair and nail genodermatoses. Arch Dermatol 2001;137(11):1465–1471.

Sybert VP. Genetic Skin Disorders. New York, Oxford University Press, 1997.

Sybert VP. Hypomelanosis of Ito: A description, not a diagnosis. J Invest Dermatol 1994;103:1415–1435.

Traupe H. The ichthyoses: A Guide to Clinical Diagnosis, Genetic Counseling, and Therapy. New York, Springer-Verlag, 1989.

Uitto J, Pulkkinen L, McLean WH. Epidermolysis bullosa: A spectrum of clinical phenotypes explained by molecular heterogeneity. Mol Med Today 1997;3:457–465.

CHAPTER 36

Pediatric Dermatology

Kimberly A. Horii, MD, and Vidya Sharma, MBBS, MPH

Skin disorders in infants and children may be different from the same diseases in older children or adults (Figs. 36-1 and 36-2). Certain skin conditions such as diaper dermatitis are typically seen only in infants; other conditions such as atopic dermatitis may appear different in children when compared with adults. Pediatric dermatology can be divided into neonatal dermatoses and dermatoses of infants and children. It is useful to describe a lesion by its morphology to develop a differential diagnosis of what the disorder might be.

Neonatal Dermatoses (Birth to 1 Month)

A few lesions may be noted at birth or shortly thereafter (Table 36-1). In the newborn period, an infectious etiology for a skin eruption needs to be ruled out because some neonatal infections can be life threatening.

Blistering (Vesiculobullous) Lesions

Blistering lesions can be mechanically induced or caused by infections.

- *Sucking blisters:* usually seen as oval bullae on the hand or forearm thought to be caused by sucking in utero. They resolve rapidly.
- *Epidermolysis bullosa* (Fig. 36-3): a group of inherited disorders with fragile skin and bullous lesions that develop spontaneously or as a result of trauma.
- *Infections* (Fig. 36-4): herpes simplex, congenital varicella, candidiasis, and congenital syphilis can present as blisters in the newborn. Herpes simplex is important to recognize because disseminated neonatal herpes infection can be fatal.

Pustular Lesions

Some pustular dermatoses are self-limited and require no treatment; others may be a result of an infection requiring therapy.

- *Candidiasis* (see Fig. 36-4): aside from blisters, candidiasis may also present with erythematous papules and pustules.
- *Erythema toxicum:* a common, benign, and self-limited condition of the newborn. Erythematous macules, papules, and pustules can occur anywhere on the body.
- *Transient neonatal pustular melanosis* (Fig. 36-5): a benign, self-limited disorder characterized by vesiculopustular lesions that rupture and evolve into hyperpigmented macules.
- *Neonatal acne:* papules and pustules develop at 2 to 4 weeks of age. It is self-limited and usually does not scar. Topical erythromycin or benzoyl peroxide may be helpful.
- *Milia:* occurs commonly on the cheeks, nose, chin, and forehead. It presents as 1- to 2-mm white or yellow papules which are frequently grouped. The lesions resolve without therapy.

Birthmarks

Newborns may have many different types of birthmarks that can be categorized by color.

White

- *Albinism:* an uncommon inherited disorder with lack of pigment in the skin, hair, and eyes. A partial lack of pigmentation is termed *piebaldism* or *partial albinism*
- *Ash leaf macules:* lance-shaped hypopigmented macules on the trunk, arms, or legs, usually associated with tuberous sclerosis.
- *Nevus anemicus:* a solitary hypopigmented macule resulting from a localized vascular reaction. The surrounding borders classically blanch with pressure.
- *Nevus depigmentosus:* a unilateral hypopigmented patch with poorly defined borders.

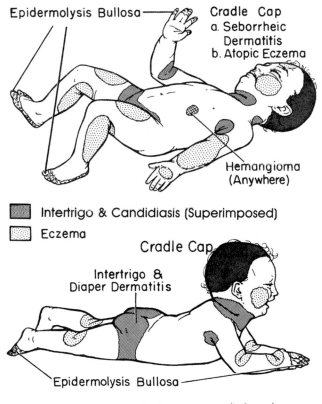

FIGURE 36-1 ■ Pediatric dermograms (infancy).

Brown

- *Café-au-lait spots* (Fig. 36-6): light brown round or oval macules. These can be normal findings, but may be seen in association with neurofibromatosis type I. This condition should be suspected if six or more café-au-lait spots greater than 0.5 cm in diameter are present in association with other clinical findings.
- *Congenital melanocytic nevus* (Fig. 36-7): a tan to dark brown well-circumscribed papule or plaque. Nevi vary in size from small to large, and often have associated hypertrichosis. Congenital nevi have the potential of developing into a melanoma depending on their size (especially >20 cm), location, border (irregular), color (especially black and multicolored), and texture (nodules).
- *Mongolian spots* (Fig. 36-8): deep brown, slate gray, or blue-black macules found mostly over the lumbosacral area and buttocks in darker pigmented infants. These are benign and self-limited.
- *Epidermal nevus* (Fig. 36-9): tan to brown verrucous linear lesions noted at birth. They may

rarely have other associated neurologic or skeletal abnormalities.

Vascular

- *Nevus simplex (Salmon patch)* (Fig. 36-10): dull pink macules on the glabella, upper eyelids, nasolabial regions (also referred to as angel kisses), or nape of the neck (also referred to as a *stork bite*). These lesions usually fade when present on the face.
- *Nevus flammeus (Port-wine stain)* (Fig. 36-11): a congenital vascular malformation composed of dilated capillaries. These are reddish-purple macules or patches that do not involute; laser therapy is a treatment option. Neurologic and ophthalmologic abnormalities (Sturge-Weber syndrome) may accompany a port-wine stain located on the face above the palpebral fissure.
- *Hemangioma of infancy* (Fig. 36-12): benign tumors of infancy composed of proliferating vascular endothelium. They grow rapidly in infancy, stabilize, and involute in childhood, most resolving by 10 years of age. They may be superficial, deep, or

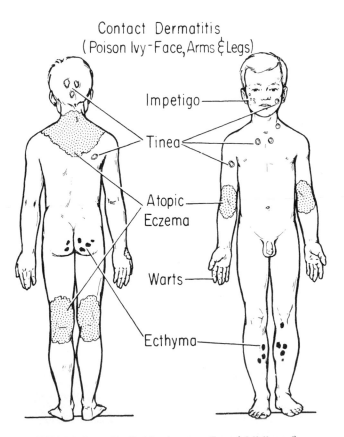

FIGURE 36-2 ■ Pediatric dermograms (childhood).

TABLE 36-1 ■ Neonatal Dermatoses (Birth to 1 Month)

Blistering (vesiculobullous lesions)

Mechanical

  Sucking blisters
  Epidermolysis bullosa
  Bullous ichthyosiform erythroderma (ichthyosis)

Infectious

  Herpes simplex
  Congenital varicella
  Candidiasis
  Congenital syphilis

Pustular Lesions

Candidiasis
Erythema toxicum
Transient neonatal pustular melanosis
Neonatal acne
Milia

Birthmarks

White

  Albinism
  Piebaldism
  Ash leaf macules
  Nevus anemicus
  Nevus depigmentosus

Brown

  Café-au-lait spots
  Congenital melanocytic nevus
  Dermal melanosis
  Epidermal nevus

Vascular

  Nevus simplex (Salmon patch)
  Nevus flammeus (Port-wine stain)
  Hemangioma of infancy—superficial, deep, or mixed

Yellow

  Nevus sebaceous

Papulosquamous Lesions

Ichthyosis
Neonatal lupus erythematosus

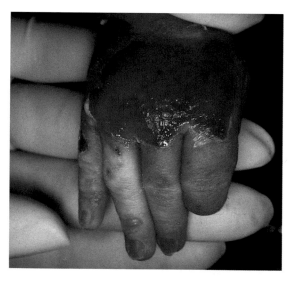

FIGURE 36-3 ■ Epidermolysis bullosa. Junctional type.

mixed. Numerous cutaneous lesions may be associated with hemangiomas in the viscera (diffuse neonatal hemangiomatosis). Large facial hemangiomas may be associated with neurologic, ophthalmologic, and cardiac abnormalities (PHACE syndrome). Management may consist of observation alone, oral prednisone, laser treatment, α interferon, or surgery.

Yellow

■ *Nevus sebaceous:* noted at birth as a yellow orange oval or linear area of alopecia on the scalp. At puberty they become raised and warty. Basal cell carcinomas can rarely develop within the nevus later in life. A benign warty tumor called *syringocystadenoma papilliferum* may occur in conjunction with a nevus sebaceous.

Papulosquamous Lesions

■ *Ichthyosis* (Fig. 36-13): associated with dry, fish-like adherent scales. The rarer lamellar form and

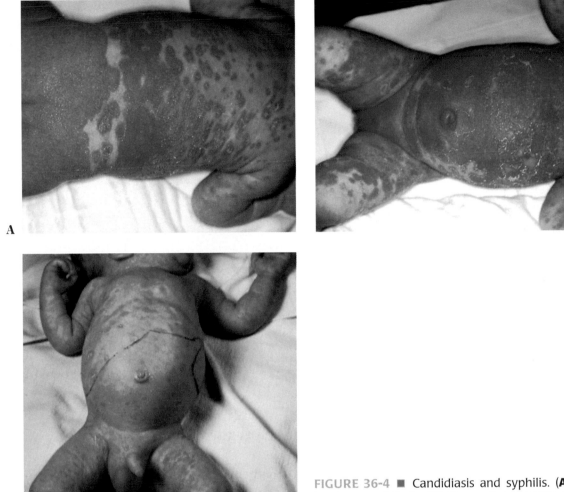

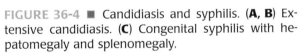

FIGURE 36-4 ■ Candidiasis and syphilis. (**A, B**) Extensive candidiasis. (**C**) Congenital syphilis with hepatomegaly and splenomegaly.

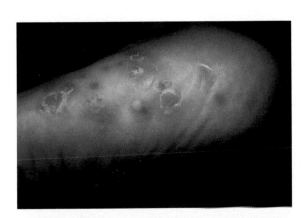

FIGURE 36-5 ■ Transient neonatal pustular melanosis.

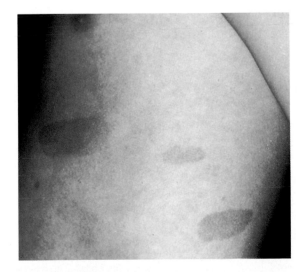

FIGURE 36-6 ■ Café-au-lait lesions.

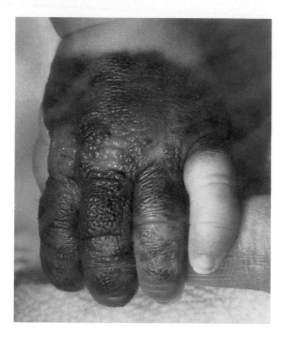

FIGURE 36-7 ■ Congenital melanocytic nevus.

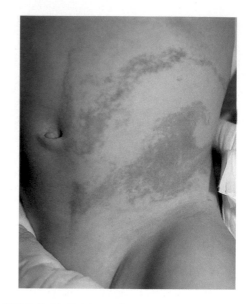

FIGURE 36-9 ■ Epidermal nevus.

congenital ichthyosiform erythroderma, both bullous and nonbullous types, are present at birth and may present with a shiny, tight layer of skin called a *collodion membrane.* Ichthyosis vulgaris and X-linked ichthyosis are usually not present at birth.

■ *Neonatal lupus erythematosus* (Fig. 36-14): characterized by heart block and annular papulosquamous skin lesions on the forehead and cheeks. The skin lesions usually fade by 6 to 7 months of age while the heart block persists. Because this is maternally transmitted, the mother also needs to be evaluated for lupus. Anti-Ro or SSA antibodies may be present in mother or newborn.

Dermatoses of Infants and Children

See Tables 36-2 and 36-3 for a summary of these dermatoses.

Blistering Lesions (Vesiculobullous)

■ *Impetigo* (Fig. 36-15): Typically presents as small vesicles or pustules which may develop into large,

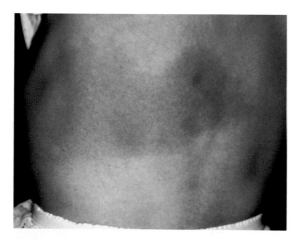

FIGURE 36-8 ■ Mongolian spot on back.

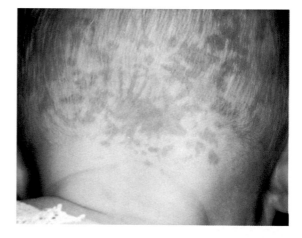

FIGURE 36-10 ■ Nevus simplex (Salmon patch).

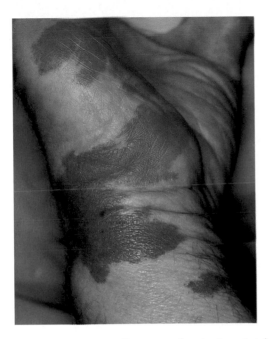

FIGURE 36-11 ■ Nevus flammeus (port-wine stain).

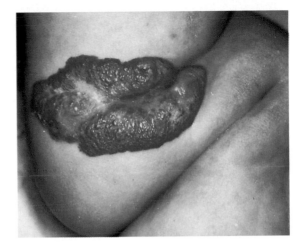

FIGURE 36-12 ■ Hemangioma of infancy—superficial.

flaccid bullae (bullous impetigo). The vesicles eventually rupture leaving erosions covered by a honey-colored crust. Impetigo is usually caused by *Staphylococcus aureus* and less commonly by *Streptococcus pyogenes*. Staphylococcal scalded skin syndrome is a desquamating disorder caused by an exfoliative toxin that results in perioral crusting and superficial desquamation most prominent in the intertriginous and flexural regions. In the newborn it is known as Ritter's disease.

■ *Viral blisters* (Fig. 36-16): herpes simplex, varicella (chicken pox), and Coxsackie (hand–foot–mouth disease) can present with vesicles on an erythematous base.

■ *Bullous disease of childhood (linear IgA dermatoses)*: sausage-shaped bullae in a "string of pearls" configuration most commonly noted on the buttocks, groin, and lower extremities. It is usually a self-limited disease. Rarely, when treatment is needed, it responds well to dapsone. Direct immunofluorescence is positive for IgA noted at the dermal-epidermal junction.

■ *Dermatitis herpetiformis*: recurrent crops of severely pruritic grouped vesicles or bullae on the extensor surfaces of the extremities, shoulders, and

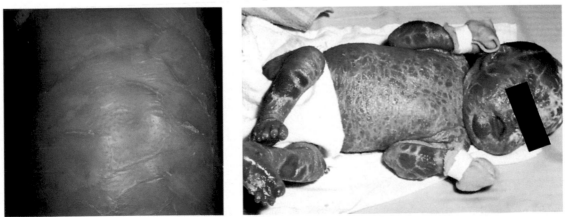

A **B**

FIGURE 36-13 ■ Ichthyosis. (**A**) Lamellar ichthyosis. (**B**) Harlequin fetus, fatal.

TABLE 36-2 ■ Dermatoses of Infants and Children

Blistering Lesions

Impetigo
Viral blisters
Bullous disease of childhood
Dermatitis herpetiformis
Incontinentia pigmenti

Pustular Lesions

Acropustulosis of infancy
Impetigo
Candidiasis

Papules/Nodules

Skin color

   Warts
   Molluscum contagiosum
   Keratosis pilaris
   Granuloma annulare
   Angiofibroma

Brown

   Melanocytic nevi
   Urticaria pigmentosa

Yellow papules

   Juvenile xanthogranuloma
   Nevus sebaceous

Red papules

   Papular acrodermatitis
   Papular urticaria
   Urticaria
   Erythema multiforme
   Pyogenic granuloma
   Viral exanthems
   Drug eruption

Vascular Lesions

Blanching

   Spider angioma

Nonblanching

   Idiopathic thrombocytopenic purpura
   Henoch-Schönlein purpura
   Meningococcemia
   Vasculitis

TABLE 36-3 ■ Dermatoses of Infants and Children

Papulosquamous

Psoriasis
Pityriasis rosea
Tinea versicolor

Eczematous Lesions

Atopic dermatitis
Seborrheic dermatitis
Immunodeficiency
Allergic contact dermatitis
Diaper dermatitis

Diseases Affecting the Hair

   Congenital/hereditary hair defects
   Alopecia areata
   Tinea capitis
   Trichotillomania

Diseases Affecting the Nails

Congenital nail defects
Twenty-nail dystrophy
Psoriasis/atopic dermatitis
Warts
Paronychia

Dermatoses Owing to Physical Agents and Photosensitivity Dermatoses

Sunburn
Thermal burn
Child abuse
Polymorphous light eruption (PMLE)
Phytophotodermatitis

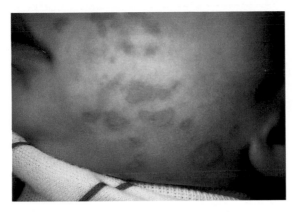

FIGURE 36-14 ■ Neonatal lupus erythematosus.

buttocks. The eruption may improve with a gluten-free diet.

■ *Incontinentia pigmenti* (Fig. 36-17): an inherited disorder presenting with vesicles in a linear distribution during the first few months of life. The vesicles are replaced by a warty stage followed by a pigmented stage. There may be associated ophthalmologic and dental abnormalities.

Pustular Lesions

■ *Acropustulosis of infancy:* noted between birth and 2 years of age predominantly in African-American infants. Recurrent crops of pruritic papulopustules or vesiculopustular lesions develop on the palms, soles, dorsum of hands, and feet. It is self-limited and often misdiagnosed as scabies.

■ *Impetigo:* (see earlier) may also be pustular.

■ *Candidiasis* (Fig. 36-18): can present with pustules and erythematous papules in the diaper and intertriginous regions.

Papules/Nodules

Skin Color

■ *Warts:* verrucous papules caused by the human papilloma virus and transmitted by skin contact. The may resolve without therapy. In children, they are common on the face, hands, and feet. When they are noted in the genitalia, sexual abuse should be considered.

■ *Molluscum contagiosum:* viral disease caused by a member of the pox virus group. They present as single or multiple dome-shaped umbilicated papules found anywhere on the body. Spread by skin contact or autoinoculation, molluscum are more common in individuals with atopic dermatitis. They may dissipate without therapy.

■ *Keratosis pilaris:* an autosomal dominant disorder characterized by minute follicular papules on the outer aspects of arms, thighs, and cheeks. It is often seen in association with atopy and dry skin. Improvement may be seen around puberty. Topical keratolytic creams may be helpful.

■ *Granuloma annulare* (Fig. 36-19): asymptomatic skin-colored or dull red papules that spread peripherally forming a ring with a normal appearing center. These are usually found on the dorsum of hands and feet. The cause is unknown and spontaneous resolution without treatment occurs in months to years.

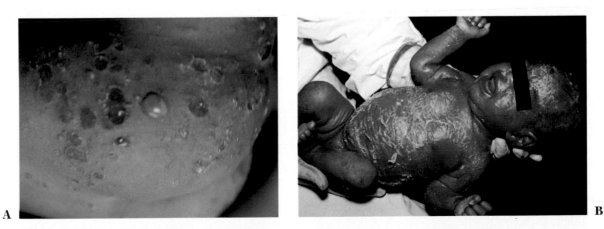

A   B

FIGURE 36-15 ■ Impetigo. **(A)** Impetigo. **(B)** Ritter's disease or Staphylococcal-scalded skin syndrome in a neonate.

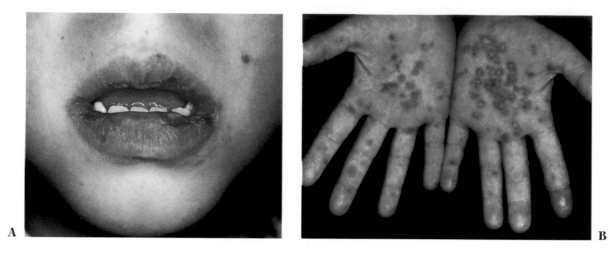

FIGURE 36-16 ■ Viral exanthem. (**A**) Erosions of lips. (**B**) Blisters on palms.

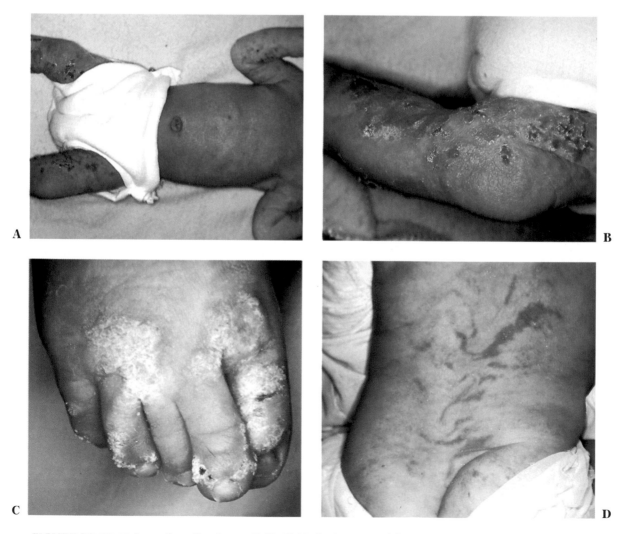

FIGURE 36-17 ■ Incontinentia pigmenti. (**A, B**) Vesicular stage. (**C**) Warty stage. (**D**) Pigmented stage.

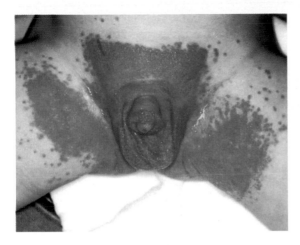

FIGURE 36-18 ■ Candidal rash.

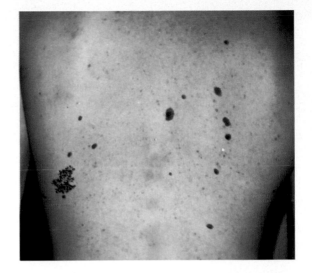

FIGURE 36-20 ■ Melanocytic nevi. Junctional nevi on the back and speckled lentiginous nevus far left midback.

■ *Angiofibroma:* firm skin colored papules. They may be associated with tuberous sclerosis when seen in a symmetrical distribution on the face.

Brown

■ *Melanocytic nevi* (Fig. 36-20): depending on the location of the nevus cells, these may be called junctional (at the border of the dermal-epidermal junction, usually flat and brown in color), intra-dermal (within the dermis, usually flesh colored and elevated), or compound nevi (both at the dermal-epidermal junction and in the dermis,

usually elevated and brown). They occur anywhere on the body and may be flat, elevated, verrucous, or papillomatous. If they are black, multicolored, large (>6 mm), or have an irregular border, an excisional biopsy should be considered.

■ *Urticaria pigmentosa* (Fig. 36-21): tan to brown macules and papules that urticate when stroked (Darier's sign). It usually has an excellent progno-sis if there is no systemic involvement. Lesions eventually resolve without therapy.

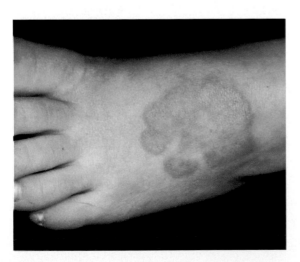

FIGURE 36-19 ■ Granuloma annulare. Dorsum of foot.

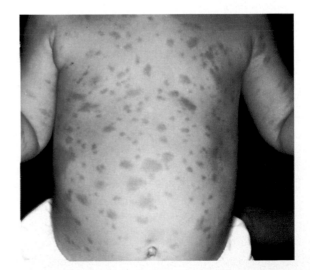

FIGURE 36-21 ■ Urticaria pigmentosa. Urticaria pigmen-tosa in a 2-year-old patient (note the red, urticating lesion below the left nipple indicating a positive Darier's sign).

Yellow

- *Juvenile xanthogranuloma:* usually develops in the first year of life and disappears around 5 years of age. They present as either solitary or multiple small yellow papules on the scalp or body. There may be associated ocular involvement if multiple lesions are present.
- *Nevus sebaceous:* see earlier.

Red

- *Papular acrodermatitis (Gianotti-Crosti syndrome):* nonpruritic flat-topped papules on the acral surfaces, especially elbows and knees. Originally associated with the hepatitis B virus, but recently other viruses have been implicated. Usually it is benign and self-limited.
- *Papular urticaria:* a delayed hypersensitivity reaction to a variety of arthropod bites. It presents as pruritic erythematous papules with a surrounding wheal. Recurrent crops occur in the summer.
- *Urticaria:* commonly seen in infants and children associated with an underlying infection or a reaction to a medication or food. It presents as pruritic, erythematous, and edematous wheals that migrate over a 24-hour period.
- *Erythema multiforme (EM):* acute hypersensitivity syndrome presenting with macular, urticarial, or vesiculobullous lesions commonly on the palms and soles. Target or "bull's eye" lesions are the hallmark of this condition with a central dusky hue and surrounding concentric erythema. It is commonly divided into erythema multiforme minor, which is a benign, recurrent, and self-limited condition also involving one mucus membrane surface. EM minor is often associated with a recurrent herpes simplex virus infection. Erythema multiforme major presents with the involvement of at least two mucous membrane surfaces, widespread bullous lesions, and more systemic symptoms. EM major is frequently associated with mycoplasma pneumoniae infection or drugs.
- *Pyogenic granuloma:* bright red papule that bleeds easily. It may arise spontaneously or at sites of trauma. Laser may be helpful for smaller lesions, but excision is usually required.
- *Viral exanthems:* roseola, rubeola, rubella, adenovirus, erythema infectiousum, and enterovirus infections may present with erythematous macules and papules. Fever may also accompany the cutaneous manifestations.

- *Drug eruption:* multiple medications may cause a diffuse cutaneous eruption consisting of erythematous macules and papules.

Vascular Lesions

Blanching

- *Spider angioma:* small telangiectatic lesion on the cheeks, nose, dorsum of hands, or sun-exposed areas. Lesions are benign and resolve spontaneously.

Nonblanching (Petechiae and Purpura)

- *Idiopathic thrombocytopenic purpura:* low platelet disorder presenting with nonblanching petechiae and purpura especially on areas of trauma. Intravenous immunoglobulin is the treatment of choice.
- *Henoch-Schönlein purpura* (Fig. 36-22): vasculitis presenting with nonblanching erythematous papules followed by palpable purpura on the buttocks and lower extremities. Abdominal pain, joint swelling, and renal involvement may occur.
- *Meningococcemia:* presents with nonblanching petechiae and purpura along with fever and signs of meningitis. Early diagnosis and treatment can be life saving.
- *Vasculitis:* nonblanching palpable petechiae and purpura commonly found on the extremities. Associated causes can include underlying medication, infection, and rarely a collagen vascular disease.

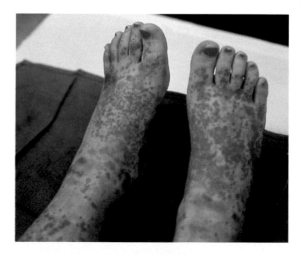

FIGURE 36-22 ■ Henoch-Schönlein purpura.

Papulosquamous

- *Psoriasis* (Fig. 36-23): seen fairly frequently in children, especially "guttate psoriasis," which is often associated with an underlying streptococcal infection.
- *Pityriasis rosea:* commonly seen in the spring and fall. A large herald patch often precedes the development of truncal lesions by 1 to 2 weeks. Lesions are oval, along Langer's lines of cleavage, with a fine, dry collorette of scale just inside the border of the plaques. An unusual form called "inverse pityriasis rosea" is seen in children with lesions located mainly in the groin and axilla.

- *Tinea versicolor:* a superficial yeast infection *(Pityrosporum orbiculare)* with hypopigmented or hyperpigmented scaly plaques on the upper chest and back and occasionally on the neck and face. Fine, dry, adherent scale is revealed upon scratching. Potassium hydroxide mount can be diagnostic.

Eczematous Lesions

- *Atopic dermatitis* (Fig. 36-24): hereditary disorder usually beginning around 1 to 4 months of age. In infants, the involvement is usually of the face, scalp, trunk, and extensor extremities. Toddlers have involvement of flexural skin surfaces and

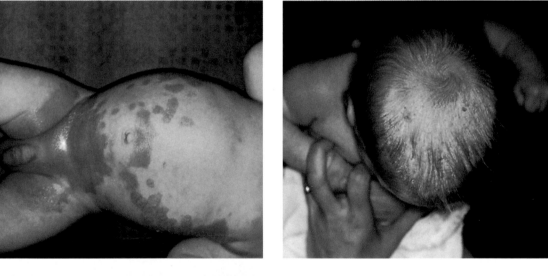

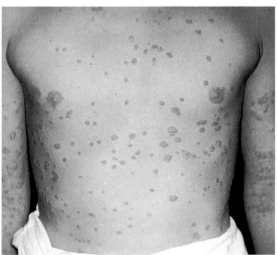

FIGURE 36-23 ■ Psoriasis. (**A, B**) Psoriasis in a 2.5 month-old child. (**C**) Guttate psoriasis following a streptococcal pharyngitis.

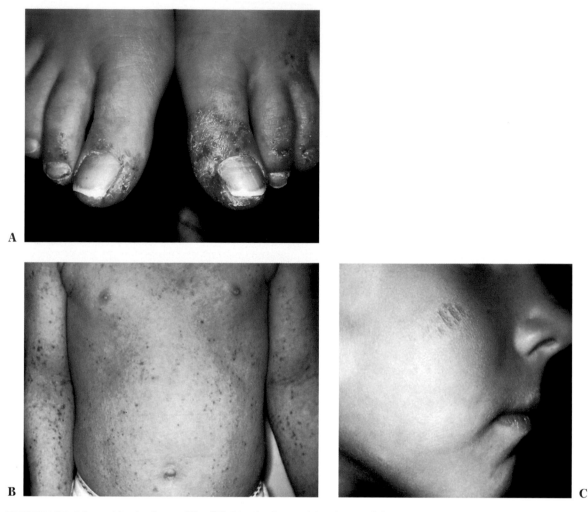

FIGURE 36-24 ■ Atopic dermatitis. (**A**) Atopic dermatitis of toes. (**B**) Atopic dermatitis of chest and antecubital fossae in a 9-year-old child. (**C**) Hypopigmented patches on cheeks (pityriasis alba).

adolescents have more severe involvement of the hands and feet. Individuals with atopic dermatitis may also have hypopigmented scaly patches on the cheeks and extensor arms referred to as *pityriasis alba.* First-line therapy continues to be emollients, antihistamines, and topical steroids. The new topical immunomodulators are second-line therapeutic options for the treatment of children 2 years of age and older.

■ *Seborrheic dermatitis* (Fig. 36-25): scaly, erythematous eruption in the "seborrheic areas," which include the scalp, face, post auricular, groin, and intertriginous areas. It appears in infancy and usually clears spontaneously. It is also seen in adolescents. Langerhans cell histiocytosis may be misdiagnosed as seborrheic dermatitis.

■ *Immunodeficiency:* severe combined immunodeficiency (SCID), Omenn's syndrome (familial reticuloendotheliosis with eosinophilia), HIV infection, and other rare immunodeficiencies can present with a widespread erythematous scaly eruption.

■ *Allergic contact dermatitis* (Fig. 36-26): the distribution and shape of these pruritic lesions is helpful in making the diagnosis. The lesions can range from vesicles to erythematous papules and eczematous plaques. Generalized reactions to poison ivy/oak are common in children. A hyperpigmented eczematoid rash in the infraumbilical area may be seen in association with a "nickel" contact dermatitis to belt buckles and/or metal snaps on pants.

■ *Diaper dermatitis* (Fig. 36-27): Irritant (secondary to stool or urine) or contact dermatitis is usually

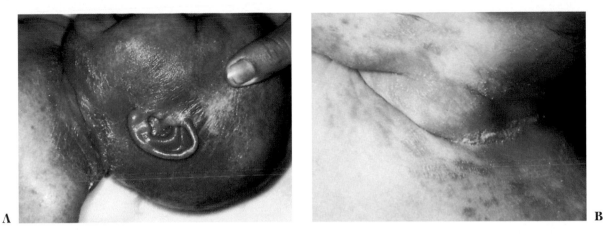

A

B

FIGURE 36-25 ■ Seborrheic dermatitis.

confined to the buttocks and perineal areas and typically spares the creases. Pustular eruptions are often seen secondary to *Candida albicans* or staphylococcal infections. "Punched out" erosions can be seen in a severe form of irritant diaper dermatitis (Jacquet's dermatitis). Atopic dermatitis usually spares the diaper region.

Disease Affecting the Hair

■ *Congenital/hereditary hair defects* (Fig. 36-28): congenital hair shaft defects can present with broken off hairs, twisted, or spun-glass appearing hair. There is no satisfactory treatment for these conditions. Abnormal hair findings may be suggestive of other underlying disorders.

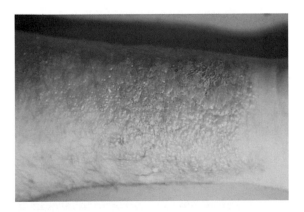

FIGURE 36-26 ■ Allergic contact dermatitis.

■ *Alopecia areata* (Fig. 36-29): common disorder presenting with the sudden appearance of patches of smooth, sharply defined alopecia. Short, tapered, "exclamation point" hairs tend to narrow as they enter the scalp. It is considered to be an autoimmune process involving the hair follicle and has been associated with thyroiditis. The prognosis depends on the extent of the hair loss (the less the better), the area involved, and chronicity. There may be associated nail pitting. Most commonly prescribed therapy remains topical or intralesional corticosteroids.

■ *Tinea capitis* (Fig. 36-30): common organisms are *Trichrophyton tonsurans* (the most common cause of tinea capitis in the United States) and *Microsporum canis.* "Black dot" tinea, caused by *T. tonsurans,* often presents with broken-off hairs and minimal inflammation. Tinea capitis may be asymptomatic or can present with scale, pruritus, alopecia, or pustules. A kerion, which is an inflammatory, pus-filled, boggy mass with associated hair loss can be seen in more severe cases. Occipital lymphadenopathy is commonly noted in patients with tinea capitis. Fungal culture and potassium hydroxide mount can be diagnostic. Treatment is with oral griseofulvin for at least 2 months. Newer antifungals (fluconazole, itraconazole, and terbinafine) are also showing promise and may begin to replace griseofulvin.

■ *Trichotillomania* (Fig. 36-31): commonly seen between 4 and 10 years of age in both genders. Patients pluck, twirl, or rub hair-bearing areas either consciously or subconsciously as a result of a habit. It usually affects the scalp, but may

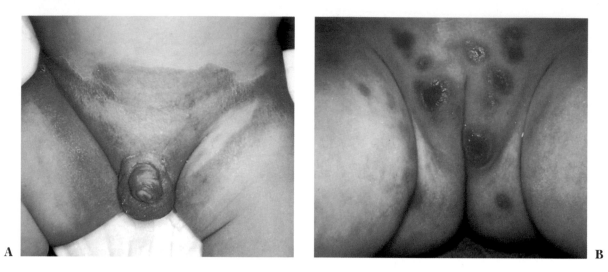

FIGURE 36-27 ■ Diaper dermatitis. (**A**) Seborrheic diaper dermatitis. (**B**) Jacquet's diaper dermatitis.

also involve eyebrows and eyelashes. It is usually self-limited.

Disease Affecting the Nails

- *Congenital nail defects:* absent or poorly developed nails are associated with many syndromes, usually representing nail matrix disorders. Ectodermal dysplasias are syndromes associated with abnormal nails, skin, hair, and teeth.
- *Twenty-nail dystrophy:* presents as thickened nails with exaggerated longitudinal ridges, noted in all

nails of the hand (ten-nail dystrophy) (Fig. 36-32) or hands and feet (twenty-nail dystrophy). This dystrophy is self-limited and may resolve over time.

- *Psoriasis/atopic dermatitis:* nails may be thickened, shiny, and contain ridges or pitting with these conditions.

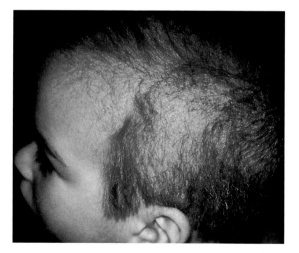

FIGURE 36-28 ■ Diffuse alopecia with ectodermal defect in 3-year-old child.

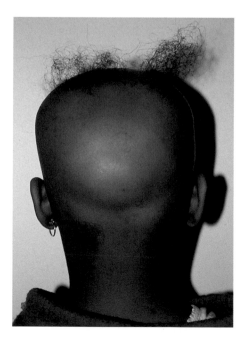

FIGURE 36-29 ■ Alopecia areata. Note completely smooth bald area.

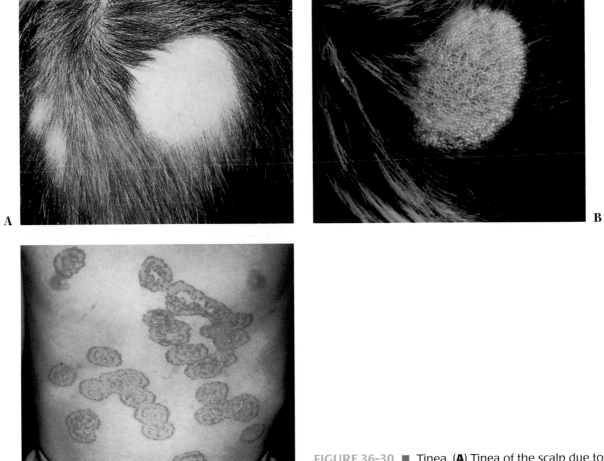

FIGURE 36-30 ■ Tinea. (**A**) Tinea of the scalp due to *M. audouinii*. (**B**) Tinea hairs fluorescing under Wood's light. (**C**) Tinea of body due to *M. canis*.

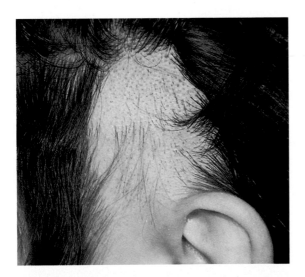

FIGURE 36-31 ■ Trichotillomania of the scalp. Note there is not complete baldness and hairs are of varying lengths.

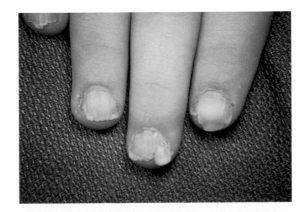

FIGURE 36-32 ■ Ten-nail dystrophy.

- *Warts:* children frequently develop warts around (periungual) and under the nail (subungual). These warts can pose a therapeutic challenge.
- *Paronychia:* usually presents as a red, painful, inflamed lesion around the nail fold, which may drain pus. It can be acute or chronic. *S. aureus* is the most common organism causing acute infection. The chronic form is often seen in thumb suckers, nail biters, and nail pickers and is commonly associated with *C. albicans.*

Dermatoses Owing to Physical Agents and Photosensitivity Dermatoses

- *Sunburn:* on the first sunny days, parents tend to underestimate the effects of the sun rays and overexpose their children. Parents should be taught the ABCs of sun exposure. *A*lways stay out of the sun between 10 AM and 4 PM. *B*lock the sun with sunscreens that protect against both UVA and UVB rays with a sun protection factor (SPF) of at least 30. *C*lothes, especially a hat and shirt, should be worn when outside. Adolescents should also be cautioned to avoid tanning salons.
- *Thermal burn:* may be partial thickness with erythema and blisters, or full thickness with loss of skin and subsequent scar formation.
- *Child abuse:* well-demarcated atypical appearing purpura, erosions, or scars should raise the suspicion of possible child abuse.
- *Polymorphous light eruption (PMLE):* idiopathic sensitivity to UV rays characterized by pruritic, eczematous, papulovesicular, or plaque-like lesions on sun exposed areas such as the cheeks, ears, nose, neck, or dorsum of the hands. If no additional sunlight exposure occurs, lesions will involute spontaneously in 1 to 2 weeks. Broad-spectrum sunscreens providing protection against UVB and UVA are helpful.
- *Phytophotodermatitis:* well-demarcated erythema (often linear) with residual hyperpigmentation on sun exposed skin. This dermatitis is more common in the spring and summer in children who have been exposed to a plant that contains furocoumarin psoralen, a photosensitizing agent. The hyperpigmentation can last for several months.

Suggested Reading

American Academy of Pediatrics. Ultraviolet light: A hazard to children. Pediatrics 1999;104:328–333.

Bruckner AL, Frieden IJ. Hemangiomas of infancy. J Am Acad Dermatol 2003;48:477–493.

Chamlin SL, Williams ML. Pigmented lesions in adolescents. Adolesc Med 2001;12:195–212.

Eichenfield LF, Hanifin JM, Luger TA, et al. Consensus conference on pediatric atopic dermatitis. J Am Acad Dermatol 2003;49:1088–1095.

Harrison S, Sinclair R. Optimal management of hair loss (alopecia) in children. Am J Clin Dermatol 2003;4:757–770.

Hurwitz, S (ed.). Clinical pediatric dermatology, ed 3. Philadelphia: Elsevier, 2005.

Kohl S. The diagnosis and treatment of neonatal herpes simplex virus infection. Pediatr Ann 2002;31:726–732.

Mancini AJ. Childhood exanthems: A primer and update for the dermatologist. Adv Dermatol 2000;16:3–37.

Makkar HS, Frieden IJ. Congenital melanocytic nevi: an update for the pediatrician. Curr Opin Pediatr 2002;14:397–403.

Pomeranz AJ, Sabnis SS. Tinea capis: Epidemiology, diagnosis and management strategies. Paediatr Drugs 2002;4:779–783.

Sanfilippo AM, Barrio V, Kulp-Shorten C, et al. Common pediatric and adolescent skin conditions. J Pediatr Adolesc Gynecol 2003;16:269–283.

Schachner LA, Hansen RC. Pediatric Dermatology, ed 3. Philadelphia, WB Saunders, 2003.

Wagner A. Distinguishing vesicular and pustular disorders in the neonate. Curr Opin Pediatr 1997;9:396–405.

Wallach D. Diagnosis of common, benign neonatal dermatoses. Clin Dermatol 2003;21:264–268.

Weston WL, Lane AT. Color Textbook of Pediatric Dermatology, ed 3. St. Louis, Mosby Yearbook, 2002.

CHAPTER 37

Geriatric Dermatology

John C. Hall

Life Stages and the Skin

A brief review of important life stages and their influence on the skin is as follows.

Puberty

At puberty, facial hair, pubic hair, and other body hair begin to grow in characteristic patterns that differ between girls and boys. Both sexes, at this time, notice increased activity of the apocrine glands, with axillary perspiration and body odor and increased development of the sebaceous glands, with the formation of varying degrees of seborrhea and the comedones, papules, and pustules of acne. Certain skin diseases tend to disappear around the onset of puberty, such as the infantile form of atopic eczema, keratosis pilaris, tinea of the scalp, and urticaria pigmentosa.

Pregnancy

Certain physiologic skin changes occur during pregnancy. Perspiration is increased. Hyperpigmentation of the abdominal midline, nipples, vulva, and face (chloasma) is seen, and nevi and freckles also become more prominent and more pigmented. Malignant melanoma is not more common during pregnancy. Hypertrichosis of the scalp may occur and then telogen effluvium hair loss of the scalp appears 3 to 6 months after delivery or after cessation of breastfeeding. Striae of breasts, abdomen, and thighs appear. The skin diseases of pregnancy are:

- herpes gestationis,
- impetigo herpetiformis,
- vulvar pruritus (often owing to candidal infection),
- palmar erythema,
- spider hemangiomas,
- pyogenic granulomas,
- rarely erythema multiforme, and
- pedunculated fibromas (skin tags).

The following dermatoses usually improve or disappear during pregnancy:

- psoriasis,
- acne (can be worse),
- alopecia areata, and
- possibly systemic scleroderma.

Menopause

Common physiologic changes in the skin of women during menopause include hot flashes, increased perspiration, increased hair growth on the face, and varying degrees of scalp hair loss. Other skin conditions associated with menopause are:

- chloasma,
- pedunculated fibromas (skin tags),
- lichen simplex chronicus,
- vulvar pruritus,
- keratoderma climacterium (palmar psoriasis), and
- rosacea.

Geriatric State

The diffuse atrophy of the skin that occurs in the aged person is partially responsible for the dryness that results in senile pruritus and winter itch. Other changes include excessive wrinkling and hyperpigmentation of the skin. Specific dermatoses noted with increased frequency are:

- seborrheic and actinic keratoses,
- basal cell and squamous cell carcinomas,
- senile purpura,
- pedunculated fibromas (skin tags), and
- capillary senile hemangiomas (cherry angiomas).

Geriatric Dermatology

Humans age gradually. Although the entire body changes slowly with advancing years, aging of the skin is readily visible and noticed by both men and women. If the sale of cosmetics (*e.g.,* moisturizing creams, "age spot" removers, wrinkle creams, wigs, hair dyes for men and women) is any sign, it would seem obvious that the constant search for the "elixir of youth" is mainly directed toward maintaining a youthful-looking skin. Consider the interest in retinoic acid (Retin-A, Renova), α-hydroxy acids, chemical peels, botulinum toxin, microdermabrasion, filler substances, and laser skin resurfacing for wrinkles and aging skin.

The two most important skin care strategies to avoid signs of aging are to protect the skin from ultraviolet light and avoid exposure to tobacco smoke.

For the trained and careful observer, the elderly patient with even "normal skin" presents a wealth of skin changes, some obvious and others less obvious (Fig. 37-1). Some of the earliest signs of aging of the skin are the development of the hyperpigmented macular lesions known as *freckles* and *lentigines* (Fig. 37-2). These can begin in persons in their 40s. They develop most commonly on the dorsa of the hands and on the face, in direct proportion to the genetically determined fair complexion of the person and the dosage of sun gained through the earlier years of life.

On the face, and to a lesser extent on the rest of the body, wrinkling of the skin also progresses with age. This is much more apparent in fair-skinned individuals. Diffuse hyperpigmentation of the face and hands, again in the sun-exposed areas, becomes more definite with age. The quite common hyperpigmentation on the side of the neck, which is a combination of brown and red discoloration, seen particularly in women, is called *poikiloderma of Civatte* (Fig. 37-3).

Actinic keratoses (see Fig. 26-6) have a definite predilection for the sun-exposed area of the body and also are related to the genetically determined complexion of the person and the environmental sun exposure.

The very common seborrheic keratoses (Fig. 37-4; see Fig. 26-1) can also be on the face but are most commonly seen on the neck, back, chest, and even in the crural area. These lesions can be so black and angry looking as to make one believe that one is dealing with a malignant melanoma. A biopsy may be necessary.

Another manifestation of aging is the development of large, open comedones on the face lateral to the orbicular area (Fig. 37-5). This is called *Favre-Racouchot syndrome.*

Pedunculated fibromas and pedunculated seborrheic keratoses are extremely common on the neck and axilla. These can begin in the 40s and 50s.

Moving down to the trunk, practically every elderly person has small, bright red capillary hemangiomas (see Fig. 26-15). These are of no clinical significance but can sometimes be disturbing for vain persons.

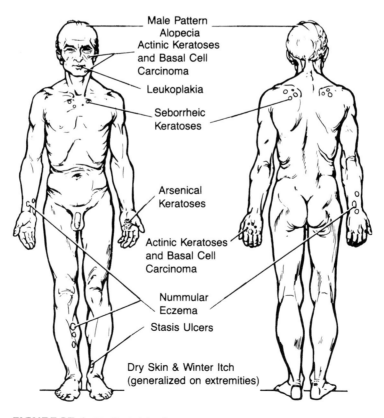

Male Pattern Alopecia
Actinic Keratoses and Basal Cell Carcinoma
Leukoplakia
Seborrheic Keratoses
Arsenical Keratoses
Actinic Keratoses and Basal Cell Carcinoma
Nummular Eczema
Stasis Ulcers
Dry Skin & Winter Itch (generalized on extremities)

FIGURE 37-1 ■ Geriatric dermograms.

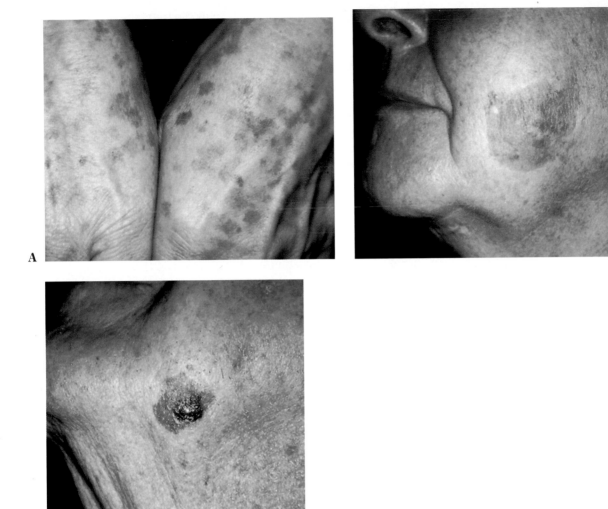

FIGURE 37-2 ■ **(A)** Senile freckles on dorsum of hands. **(B)** Lentigo on cheek. **(C)** Malignant melanoma in lentigo, on jaw area. *(Syntex Laboratories, Inc.)*

On the legs, and to a lesser extent on the arms and body, it is common to see dry skin and xerosis (Fig. 37-6). Most persons are not aware of the fact that as they age, they need to decrease their frequency of bathing, or, more importantly, increase skin lubrication immediately after bathing, especially in the winter. Winter itch is quite common on the legs and can make the patient miserable, yet the treatment is simple, involving less frequent bathing and a corticosteroid ointment or lubricant.

Bruising occurs much more frequently in the aged skin and is most commonly seen on the extremities. This is referred to as *senile purpura*. Ecchymoses occur at sites where the patient often does not even remember any trauma.

In general, the color of the entire skin becomes pale and opaque.

The appendages of the skin change also. The most obvious and common changes are in the scalp, where the hair develops varying shades, from grayness to pure white color in certain persons.

Male-pattern alopecia, which can begin in the late teens, becomes more progressive through life. For the elderly patient, though, who has not had this hereditary balding problem, another form of hair loss, manifested as a diffuse thinning of the scalp hair, can develop. This senile alopecia can occur in both men and women. Diffuse hair loss is also obvious in the axillae and the pubic area.

Excess facial hair is commonly seen in the elderly woman and can require shaving.

The nails do not change tremendously with age, but there is an increase in the longitudinal ridging. The toenails

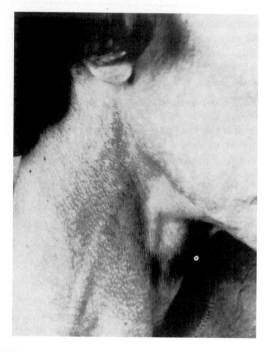

FIGURE 37-3 ■ Poikiloderma of Civatte. Very common reddish brown discoloration on sides of neck, seen mainly in women.

commonly become discolored, usually yellowish or brownish and often accompanied by onychomycosis (see Chap. 25).

The sebaceous glands and sweat glands become less active in the older person. For the unfortunate persons who have had acne for years, age can be pleasant for them, with a clearing of this problem. If a patient does present with a complaint of the recent development of acne, the patient should be asked carefully about the administration of testosterone, either orally or by injection. The decrease in the secretion of oil and sweat glands contributes directly to the development of the dry skin or xerosis mentioned.

The mucous membranes become drier. Patients complain of dry lips and tongue. The mucous membranes of the vaginal orifice also become dry, atrophic, and fragile.

Thus, essentially every elderly person has some evidence, however mild, of a skin problem.

Incidence of Geriatric Skin Diseases

For a study of the incidence of true skin diseases in a group of geriatric patients, there is a summary of a report in a classic study by Gip and Molin (see Suggested Reading). These investigators studied 286 patients older than the age of 60 years who were hospitalized in a Swedish geriatric clinic. The skin of each patient was examined carefully. Histopathologic, bacteriologic, or mycologic examinations

were undertaken in some cases. In the 107 men there were 231 skin diagnoses (2.2 per person), and in the 179 women 372 skin diagnoses were made (2.1 per person). The number of skin diagnoses per person ranged from 1 to 5. No skin diagnoses were registered in 22 cases (only 8%) (5 men and 17 women). All of the skin diagnoses were recorded. The following list contains the 10 most frequent dermatologic disorders registered (the numbers refer to the total number of dermatologic disorders found in the 286 men and women examined):

- pigmented nevus (143),
- discoloration of the toenails (133),
- seborrheic keratosis (84),
- plantar hyperkeratosis (36),
- stasis dermatitis of the legs (31),
- seborrheic dermatitis (27),
- dermatitis of the legs (unspecified) (23),
- marked atrophy of the skin (19),
- xanthelasma (12), and
- capillary hemangiomas (10).

They attributed most of the cases of discoloration of the nails to bacterial and fungal infections, related to air content of the nail plate, or hemorrhage.

Management of Geriatric Skin Problems

The dermatologic management of an elderly patient is considerably complicated, however, by the patient's physical and mental ability to understand and carry out instructions. Writing out instructions carefully and legibly can be very helpful. Carefully explaining instructions for skin care to a relative or care giver can be valuable. The correct application of wet dressings, coping with tub bathing, and even the simple application of creams and ointments can be complex processes for elderly patients. And as age progresses and debility increases, this care is further complicated by having to be administered by another person, such as a family member or nurse; this, additionally, has aesthetic and economic limitations.

SAUER'S NOTES

1. Nowhere is the broadness of the term *management* more meaningful than when it is used in reference to the handling of the skin problem for an elderly patient.
2. Management implies the imparting of much more information and instruction than the simple prescribing of "treatment."

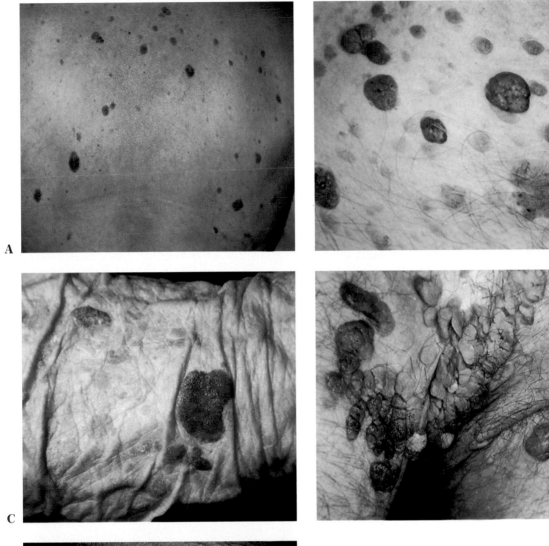

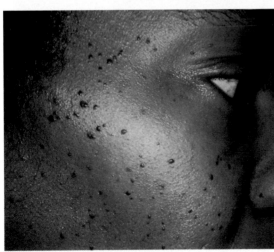

FIGURE 37-4 ■ **(A)** Seborrheic keratoses over back of 71-year-old man. **(B)** Seborrheic keratoses, close-up. **(C)** Large seborrheic keratosis on hand in 84-year-old woman. **(D)** Multiple seborrheic keratoses of crural area. **(E)** Seborrheic keratoses or dermatosis papulosa nigra on face.

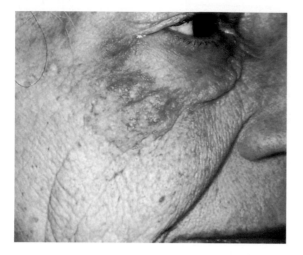

FIGURE 37-5 ■ Senile elastosis with cysts and comedones of cheek (Favre-Racouchat syndrome). *(Courtesy of Syntex Laboratories, Inc.)*

Most elderly patients can be treated at home, but some of the more severe skin problems are seen in institutionalized persons. Depending on the care available and the extent of the dermatosis, hospitalization may be necessary. The role of both corticosteroids and antibiotics in decreasing the number of elderly patients needing hospitalization is enormous and is most fortuitous.

Classification of Geriatric Dermatoses

The elderly patient is subject to the regular skin ills. However, as with the other age extreme, the child, there can be a different reaction by the aged skin to a given skin problem by virtue of the presence of fragility, dryness, and atrophy.

It is unusual to see certain skin problems in the aged, such as atopic eczema, acne, pityriasis rosea, impetigo, primary and secondary syphilis, herpes simplex, warts, exanthems, chloasma, and sunburn (Fig. 37-7). A compilation of the more common problems of the geriatric patient is as follows, listed according to chapter groupings.

Dermatologic Allergy

Allergies are discussed in Chapter 9.

Contact Dermatitis

For the geriatric patient this commonly is a dermatitis caused by the use of too harsh a local medication (Figs. 9-1 through 9-4). This is seen quite frequently where too strong or too drying a salve is used in the treatment of itching legs.

Nummular Eczema

Nummular eczema is quite a common problem, seen particularly in the winter and characterized clinically by coin-shaped vesicular areas on the arms, the legs, and, less frequently, the buttocks (Fig. 37-8; see also Figs. 9-11, 26-3, and 26-5).

Drug Eruptions

Drug eruptions are not uncommon and can be seen as a photosensitivity-type dermatitis when the patient is on a

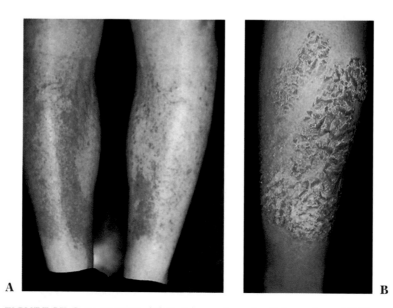

FIGURE 37-6 ■ Xerosis. **(A)** Redness of winter itch on legs. **(B)** Xerosis with secondary infection on legs. *(Courtesy of Johnson & Johnson.)*

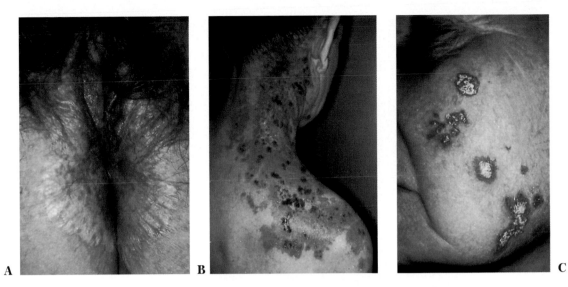

A   B   C

FIGURE 37-7 ■ **(A)** Lichen sclerosus et atrophicus of vulva (not leukoplakia). **(B)** Herpes zoster of shoulder and neck. **(C)** Discoid lupus erythematosus of cheek in 77-year-old woman.

diuretic or a phenothiazine-type tranquilizer, as a side effect of nonsteroidal anti-inflammatory drugs to treat arthritis or as an acne-like picture, due to the administration of testosterone (Fig. 37-9; see also Fig. 9-12).

Pruritic Dermatoses

Pruritic dermatoses are discussed in Chapter 11.

Generalized Pruritus

This is quite common and can defy adequate therapy (Fig. 37-10). Careful examination of the patient is necessary to rule out any internal cause of the generalized pruritus. Rather frequently, and rather unfortunately, no apparent cause is ascertainable. Scalp and face itching can be a real problem.

Xerosis

As a cause of the generalized itching in the winter, this is rather easily managed by decreasing bathing and applying an emollient lotion or even a mild corticosteroid ointment immediately after bathing (see Fig. 37-6B). See Chapter 11 for a more detailed discussion of this problem in the elderly patient.

Localized Pruritic Dermatoses

These are not as common as the more generalized pruritic dermatoses.

Vascular Dermatoses

Vascular dermatoses are considered in Chapter 12.

Urticaria

This is not commonly seen.

Stasis Dermatitis

This is rather common in elderly patients and is almost always associated with venous insufficiency owing to varicose veins or other circulatory problems. It is important to stress that circulatory support dressings (Ace wrap) or garments (Jobst or Compass) are indicated on a continuing basis after the dermatitis has responded to therapy. This can prevent the development of stasis ulcers (Fig. 37-11).

Atrophie Blanche

Arterial insufficiency of the legs from several causes can produce redness, scaling, ulcers, and, eventually, stellate scars. It occurs mainly over the ankles.

Seborrheic Dermatitis, Acne, and Rosacea

These condition are reviewed in detail in Chapter 13.

Seborrheic Dermatitis

This becomes less bothersome with age but can recur following a cerebrovascular accident, stroke, or Parkinson's disease (see Figs. 13-1 through 13-3).

Acne

This is rarely seen in the elderly patient. If it is present, the patient should be asked about intake of testosterone and

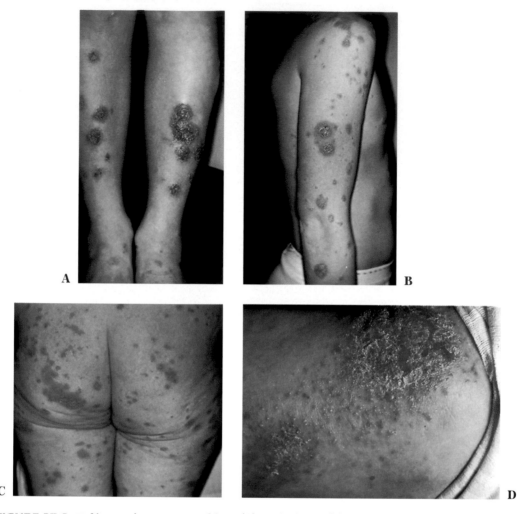

FIGURE 37-8 ■ Nummular eczema of legs (**A**) and of arm (**B**) of same patient. (**C**) Nummular eczema of buttocks. (**D**) Close-up showing oozing in nummular eczema of leg. *(Johnson & Johnson.)*

corticosteroid drugs (especially if used more than 1 month), which can produce acne.

Papulosquamous Dermatoses

Chapters 14 and 15 cover papulosquamous dermatoses in depth.

Psoriasis

It is rare to see psoriasis (see Figs. 14-1, 14-2, and 36-23) develop as a new problem in an elderly person. Thus, most elderly persons who have psoriasis have learned to live with the disease.

Dermatologic Bacteriology

Dermatologic bacteriology is covered in Chapter 21.

Furuncles and Carbuncles

These lesions are not too common.

Decubital Ulcers

The alternate term *bedsore* describes the pathogenesis of these chronic, painful, and debilitating ulcerations. They occur on pressure sites, mainly the buttocks and posterior aspect of heels. The patient is usually bedridden. Prophylactic measures are extremely important. Good nursing care can prevent some of these ulcers. The care should include turning the patient frequently, keeping the patient clean and dry, and applying powder to the bed. Once an ulcer has developed, the care is compounded. Donut-type sponge-cushion supports and special mattresses are indicated, with local application of povidone–iodine (Betadine) solution

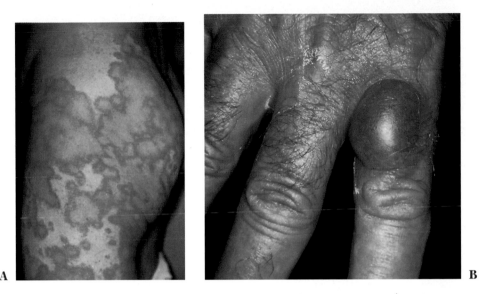

FIGURE 37-9 ■ **(A)** Drug eruption from phenacetin. **(B)** Fixed bullous drug eruption due to tetracycline. *(Courtesy of Johnson & Johnson.)*

and continued good nursing care. Surgical dressings such as Opsite, Duoderm, Tegaderm, and Polymem may be helpful. Plastic surgery may be necessary.

Stasis Ulcers

These (see Fig. 37-11B) are the cause of marked disability in the elderly patient. The ulcers heal slowly and, even when large in size, may be relatively nonpainful. The care required to heal these ulcers, or even prevent them from spreading, can be considerable. More often than not, other members of the family or nursing personnel must take over the management of these chronic sores.

Syphilology

Tertiary syphilis of the skin or other organs is now rarely seen (see Chap. 22). The most common problem seen in the elderly patient in relation to syphilis is the persistently positive serology that occurs after adequate therapy. Some syphilologists are alarmed that dormant but persistent spirochetal infections can become clinically

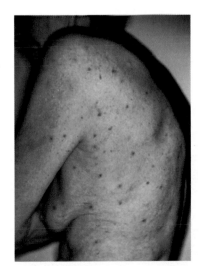

FIGURE 37-10 ■ Senile pruritus in 74-year-old woman. *(Courtesy of Johnson & Johnson.)*

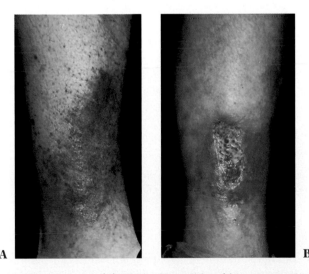

FIGURE 37-11 ■ **(A)** Stasis dermatitis of leg aggravated by contact allergy to neomycin. **(B)** Stasis ulcer of leg with varicose veins.

significant, with involvement of the eye and central nervous system.

Dermatologic Mycology

Dermatologic mycology is discussed in depth in Chapter 25.

- *Candidal infections:* the most common mycologic infections seen in the elderly patient, particularly if the patient is obese. Lack of bathing and cleansing is a major factor. Prolonged antibiotic therapy may also be contributory as well as prolonged bedrest and incontinence of urine and feces.

Dermatologic Parasitology

Chapter 17 covers dermatologic parasitology in detail.

- *Scabies:* As an epidemic in a nursing home, scabies can be a difficult management problem. The elderly, especially if mentally confused, present a challenge for basic hygiene. When they itch, this itch is usually attributed to dry skin or senile pruritus. Only when several residents in the nursing home, and the personnel, begin to itch does one think of scabies as a cause. Then the therapy is difficult because so many persons are affected (and for personnel, possibly their families) that a basic simple therapy becomes a major management problem. All persons affected must be treated at the same time.

Bullous Dermatoses

Bullous dermatoses are discussed in Chapter 18.

- *Pemphigoid* (see Fig. 36-15): This is probably the most common bullous condition seen in elderly patients. Unfortunately, the potent medications needed to treat this disease are often a major problem. Bullous pemphigoid (Fig. 37-12A) in the elderly should prompt a careful workup to rule out an internal malignancy.

Exfoliative Dermatitis

This is a miserable disease (see Chap. 19 and Fig. 19-1), and the cause can be difficult to determine. An axiom is that half of the patients older than age 50 years with exfoliative dermatitis have a lymphoma.

Pigmentary Dermatoses

Hyperpigmentation or hypopigmentation (see Chap. 31) of the skin can occur in the elderly from many causes. Aside from a simple change in pigmentation of the skin owing to age, other pigmentary problems are uncommon.

Collagen Diseases

Discoid lupus erythematosus can begin in old age (see Chap. 32 and Fig. 37-7C).

The Skin and Internal Disease

Integumentary manifestations of systemic disease are discussed in Chapter 33.

Diabetes Mellitus

This causes a degeneration of the vascular supply, and skin changes in the diabetic are progressive with age. Ulcers, diabetic dermopathy, gangrene of the digits, and ulcerations of the mal perforans type (see Fig. 33-3) are most commonly seen.

Diseases Affecting the Hair

See Chapter 28 for a discussion of diseases affecting the hair.

- *Graying of the hair and thinning of the hair:* These were discussed earlier.
- *Hirzutism:* This excessive growth of hair is common on the face of women.

Diseases Affecting the Nails

Other than the development of increased ridging of the nail plates and the discoloration of the toenails, mentioned earlier, there are no major nail changes in the aged individual, except for onychomycosis (fungal infections of nails) of the toenails (see Chap. 29).

Diseases of the Mucous Membranes

The mucous membranes can become dry and fragile with age (see Chap. 30).

Dermatoses Owing to Physical Agents

Effects of sunlight on the skin (see Chap. 34) are extremely common and can result in simple hyperpigmentation and atrophy of the skin or can produce actinic keratoses (see Figs. 26-6, 26-7) that can occasionally eventuate as squamous cell carcinomas (Fig. 37-13; see Fig. 26-11).

Photosensitivity Dermatoses

Photosensitivity problems are rarely seen unless triggered by drugs (see Chap. 34).

Genodermatoses

The genetic inheritance of the person has considerable influence on the aging of the skin, including wrinkling, the

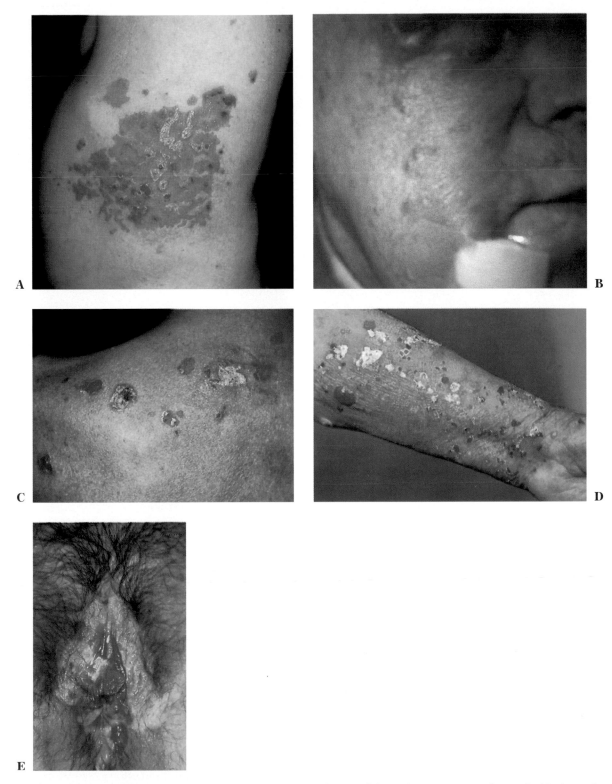

FIGURE 37-12 ■ (**A**) Pemphigoid on lateral abdominal area. (**B**) Angiosarcoma on face of elderly male. (**C**) Pemphigus vulgaris of upper back area. (**D**) Pemphigus vulgaris of forearm. (**E**) Benign mucosal pemphigoid of vulva showing erosions.

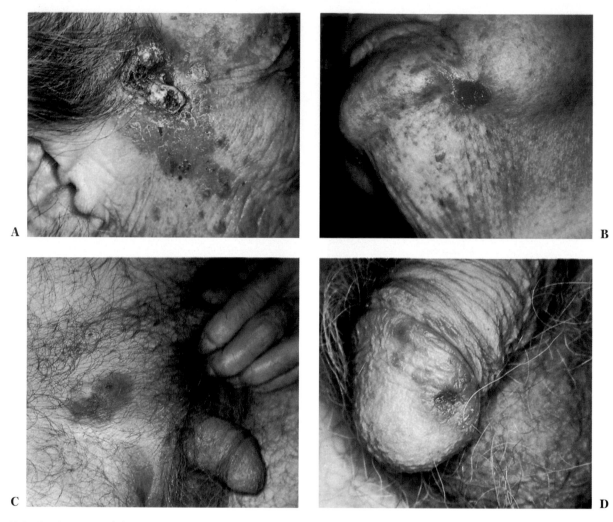

FIGURE 37-13 ■ (**A**) Squamous cell carcinoma and keratoses on aged skin. (**B**) Squamous cell carcinoma in area of chronic radiodermatitis for hypertrichosis of skin. (**C**) Paget's disease of crural area. (**D**) Erythroplasia of Queyrat on penis. *(Syntex Laboratories, Inc.)*

effect of sunlight, the activity of the oil and sweat glands, and hair changes (see Chap. 35).

Tumors of the Skin

Tumors of the skin are reviewed in Chapter 26.

- *Seborrheic keratoses* (see Figs. 26-1 and 37-4): As mentioned, these are common, seen in almost every elderly person. The number of these lesions is genetically determined.
- *Pedunculated fibromas:* Such fibromas of the neck and axilla are quite common, and, again, there is a familial tendency for these to develop.
- *Precancerous tumors:* Tumors such as senile or actinic keratoses (see Figs. 26-6 and 26-7) develop

in relation to earlier sun exposure and the genetic makeup of the skin complexion.

- *Squamous cell carcinoma* (see Figs. 26-10, 26-11, and 37-13): This can develop by itself or from degeneration of actinic keratoses.
- *Basal cell carcinomas* (Fig. 37-14; see Figs. 3-2C and 26-9): These are the most common malignancies of the skin in the elderly patient. These are characterized by waxy nodular lesions, with or without ulceration in the center.
- *Venous lake or varix:* Occurring on the lips and ears, these are common and can frighten the patient into thinking that he or she has a melanoma.
- *Capillary hemangiomas* (see Fig. 26-15): These are present on the chest and back of almost every

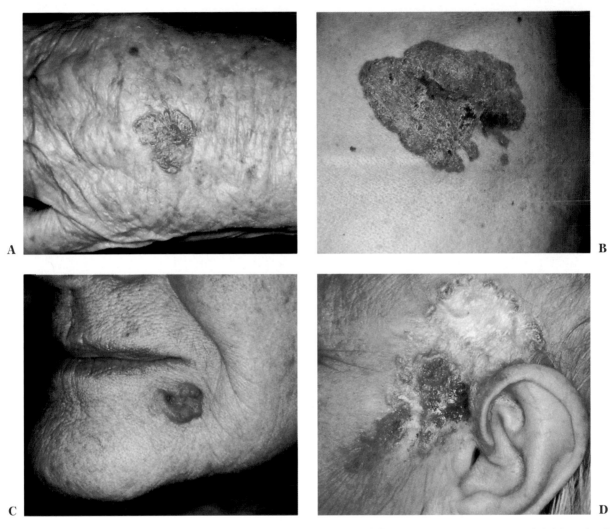

FIGURE 37-14 ■ **(A)** Basal cell carcinoma and wrinkling of hand. **(B)** Lateral view of large superficial basal cell carcinoma on back. **(C)** Basal cell carcinoma on chin. **(D)** Extensive basal cell carcinoma in a 79-year-old patient. *(Syntex Laboratories, Inc.)*

elderly person and hence the designation senile angiomas.

■ *Nevi* (Fig. 37-15; see Fig. 26-16): These mature with age, and many seem to disappear. Junctional elements are rarely seen in nevi in the geriatric patient.

■ *Malignant melanoma* (see Fig. 26-18): It can develop from a brownish-black, flat lesion known as a lentigo, which is usually seen on the face and arms. The result is a *lentigo maligna melanoma which develops on chronically sunexposed skin* (see Fig. 37-3C).

Vitamin Deficiencies

As the aged population continues to become a higher percentage of the total population and life expectancy increases, the nutritional status of this elderly population becomes increasingly important. The vitamin deficiencies are therefore discussed as follows.

Dermatoses owing to lack of vitamins are rare in the United States. However, a common question asked by many patients is, "Doctor, don't you think my trouble is caused by a lack of vitamins?" The answer in 99% of cases is "No!"

Vitamin A

Phrynoderma is the name for generalized dry hyperkeratoses of the skin owing to chronic and significant lack of vitamin A. Clinically, the texture of the skin resembles the surface of a nutmeg grater. Eye changes are often present, including night blindness and dryness of the eyeball.

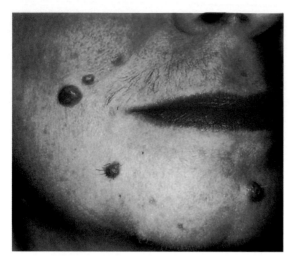

FIGURE 37-15 ■ Compound nevi on face.

Large doses of vitamin A (25,000 to 50,000 international units t.i.d.) are used in the treatment of patients with Darier's disease, pityriasis rubra pilaris, comedonal acne, and xerosis (dry skin). The value of this therapy has not been proved. Vitamin A therapy in high doses should be for only 4 to 6 months at a time, with cessation of therapy for 6 to 8 weeks before resuming it again because of hepatotoxicity.

Hypervitaminosis A, caused by excessively high and persistent intake of vitamin A in drug or food form, causes hair loss, dry skin, irritability, weight loss, and enlargement of the liver and spleen.

Isotretinoin (Accutane) is a vitamin A acid preparation that is beneficial for severe cystic acne and a few other rarer conditions.

Acitretin (Soriatane), another synthetic derivative of vitamin A, is useful for pustular and exfoliative psoriasis. Both Accutane and Soriatane have severe side effects, including fetal abnormalities. They should never be prescribed unless the physician and patient thoroughly understand the potential dangers of these vitamin A derivatives.

Vitamin B Group

Clinically, a patient with a true vitamin B deficiency is deficient in all of the vitamins of this group. Thus the classic diseases of this group, namely, beriberi and pellagra, have overlapping clinical signs and symptoms.

Vitamin B_1 (Thiamine)

This deficiency is clinically manifested by beriberi. The cutaneous lesions consist of edema and redness of the soles of the feet.

Vitamin B_2 (Riboflavin)

Deficiency of vitamin B_2 has been linked with red fissures at the corners of the mouth (perlèche) and glossitis. This can occur in marked vitamin B_2 deficiency, but most cases with these clinical lesions are due to contact dermatitis or malocclusion of the lips from faulty dentures.

Nicotinic Acid

This deficiency leads to pellagra, but other vitamins of the B group are contributory. The skin lesions are a prominent part of pellagra and include redness of the exposed areas of hands, face, neck, and feet, which can go on to a fissured, scaling, infected dermatitis. Local trauma may spread the disease to other areas of the body. The disease is worse in the summer and heals with hyperpigmentation and mild scarring. Gastrointestinal and neurologic complications are serious. Dementia, dermatitis, and diarrhea are the "three Ds" of pellagra.

Vitamin C (Ascorbic Acid)

Scurvy is now a rare disease, and the skin lesions are not specific. They include a follicular papular eruption, petechiae, and purpura.

Vitamin D

No skin lesions have been attributed to lack of this vitamin. Vitamin D and vitamin D_2 (calciferol) have been used orally in the treatment of lupus vulgaris. Vitamin D_3 (Dovonex ointment) is used topically for psoriasis.

Vitamin E

It has been reported that vitamin E is effective in treating yellow nail syndrome.

Vitamin K

Hypoprothrombinemia with purpura from various causes responds to vitamin K therapy.

Lipidoses

The manifestations of fat deposition in the skin are seen often in the elderly population, and that is why it is included in this chapter.

This complex group of metabolic diseases causes varying skin lesions, depending somewhat on the basic metabolic fault. The most common skin lesions are xanthomas, which are characterized by yellowish plaques or nodules readily seen on the skin surface (Fig. 37-16). Xanthomatous lesions are either due to primary hyperlipidemia or the secondary

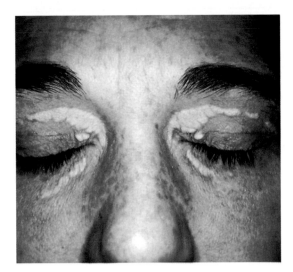

FIGURE 37-16 ■ Xanthelasma.

result of a primary disease such as alcoholism, diabetes mellitus, hypothyroidism, or, less commonly, obstructive jaundice, nephrotic syndrome, and dysproteinemia.

The diagnosis of a patient with a xanthoma begins with tests for fasting plasma cholesterol and triglycerides. These tests should uncover 95% of the patients with hyperlipidemia. If these tests are abnormal, then plasma turbidity studies and plasma lipoprotein electrophoresis should be performed. On the basis of abnormal lipoprotein patterns, five types of familial hyperlipidemia can be recognized: tendinous xanthomas, planar xanthomas (most common form is xanthelasma or xanthelasma palpebrarum), tuberous xanthomas, eruptive xanthomas, and xanthoma disseminatum. These can usually be correlated with specific lipoproteins.

For secondary hyperlipidemia, therapy would be aimed at the primary disease. For familial hyperlipidemia, diet therapy and drug therapy must be considered, based on the type of disease.

Xanthoma-like deposits in the skin occur in several other diseases, namely, the histiocytosis group of diseases, which are Schüller-Christian syndrome, Letterer-Siwe disease, and eosinophilic granuloma. Vesicular lesions can be seen in cases of Schüller-Christian syndrome, and a seborrheic dermatitis–like picture is evident in Letterer-Siwe disease (see Dictionary–Index, Fig. 2A).

Extracellular lipid accumulations occur in lipoid proteinosis, extracellular cholesterosis, and necrobiosis lipoidica diabeticorum. Skin lesions of the latter occur mostly in women, on the anterior tibial area of the leg, and are characterized by sharply circumscribed, yellowish plaques with a bluish border. Diabetes is present in the majority of patients.

Disturbances of phospholipid metabolism include Niemann-Pick disease and Gaucher's disease. Patients with both disorders develop a yellowish discoloration of the skin.

Neuroses and Psychoses

The aging population frequently falls victim to psychiatrically induced skin diseases. We have, therefore, put this review in this chapter.

A common belief among many members of the medical profession is that the majority of skin diseases are caused by "nerves" or are a neurotic manifestation. This old idea is undoubtedly based on the familiar sight of the scratching skin patient; he just looks "nervous," and it makes one nervous and itchy merely to look at him. It is hard to know which came first for most patients, the itching or the nervousness. In practice, it is good to deemphasize the nervous element, but not to ignore it. An answer to patients and physicians who question the role of nerves in a particular case is to say that they play a definite role in many skin eruptions, but rarely are nerves the precipitating cause of a dermatosis. If a patient has an emotional problem and also has an itching dermatitis, a flare-up of the problem intensifies the itch, just as it aggravates another patient's blood pressure or migraine headache.

Therapy for patients with skin disease in which "nerves" are believed to play a dominant part can be handled well by the calm, receptive, attentive, interested general physician. Simple local therapy prescribed with the confidence of a competent physician often establishes in the patient the necessary faith to cure the complaint. Occasionally, these patients do not respond to such therapy, and in rare cases the patient might benefit from special psychiatric care.

The following list divides the psychocutaneous diseases into those believed to be (1) related to psychoses, (2) related to neuroses, and (3) of questionable psychic relationship.

Dermatoses Related to Psychoses

- *Factitial dermatitis:* The patient denies that he or she is producing the skin disease. This is not to be confused with neurotic excoriations.
- *Skin lesions owing to compulsive movements:* An example is the chronic biting of an arm in a dementia patient.
- *Delusions:* Of parasitism, cancer, syphilis, and so on (see Fig. 33-1A); various "proofs" are often presented by the patient to substantiate his or her existing belief. Pimozide (Orap) therapy is useful in some cases.

■ *Dysmorphic syndrome:* Patients have symptoms of cutaneous pain, burning, or other dysesthesias or, alternatively, have concerns about the structure and function of the skin (see Fig. 33-1A) or body contour. This is a common problem in the adult population. This is also called *cutaneous nondisease.* Symptoms most commonly involve the face, scalp, and genitals (*vulvodynia*). Do not confuse with lichen sclerosis et atrophicus (see Fig. 37-7A). This is a psychotic problem. Haloperidol (Haldol) in a low dosage of 1 to 2 mg twice daily can be helpful.

■ *Trichotillomania in adults:* This is a rare cause of hair loss.

Dermatoses Related to Neuroses

■ *Neurotic excoriations* (see Fig. 33-1): The patient admits picking or scratching the lesions.

■ *Phobias:* The patient fears contraction of a disease (*e.g.,* syphilophobia, acarophobia, cancerophobia, bacteriophobia).

■ *Trichotillomania of children:* This is not as serious as it is in adults. The physician's index of suspicion must be high to diagnose this disease (see Chap. 28).

■ *Lichen simplex chronicus* (see Figs. 11-1 and 11-2): The primary cause can be an insect bite, contact dermatitis from a permanent wave, psoriasis, stasis dermatitis, or one of many other conditions that can initiate the scratching habit. The habit then outlives the disease, and the lichen simplex cycle develops.

Dermatoses of Questionable Psychic Causes

■ hyperhidrosis of palms and soles,
■ dyshidrosis,
■ alopecia areata,
■ lichen planus,
■ chronic urticaria,
■ rosacea,
■ atopic eczema,
■ psoriasis,
■ aphthous stomatitis, and
■ primary pruritus, local or generalized.

Internal Cancer

A final word on the geriatric population concerns the association of internal cancer and skin disease (see Figs. 33-2 and 33-11). Skin lesions may develop from internal malignancies either by metastatic spread or by the occurrence of nonspecific eruptions. The most interesting of the nonspecific

dermatoses is the rare entity acanthosis nigricans. The presence of the velvety, papillary, pigmented hypertrophies of this disease in the axillae, the groin, and other moist areas of an adult indicates an internal cancer, usually of the abdominal viscera, in over 50% of cases. A benign form of acanthosis nigricans exists in children and becomes most manifest at puberty. As in older adults there is an association with obesity and the metabolic syndrome, which is a condition of insulin resistance. This benign form is not associated with cancer.

Herpes zoster (see Fig. 37-7B) can be severe, painful, and at times, especially when severe or generalized, associated with underlying cancer.

A dermatitis herpetiformis–like eruption with vesicles and intense pruritus is seen occasionally in patients with an internal malignancy or lymphoma.

Purpuric lesions and pyodermas also occur as nonspecific changes in patients with malignancies (see Fig. 33-2).

Specific skin lesions showing the malignancy or lymphoma on biopsy occur in mycosis fungoides, leukemia, lymphomas, and metastatic skin lesions from internal malignancies.

A severe form of pemphigus, called *paraneoplastic pemphigus,* is associated with underlying cancer.

Suggested Reading

Arlian LG, Estes SA, Vyszenski-Moher DL. Prevalence of *Sarcoptes scabiei* in the homes and nursing homes of scabietic patients. J Am Acad Dermatol 1988;19:806.

Barthelemy H, Chouvet B, Cambazard F. Skin and mucosal manifestations in vitamin deficiency. J Am Acad Dermatol 1986;15:1263.

Black MM, McKay M, Braude P, et al. Obstetric and Gynecologic Dermatology, ed 2. St Louis, Mosby, 2001.

Castanet J, Ortonne J. Pigmentary changes in aged and photoaged skin. Arch Dermatol 1997;133:1296.

Cohen PR, Scher RK. Nail changes in the elderly. J Geriatr Dermatol 1993;1:45.

Cook JL, Dzubow LM. Aging of the skin. Arch Dermatol 1997;133:1273.

Drake LA, et al. Guidelines of care for photoaging/photodamage. J Am Acad Dermatol 1996;35:3.

Fleischer AB, Feldman SR, Bradham DD. Office-based dermatologic services provided to the elderly by physicians in the United States in 1990. J Geriatr Dermatol 1993;1:146.

Fleischer AB. Pruritus in the elderly: Management by senior dermatologists. J Am Acad Dermatol 1993;28:603.

Fosko SW. Management of photoaging in the elderly. J Geriatr Dermatol 1993;1:38.

Gip L, Molin L. Skin diseases in geriatrics. Cutis 1970;6:771.

Hurley HJ. Skin in senescence: A summation. J Geriatr Dermatol 1993;1:55.

Kantor GR. Investigation of the elderly patient with pruritus. J Geriatr Dermatol 1995;3:1.

Kligman AM. Psychologic aspects of skin disorders in the elderly. J Geriatr Dermatol 1993;1:15.

Kligman AM. An overview of cutaneous geriatrics. J Geriatr Dermatol 1994;2:6.

Marks R. Skin Disease in Old Age, ed 2. London, Martin Dunitz Ltd., 1999.

Norman RA. Geriatric Dermatology. Boca Raton, FL, CRC Press, 2001.

Parish LC, Brenner S, Ramos e Silva M, Parish JL. Women's dermatology from infancy to maturity. Boca Raton, FL, CRC Press, 2001.

Rousseau P. Pressure sores in the elderly. Geriatr Med Today 1988;7:28.

Warren R, Gartstein V, Kligman AM, et al. Age, sunlight, and facial skin. J Am Acad Dermatol 1991;25:751.

CHAPTER 38

Tropical Diseases of the Skin

Francisco G. Bravo, MD, and Alejandro Morales, MD

A chapter on tropical disease usually implies infectious diseases not usually seen in cities of the developed world. However, that is no longer true if one considers the migratory trends affecting almost any large metropolis around the world. Add to that effect the development of better and faster communications that may allow somebody living in Los Angeles to reach a far post in the Amazon jungle in less than 36 hours, and vice versa. Today, city dwellers want to go and visit far away places to enjoy the beauty of nature, but, in so doing, they also, expose themselves to infectious diseases their local doctors never heard of, until now. This chapter presents a quick overview of some of those diseases a physician may encounter, either in travelers or immigrants to large cities.

Viral Diseases

HTLV-1

The human T-cell lymphotropic virus, type I, (HTLV-1) is a retrovirus of the subfamily *Oncovirnae,* with the ability to infect CD4 cells and induce different degrees of immunosuppression. An estimated 10 to 20 million persons are infected with the virus worldwide. There are multiple endemic areas in the world, including Gabon, Zaire, Ivory Coast, Japan, as well as specific populations such as the Australian aborigines. Its presence is well established in Caribbean countries such as Jamaica, Trinidad, Barbados, and Haiti. In South America, countries affected include Brazil, Colombia, and Peru, although some manifestations of the disease have also been reported in Chile, Argentina, and Uruguay. In the United States, Canada, and Europe, the incidence of seroprevalence is low, but when one looks at specific migratory populations, the number can increase dramatically.

The infection disseminated to Central and South America from two different sources of migration: the trade of African slaves in the 19th century and migration of Japanese as labor force in the 19th and 20th centuries. Incidence of seroprevalence in places like Peru may be as high

as 1% to 2%, whereas in place like the United States, seroprevalence among blood donors is about 0.025%.

Presentation and Characteristics

The most common routes of transmission are breastfeeding, sexual contact, and blood transfusions. As opposed to HIV infection (the other well-known retrovirus) most HTLV-1–infected patients remain asymptomatic for the rest of their life, and no more that 5% develop some clinical manifestations.

HTLV-1 infection can induce disease secondary to immunosuppression (infective dermatitis, crusted scabies, and disseminated dermatophyte infections), autoimmunity (tropical spastic paraparesis, uveitis), and neoplasia (leukemia-lymphoma). Most dermatologists may have heard of the cutaneous T-cell lymphomas, but, in fact, cutaneous disease caused by immunosuppression may be more common.

- *Infective dermatitis* was first described in Jamaican children in 1966. Its relation to HTLV-1 infection was described in 1970 by Louis La Grenade. The clinical picture is that of a chronic eczematous dermatitis affecting the scalp and intertriginous areas, such as neck folds, axilae, and groin. On the face it may follow a seborrheic dermatitis–like distribution. The main affected population is children, although the disease may be seen in adulthood. An important component is the constant degree of superinfection by *Staphylococcus aureus* and β-hemolytic *Streptococcus*. One can describe this condition as an "oozing, honey crusted seborrheic dermatitis or intertrigo," as an "always impetiginized scalp psoriasis," or as "atopic dermatitis with predominantly scalp involvement." This is in fact a virus-induced dermatitis and a model for atopic dermatitis. Most patients with infective dermatitis dry their eczema when treated with antibiotics, but the disease recurs when the treatment is discontinued, following a chronic course. Many children affected go into remission when reaching puberty, similar to atopics. Some consider infective dermatitis a marker for a higher risk of developing lymphoma.

- *Crusted scabies* have been described in populations who are known to be endemic for HTLV-1, such as Australian aborigines. Also in places with high prevalence, like Lima, Peru (estimated incidence 2%), data in the literature have shown that most cases are related to the retrovirus infection, even more commonly than immunosuppression owing to HIV infection or chronic steroid therapy.
- *Pruritus, xerosis,* and *ichthyosis* are considered by some researchers as the most common HTLV-1 manifestations, although not very specific.
- *Adult T-cell leukemia-lymphoma* was linked to HTLV-1 in Japanese population in 1977. The malignancy may follow either an acute course with multiple organ involvement, or a localized, purely cutaneous disease similar to mycosis fungoides. The skin lesions may vary, from plaques to nodules or tumors and even erythroderma. Four subtypes have been described: smoldering, chronic, lymphoma type, and acute prototypic type. Hypercalcemia may be part of the systemic involvement.

Dengue

Presentation and Characteristics

Dengue, or breakbone fever, is one of the most prevalent viral diseases in the world, causing a systemic illness that can be either a neurologic infection, acute febrile disease with arthropathy, or hemorrhagic fever. It is caused by a RNA flavivirus, with four described serotypes. It is present around the world (100 million cases per year) in tropical and subtropical areas of Africa and Asia, and it is also becoming an increasing public health problem for some countries in South and Central America.

The disease is transmitted by a bite of mosquitoes belonging to the genera *Aedes,* mainly *A. aegypti,* also a carrier of yellow fever. For the most part, dengue is present in urban areas with poor sanitary systems. The mosquitoes thrive whenever they find open reservoirs of water. The *Aedes* also works as the main living reservoir for the virus.

The disease may adopt various clinical forms, from mild to classic to a more severe and dangerous hemorrhagic form, the so-called dengue hemorrhagic fever (DHF). Whereas the classical form is more common in new arrivals to endemic areas, the more severe DHF is the more likely it is to affect children, residents of endemic areas, and those who already had dengue in the past.

Clinical Appearance

The classical form starts as a sudden fever, lasting 2 to 5 days, associated with headache, intense myalgias, arthralgia, and retro-orbital pain. Cutaneous involvement varies, from facial flushing to a more diffuse, macular or maculopapular morbiliform eruption. The erythematous areas become confluent, leaving small spared areas of normal skin, similar to that seen in pityriasis rubra pilaris, although lacking its roughness. The main area on involvement is the trunk and spreading centrifugally toward the extremities. Petechial eruptions affecting the lower extremities also have been described. Pruritus may be present, and a later state of desquamation may follow.

DHF presents with a more severe course, including vomiting, facial flushing, circumoral cyanosis, and weakness. Extremities feel cool and clammy. Hemorrhagic complications, such as gastrointestinal and genital bleeding, appear, and the patient may go into a dengue shock syndrome. This state may have a mortality rate as high as 10% if not given the appropriate support.

Differential Diagnosis

- Yellow fever
- Malaria
- Typhoid (with roseola)
- Hemorrhagic viral fevers
- Viral hepatitis
- Drug eruptions
- Poisoning

Bacterial Infections

Bartonellas and Verruga Peruana

Until the AIDS era, bartonellosis (Fig. 38-1) was one of those exotic diseases that may have only been studied for board examinations. The first description of the disease were at the beginning of this century and came from endemic areas in the Peruvians Andes under two different names, *Carrion's disease* and *verruga peruana*; it was caused by *Bartonella bacilifomes*. The bacteria, a gram-negative rod, was transmitted from the natural reservoirs to human by the bite of mosquitoes belonging to the *Lutzomya* family.

Presentation and Characteristics

The disease has two characteristic phases. At first, its produces an impressive bacteremia and parasitism of the

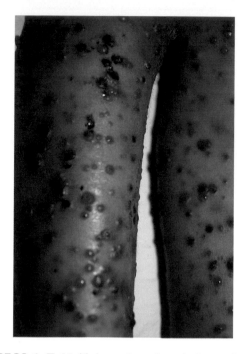

FIGURE 38-1 ■ Multiple angiomatous lesions of verruga peruana.

reticuloendothelial system (Carrion's disease), in which the microorganism may be seen inside red blood cells on peripheral smears. The clinical picture is a systemic disease with fever, malaise, and high susceptibility to other bacterial infections, such as salmonellosis.

The most distinct and relevant phase for dermatology is the eruptive phase, known as *verruga peruana*. It may follow the bacteremia or it may present de novo. Characteristically, an eruption of multiple papules, nodules, and tumors appears over a period of weeks. The more superficial lesions have an angiomatous appearance, resembling pyogenic granulomas. No systemic symptoms are seen during this phase. The natural course of the disease is toward spontaneous involution, although antibiotic treatment may induce a more prompt remission.

At the beginning of the 1980s, some patients with AIDS presented with a clinical picture very similar to the eruptive phase of verruga peruana. This new disease was named *bacillary angiomatosis*. The histologic descriptions of the eruptive lesions of bacillary angiomatosis were identical to those described in verruga peruana, the only bartonellosis known at that time. The initial thought was to associate this new entity to cat-scratch disease, and to what was supposed to be its etiology, a new bacteria called *Afipia felis*. At a later time, isolation of a gram-negative rod from the lesions lead to classifying it under a new family of bacteria called *Rochalimaea*. When genetic studies where performed comparing the genes of *Bartonella baciliformes* and the new *R*ochalimaea family, it became evident that they were closely related, and they were renamed under the *Bartonella* family. The new *Bartonella* species include *B. henselae, B. quintana* (both cause bacillary angiomatosis, cat-scratch fever, and systemic disease associated with fever), and *B. elizabethian,* which causes septicemia and endocarditis in alcoholics.

Bacillary angiomatosis is now recognized as a disease characteristic of immunosuppressed patients of all kinds, although it has been reported in immunocompetent patients. The most likely natural reservoir are domestic animal such as cats. It is cosmopolitan, as opposed to verruga peruana, which is still endemic to Andean areas of Peru and Ecuador.

Anthrax

Anthrax is an infection caused by *Bacillus anthraces,* an encapsulated gram-positive bacteria that can survive for up to 20 years in dry grass. It is a disease that occurs in people who work with cattle. Its contagiousness is favored by a preexisting lesion on the skin and can even be caused by the simple inhalation of spores. The cutaneous lesion is called *malignant pustule;* it occurs in exposed areas of the skin, especially the face, neck, arms or hands, and is usually a solitary lesion (Fig. 38-2). One to 5 days after inoculation, a papule grows, a blister then forms on a edematous base that eventually breaks, leaving a hemorrhagic crust. Redness and edema may be very marked. General symptoms appear on the third or fourth day; the condition can be very toxic and even lead to death.

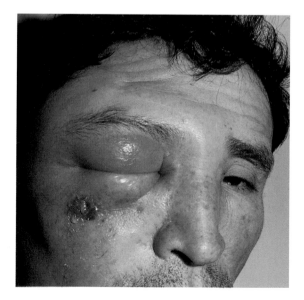

FIGURE 38-2 ■ Anthrax, 48 hours after infection.

Treatment

Treatment options include penicillin, doxycycline, and quinolones.

Rhinoscleroma

Presentation and Characteristics

Rhinoscleroma, also known as *scleroma*, is a chronic disease of very slow progression that is potentially fatal. It is caused by *Klebsiella rhinoscleromatis* (Frish Bacillus).

- The first symptoms are generally nasopharyngeal; the lesions grow slowly, and often the patient does not seek medical attention for years. The initial stage is that of rhinitis. This is an exudating stage, with symptoms similar to a common cold, including headache and difficulty breathing. There is a very purulent, fetid secretion with crusts and occasional epistaxis.
- The second stage has a proliferating pattern, with improvement of the cold-like symptoms; however, obstruction and infiltration of nasal tissues by a friable granulomatous tissue may extend into the pharynx and the larynx, causing a change in the tone of voice with hoarseness. Later, during a nodular period, the nose takes on the size and shape similar to that of a "tapir." Respiration becomes difficult, and it may be necessary to do a tracheotomy.
- The third stage is fibrotic sclerosis, and although there may be clinical improvement and occasionally a spontaneous cure, usually there is a very heavy distortion of the anatomic structures. Invasion of the bone and opacification of the nasal sinuses, with eventual destruction of bone tissue, may occur. The diagnosis is based on the clinical and histologic picture and the presence of bacillus of Frish.

Treatment

Treatment includes antibiotics such as tetracycline, azithromycin, cephalosporins, and trimethoprim. It does not respond to sulfa preparations or penicillin. The best medication is tetracycline, 2 g/d, in divided doses for 6 months.

Pinta

Pinta is a treponemal disease of endemic behavior, caused by *Treponema carateum* (Fig. 38-3). Its occurrence has been restricted to low land tropical areas of Central and South

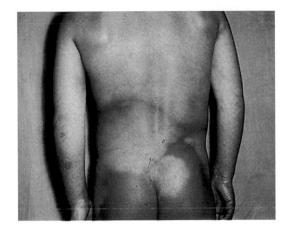

FIGURE 38-3 ■ Pinta showing early hyperpigmentation and depigmented patches on the back.

America, specially in the Amazon region. It is still reported in some aborigine populations of the Brazilian and Venezuelan Amazon.

Presentation and Characteristics

Pinta has some characteristics similar to syphilis, but aside from an occasional juxta-articular lymph node, it is a purely cutaneous disease. Pinta is transmitted during childhood by direct contact with lesions from infected individuals, but is not transmitted by sexual contact.

Patients go through three different stages, with early, secondary, and late lesions. The early or primary lesion is a erythematous papule that becomes scaly, psoriasiform, and even lichenified. It is usually located on lower extremities and becomes dyschromic with time.

Secondary lesions appear about 2 months after the primary lesion. They are multiple, with morphology similar to the primary lesion, although smaller in size. They are bilateral and symmetrical, and rarely located on the palms and soles. The most prominent change is again the dyschromia, with hyper- and hypopigmentation mixed in single lesions. They are mostly located over bony prominence. The late lesions consist of extensive areas of hypopigmentation and achromia, resembling vitiligo.

Spirochetes can be easily detected on deep scraping of lesions at any stage. All serologic tests for syphilis are positive, and the distinction from *T. palidum* infection is impossible.

Diagnosis

The diagnosis should be suspected in patients from endemic areas with extensive dyschromias.

Treatment

Treatment is based on penicillin therapy. The changes in color do not reverse with antibiotic therapy.

Yaws and Bejel

These two treponematoses are related to syphilis, although epidemiologically they behave in an endemic fashion.

- Yaws, also called *pian or frambesia,* is a disease caused by *T. pertenue,* with identical morphology to *T. pallidum.* It is endemic to all tropical areas around the world, from Central and South America, to Africa, Asia, Australia, and the Pacific Islands. It is acquired during childhood. The clinical manifestations go through the three classical stages of early, secondary, and late lesions. The primary lesion is chancroid in appearance, whereas the secondary lesions are papillomatous verrucous, similar to condylomas. On skin they resemble raspberries, giving origin to its French name, *frambesia.* Bone involvement can be rather destructive, resulting in severe deformities and mutilations. Tertiary lesions can be gumma-like, and achromic, as in pinta, and can produce palmoplantar hyperkeratosis. Treatment is based on the use of penicillin.
- Bejel is an endemic form of treponemal disease, produced by a variant of *T. pallidum.* At present, it is still reported in the Middle East, the African Sahara, and some areas of the tropical belt. Like the other endemic treponematosis, it is a disease of infants and children. The clinical manifestations are similar to the mucosal lesions of secondary syphilis, with a condylomatous appearance. Tertiary lesions are similar to yaws.

Mycobacterial Infections

Tuberculosis and leprosy are two diseases caused by mycobacteria, but these are discussed in Chapter 21.

Infections Caused by Atypical Mycobacteria

Mycobacterium marinum *Infection (Swimming Pool Granulomas)*

Mycobacterium marinum (formerly called *Mycobacteria balnei*) infection is characterized by the presence of an indolent verrucous papule that later evolves into a plaque or a nodule, with central scarring that may eventually ulcerate (Fig. 38-4).

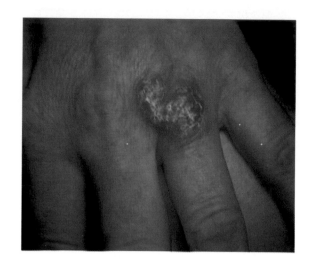

FIGURE 38-4 ■ Swimming pool granuloma.

Presentation and Characteristics. It is commonly located on the extremities, especially at points of trauma (hands, elbows). It is classically associated with exposure to water, in fish tanks, in swimming pools, or in seawater-related workers, such as divers. The incubation period ranges from approximately 2 to 6 weeks. The lesion is usually solitary and there is no systemic reaction. Satellite lesions may appear and may simulate sporotrichosis. Isolated lesions may also be confused with lupus vulgaris, tuberculous leprosy, and leishmaniasis. Either visualization of the bacteria on skin tissue or its isolation by culture are rather difficult.

Treatment. Minocycline seems to be the drug of choice, although clarythromicyn, rifampin, tetracycline, and doxycycline are alternative therapies. Surgical excision, or thermal therapy, has been employed with relative success.

Mycobacterium ulcerans *Infection (Buruli Ulcer)*

This mycobacterial infection was first described in southern Australia as Bairnsdale ulcer and later, endemic areas were also reported in Africa (from the Buruli valley in Uganda), and South America. In West and Central Africa, it is considered a public health problem. This is, in fact, the third most common worldwide mycobacterium infection in immunocompetent patients, only after tuberculosis and leprosy.

Presentation and Characteristics. The bacteria lives in the environment, and is acquired by humans through contamination of traumatic wounds. The classical clinical presentation is an ulcer, located most commonly in extremities. The cavity extends laterally, undermining the edges of the lesion, so the defect is always larger than what is seen at first glance. The ulceration continues to enlarge, producing marked destruction and mutilation of the affected areas. The morbidity of the disease is directly related to the skin lesion, with no systemic symptoms.

There is no granuloma formation, as opposed to other common mycobacterioses. On special stains such as Ziehl-Nielsen, a huge amount of bacteria is seen in the necrotic areas. The necrosis is a direct effect of a bacterial toxin, micolactone, a soluble polyketide causing immunosuppression and cytotoxicity.

Diagnosis. The diagnosis is made on the basis of the clinical and histologic findings. The bacteria is difficult to isolate, although it can be done on special mycobacterial media. New diagnostic techniques, including PCR, will allow early diagnosis in smaller lesions, that are more susceptible to surgical excision, which is the definitive treatment.

Rapidly Growing Mycobaterium (M. fortuitum group)

This group includes a series of microorganisms causing chronic infections after traumatic, surgical, cosmetic, or therapeutic inoculation. A growing number of cases presenting are been reported in South America as late complications of liposuctions or mesotherapy. Mycobacterium species implicated include *M. fortuitum, M. abscessus,* and *M. chelonae.*

Presentation and Characteristics. Patients present with cold abscesses at the site of trauma, injection or surgery, weeks to months after the precipitating event. Upon drainage, a purulent fluid may be obtained. Direct exami-

nation shows the presence of acid-fast staining bacilli. Unless suspected, the lesion becomes chronic, with posterior appearance of fistula and progressive infiltration of surrounding tissues. Although they are called rapid growers, that is not always the case, either requiring special media or lower temperatures. *M. abscessus* is able to grow for more than a year in distilled water; contamination of surgical material or substances to be injected should be considered as potential sources of infections when dealing with epidemic outbreaks.

Treatment. Treatment of choice includes clarithromycin and minocycline.

Parasitic Diseases

Protozoal Dermatosis

Leishmaniasis

Leishmaniasis is an infectious process caused by intracellular parasites of the *Leishmania* family (Fig. 38-5). The disease is transmitted from natural reservoirs to humans by mosquito bites.

Presentation and Characteristics. The different forms of cutaneous disease are produced by species of *Leishmania* specific for certain regions in the world, like those seen in the Middle East (*L. tropica*), Central America (*L. mexicana*), and South America (*L. peruviana* and *L. brazilensis*). There is even an endemic area of leishmaniasis in the state of Texas. Different names are given to the disease depending on the geographic location: *oriental sore* in Asia, *Chiclero's*

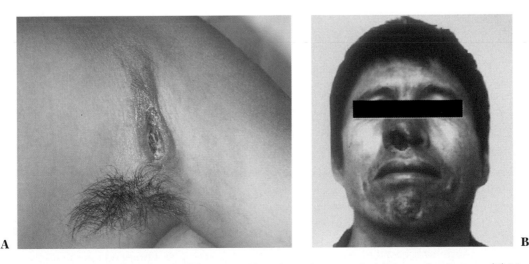

FIGURE 38-5 ■ Leischmaniasis. (**A**) Unusual location after recent visit to endemic area. (**B**) Mucocutaneous form. The septum is involved.

ulcer in Mexico, *Uta* in the Andes, and *Espundia* in the Amazon basin.

The classical cutaneous lesion consists of a round, isolated ulceration, with slightly elevated and indurate borders, which are asymptomatic. The classical location is in areas of the body not covered by clothing and, therefore, exposed to the mosquito bite, namely, the face, neck and extremities. The lesion itself is painless and tends to regress spontaneously.

The variety known as *mucocutaneous leishmaniasis*, which is produced by *L. brazilensis,* is characterized by its ability to produce, after a dormant period, an ulceration on the mucosa of the nasal septum, that can progress externally mutilating the whole nose and nasolabial area. When the progression is on the mucosal side, it may destroy the palate, producing a granulomatous infiltration of the pharynx, the larynx, and even the upper respiratory airway.

The tissue destruction seen in leishmaniasis is in fact a result of the great inflammatory reaction induced by the parasite, rather than the virulence effect of the microorganism itself. In an early lesion, there is a heavy infiltration of histiocytes, many of them engulfing the *leishmania* organism. The more organized, the less likely that *leishmanias* is seen on the biopsy specimens.

Diagnosis. Methods of diagnosis include direct examination of aspirate from the ulcer, culture in specific media, and PCR techniques. The leishmanina test, an intradermal reaction to fragments of the parasite, is useful when working up a diagnosis in someone who is just an occasional visitor to endemic areas. The high sensitivity of the test makes it very useful to rule out rather than to confirm the diagnosis.

Treatment. Treatment, when indicated, is based on use of antimonial preparations, and in difficult cases, amphotericin B. Always consider leishmaniasis in the differential diagnosis of chronic cutaneous ulcerations, especially when there is a history of living in or traveling to endemic areas, some of them very popular among the ecotourist. Soldiers in Iraq have been infected in significant numbers.

Trypanosomiasis Sudamericana (Chagas Disease)

Trypanosomiasis sudamericana is caused by *Trypanosoma cruzi* and is transmitted by a reduviid, *Triatoma infestans* (kissing bug). In most cases, the portal of entry is the conjunctiva, causing unilateral edema of the eyelids and inflammation of the lacrimal gland (Romaña sign). There are general manifestations such as headache, fever, myalgia, and hepatosplenomegaly. Fatal cases occur due to meningoencephalitis or myocarditis.

Amebiasis, Including Free-Living Amebas and Entamoeba histolytica

Free-living amebas are usually associated with disease of the central nervous system (Fig. 38-6). The infection is acquired by swimming in ponds and streams with still water. There are two types of meningo encephalitis produced by these organisms. The *Naegleria* species causes an acute form, with no skin manifestations. The subacute, granulomatous form is produced by two families, *Acanthamoeba* and *Balamuthia*. *Acanthamoeba* infection is known to induce chronic ulcerative lesions in AIDS patients, and rarely isolated, centrofacial plaques in immunocompetent hosts. In the 1990s, a new variety, named *Balamuthia mandrillaris,* has been recognized as the causative agent on many of the cases of free-living amoeba granulomatous meningo encephalitis around the world, especially in South America and Australia. Cases have been reported in the United States, mainly in California and Texas.

Many cases have a primary skin lesion, a central face plaque, of granulomatous appearance, usually located on the nose, but also in the trunk and extremities. In the months following cutaneous involvement, all patients develop focal CNS symptoms, marking the beginning of a necrotizing encephalitis. Except for few cases reported in the last years, the outcome is always fatal. However, the early recognition of the skin lesion as a marker of the infection may allow early treatment with combination of antiparasitic and antifungal drugs with subsequent improvement of the survival rates.

Ameba histolytica can produce cutaneous lesions, most commonly in the anal margin and genital region, but also in skin that is not periorificial. The elementary lesions are large cutaneous ulcerations, vegetative lesions, and even abscesses.

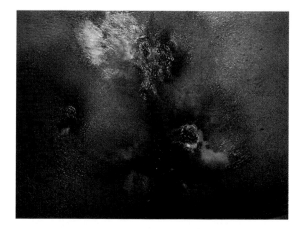

FIGURE 38-6 ■ Cutaneous amebiasis with deep ulcers of the buttocks caused by direct extension following amebic dysentery. *(Courtesy of Dr. A. Gonzalez-Orchoa.)*

Helminthic Dermatosis (roundworm)

Cutaneous Larva Migrans

Presentation and Characteristics. This is a disease caused by hookworms, usually parasites of dogs and cats. The ova are excreted through the feces and they remain viable in sandy, moist ground. The larva then penetrate the skin of bathers or people who walk on the contaminated ground. Usually, the "culprits" are *Ancylostoma duodenale, Necator americanus,* and other hookworms. Clinically, the parasite causes a serpentine, erythematous, papular, pruritic eruption in the skin (Fig. 38-7). The parasite is usually ahead of the tract. Vesicles, excoriations, and crusts are present.

Treatment. Treatment includes topical thiabendazole or albendazole by mouth 200 mg twice a day for 3 days.

Larva Currens

As opposed to cutaneous larva migrans, in which lesions move over a period of days, the cutaneous form of *Strongiloidiasis* moves over a period of hours, which is the reason for the "currens" denomination. This is more common among immunosuppressed patients, in whom multiple tracts can be seen. At the present time, ivermectin is the treatment of choice, 200 µg/kg, and in these immunosuppressed patients, it can actually be life saving.

Gnathostomiasis

This condition was described initially as a parasite of large felines by Owen in 1886.

Presentation and Characteristics. It is caused by *Gnathostoma spinigerum.* Clinically, it produces a nodular migratory eosinophilic panniculitis. This parasite normally inhabits the stomach of domestic animals such as dogs and cats. The eggs are excreted in the stools of these animals. They then reach the rivers, hatch in the water, and are ingested by organisms of a *Cyclops* species, developing into the second larval stage. This is later ingested by fish, forming a third larval stage in their muscular tissue, which in turn is eaten by a definitive host. Humans, who are not the definitive host, could develop the characteristic panniculitis of this disease from eating raw fish, such as in cebiche or sushi. The parasite migrates through the tissues, most commonly to the skin, but it may go to any of the internal organs. Clinically, after a variable incubation period of 4 weeks to 3 years, patients develop the classical symptom of pruritic, migratory, edematous, cutaneous plaques. Exceptionally, the parasite may be seen, measuring around 0.4 mm in diameter and no more than 4 mm long.

Treatment. Treatment alternatives include albendazol 200 mg, twice daily for 2 to 3 weeks or ivermectin 200 µg/kg in a single dose, that can be repeated every 2 weeks.

Filariasis

Filariasis are systemic infections caused by different species of nematodes, all transmitted by mosquito bites, with hematogenous (rather than cutaneous, as in onchocerciasis) spreading of microfilaria.

Presentation and Characteristics. The symptoms are related to chronic inflammation of the lymphatic system. They commonly occur in tropical areas of the world. Loa loa infection is reported in West Africa. *Wuchereria bancrofti* and *Brugia malayi* are more common in Asia and tropical Africa.

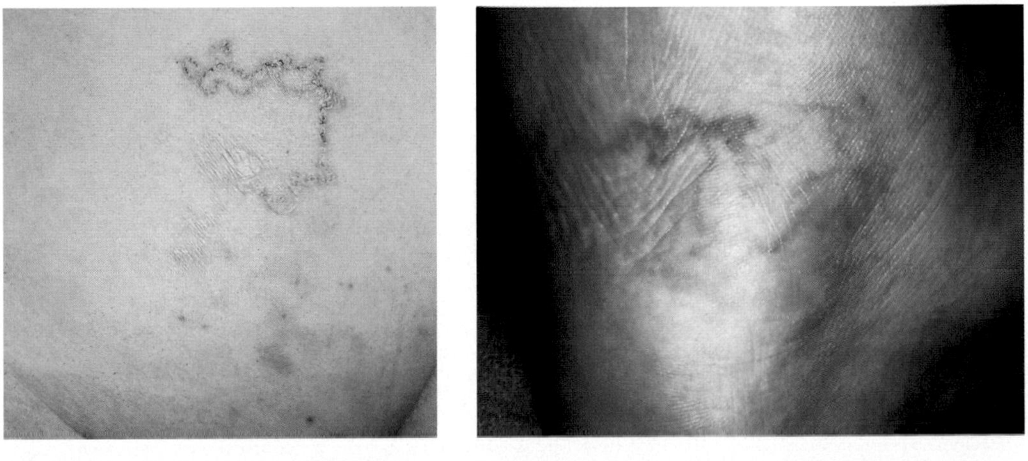

FIGURE 38-7 ■ **(A)** Larva migrans. **(B)** Creeping eruption of larva migrans on sole of foot.

Symptoms vary according to the stage of disease. During the hematogenous spread, microphilarias are abundant in blood, producing temporary migratory swelling on extremities that are self-limited and recurrent. Acute lymphangitis and lymphadenitis may affect groin and axillae. Genital involvement includes acute orchitis, epididymitis, and funiculitis, which are very painful. They also can be recurrent, and evolve into fibrosis. Urticaria may be part of the clinical presentation. Late changes are caused by obstruction of lymphatics, giving rise to different forms of elephantiasis, affecting extremities and scrotum with massive edemas.

Diagnosis. Diagnosis is reached by the presence of microphilaria in blood smears and serologic testing.

Treatment. Treatment is based on use of diethylcarbamazine. Recent reports on the use of ivermectin seem very promising.

Onchocerciasis

Onchocerciasis is a chronic infestation of the skin by *Onchocera volvulus*. This is a microfilarial nematode whose natural hosts are men and flies from the genus *Simuliun*.

The disease was first described in Africa and later in Central America. Recently, the reports extend the disease to the northern countries of South America.

Presentation and Characteristics. The transmission occurs when flies became infected by biting sick people. After a short period of maturation the microfilaria moves to the buccal apparatus of the insect and enters the skin of a noninfected human with the next blood meal.

The infective forms become adults in 6 to 8 months inside cutaneous nodules, where they begin producing microfilariae.

Cutaneous involvement includes the characteristic nodules containing adult forms. They tend to locate on scalp in Central American patients and on extensor surfaces in Africans patients. Other clinical presentations include facial erythema, facial livedoid discoloration, and prurigo-like eruption on buttocks and extremities. Later signs are extensive lichenification, dischromia, elephantiasis of extremities, scrotum, and the so-called hanging groin.

Ocular involvement is related to the direct invasion of eye structures by the microfilaria, resulting in complete and permanent loss of vision; this is the reason the disease has been called *river blindness*.

Diagnosis. Diagnosis is easy to confirm either by direct scraping or histologic analysis of skin lesions in which the adult form and microfilaria are identified.

Treatment. This disease is particularly worthy of mention because a specific treatment is now available. It consist of the oral administration of ivermectin, extremely effective even as a single-dose therapy.

Trematodes Dermatosis (Flukes)

Cercarial Dermatitis. *Cercarial dermatitis,* or swimmer´s itch, is caused by the penetration of the skin by schistosoma of birds or mammals. The cercaria are found in bodies of water; they can penetrate the skin of a mammal and, if the host is receptive, reach the bloodstream and spread to other organs. In humans, who are not the definitive host, the cercaria are unsuccessful in reaching the blood; they are retained in the epithelial layers and finally destroyed, resulting in dermatitis. Clinically, pruritic macules, papules, hemorrhages, and excoriations develop in the exposed areas. This resulting dermatitis is a product of the sensitization to the cercarial proteins. In massive or repeated infestations, the signs and symptoms are consequently more severe.

Seabather's eruption generally occurs in the area under swimwear after bathing in the ocean; however, it may also be seen in the axilla, neck, and flexor areas (Fig. 38-8). It is pruritic and papular, and occurs within hours after leaving affected waters. Occasionally, the skin eruption is complicated by fatigue, malaise, fever, chills, nausea, and gastrointestinal complaints. These episodes appear to be more severe after repeated attacks. This condition is caused by the cnidarian larvae of *Linuche unguiculata* (thimble jellyfish). This larva has been found in water samples, and in affected patients there have been demonstrated high IgG levels specific to

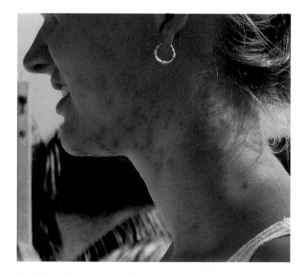

FIGURE 38-8 ■ Seabather's eruption, caused by thimble jellyfish off coast of Belize. *(Courtesy of Dr. Kate Schafer.)*

L. unguiculata. Symptomatic treatment is accomplished with antihistamines, topical corticosteroids, and even oral steroid therapy. It is a self-limiting condition that lasts about 12 days even without therapy.

Schistosomiasis or Bilharziasis

In South America, schistosomiasis is caused by *Schistosoma mansoni.* The reservoir is usually water contaminated with feces from infected people, containing ova and free-swimming cercaria capable of penetrating human skin. The organisms pass rapidly through the epidermis and are carried by the blood and eventually mature into flukes in the intrahepatic portion of the portal system. The mature fluke migrates to the pelvic veins where eggs are laid. In the skin, one may see a papular eruption identical to swimmer's itch or even urticarial reactions on occasion. In areas of high endemicity, there is granulomatous inflammation of the skin of the perineum resulting in nodular masses, fistulae, and sinus tracts.

Dermatosis Caused by Arthropods

Human Scabies

Presentation and Characteristics

This disease is usually transmitted through prolonged personal contact, and less often by clothing and bed linens. The mite's location is in a "burrow" in the stratum corneum where it deposits its eggs. An allergic sensitization to the mite and or its products causes the clinical picture (Fig. 38-9). Itching appears 2 to 4 weeks after the infestation and is classically more severe at night. As a clinical finding, the burrow is pathognomonic and diagnostic. The remaining lesions are caused by scratching, secondary infections, and allergic reaction. The burrow is a skin-colored, tortuous, elevated line of 1 to 1.5 cm in length. They are usually found in the finger webs, flexor surface of the wrist, nipples, and elbows. In children, they are common in the palms and soles.

Diagnosis

Diagnosis is confirmed by a potassium hydroxide (KOH) preparation of the skin and the identification of the parasite.

Treatment

For treatment, permethrin 5% solution, one 8-hour application at night is considered the standard treatment today. The γ-isomer of hexachlorobenzene (Lindane), 1% in a vanishing cream, was used for years, but it is used less commonly today because of its toxicity and should not be used in pregnant women or infants. With both medications, a second application is made after 1 week. Note that this application should cover the entire body completely. A 6% sulfur precipitate in Vaseline for 3 consecutive days is employed in infants and pregnant women. Recently, ivermectin 200 μg/kg, in a single dose, has been found to be very effective. The nails should be cut short and scrubbed vigorously. Clothing and bed linen should be washed thoroughly.

Variations

Norwegian scabies, also known as *crusted scabies,* is the same disease but in an immunosuppressed individual. Typically, extensive, crusted hyperkeratotic plaques are seen, but itching may not be as prominent. The KOH examination shows severe infestation, and the patient is much more contagious. Treatment should include exfoliants such as 20% urea or

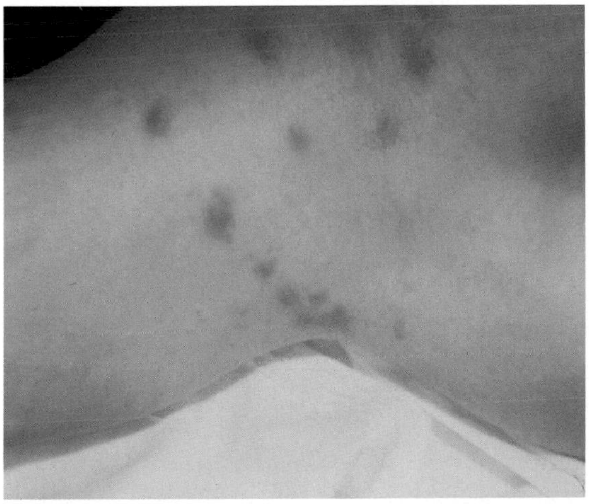

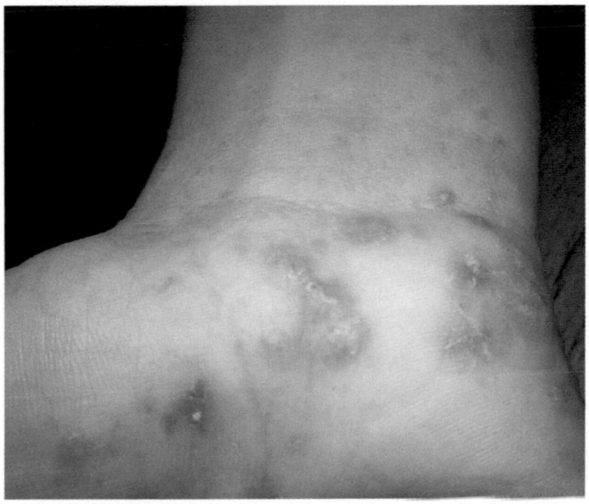

FIGURE 38-9 ■ **(A, B)** Scabies.

20% salicilic acid in an ointment base. Nodular scabies consists of brown or red firm nodules on the penis, scrotum, or buttocks; such lesions may persist for months despite specific antimite treatment. It is a delayed allergic reaction with no mite present.

Animal Scabies

In this disease, very similar to papular urticaria, the mites invade human skin but they do not become established in it. There are varieties from dogs, sheep, birds, and so forth. Excoriated, crusted papules can be seen and pruritus can be very severe, especially in the evening.

Arachnidism

Latrodectism

Latrodectus mactans are small, dark spiders called *black widows.* They have a black or brown underside with a red, orange, or white hourglass marking on the back. They are commonly found in fields, under stones, and in outhouses.

Their venom is neurotoxic and they bite usually on the genitalia or buttocks. Pain develops within 1 hour with accompanying reddening and swelling (Figs. 38-10 and 38-11). Systemic symptoms include muscle cramping, rigidity, and later weakness, sweating, bradycardia, hypothermia and hypotension. The mortality rate is about 5% in children.

Treatment. Treatment includes intravenous 10% calcium gluconate and corticosteroids; however, the most effective therapy is systemic antivenom.

Loxoscelism

Loxosceles reclusa is found in the United States, and *Loxosceles laeta* is found in Central and South America. The *Loxosceles* spiders are light brown to chocolate in color, with nocturnal habits, and are commonly found seeking warmth in discarded clothing.

Presentation and Characteristics. Usually affected areas include the arm and thigh of adults or the face in children.

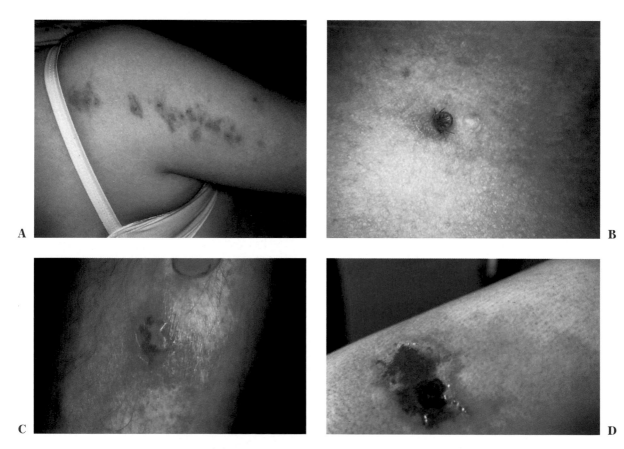

FIGURE 38-10 ■ Arthropod bites. (**A**) Bedbug bites on the arm. (**B**) Tick imbedded in the skin, presented as a tumor by patient. (**C**) Brown recluse spider bite on leg. (**D**) Severe brown recluse spider bite on thigh.

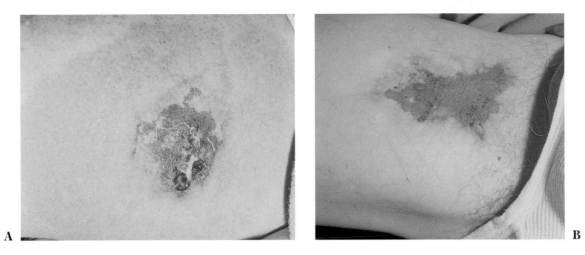

FIGURE 38-11 ■ **(A)** Spider bite (*Loxosceles laeta*), erythema, central necrosis, and blister formation. **(B)** Spider bite (*Loxosceles laeta*), with vertical extension of necrosis due to gravity.

Pain develops 2 to 8 hours after the bite. The lesion becomes indurated and red, with a central blister and subsequent necrosis that can be quite large. The necrotic area eventually becomes mummified; around the 14th day the eschar sloughs off. General symptoms include fever, chills, vomiting, petechiae on the skin, as well as thrombocytopenia and hemolytic anemia, especially in children.

Treatment. Treatment is with corticosteroids and dapsone, which may be effective in limiting the size and extension of the necrosis.

Diseases Caused by Chiggers

These mites, also known as *harvest mites,* are the cause of the infestation known as *trombiculiasis.* It is seen worldwide, although most frequently in tropical areas. The disease is acquired while walking through vegetation, and the affected area is usually on exposed skin depending on the clothing used. The offender chigger is the larval stage of the mite, 0.25 to 0.4 mm in diameter, orange to red in color, with three pairs of legs. It gets fixed to the skin by its buccal apparatus and starts a process of liquefying and sucking the skin elements. As a consequence, it produces a type of papular urticaria: multiple red itchy papules, sometime s purpuric or vesicular, which are extremely pruritic (Fig. 38-12).

Treatment

Topical treatment is with steroids and antipruritic lotions; occasionally this condition requires systemic antibiotic therapy as well as steroids.

Diseases Caused by Nigua

Tungiasis is a human infestation produced by *Tunga penetrans*, a sand-flea that thrives on moist, sandy ground near pigsties and cowsheds. It is widely distributed in tropical and subtropical areas of South America and Africa. It is known by various names (*pique, nigua, bicho dos pes*). It is commonly acquired when walking bare-foot in contaminated areas, including residential gardens recently fertilized with cattle manure.

Presentation and Characteristics

The infection is produced by the female flea, who burrows the skin of toeweb spaces and near the nail. The flea inserts her body full of eggs, to die at a later time. The initial clinical manifestations is a black dot, representing the burrow full of eggs that can later be seen on top of a papule or vesicle (Fig. 38-13). Its walls are horny tissue from the epidermis itself. The lesion becomes infected or simply produces a foreign-body reaction that terminates in suppuration and opening of the cavity, forming a coalescing lesion that may form a honeycomb plaque. It may serve as a port of entry for a more severe infection, and even gangrene.

Treatment

The best treatment is the extraction of all the insect part, and, of course, the best prevention is to wear closed shoes.

Paederus Dermatitis

Blister beetle or *paederus dermatitis* is caused by contact with the body fluids of *Paederus irritans,* a member of the

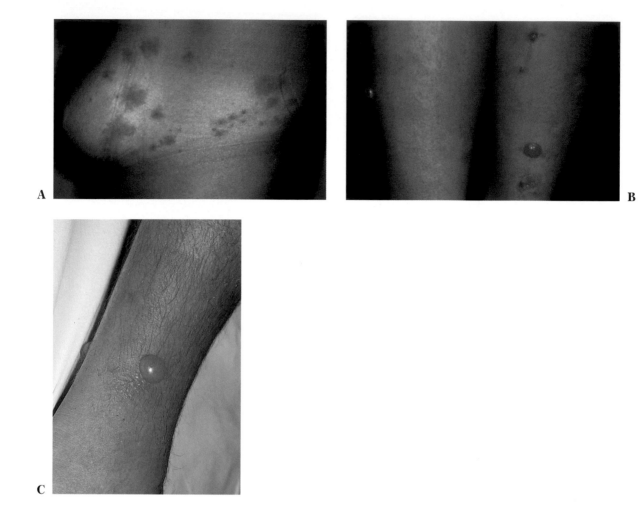

FIGURE 38-12 ■ **(A)** Chigger bites collected under bra. **(B)** Bullous chigger bites on the legs. **(C)** Chigger bite, blister formation.

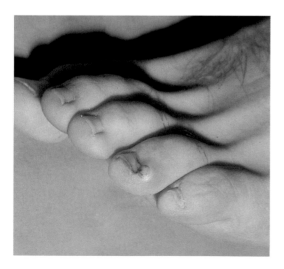

FIGURE 38-13 ■ Nigua. Most common location by toenail.

order *Coleopteran*, family *Staphylinidae*. An increase incidence has been seen in Peru and Ecuador with the El Niño phenomenon. The same disease, following an identical cycle during "El Niño" years, is seen in other continents like Africa. In Kenya, different species of Paederus, mainly *P. crebinpunctatis* and *P. sabaeus*, are responsible for the disease (*Nairobi Fly*). Clinically, an initial burning is felt, followed by erythema and, later, the appearance of a blister usually in a linear fashion ("latigazo" or whiplash) in exposed parts of the body (Fig. 38-14). The vesication is produced by paederin, a protein from the exoskeleton of the insect.

Treatment

Treatment includes compresses, topical corticosteroids, and in some serious cases, oral prednisone and antibiotics.

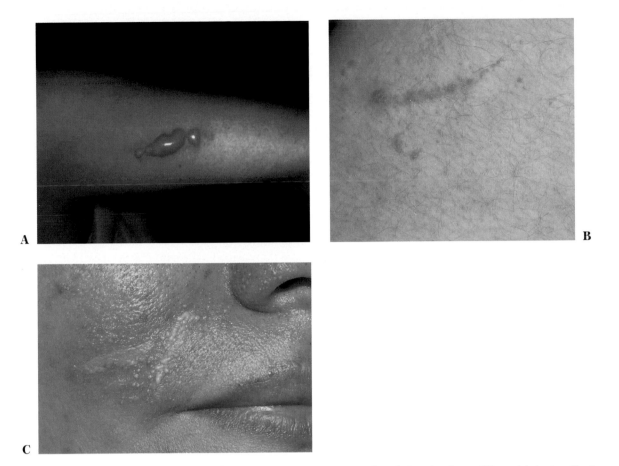

FIGURE 38-14 ■ **(A)** Blister beetle bullous reaction on arm. **(B, C)** Beetle dermatitis, whiplash effect (latigazo).

Deep Fungi

Histoplasmosis

This disease is caused by *Histoplasma capsulatum*. Found throughout the world in temperate areas, *H. capsulatum* is a saprofitic fungus that grows in the soil, prevalently in soil of caves inhabited by bats. The disease is transmitted by the inadvertent inhalation of the spores. Epidemics have occurred while exploring infested caves or cleaning sites where chicken excrement (guano) may be present.

Presentation and Characteristics

A benign clinical form mimicking a common cold, may leave a calcified nodule in the lung similar to that of tuberculosis. In its most severe form, the disease can disseminate, involving the reticuloendothelial system. Mucocutaneous nodules and granulomas may be seen. In AIDS, the disease is seen in its most severe form. Primary cutaneous

histoplasmosis occurs and is caused by direct inoculation. It is a nodular or indurated ulcer (Fig. 38-15) with accompanying lymphadenopathy. Occasionally an allergic response has been seen appearing as urticaria or as erythema annularis centrifigum.

Diagnosis

The diagnosis is accomplished by demonstrating the small intracellular histoplasma capsulatums in sputum, bone marrow, or biopsy specimens.

Treatment

Treatment is with ketoconazole or itraconazole.

Coccidiodomicosis or San Joaquin Valley Fever

This disease is caused by *Coccidiodes inmitis*, a soil inhabitant. Infection in both humans and animals is acquired by

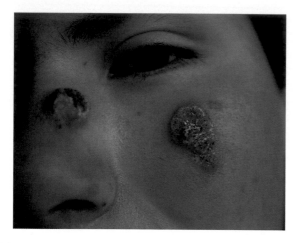

FIGURE 38-15 ■ Ulceration owing to histoplasmosis.

the inhalation of fungus-laden dust particles, or rarely, through a primary infection of the skin.

Presentation and Characteristics

The severity of coccidiodomicosis can range from very mild, simulating a common cold, to an acute disseminated fatal disease, especially in patients with AIDS. An allergic reaction with erythema multiforme or erythema nodosum occurs in some cases. The basic symptoms of malaise and fever may suggest coccidiodomicosis if the patient has traveled through an endemic area.

Diagnosis

Diagnosis is made by KOH mounts of sputum or isolation of the fungus in a culture. Colonies of the coccidiodomicosis fast-growing phase are dangerous to handle and the greatest care should be implemented when manipulating cultures.

Treatment

Treatment includes amphotericin B, ketoconazole, and itraconazole.

Chromoblastomycosis

Chromoblastomycosis is a chronic cutaneous mycosis, characterized by a distinct clinical presentation and the presence of the so-called sclerotic bodies on tissue cuts. A great variety of fungi are able to cause the disease, including *Phialofora verrucosa, Fonsecaea pedrosoi, Fonsecae compacta, Cladosporium carrionii, Rhinocladiella aquaspersa,* and *Botryomyces caespitosus.* The disease has been reported worldwide, with most cases coming from the tropical and subtropical areas of South America and Africa. Some fungi

have a preference for certain climates. *F. pedrosoi* is most common in wet and humid areas within the torrid zones, whereas *C. carrionii* prefers dry and semidesert regions of the tropical-intertropical zones.

Presentation and Characteristics

The most common affected area are the lower extremities, although in some geographic locations, like the arid plains of Venezuela, the upper girdle (shoulder, arm, back) is the prevalent site of infection.

The primary process occurs at the site of inoculation, most probably through traumatized skin. The fungus is acquired from the environment, where lives as saprophytes of woods, vegetable debris, or soil. The disease is not transmitted from person to person. The primary lesion is exophytic, either a papule, a nodule, or a tumor. The lesions multiply and tend to coalesce, forming plaques with a verrucous surface (Fig. 38-16). Ulceration may develop, but there is no fistula formation, as in mycetoma, and the bone and muscle are spared. The affected limb may end up in elephantiasis.

Diagnosis

The diagnosis is easily made by direct examination with KOH of scrapings from the lesion. The morphology adopted by the fungus is a cluster of oblong round cells with thick walls and flattened abutting surfaces, divide by septation in more than one plane; they are known as *sclerotic bodies* or *muriform cells.* The histopathology shows pseudocarcinomatous hyperplasia with a granulomatous suppurative reaction in the dermis. The sclerotic bodies have a brown color, and are easily identified by size (4 to 12 μm) and looking like copper pennies. Species identification is only possible after culture isolation on Sabouraud's media, after 4 to 6 weeks.

Treatment

Treatment options includes surgical excision when the lesion is small. Pharmacologic agents, reported to be useful, but probably not curative by themselves include 5-fluocytosine, itraconazole, and sarpeconazole.

Mycetoma or Maduromycosis

Also known as Madura foot, mycetoma is a chronic subcutaneous infection with a distinct clinical picture of edema with fistula formation and draining of grains (Fig. 38-17). The disease is caused by at least 20 different species of fungi (eumycetoma) and actinomycete (actinomycetoma). Among the true fungi are *Madurella mycetomatis, Madurella grisea, Pseudallescheria boydii, Acremonium*

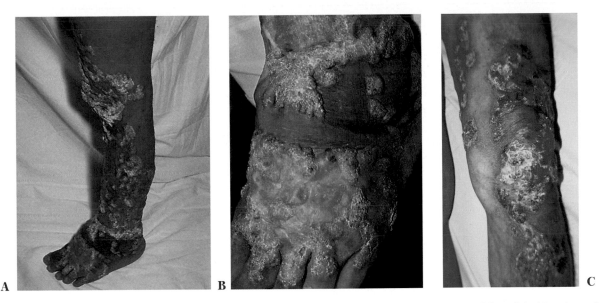

FIGURE 38-16 ■ Chromoblastomycosis cauliflower-like leg lesion (**A**), with close-up of foot (**B**). *(Courtesy of Dr. W. Schorr.)* (**C**) Chromoblastomycosis, with verrucous surface.

kiliensi, Leptosphaeria tompkinsii, Exophilia jeanselmei, Neostudina rosati, Curvularia lunata, Aspergillus nidulans, Fusarium moniliforme, and *Phialophora cyanescens.* Actinomycetomas may be caused by *Actinomadura madurae, Streptomyces somaliensis, Nocardia asteroides,* and *Nocardia*

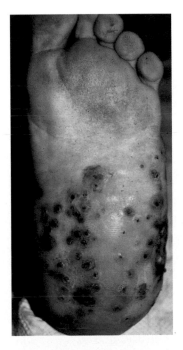

FIGURE 38-17 ■ Mycetoma. The black granules are indicative of a fungal rather than an actinomycotic etiology.

brazilensis. The disease has a worldwide distribution. Originally described in India, with a high incidence in the region of Madura, it is typically seen in dry tropical areas. Endemic areas include Sudan, India, Somalia, Mexico, and the Amazon region. Whereas in Mexico cases are predominantly caused by *Nocardia* species, in South America the predominant agent is *M. grisea.* The organisms gain entry into the body at points of trauma and it is most common among men who work outdoors barefoot or who exposed large areas of the skin, as would stevedores. The clinical picture manifests over a period of months or years as nodule that later evolves into edematous areas with marked fibrosis, followed by formation of fistula that drain or expel "grains." Bone involvement is characterized by periostal erosion and proliferation as well as the development of lytic lesions; otherwise, there is no systemic involvement. Morphology of the grains may give an idea of the specific etiological agent, but precise identification requires culture isolation. Dark grains are usually caused by fungi, and white to yellow grains can be caused by either actinomyces or fungi.

Treatment

Treatment depends on the organism isolated; for cases where actinomycetes are isolated, therapy should include streptomycin, dapsone, sulfamethoxazole-trimethoprim, rifampin, and amikacin. Eumycetoma are more difficult to treat, with some response to oral imidazoles reported, including ketoconazole, itraconazole, and voriconazole. Surgery should be considered for more advanced cases.

Sporotricosis

Sporotricosis is a mycotic infection produce by the environmental fungus *Sporotrix schenkii* (Fig. 38-18). It has a worldwide distribution, although endemic areas do exist, for example, in the Peruvian Andes. It is commonly associated with trauma from a rose thorn and is an occupational hazard for florists and gardeners.

Presentation and Characteristics

The classical picture (about 70% of the cases) is the so-called lymphocutaneous or sporotricoid pattern, characterized by a primary lesion, mostly an ulcerated plaque, followed by several satellite lesions, either papular, nodular, or crusted, in a linear lymphatic distribution. It is commonly located on an extremity and, in children, on the face. There is a second type of presentation with only one isolated lesion, either a plaque, nodule, or ulcer. This is known as the fixed cutaneous form of sporotricosis. Rarely, the infection can disseminate to involve multiple sites and organs; the most common extracutaneous site is a joint. On histology, the findings are those of a granulomatous reaction, often with a suppurative component.

Diagnosis

The fungus is rarely seen on direct examination or on tissue cuts, even with special stains. When visible, it has a levaduriform morphology. Fortunately, the fungus easily grows on Sauboroud media, which is the easiest and most reliable

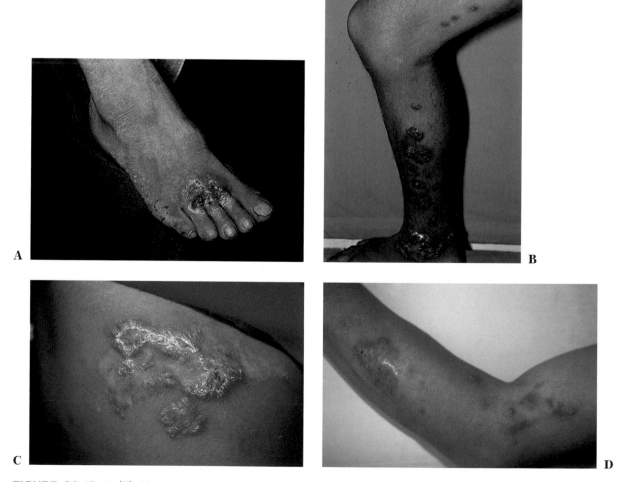

FIGURE 38-18 ■ **(A)** Verrucous sporotrichosis on dorsum of foot. (*Courtesy of Dr. A. Gonzalez-Ochoa.*) **(B)** Sporotrichosis with lymphatic spread on leg. (*Courtesy of Dr. A. Gonzalez-Ochoa.*) **(C)** Sporotrichosis, fixed lesion. **(D)** Sporotrichosis with classic pattern.

way to make the diagnosis. The intradermal reaction known as the sporotriquin test may help to confirm the diagnosis.

Treatment

Treatment options include the use of potassium iodide solution and itraconazole.

Paracoccidioidomycosis

As opposed to sporotricosis and chromoblastomycosis, in which the disease is located at the inoculation site, paracoccidioidomycosis is a systemic disease with hematogenous spreading from a primary pulmonary focus (Fig. 38 19).

Presentation and Characteristics

The infection has a specific geographic distribution through Central and South America. In some countries, such as Brazil, it reaches the status of public health problem. The agent, *Paracoccidioides brazilensis*, is a dimorphic fungus with special preference for tropical and subtropical forest with mild temperature and high humidity.

The infection is acquired by inhalation, with a primary lesion in the lung. From there, it may take two courses: an aggressive form with an acute severe pneumonia and rapidly progressive systemic disease or a relentless course with chronic pulmonary disease. The typical patient is a middle-aged male agricultural worker. They may present themselves to the dermatologist with involvement of the mucosae and skin. The lesions on lips, buccal mucosae, gums, palate, and pharynx are infiltrating ulcerated plaques and nodules, with subsequent destruction and scarring deformities of those structures.

On the skin the lesions vary widely. They may begin as small acneiform pustules 2 to 3 mm in size that later ulcerate, or they can adopt a pattern related to affected lymph nodes. Cold abscess may develop. In some instances, multiple symmetric papules either with verrucous or umbilicated surfaces may be present. On soles, they could be easily misinterpreted as warts, whereas on the face, they may look like moluscum.

Diagnosis

The size of the fungus and its characteristic morphology allow easy identification on sputum preparation and scrapings from the mucosal and cutaneous lesions. It is easy to recognize the blastospores with multiple gemations, giving the "pilot wheel" appearance. Identical structures are seen on histologic examination of the affected tissues. The reaction pattern seen on biopsy is a granulomatous reaction with multiple giant cells, some of them engulfing the budding elements. The fungus grows on Sabouraud's medium in 4 or more weeks, as a mold at 20 to 26°C and as a yeast at 34 to 37°C.

Treatment

Treatment choices have evolved, from sulfonamides to ketoconazole up to the new triazoles (itraconazole and fluconazole). At present, itraconazole is considered the drug of choice because of the lower doses required, shorter period of treatment, and fewer side effects.

Lobomycosis

This chronic skin infection is produced by *Lacazia loboi* (formerly *Loboa loboi*), a large fungus with a levadurifom morphology. The disease is endemic in tropical areas of South America.

Presentation and Characteristics

The disease is acquired by primary inoculation from the environment through traumatized skin. The clinical lesions take years to develop. The classical clinical manifestation is the formation of nodules with a keloid appearance, usually located on extremities, ears, face and neck, with the scalp being spared in most cases (Fig. 38-20). Other elementary lesions include infiltrated plaques, gummas, ulcers, and verrucoid nodules. The histology consists of a massive histiocytic infiltrate, without the pseudocarcinomatous hyperplasia commonly seen in chromoblastomycosis. This is the reason why in lobomycosis the nodules tend to have a smooth surface, as opposite to the verrucous surface of chromomycosis.

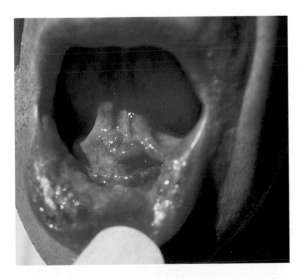

FIGURE 38-19 ■ Infiltrative deforming lesion of paracoccidioidomycosis.

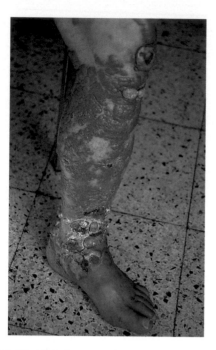

FIGURE 38-20 ■ Lobomycosis. Note the smooth surface and compare to chromoblastomycosis (Figure 38-16C).

The morphology of the fungus is quite distinctive, with globose, lemon-shaped buds, 9 to 10 μm in diameter, organized in short and long chains of uniform beads. The organism is easily seen in KOH preparations from lesions. The fungus has not been grown in culture media.

Treatment

The only effective treatment is wide surgical excision. Recurrences are very common. A recent report suggests that the combination of itraconazole and clofazimine may be of some benefit.

Noninfectious Miscellaneous Dermatosis

Pityriasis Alba

This is very common in children and consists of hypopigmented, poorly defined, scaly macules and plaques found on the face and upper outer arms. It is believed to be a mild form of atopic eczema. Lesions are first noticed after exposure to sunshine where the surrounding sun-affected skin appears quite tan.

Treatment

Treatment consists of topical 1% hydrocortisone ointment at night and sunscreens during the day.

Papular Urticaria

This term defines an exuberant reaction to arthropod bites (Fig. 38-21). Initially, there is an irritated weal, and, later, an intensely pruritic papule develops at the site of the bite. There may be a central hemorrhagic puncture, a vesicle, or even a blister, especially in children. The number and localization of the lesions depend on the type of exposure and feeding habits of the arthropod. New bites may exacerbate quiescent old bites. Because of scratching, lesions can become infected and crusted. Localization of the affected areas helps to reveal the causative arthropod: involvement of the legs suggests fleas, of the waist and thighs suggest chiggers, of the abdomen and arms suggest sarcoptic mange of dogs, and a generalized eruption suggests bird mites.

Treatment

Treatment consists of oral antihistamines, topical corticosteroids, and fumigation of the dwelling.

Miliaria

Also known as *prickly heat* (Fig. 38-22), *sudamina,* or *lichen tropicus,* this condition results from the obstruction of the sweat ducts caused by a combination of extreme heat and humidity. Depending on the level of obstruction, different clinical pictures can be seen. In *miliaria crystallina,* obstruction is very superficial; in *miliaria rubra,* the obstruction is deeper and clinically more puritic. The lesions have an erythematous base and consist of tiny, red papules. In *miliaria profunda,* there can be associated anhidrosis, compensatory

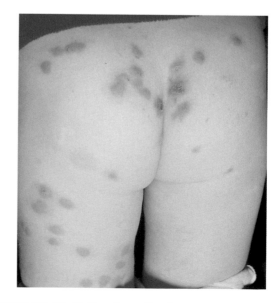

FIGURE 38-21 ■ Papular urticaria.

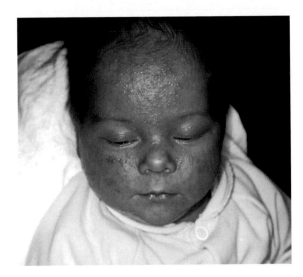

FIGURE 38-22 ■ Prickly heat at 3 weeks.

hyperhidrosis, and so-called tropical asthenia. Secondary infections are common.

Treatment

Treatment consists of seeking a cooler environment, loose clothing, fluids by mouth, and antibiotics where indicated for secondary infection.

Pemphigus Foliceaous (Fogo Selvagem)

Fogo selvagem is an endemic type of pemphigus foliaceous, described in the Amazonic regions of Brazil, and to a lesser degree in other countries in South America. It is clinically identical to the common type of pemphigus foliaceous, except for the young age of the population affected, and its common presentation in families.

An infectious agent has been postulated as the possible cause. The role of viruses, streptococcus variants, and transmission of the disease by a *Simulidae* species of fly have been the subject of debate. The areas of prevalence are located in regions of wild jungle that have become agricultural. The disease may take a self-limited course or, most likely, progress to a generalized form that otherwise is identical to the cosmopolitan forms of pemphigus. The patient may become erythrodermic. It is chronic and treatment is based on high-dose corticosteroid therapy, as well as other forms of immunosuppressive therapy

A Final Word

Tropical dermatology is not exotic medicine anymore. The patient that one might see in a clinic in a Midwestern city may have just returned from a trip to the Amazon—less than a 23-hour flight—and the little ulceration he has on his right arm may not be just a simple impetigo, but a cutaneous form of leishmaniasis or another heretofore remote condition. A global world means global patients and, thus, requires global thinking. A sufficient history for the dermatology patient should include questions about the faraway places to which he or she may have traveled and the surroundings to he or she may have been exposed. In jet-age dermatology, just looking may no longer be enough.

Acknowledgments

We are grateful to Dr. Beatriz Bustamante, Dr. Carlos Seas, and the Leishmania Group of the Instituto de Medicina Tropical Alexander von Humboldt of the Universidad Peruana Cayetano Heredia, for allowing us to use some of their clinical photos.

Suggested Reading

Bravo F, Sanchez MR. New and re-emerging cutaneous infectious diseases in Latin America and other geographic areas. Dermatol Clin 2003 Oct;21(4):655.

Canizares O, Harman R. Clinical Tropical Dermatology, ed 2. Boston, Blackwell Scientific, 1992.

Fisher AA. Atlas of Aquatic Dermatology. Orlando, FL, Grune & Stratton, 1978.

Grevelink SA, Lerner EA. Leishmaniasis. J Am Acad Dermatol 1996;34:257.

Lotti T, Hautmann G. Atypical mycobacterial infections: A difficult and emerging group of infectious dermatosis. Int J Dermatol 1993;321:499.

Lucchina LC, Wilson ME, Drake LA. Dermatology and the recently returned traveler: Infectious diseases with dermatologic manifestations. Int J Dermatol 1997; 36:167.

Lupi O, Tyring SK. Tropical dermatology: Viral tropical diseases. J Am Acad Dermatol 2003;49(6):979.

Schaller KF. Colour Atlas of Tropical Dermatology and Venerology. New York, Springer-Verlag, 1994.

Vetter RS, Visscher PK. Bites and stings of medically important venomous arthropods. Int J Dermatol 1998; 37:481.

CHAPTER 39

Cutaneous Signs of Bioterrorism

Scott A. Norton, MD, MPH

Previous editions of this book did not include a chapter on dermatologic manifestations of bioterrorism, but the world changed on the day we now know as "9/11." In this new era, physicians in the United States and worldwide have a new responsibility to know the fundamentals of recognizing and diagnosing an outbreak associated with biological agents. In this regard, the dermatologist has a particularly important role because most illnesses that arise from biological agents have a cutaneous component. In some, for example smallpox, skin involvement is the most dramatic feature of the disease; in others, cutaneous manifestations are not a central feature but it is possible, even likely, that the diagnosis of the index case will be made from cutaneous findings, subtle or obvious. For this reason, a discussion of the most important of these agents, smallpox and anthrax, is included in the text.

The Centers for Disease Control and Prevention (CDC) identifies six biological agents as posing the greatest risk for use in terrorism (Table 39-1), based on ease of manufacture, ease of dissemination, rate of subsequent person-to-person transmission, lethality, and psychosocial effects (literally, how terrified the community will be).

Smallpox

> The patient [with smallpox] presents a terrible picture, unequalled in any other disease, one which fully justifies the horror and fright with which small-pox is associated in the public mind.
>
> William Osler from *The Principles and Practice of Medicine*

Historical Aspects

The World Health Organization (WHO) regards smallpox, also called *variola,* as humankind's deadliest disease. Indeed, smallpox has caused perhaps 10% of all human deaths and, even during its waning years in the twentieth century, smallpox killed half a billion people. One third of its victims die; survivors are usually maimed for life with pocked scars or blindness. Because of the mortality and morbidity associated with smallpox, people long sought ways to prevent, ameliorate, or cure the disease. Fortunately for humankind, smallpox had several characteristics that made it vulnerable to eradication: there is no subclinical carrier state in humans, the disease is not transmitted by food or water, and there are no animal reservoirs or vectors. The disease occurs only in humans and, during the smallpox era, it was readily diagnosed on a clinical basis alone. A person who survived a bout of smallpox achieved lifelong immunity, but most important, smallpox was preventable through vaccination.

The cowpox vaccine, which Edward Jenner used, and the vaccine that replaced it, one derived from the closely related vaccinia virus, confer near complete immunity against smallpox. A concerted global vaccination program, led by the health organizations and governments around the world, used the vaccine to quell this disease. The last naturally occurring cases were in Bangladesh and Somalia during the mid-1970s, and a few years later the WHO proclaimed the eradication of smallpox. Shortly afterward, all laboratory stocks of variola virus were destroyed except for a few laboratories that maintained small amounts of the virus, putatively for research purposes. There is speculation, however, that unmonitored stocks of virus are in the hands of rogue states or terrorist organizations. Consequently, there is a risk, at least theoretically, that smallpox might recur. If so, the reappearance of this disease will mark one of the most catastrophic medical, public health, and criminal events that our species has witnessed. For this reason, it is worth bringing smallpox out of the history books and into our current textbooks.

Presentation and Characteristics

Virology

Smallpox is caused by the variola virus, a member of the *Orthopoxvirus* genus within the Poxvirus family. This

TABLE 39-1 ■ Biologic Agents Most Likely to Be Used in Terrorism or Warfare*

Disease	Pathogen	Likely Presentation When Used as a Bioweapon	Cutaneous Manifestations	% of Patients in a Bioterrorism Setting Who Have Cutaneous Manifestations
Smallpox	*Variola*, an orthopoxvirus	Classic illness described in chapter	Exanthem followed by classic vesicopustular eruption predominantly on acral surfaces; "pearls of pus"	All
Anthrax	*Bacillus anthracis*, an aerobic encapsulated spore-forming gram-positive rod	Inhalational disease starts with flulike presentation and progresses	Edematous papule or plaque evolving into an ulcer surmounted by a black eschar	Roughly 50%
Plague	*Yersinia pestis*, an aerobic gram-negative rod with safety-pin bipolar staining	Fever, weakness, and rapidly developing pneumonia with dyspnea, chest pain, and bloody cough, leading to respiratory failure, shock, and rapid death	Bubonic form from fleabites produces painful tender enlarged lymph nodes (buboes); pneumonic plague may cause DIC with purpura	Not known
Tularemia	*Francisella tularensis*, an aerobic pleomorphic gram-negative coccobacillus	Hemorrhagic bronchopneumonia with fever	If acquired transcutaneously, then an ulceroglandular or lymphocutaneous presentation	Not known
Botulism	Toxin produced by the anaerobic gram-positive rod, *Clostridium botulinum*	Rapid onset of symmetric descending flaccid paralysis, starting in bulbar muscles; afebrile, normal mental status, and no sensory deficits	Facial nerve paralysis, dilated pupils, dry oral mucosa	Presumably most
Viral hemorrhagic fevers	Examples include arenaviruses (e.g., Lassa), filoviruses (Marburg and Ebola)	Flulike illness with fever, myalgias, and extreme fatigue; severe cases have uncontrolled internal and orofacial bleeding	Petechiae, purpura, and hemorrhage	Presumably most

*Biological warfare is defined as the intentional use of microorganisms or toxins to produce death or disease in humans, animals, or plants.
Abbreviation: DIC, disseminated intravascular coagulation.

genus also includes cowpox, vaccinia, monkeypox, and a few other viruses that cause mostly non-human disease. The Poxvirus family has two other genera, one with the familiar molluscum contagiosum, and the other with the zoonotic disorders of orf and milker's nodules. All members in the Poxvirus family are DNA viruses that replicate within the host cell's cytoplasm, unlike nearly all other viruses, which replicate inside the nuclei.

Clinical Disease

Smallpox is transmitted primarily in a respiratory manner by droplets from close contact with infected individuals. Fomite transmission, for example from skin crusts, can occur but it is rare. Weaponized smallpox, on the other hand, is likely to be spread long distance through aerosolization of the virus.

Smallpox has three clinical stages. The first, the incubation phase, starts when a person is initially infected with the virus. Incubation lasts approximately 12 to 14 days (range, 7 to 17 days) and during this time, individuals are unaware they are infected. They feel well, have no clinical manifestations, and cannot transmit the virus to others. The second stage, the prodrome, begins with a sudden high fever (typically 102 to 104°F) accompanied by severe headache and backache. During the prodrome, the patient is viremic, appears toxic, is often prostrate with pain, and may be delirious. After 2 to 4 days, the prodrome ends with a slight defervescence and the appearance of an oropharyngeal enanthem. This marks the beginning of the eruptive stage and now the patient is infectious. The classic exanthem has several distinctive features (Fig. 39-1). Individual lesions evolve gradually through several morphologic forms over 14 to 18 days. Lesions progress from macules to papules to vesicles to umbilicated vesicles to pustules to crusted scabs, with each form lasting 1 to 2 days. An important diagnostic feature of smallpox is that at any one time, all lesions are in the same morphologic stage of development. In contrast, chickenpox lesions progress rapidly and asynchronously, thus all morphologic

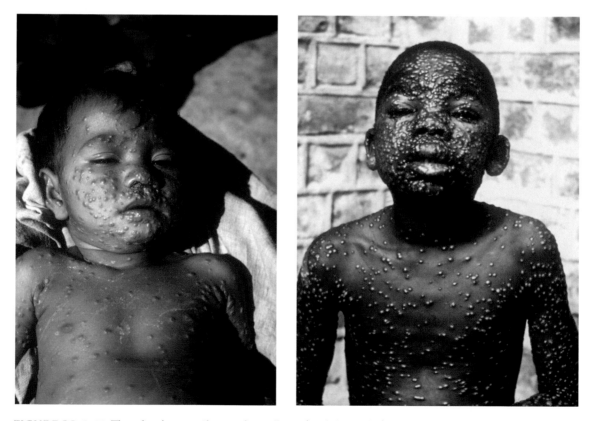

FIGURE 39-1 ■ The classic exanthem of smallpox (variola major) shows pustules with uniform morphology, more prominent on acral surfaces. In the past, one third of unvaccinated individuals who acquired smallpox died of the disease. The survivors were usually marked with pitted scars called *pocks,* and many were blinded by smallpox as well. *(Courtesy of the Public Health Image Library of the Centers for Disease Control and Prevention.)*

forms (e.g., papules, vesicles, pustules, and crusts) are typically present at any moment.

Another distinction between classic smallpox and chickenpox is that in the former disease, lesions are most abundant on acral surfaces (face, palms, and soles) (Fig. 39-2, left), whereas in the latter, lesions are most abundant centrally (on the trunk). Furthermore, the delicate lesions of classic chickenpox are described as "dewdrops on a rose petal," but firm smallpox lesions can be described as "pearls of pus"—they are deep-seated, globose, opalescent papules and pustules (Fig. 39-2, right). The smallpox patient is infectious from the onset of the enanthem until all scabs have separated, roughly 20 to 25 days later. Historical records show that the disease killed roughly 30% of unvaccinated individuals, and produced pocks (depressed facial scars) on most survivors. In people who received vaccinations less than 10 years before exposure to smallpox, historical case fatality rates were 1% to 3%.

Types of Smallpox

About 90% of patients with smallpox present with classic disease (see Fig. 39-1) in which individual pustules are either discrete (surrounded by normal-appearing skin) or coalesce perhaps with one or two neighboring pustules. Two variants of smallpox, the hemorrhagic type and malignant (or flat) type, have especially poor prognoses. *Hemorrhagic smallpox* is characterized by disseminated intravascular coagulation and purpura. It occurs more frequently in pregnant women. *Malignant smallpox* is characterized by innumerable flat lesions that cover the entire skin, producing an edematous appearance that resembles anasarca. *Flat-type smallpox* produces neither classic pustules nor scabs. Both of these variants, hemorrhagic and flat smallpox, have mortality rates of more than 95%.

Diagnosis

Naturally occurring disease has not existed since 1977 and there is no absolute confirmation that stocks of smallpox virus are in the hands of terrorists. Therefore, practitioners confronted by a patient with fever and pustules should remind themselves to look for alternative explanations. The CDC has an algorithm for the evaluation of suspected smallpox and offers the differential diagnosis shown Table 39-2. The algorithm, *Evaluating patients for smallpox: acute, generalized vesicular or pustular rash illness protocol* is available on the CDC's web site (www.bt.cdc.gov/agent/smallpox/diagnosis/pdf/spox-poster-full.pdf).

A thousand years ago or today, the disease that most resembles smallpox is chickenpox. A classic presentation of chickenpox will not resemble smallpox, but a variant presentation, one perhaps with a few more acral lesions and a higher temperature, might. If faced with a patient in whom smallpox is in the differential diagnosis, the physician should institute the same infection control precautions used for chickenpox or other respiratory diseases, then review the key clinical differences between the two diseases

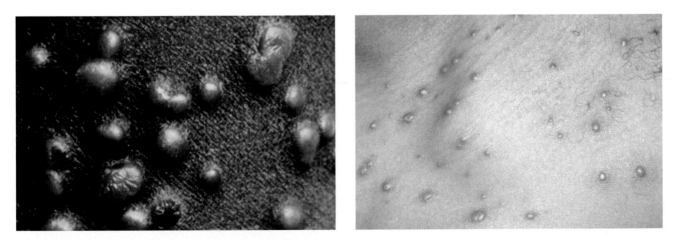

FIGURE 39-2 ■ Smallpox lesions (*left*) can be described as "pearls of pus"—they are firm, deep-seated, globose, opalescent papules and pustules. These lesions are from the sixth day of the exanthem, just before the pustules begin to umbilicate. Lesions of chickenpox or varicella (*right*) are more delicate, typically described as a "dew drop on a rose petal" in which the fragile vesicle sits atop a reddish area. Note that varicella lesions are in various stages from macules, papules, vesicles, and pustules. (*Image on left courtesy of the Public Health Image Library of the Centers for Disease Control and Prevention.*)

TABLE 39-2 ■ Differential Diagnosis for Febrile Patient With Vesicles and Pustules

Chickenpox

Disseminated herpes zoster

Disseminated herpes simplex

Impetigo

Pustular drug eruptions

Erythema multiforme

Enteroviral infections (especially hand, foot, and mouth disease)

Infected arthropod bites

Contact dermatitis

Monkeypox

Molluscum contagiosum (in immunocompromised patients)

(see Table 39-2), consult the CDC algorithm, and attempt to establish the diagnosis of a some other disease (Table 39-3). In other words, by ruling in chickenpox or another disease, one can rule out smallpox.

According to the CDC algorithm, if one cannot rule out smallpox, then local public health authorities must be notified. One should continue to follow the algorithm. The CDC reminds us that once an index case of smallpox has laboratory confirmation, the clinical case definition changes. At that point, the clinical definition becomes a febrile patient with an exanthem and an epidemiologic risk of exposure has smallpox until proven otherwise. Unvaccinated health care workers who are exposed to a patient with smallpox can take

TABLE 39-3 ■ Clinical Presentations of Classic Chickenpox and Smallpox

Chickenpox	Smallpox
Mild or no prodrome	Febrile prodrome
Superficial vesicles "dew drops on a rose petal"	Deep pustules "Pearls of pus"
Individual lesions evolve rapidly	Individual lesions evolve gradually
Lesions with different morphologies	Lesions with same morphology
Central predominance	Acral predominance
Spares palms and soles	Involves palms and soles
Patient is rarely toxic	Patient is usually toxic or moribund

reassurance in the rapid efficacy of the smallpox vaccine. It works so quickly that postexposure vaccination, even up to 4 to 5 days after exposure, prevents the disease from progressing through the 12-day asymptomatic incubation stage into the symptomatic or infectious stages of the disease.

Vaccination

In the United States, compulsory vaccination against smallpox ceased in the early 1970s. It is clearly the most successful vaccine ever devised but with the declared demise of smallpox, there was no further need to vaccinate individuals. Since the time of the attacks of September 11, 2001, however, smallpox vaccination is available for certain emergency response personnel, medical staff, and military personnel. Because the vaccine contains a live virus, it should not be administered to persons who are pregnant or immunocompromised. Furthermore, people with atopic dermatitis, active or quiescent—or who have a remote history of atopic dermatitis—should not be vaccinated because of the risk of eczema vaccinatum. In this condition, the specific immunologic defects associated with atopic dermatitis render these individuals exquisitely vulnerable to a virulent and unchecked replication of the live vaccinia virus over the entire skin. Eczema vaccinatum can be fatal. Another possibly fatal condition is progressive or necrotizing vaccinia. In this example, a severely immunocompromised person is vaccinated (or is exposed inadvertently to vaccinia) and is unable to mount an immune response to control the live virus. It can spread inexorably through the compromised person's skin and organs.

Anthrax

Anthrax is one of the oldest diseases known to humankind. It is a naturally occurring bacterial disease caused by the aerobic gram-positive rod, *Bacillus anthracis*. Typically, anthrax occurs in rural areas where it is associated with domesticated ruminants (sheep, cattle, and goats). Its historical importance includes several "firsts." It was the first bacterium seen under the microscope, the first organism to satisfy Koch's postulates, the first bacterial disease to have an effective vaccine, and the first bioterrorism agent of the twenty-first century.

When exposed to harsh environmental conditions, the rods of *B. anthracis* transform into spores that can remain dormant in soil for decades, impervious to heat, cold, desiccation, and solar radiation. These hardy spores are 1 to 2 μm in diameter and can be easily aerosolized and inhaled. *Woolsorter's disease* is the name for the occupational illness caused by the inhalation of anthrax spores aerosolized during the handling of unprocessed wool and animal hides. The mortality rate of untreated inhalational anthrax exceeds 90%. Thus, easy weaponization of this highly lethal agent makes it one of the most feared biological weapons. During the Cold War, several nations produced massive quantities of weaponized anthrax, evidence of which became well known after a mishap at a Soviet bioweapons facility. A cloud of anthrax spores was accidentally released and dozens of people downwind in the town of Sverdlosk died from inhalational anthrax.

Perhaps 95% of naturally occurring anthrax manifests as cutaneous disease, usually in agrarian settings. The Sverdlosk disaster, however, led to the notion that weaponized anthrax caused only inhalational illness. The letter-borne anthrax incidents of late 2001 in the United States showed otherwise: only 11 of the 22 victims had inhalational disease. The other 11 had cutaneous anthrax.

Clinical Features

Cutaneous anthrax develops when spores enter minor, often unnoticed, breaks in the skin. The most typical sites are exposed surfaces of the hands, legs, and face (Fig. 39-3). In the hospitable environment of the skin of a mammal (such as a human), the spores are activated, revert into rods, and begin producing toxins. A dermal papule, often resembling an arthropod bite reaction, develops over several days and soon evolves into a painless edematous ulcer with a central black eschar. One to several lesions may appear, depending on the manner of inoculation. There may be regional lymphadenitis, malaise, and fever. Individual lesions often look pustular, leading to the phrase "malignant pustule";

nevertheless, they contain no pus. In fact, histologic examination of cutaneous anthrax shows edema and necrosis with no inflammatory infiltrate. This is because anthrax is a toxin-mediated disease, an important point because antibiotic treatment of anthrax kills the bacteria but does not alter the course of already produced toxins.

Diagnosis

The acute onset of a painless edematous noduloulcerative lesion with a black eschar should invoke the clinical diagnosis of cutaneous anthrax. Other entities to consider are listed in Table 39-4. The CDC requests that practitioners notify local or state health departments before attempting a laboratory diagnosis of cutaneous anthrax. The American Academy of Dermatology's *Cutaneous Anthrax Management Algorithm,* (available at www.aad.org/professionals/educationcme/bioterrorism/CutaneousAnthrax.htm) leads one through the proper steps to swab exudates for gram stain and culture, to obtain biopsy specimens for histopathology and immunohistochemical staining, and to draw blood samples for culture and serology.

Patients with inhalational anthrax often present initially with a flulike illness that progresses virulently into severe illness. A distinctive radiographic feature of inhalational disease is a widened mediastinum without evidence of a primary pulmonary disorder such as pneumonia.

Treatment

Naturally occurring anthrax is susceptible to penicillin and doxycycline but weaponized anthrax may have been

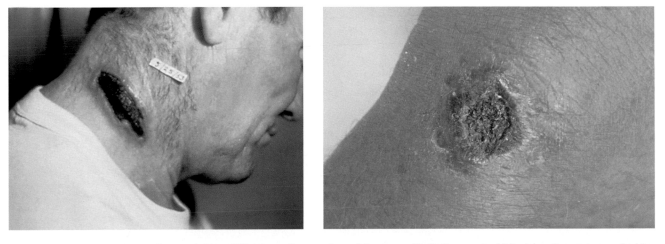

FIGURE 39-3 ■ Lesions of cutaneous anthrax on the neck and forearm. Note the central black eschar surrounded by a red rim. The word *anthrax* derives from the Greek term for burning coal, *anthracis. (Courtesy of the Public Health Image Library of the Centers for Disease Control and Prevention.)*

TABLE 39-4 ■ Differential Diagnosis for Cutaneous Anthrax

Differential Diagnosis of Eschar and Ulceration

Cutaneous anthrax	Cutaneous diphtheria
Brown recluse spider bite	Orf/Milker's nodule
Coumadin necrosis	Plague
Cutaneous leishmaniasis	Rat bite fever
Cutaneous tuberculosis	Pyoderma gangrenosum
Ecthyma gangrenosum	Staphylococcal/
Glanders	Streptococcal ecthyma
Heparin necrosis	Tropical ulcer
	Tularemia

Anti-phospholipid antibody syndrome ulcers

Opportunistic fungal infections (eg, due to aspergillosis or mucormycosis)

Scrub typhus, tick typhus, and rickettsialpox

Differential Diagnosis for Ulceroglandular Syndromes

Cat scratch disease	Melioidosis
Chancroid	Plague
Glanders	Staphylococcal/
Herpes simplex infection	streptococcal adenitis
Lymphogranuloma venereum	Tuberculous adenitis
	Tularemia

engineered to be resistant to these antibiotics. Therefore, a fluoroquinolone such as ciprofloxacin, is recommended for initial treatment of confirmed or suspected anthrax, even in pregnant women and children in whom this class of antibiotic is rarely administered. Once drug sensitivities have been established, the patient may be switched to another antibiotic as clinically indicated. As mentioned, antibiotics kill activated *B. anthracis* rods but do not reverse the effects of toxins that have been produced.

Although cutaneous anthrax is usually an uncomplicated and readily treatable infection, public health ramifications warrant hospitalization. Standard universal precautions are appropriate, but specific measures against secondary respiratory transmission are unnecessary. Unlike smallpox, anthrax cannot be transmitted person to person; it is acquired only via exposure to spores, not to the activated bacilli found in people with clinical disease.

Suggested Readings

Carucci JA, McGovern TW, Norton SA, et al. Cutaneous anthrax management algorithm. *J Am Acad Dermatol* 2002;47:766.

Cieslak TJ, Christopher GW, Ottolini MG. Biological warfare and the skin II: viruses. *Clin Dermatol* 2002; 20(4):355.

Cieslak TJ, Talbot TB, Hartstein BH. Biological warfare and the skin I: bacteria and toxins. *Clin Dermatol* 2002;20(4):346.

Fenner F, Henderson DA, Arita I, et al: *Smallpox and its eradication.* Geneva, World Health Organization, 1988.

McGovern TW, Christopher GW, Eitzen EM. Cutaneous manifestations of biological warfare and related threat agents. *Arch Dermatol* 1999;135:311.

Meffert JJ. Biological warfare from a dermatologic perspective. *Curr Allergy Asthma Rep* 2003;3:304.

Seward JF, Galil K, Damon I, et al. Development and experience with an algorithm to evaluate suspected smallpox cases in the United States, 2002-2004. *Clin Infect Dis* 2004;39:1477.

CHAPTER 40

Sports Medicine Dermatology

Rodney S. W. Basler, MD

Parallel to the burgeoning interest of the general population in establishing personal fitness programs, sports-related conditions of the skin resulting from injury, infection, and exacerbation of preexisting dermatosis are presenting with increasing frequency in the offices of dermatologists across the country. In addition, athletes at all levels of competition from junior high school through professional sports are in need of the services of dermatologic practitioners who are well informed in this subset of cutaneous problems. By classifying the various categories of dermatologic issues related to sports medicine into these groupings, a problem-oriented approach to dermatology and sports medicine emerges that will enable the clinician to approach these problems in a direct organized manner (Table 40-1).

Athletic Injuries

The integument, positioned at the interface between the athlete and the sporting environment, is the body organ that experiences disruption both from acute and long-term application of sports-related external forces. Preventing these injuries, or treating them aggressively to bring about an immediate resolution, greatly enhances a participant's ability to return to workouts and competition.

Friction Injuries

Abrasions

Presentation and Characteristics. Abrasions occur when the granular and keratinocized cells of the outer layers of skin are abruptly removed from the underlying dermis or "true skin." This trauma exposes the lower papillary and reticular dermis, causing punctate bleeding from the severed arterials of the dermal papilla. These pinpoint areas of bleeding within a larger patch of tissue exudate produce the appearance of a lesion referred to in the vernacular as "raspberry" or "strawberry" (Fig. 40-1).

Treatment. The treatment of acute abrasions, as with all other forms of injury, is determined by its severity. Minor abrasions can be treated by gentle cleansing with a mild detergent or soapless cleanser such as Cetaphil antibacterial bar. A trick used by many trainers is to have a can of mentholated shaving gel in their treatment kit, which also works well for cleansing minor lesions and precludes the need for having clean water on the sideline, although the latter is usually present for preventing dehydration. Bacitracin ointment and a dry dressing can then be applied; this provides a moist environment promoting healing with a minimum of scarring. Larger abrasions, especially those that have been contaminated by the environment, require more aggressive immediate care. Treatments must minimize additional trauma, and aggressive scrubbing, especially with cleansers such as hydrogen peroxide or povidone iodine, which may be cytotoxic should be avoided. A large "pistol-type" or plunger syringe should be used to irrigate the lesion; nontoxic surfactant cleansers are the wash of choice.

Proper cleansing is followed by the application of a hydrocolloid or semiocclusive hydrogel dressing that provides a moist healing environment allowing for epithelial migration and preventing the formation of crust or eschar (Fig. 40-2) These artificial barriers can remain in place for 5 to 7 days, and may be covered with padding and tape to allow for continued participation in practice or competition.

Prevention. Preventing abrasions requires little more than a common sense approach to protecting skin potentially exposed to acute trauma. Areas at risk should be covered with protective equipment such as sliding pads, long-sleeved shirts, long socks, "biker" shorts, or a self-adhesive bandage such as Coban.

Turf Burn

Presentation and Characteristics. Turf burn is a related injury that develops when an athlete, most commonly a

TABLE 40-1 ■ Classification of Dermatologic Issues Related to Sports Medicine

Injury

Friction
Abrasions
    Acute traumatic
    Turf burn
    Chronic
        Calluses
        Blisters
        Chafing
        Jogger's nipples
Pressure
    Tennis toe
    Acne mechanica
    Talon noir
Ultraviolet damage

Infections

Bacterial
    Impetigo
    Occlusive folliculitis
    Bikini bottom
    Pitted keratolysis
Fungal
    Tinea cruris
    Tinea pedis
Viral
    Plantar warts
    Herpes gladiatorum
    Molluscum contagiosum

Preexisting Dermatosis

Physical urticaria
Eczema

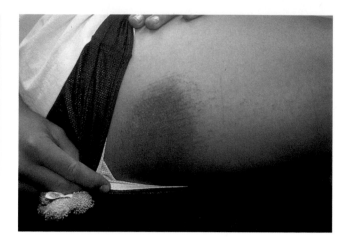

FIGURE 40-1 ■ Abrasion from sliding into plate: collegiate softball player. *(From Basler RSW, Garcia MA, Gooding PA: Immediate Steps for Treating Abrasions. Phys Sportsmed 2001;29(4):69-70).*

Prevention. As with other forms of abrasion, turf burns are best prevented by having equipment or athletic tape, or Coban applied to areas of potential injury.

Chronic Friction Injury

Calluses

Presentation and Characteristics. Calluses present as thick hypertrophied stratum corneum without the characteristic puncta noted with clavi or "hard corns." They represent a compensatory protective response that forms a keratin shield between the outer layers of the skin and an

football or soccer player, has an exposed area of skin slide across artificial turf. Interestingly, the injury is also seen, with some frequency in an ancillary group of athletes, particularly at a collegiate or professional level, namely cheerleaders. As the name implies, the injury results as much from the generation of heat in the skin as from friction, producing an injury that is part abrasion and part burn (Fig. 40-3); artificial turf has a lower coefficient of friction than natural grass, especially when wet.

Treatment. Because the injury is not as deep as seen with most acute traumatic abrasions, treatment can be less aggressive with cleansing of the area and the application of an antibiotic ointment, such as mupirocin or silver sulfadiazine (Silvadene).

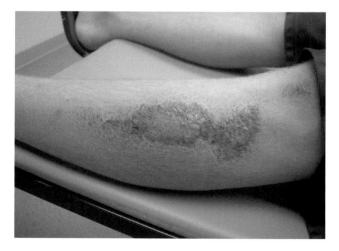

FIGURE 40-2 ■ Resolving deep abrasion treated with hydrocolloid dressing.

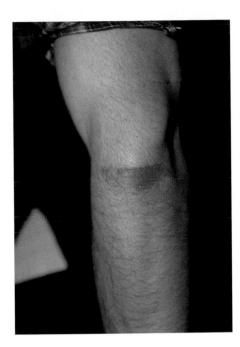

FIGURE 40-3 ■ Turn burn in collegiate football player. *(From Basler RSW, Garcia MA, Gooding PA: Immediate Steps for Treating Abrasions. Phys Sportsmed 2001;29(4):69-70).*

article of equipment, by far the most common being athletic shoes. There often is a history or recently appearing clinical evidence of an anatomic defect underlying the callus. Significant calluses also may be observed on the palmar surface of the hands of golfers, oarsmen, tennis players (Fig. 40-4), and gymnasts. Gymnasts consider calluses to be a competitive advantage, and for that reason, generally do not treat them.

Treatment. Because calluses often represent a protective mechanism of the skin, treatment is usually not necessary. The main reason to approach the lesions is to prevent the formation of painful blisters near the edges of the calluses. Careful paring, usually after soaking, followed by smoothing with a pumice stone or file, usually eliminates the calluses.

Prevention. To a certain extent, calluses are not preventable, and there is no particular reason for concern, unless they interfere with athletic performance or blister formation is a problem. Modification of footwear and the addition of gloves for tennis players and weightlifters are sometimes helpful.

Blisters

Presentation and Characteristics. The appearance of a tender vesicle or bullae, sometimes tinged with blood, over the site of the application of applied force does not usually represent a diagnostic quandary (Fig. 40-5). Unfortunately, especially when unroofed, these lesions cause significant pain and tenderness to the athlete, and may seriously curtail the length or level of competitive activity. During a recent playing of the U.S. Open tennis tournament, it was noted that more participants visited the first aid tent for skin-related problems than all other injuries combined, and the great majority of the problems were blisters.

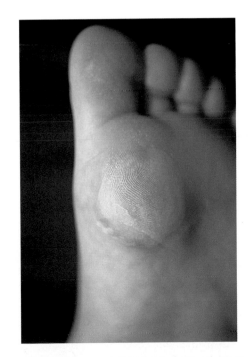

FIGURE 40-5 ■ Large blister on foot of high school tennis player.

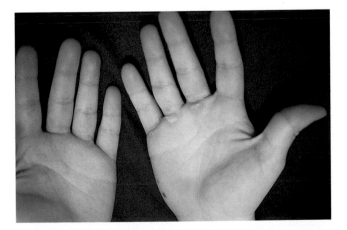

FIGURE 40-4 ■ Calluses on hand of high school tennis player.

Treatment. As with most injuries, treatment depends on the size and location of the blister. Small blisters are usually self-limiting and respond to conservative management. It has been shown that the optimal approach to the epidermal "roof" is to leave it intact when possible. The blister should be drained three times at 12-hour intervals for the first 24 hours using a flamed needle or scalpel. The blister is then covered with a hydrocolloid membrane or tape, either of which can be left in place for 5 to 7 days, allowing for reepithelialization.

Prevention. In general, to help prevent blisters, athletes should increase the length and intensity of exercise workouts gradually, especially when breaking in new shoes or rackets. Early studies in the military proved, unequivocally, that moisture is a major contributory factor, and needs to be minimized, especially over the feet. Newer acrylic-composition socks are designed to wick perspiration from the skin at the same time that they diminish friction and should be changed every 30 to 60 minutes if they become drenched in sweat. Some athletes also find the application of petroleum jelly or Aquaphor over pressure points to be of considerable benefit.

Chafing

Presentation and Characteristics. Chafing is produced by the mechanical friction between the skin covering two apposing body parts or between the skin and an article of clothing. It is a common problem, familiar to participants of nearly all sports, and presents as bright red, inflamed, abraded patches that are sensitive to the touch. In extreme cases, bleeding may be noted from the area of involvement. Although it is annoying and distracting, the condition usually does not lead to cessation of play. The upper inner thighs and axillae represent the most common distribution, and excess muscle or fat may contribute to the problem.

Treatment. The application of a lubricating ointment such as triple antibiotic or Aquaphor both relieves the symptoms and helps to prevent further chafing.

Prevention. Merely changing the athletic clothing to a fabric that generates less friction may bring about very significant improvement. Any adjustment in the area of involvement that eliminates or diminishes the friction applied to the skin surface ameliorates chafing. As mentioned, the application of petrolatum or Aquaphor may be very helpful. To decrease moisture, which may play a causative role, some athletes favor absorbent powders.

Jogger's Nipples

Presentation and Characteristics. A painful problem caused by long-term friction applied to a specific body part is the erosions that occur over the areolae and nipples of certain athletes. In extreme cases, the resulting injury may even cause hemorrhage into the clothing or uniform covering the area of involvement. Because the condition is particularly common in long-distance runners, it is usually referred to as *jogger's nipples*. Because most women athletes wear some type of soft protective sports bra, the problem is more common among men.

Treatment. Treatment is essentially the same as for all forms of superficial abrasion. The application of an antibiotic ointment covered by a simple dressing such as a Band Aid is usually sufficient.

Prevention. The most obvious preventative action, of course, is to simply have athletes who are prone to this condition run without a shirt. However, for obvious reasons, this may not be practical. Changing to a softer fabric of running shirt, especially one that does not have a logo, may be beneficial. Friction-reducing ointments may also be helpful, but often are rubbed off over time. Affixing a piece of tape cut exactly to the size and shape of the areola is probably the best preventative measure.

Pressure Injuries

Subungual Hemorrhage

Presentation and Characteristics. The appearance of pooled blood under the plate of the great toenail (Fig. 40-6) is a manifestation of acute bleeding resulting from the repeated forceful contact of the anterior nail plate, with the front part of the athletic shoe. Although the injury can be caused by shoes that are too short, it usually results from too small of a toe box. Although tennis players are more commonly affected than participants in other sports, (giving rise to the epithet *tennis toe*) the injury is also noted in other sports with the associated terms *jogger's toe* and *skier's toe*. Although acute cases may cause some pain and tenderness, symptoms are usually minimal and it is not necessary to shorten an exercise or competition schedule.

Treatment. In the acute phase, blood may be drained from beneath the nail with the time-honored flamed paperclip, or with a Geiger cautery if one is available. Soaking in warm water brings about some palliative benefit, as well, and tends to be more popular with affected athletes.

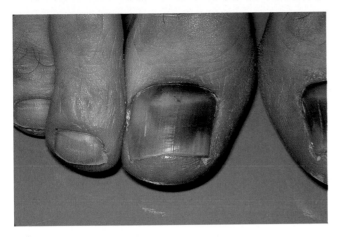

FIGURE 40-6 ■ Subungual hematoma in high school tennis player.

Prevention. Trimming the great toenail, in a straight tangential plane to the shortest point that it does not cause discomfort, is of major benefit. Careful attention to properly fitting shoes, especially ones with a generous toe box, is also recommended. Unfortunately, some athletes who are particularly prone to this condition notice some degree of involvement regardless of attempts to eliminate the problem.

Acne Mechanica

Presentation and Characteristics. Acne mechanica is a papulopustular eruption in the areas beneath heavy padding of certain contact sports, especially football and hockey. It varies in clinical presentation from acne vulgaris in that there is more inflammation, particularly around the papules, and the pustules appear to be more deep seeded. As first described by Mills and Klugman, the condition is produced by the combined factors of pressure, occlusion, friction, and heat. As would be expected, skin changes are most dramatic during the season when the equipment is worn and tend to spontaneously resolve after the season concludes.

Treatment. Acne mechanica responds to a certain, although lesser, extent to entities used to treat acne vulgaris. Rigorous cleansing with a moderately abrasive cleanser, and the use of a back brush is recommended after each practice session or game. The application of an astringent or keratolytic agent, such as adapalene or retinol, may also be of considerable benefit. Because physical factors play an important role in pathogenesis, systemic antibiotics seem to be of considerably less help in treating the condition than in treating acne vulgaris, but may still be used and be of limited value.

Prevention. The simplest form of prevention of acne mechanica is the wearing of a clean, absorbent, cotton t-shirt under the equipment causing the problem, especially shoulder pad in football players. The procedures and medications recommended for treatment might also be considered as part of prevention.

Talon Noir

Presentation and Characteristics. The skin change referred to as *talon noir* or *black heel* involves the skin over the calcaneal portion of the foot, and demonstrates asymptomatic color change due to blue to black punctate petechiae, especially on the posterolateral aspect of the heel. In uncommon cases, the condition may also be seen on the palms of weight lifters, golfers, or tennis players, where it is referred to *black palm*. For reasons that are not entirely clear, talon noir is seen almost exclusively in older teenagers and young adults.

Treatment. No treatment is available or actually warranted for this essentially cosmetic condition. It usually comes to the attention of care givers only because of the concern of the patient or their family, of the possibility of it representing a malignant melanoma.

Prevention. Although there is probably little that can be done to prevent black heel, properly fitting shoes may contribute to fewer problems during subsequent seasons.

Ultraviolet Damage

Presentation and Characteristics. Photo-injury to the skin is characterized by the all too familiar, painful, erythematous to deep red, to even violaceous changes that occur in exposed skin secondary to overexposure to ultraviolet rays of the sun. In extreme cases, vesicles, bullae, and even systemic symptoms may accompany this reaction. Participants in nearly all of the outdoor sports are at risk, especially protracted activities, such as fishing, general water sports, and golfing. Long-term ultraviolet damage includes premature aging, premalignant keratosis, and actual cutaneous malignancy, all of which are among the most preventable diseases to afflict the integument.

Treatment. Although treatment definitely takes a backseat to prevention when dealing with solar injury, nearly all people who participate in any form of outdoor sports and lack deep natural melanotic pigmentation have experienced some level of sunburn. For the milder cases, topical application of an emollient moisturizing agent, with or without minimum potency corticosteroids, usually suffices to bring about significant palliation of symptoms. Systemic over-the-counter anti-inflammatories, such as aspirin and ibuprofen are also of value, as are the more potent anti-inflammatories, such as prescription nonsteroidal anti-inflammatories and corticosteroids with more severe photo injury. Many practitioners and patients prefer spray steroids to cover the involved areas, because they preclude the need of further irritation and discomfort from application. Usually a short course, generally 5 to 7 days, of treatment is adequate in nearly all cases.

Prevention. The prevention of actinic damage of the skin in the general population is one of the most important and rigorously pursued challenges to face dermatologists. The basic recommendations of limiting outdoor athletic exposure to the hours before 10:00 AM and after 4:00 PM are sometimes impractical, but must be stated. Covering all exposed areas as much as possible with opaque clothing is equally important, but also sometimes not possible. Head covering with a brim rather than a cap is advised, but represents protection no greater than a sun protective factor (SPF) of 2. Sunscreen remains our most valuable line of defense, and should optimally be applied 20 to 30 minutes before sun exposure and every 2 to 4 hours during, depending on the amount of water or perspiration that is diluting the product. An SPF of at least 15 is required and a product with combined UVB and UVA protection is recommended. Of course, sunscreen must be applied even on cloudy days because of the penetration of damaging rays through cloud cover.

Infections

Bacterial Infections

Impetigo

Presentation and Characteristics. Superficial bacterial infection such as pyoderma or impetigo is a hazard of all contact sports. As with many of sports-related infections, wrestling probably puts its participants at greatest risk, and bacterial skin infections may reach epidemic proportions among wrestling teams and at large wrestling meets. Any thin-roofed vesicle or bullae with purulent fluid or honey-crusted plaque on exposed areas of skin, particularly those extending from a mucous membrane, are suspect for this type of infection. These may progress rapidly to sharply marginated erosions, sometimes with points of bleeding.

Treatment. Treatment should be aggressive, straightforward, and immediate with systemic antibiotics being the main line of defense. The application of a compress made of warm water and antibacterial cleanser eliminates much of the surface bacteria, and the application of an antibacterial cream usually hastens healing as well.

Prevention. Any athlete suspected of carrying bacterial infection must be prohibited from competition. In wrestling, careful and regular sterilization of the mats with an appropriate disinfectant is also a necessity. Showering with an antibacterial soap immediately after competition often prevents actual infection in athletes as well.

Occlusive Folliculitis

Presentation and Characteristics. Occlusive folliculitis is seen under heavy, protective padding in sports such as football and hockey, much in the same way as is acne mechanica. The deep infection of the follicles with furuncle production and the lack of more superficial inflammatory papules (Fig. 40-7) differentiate these entities. In addition, the area of involvement is more limited and coincides exactly with overlying equipment.

Treatment. As with other bacterial infections, aggressive systemic antibiotic therapy is warranted in occlusive folliculitis, although it may need to be prolonged over several weeks or months during which the causative equipment is in contact with the skin. The topical application of antibiotics

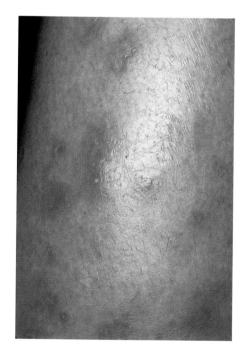

FIGURE 40-7 ■ Occlusive folliculitis under thigh pad of collegiate football player.

used to treat acne, such as clindamycin or erythromycin, with or without benzoyl peroxide is also of considerable benefit.

Prevention. The application of an absorbent powder over the areas of involvement may be of considerable value. The causative equipment or padding should be removed as quickly as possible after a workout, and any clothing or equipment that comes into direct contact with the skin should be kept as clean as possible, even disinfected if necessary.

Pitted Keratolysis

Presentation and Characteristics. Pitted keratolysis is a superficial infection of the stratum corneum accompanied by the hallmark pungent odor, which has contributed to its alternative designation of *toxic sock syndrome*. Examination of the bottom of the foot shows macerated skin, often with a faintly erythematous border and characteristic "punched out" areas. It is only mildly symptomatic to the athlete.

Treatment. The application of over-the-counter acne gels, such as 10% benzoyl peroxide may, in themselves, be curative for this condition. If this does not represent adequate treatment, prescription acne medicine such as benzoyl peroxide–clindamycin and benzoyl peroxide–erythromycin products are particularly affective.

Prevention. Careful washing of the feet with an antibacterial soap, followed by towel and air drying, is a common-sense approach to the problem. Absorbent powders inside the stocking and the regular application of a 20% aluminum chloride solution also helps to prevent the condition.

Fungal Infections

Tinea Pedis

Presentation and Characteristics. *Athlete's foot* and *jock itch* indicate the close association of fungal infections with sports. The macerating affect of perspiration in nearly every athletic environment reduces the natural barrier of the epidermis, allowing invasion of fungal elements. Toe webs are usually the first, and generally the most common, site of infection, with spread to the keratin over the soles and lateral aspects of the feet. Marginated erythema and scaling, often with vesicle formation are noted in areas of involvement. Unilateral distribution is also helpful in differentiating this entity from dyshidrotic eczema. Dystrophic onychomycosis may represent a reservoir of organisms that later spread over the skin.

Treatment. Topical antifungal creams, such as terbinafine and clotrimazole, may be effective in some early superficial cases, but systemic antifungals, such as griseofulvin, fluconazole, itraconazole, or terbinafine, are often required for treatment. When topical medications are used in the toe webs, solutions, sprays, and gels seem to work better than creams or ointments. If there is a deep commensal infection of the toe web where the infection seems to be potentiated with bacterial overgrowth, strong systemic medications such as ciprofloxacin may be indicated.

Prevention. Any procedure that helps to keep the stratum corneum dry, thereby maintaining the natural physical barrier of fungal invasion, is beneficial in preventing this infection. The application of a foot powder or aluminum chloride in patients who show significant maceration is definitely helpful, and the use of shower thongs in the locker room may help those prone to chronic recurrent infections. The long-term administration of a systemic antifungal, such as fluconazole or itraconazole with a dosage as low as 200 mg per month, may be highly affective for prophylaxis.

Tinea Cruris

Presentation and Characteristics. Another time-honored epithet that underscores the association of fungal infection with athletes is *jock itch*. Although this infection presents in the groin, the source of infection is usually an indolent infection of the feet or toenails. When the causative organism is a dermatophyte, the involved area shows erythema and scaling, with a sharp margination, and rarely progresses to the genitals because of the fungistatic affect of sebum in this area. Fungal infections also lack the deep red coloration and satellite lesions seen when yeast is involved. Individual lesions may look particularly innocuous and imitate nummular eczema in wrestlers.

Treatment. Early localized infections may respond to prescription, or even over-the-counter, topical antifungals, such as miconazole or terbinafine. Some clinicians favor the older iodochlorhydroxyquin HC preparation. Systemic antifungals may be required in stubborn, persistent cases, and high-dose (250 mg b.i.d.) terbinafine may be required in particularly virulent infections in wrestlers, especially in the hair.

Prevention. Immediate showering after any exercise session with careful attention to removing soap and towel drying intertriginous regions is strongly recommended. The daily change of sports briefs and attention to choosing those made of an absorbent fabric is also helpful. Absorbent powders in the groin as well as axillae may also prevent infection in these areas, particularly in susceptible wrestlers. Fluconazole at a dosage of 200 to 400 mg/week throughout the entire season may preclude missing important meets because of active fungal lesions.

Viral Infections

Plantar Warts

Presentation and Characteristics. Cutaneous invasion by the human papillomavirus, particularly of the skin of the feet, is relatively common among athletes. The macerating effect of perspiration is a contributing factor as with other forms of infection. In addition, the moist environment of the locker room, especially the showers, provides for a most hospitable environment for causative viruses to live and reproduce. Any area of the plantar portion of the foot may be involved with a very tender hyperkeratotic papule present, often revealing small black dots when the superficial portion is removed. Confluence of individual papules may result in relatively large mosaic warts, and lesions over the weight-bearing portions of the foot may cause considerable morbidity, especially in long-distance runners.

Treatment. In treating these localized viral infections, a conservative approach to therapy is recommended, particularly one that allows for continued practice and competition during therapy. If maceration appears to be a major contributory factor, the application of a 20% aluminum chloride solution or even stronger mixtures containing 10% to 25% formalin often bring about complete resolution with no morbidity. Some physicians and trainers favor the topical application of 50% trichloracetic acid solution under a 40% salicylic acid plaster, applied once or twice weekly, followed by vigorous paring. Aggressive ablative therapy, such as excision, electrodessication, or laser treatment, holds no curative advantage, and carries significant risk of short-term disability and even permanent scarring.

Prevention. Wearing shower thongs in the locker room decreases the likelihood of coming into contact with the causative virus; foot powders diminish maceration. The regular application of a 20% aluminum chloride solution may also be of considerable preventative value.

Herpes Gladiatorum

Presentation and Characteristics. As implied by its name, this superficial viral infection of the skin is noted almost

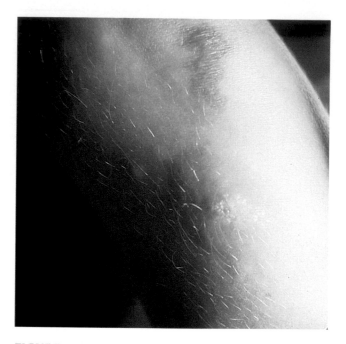

FIGURE 40-8 ■ Herpes gladiatorum in collegiate wrestler.

exclusively in wrestlers, although it may sometimes be seen in other forms of contact and noncontact sports, including basketball. The head, neck, and upper extremities, which are exposed during periods of contact, are usually those noted, with the appearance of grouped vesicles on an erythematous to violaceous base (Fig. 40-8). Dermal edema is usually present, and burning and tenderness are noted by the athlete.

Treatment. Systemic antivirals are, of course, the primary entity in the arsenal for treating this infection, and should be started immediately when symptoms occur, even before actual skin lesions are noted. Local improvement can be accelerated by unroofing the vesicles and applying benzoin topically, then injecting localized lesions intralesionally with a dilute triamcinolone solution.

Prevention. Athletes with a history of recurrent herpes lesions may greatly benefit from the prophylactic use acyclovir or valacyclovir. Adequate dosage usually is 400 mg/d of acyclovir or 500 mg/d of valacyclovir. These medications should be started before the training season begins, and continued through the course of the competitive schedule. Any athlete with active herpes must be prohibited from competition during the stage of intact or draining vesicles, usually requiring a quarantine period of 4 to 6 days, until all lesions are dry.

Molluscum Contagiosum

Presentation and Characteristics. Again, the venues of competitive wrestling seem to offer the primary athletic source of infection with the large pox virus that causes molluscum contagiosum. Less commonly, these lesions may also be seen in swimmers, and it has been speculated that the solutions used to sterilize pool water are not adequate to completely eliminate the virus. In addition, many athletes may be infected in non-sports arenas, such as "coed wrestling." Small, grouped, waxy papules are usually seen on exposed areas of skin with individual papules showing a central umbilication in some cases. A linear distribution of lesions referred to as *pseudo-koebnerization* may also be noted, especially in wrestlers.

Treatment. Lesions are easily removed by curettage, but this leads to superficial abrasions that may preclude contact for a short period of time. Curettage may be easily carried out following the application of a topical anesthetic gel. Liquid nitrogen and tape striping with highly adhesive tape may also be effective.

Prevention. The prohibition of competition by infected participants is a necessity, and removal of localized individual lesions at their first appearance also helps to prevent self-inoculation.

Preexisting Dermatoses

Physical Urticarias

Presentation and Characteristics. The physical urticarias, particularly cholinergic urticaria, are most commonly diagnosed through history, although they have a distinctive form of papular erythema with a more punctate dermal edema than seen with acute allergic urticaria. The erythematous papules are smaller and more distinct; wheal is formation much less pronounced. The inner aspects of the arms and legs as well as the lateral flanks are common areas of involvement. By history, factors that induce physical urticaria are those indigenous to athletic endeavor, such as rapid temperature changes, especially cold to hot, physical exertion, and emotional stress. Cold urticaria and aquagenic urticaria also fall into this category, and can be disabling to swimmers. Pressure urticaria usually appears under articles of athletic equipment.

Treatment. Because of its anti-serotonin affect, cyproheptadine is particularly helpful in the physical urticarias. A dosage of 4 mg at bedtime may, in fact, be essentially curative in milder cases. Unfortunately, this antihistamine is quite sedating, and taking the drug the night before a morning competition may leave the athlete in less than prime condition, especially in terms of competitive alertness. Combination therapy with H_1-H_2–inhibiting antihistamines usually works better than a single drug regimen. In especially difficult cases, corticosteroids, sometimes on a long-term alternate-day schedule, may be required to eliminate the problem. Athletes being administered this course of treatment must be aware of the fact that the older, less specific means of steroid screening may reveal this use of corticosteroids, causing them to test positive.

Prevention. The use of prophylactic antihistamines, especially cyproheptadine, as noted, is probably the best precaution to take for people who are prone to developing physical urticaria. Otherwise, elimination of the problem may be particularly difficult, short of complete cessation of athletic activity. If the reaction is seen secondary to changes in the temperature, gradual warming or cooling the body may diminish the severity to a limited extent.

Atopic Eczema

Presentation and Characteristics. Most atopes have a lifelong history of skin sensitivity with the characteristic flexural (Fig. 40-9) and facial involvement, and are well aware of their problem. Poorly marginated erythema and scaling in the commonly involved areas associated with persistent itching and evidence of excoriation are the hallmark of this condition. Unfortunately, increased body heat and perspiration, which are found in nearly all forms of athletic endeavor, generally exacerbate the condition.

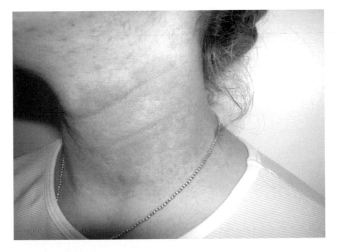

FIGURE 40-9 ■ Eczema of neck flaring during season in atopic collegiate tennis player.

Treatment. The treatment of sports-induced eczema is essentially the same as that for any patient with atopic eczema, although there may be a need to be more aggressive in athletes during their competitive seasons. Topical corticosteroids in emollient cream or ointment bases are the traditional first line of defense, with the newer immunomodulators, tacrolimus and pimecrolimus, more beneficial in patients who have a long-standing history of atopic eczema. Tacrolimus and pimecrolimus may have a significant drawback, however, in that they usually impart a sensation of heat in the skin during periods of exercise, which the athlete may find annoying or distracting. Systemic corticosteroids over varying lengths of time may ultimately be required to bring the condition under control to a point that it does not interfere with athletic performance.

Prevention. Short, tepid showers, using an oil- or cream-based soap immediately following exercise periods to remove sweat are recommended, and should be followed with lubrication with an emollient cream or lotion, or a bath oil. Any of the medications used for treatment may also be considered to be preventative, including the use of antihistamines throughout the course of the season. It is particularly important for patients suffering from eczema to have the condition under the best possible control in the off season so as to preclude the need for aggressive therapy once conditioning becomes more intense.

Conclusion

Well-informed, up-to-date medical practitioners who deal with problems of the integument need to have a basic understanding of the care and prevention of cutaneous injuries that pertain to recreational and competitive athletes. Most skin problems that arise in the course of training or general fitness regimens can be treated aggressively and directly, and prevented through thoughtful planning and preparation. When treated in an immediate and knowledgeable manner, very few of the skin conditions that arise as a result of sports participation need interfere with an active lifestyle or the pursuit of lofty competitive goals.

Suggested Reading

Basler RSW. Managing skin problems in athletes. In: Mellion MB, Walsh W, Shelton GL, eds. Team physician's handbook, ed 3. Philadelphia, Hanley & Belfus, 2002, 311–325.

Basler RSW. Acne mechanica in athletes. Cutis 1992;50: 125–128.

Basler RSW. Skin injuries in sports medicine. J Am Acad Dermatol 1989;21:1257–1262.

Basler RSW. Sports related injuries in dermatology. In: Callen JP, ed. Advances in dermatology. St Louis, Mosby, 1988, 4, 29–50.

Basler RSW. Skin lesions related to sports activity. Prim Care 1983;10:479–494.

Basler RSW, Basler DL, Basler GC, et al. Cutaneous injuries in women athletes. Dermatol Nurs 1998;10:9–18

Basler RSW, Basler GC, Palmer AH, Garcia MA. Special skin symptoms seen in swimmers. J Am Acad Dermatology 2000;43:299–305.

Basler RSW, Garcia MA. Acing common skin problems in tennis players. Phys Sportsmed 1998;25:37–44.

Basler RSW, Garcia MA, Gooding KS. Immediate steps for treating abrasions. Phys Sportsmed 2001;29:69–70.

Bergfeld WF. Dermatologic problems in athletes. Clin Sports Med 1982;1:3.

Eiland G, Ridley D. Dermatological problems in the athlete. J Orthop Sports Phys Ther 1996;23:388–402.

Levine N. Dermatologic aspects of sportsmedicine. Dermatol Nurs 1994;6:179–186.

CHAPTER 41

Dermatoses of Pregnancy

J. K. Shornick MD, MHA

The dermatoses of pregnancy can be extremely confusing. Several reported entities have not survived the scrutiny of time. It is doubtful whether perpetuating their inclusion in current classification schemes serves any useful purpose. In the end, the vast majority of rashes specific to pregnancy can be relegated to one of four categories: herpes gestationis, pruritic urticarial papules and plaques of pregnancy PUPPP, prurigo of pregnancy, or cholestasis of pregnancy.

Needless to say, the pregnant woman is subject to the entire repertoire of the dermatologist's trade. Often the first challenge is to decide whether pregnancy is relevant to the current condition or not.

Terminology

The generally accepted, current classification of skin diseases specific to pregnancy is listed in Table 41-1.

Herpes Gestationis (Pemphigoid Gestationis)

Herpes gestationis (HG) is the prototype of rashes specific to pregnancy. It is almost always associated with pregnancy. There are however multiple reports of HG in association with choriocarcinoma or trophoblastic tumors in women. There are no reports of an HG-like disease in association with choriocarcinoma in men. Thus, HG appears to be exclusively associated with the presence of placentally derived tissue.

Although the least common (occurring in approximately 1 :50,000 pregnancies), HG is the most clearly defined skin condition, and the most important to exclude. It remains idiopathic, although it is invariably associated with pregnancy (or trophoblastic tissue), carries a genetic predisposition, and is immunologically mediated.

Presentation and Characteristics

Clinical Appearance

- First onset may occur during any pregnancy, generally during the second or third trimester. Explosive onset in the immediate post partum period can occur in up to 25% of cases.
- Clinical lesions vary from intensely pruritic urticarial plaques to pemphigoid-like tense blisters. One often sees rapid evolution from the urticarial phase to clustered or arcuate tense blisters. Patients with only urticarial lesions and no progression to blisters have been reported.
- Intense, relentless pruritus is invariable.

Distribution

Onset occurs in the periumbilical area in 50% of patients, but may also first appear on palms, soles, or extremities. Facial involvement is rare and mucosal involvement essentially nonexistent.

Course

- Exacerbation at delivery occurs in approximately 75% of patients and may be dramatic.
- Generally recurs during subsequent pregnancies, although "skip pregnancies" have been reported. Flares associated with menstruation or oral contraceptives are also reported.
- Spontaneous resolution over weeks to months following delivery is the rule, although case reports of protracted disease are available.
- There is no increased maternal risk in association with HG.
- Newborns may be affected up to 10% of the time, presumably through passive transfer of the HG IgG.

TABLE 41-1 ■ **Classification of Dermatoses of Pregnancy***

Classification	Synonyms or Variants
Herpes gestationis	Pemphigoid gestationis
Pruritic urticarial papules and plaques of pregnancy (PUPPP)	Polymorphic eruption of pregnancy Toxemic rash of pregnancy Toxic erythema of pregnancy Late-onset prurigo of pregnancy
Prurigo of pregnancy	Prurigo gestationis (Besnier) Early onset prurigo of pregnancy Papular dermatitis of pregnancy Pruritic folliculitis of pregnancy Linear IgM disease of pregnancy
Cholestasis of pregnancy 1. Prurigo gravidarum 2. Jaundice of pregnancy	Obstetric cholestasis

*Preferred terminology is noted in bold.

- There is an increased risk of premature delivery associated with HG (32% before 38 weeks, 16% before 36 weeks).

Laboratory Findings

- Routine laboratory results are normal. Mild peripheral eosinophilia may occur, but is not clearly clinically relevant.
- Histopathology classically shows a subepidermal blister with eosinophils. Eosinophils are uncommon in PUPPP and suggest one should at least consider HG in the differential diagnosis.
- Direct immunofluorescence showing complement, with or without IgG deposited in a smooth, linear band along the dermal–epidermal junction is the diagnostic sine qua non, occurring in essentially 100% of cases. Split specimens show staining on the epidermal fragment. Indirect immunofluorescence reveals an IgG1 capable of avid complement activation. Titers of the HG antibody are low and historically do not correlate with the extent or severity of skin involvement. Recent, more sensitive immunoblotting and enzyme-linked immunoassays may challenge that assessment.

Cause

- The HG antigen is a 180-kD transmembrane glycoprotein with its *N*-terminal end embedded within the intracellular component of the hemidesmosome and its *C*-terminal component located extracellularly. The extracellular portion contains 15 collagenous domains interspersed by 16 noncollagenous domains. Antibodies from patients with bullous pemphigoid, mucous membrane pemphigoid, lichen planus pemphigoides, and linear IgA disease all react to specific antigens along the extracellular component of BP180. The 16th noncollagenous A domain (NC16A) is the target in HG. NC16A is also known as BP180, BPAg2, and type XVII collagen.
- Pathophysiologically, the antibody fixes to the BMZ, triggering complement activation via the classical complement pathway. Chemoattraction and degranulation of eosinophils follow. It is the release of proteolytic enzymes from eosinophilic granules, which appears to dissolve the bond between epidermis and dermis.
- Up to 80% of HG patients have HLA-DR3, approximately 50% have -DR4, and 40% to 50% have the simultaneous presence of both. HLA-DR3 shows linkage disequilibrium with the C4 null allele and a corresponding in crease in the C4 null allele has also been reported. However, neither HLA-DR3 nor -DR4 is requisite for the development of HG and there is no obvious correlation between the presence of either antigen or the extent or severity of disease.
- All patients demonstrate anti-HLA antibodies. Whether this represents phenomenon or epiphenomenon remains to be seen, but their strikingly high incidence implies the universal presence of placental compromise.
- Special stains of HG placenta have suggested a primary immunologic reaction in the villous stroma of chorionic villi, leading to the suggestion that HG is actually a primary disease of placental tissue, with secondary involvement of the skin. This hypothesis is attractive from many viewpoints, but remains to be clarified.
- Antithyroid antibodies are also increased, although their clinical relevance is unclear; the majority of patients are clinically euthyroid. On the other hand, the risk of autoimmune thyroid disease, especially Grave's disease, is clearly increased in those with a history of HG.

Differential Diagnosis

The primary differential in HG is between PUPPP and a wide variety of diseases irrelevant to pregnancy. Urticaria and arthropod bites can be difficult to differentiate. Immunofluorescence is the key to separating HG from the rest, but is hardly reasonable in all cases of pruritic rashes during pregnancy. Most typically, the relentless progression of unbearable itch associated with urticarial lesions, rapidly progressing to tense blisters, is characteristic of HG.

Treatment

- HG is sufficiently rare that treatment guidelines are all driven by expert opinion.
- Because HG is not associated with significant maternal or fetal risk, it is imperative not to create risk from therapy.
- Topical steroids and antihistamines are rarely of benefit.
- Systemic steroids, beginning at 0.5 mg/kg/d, remain the cornerstone of effective therapy. Many patients improve during the later part of pregnancy, only to flare at the time of delivery. Because profound flares at the time of delivery are common, one should be prepared to initiate or increase steroids during the immediate postpartum period.
- There has been no clear evidence that HG is associated with increased fetal morbidity or mortality (other than premature birth) in the largest studies available, although that impression certainly remains from a review of individual case reports.
- There is no evidence that systemic steroids decrease the risk of premature delivery.

Pruritic Urticarial Papules and Plaques of Pregnancy (Polymorphic Eruption of Pregnancy)

Polymorphic eruption of pregnancy (pruritic urticarial papules and plaques of pregnancy [PUPP]) is the most common of the specific dermatoses of pregnancy, estimated to occur in 1:130 to 1:300 pregnancies. It is idiopathic, defined clinically, has negative immunofluorescence, and tends not recur during subsequent gestations.

Presentation and Characteristics

Clinical Appearance

- Most cases (75% to 85%) develop during the first pregnancy, but first onset after multiple pregnancies has been reported.
- There is an abrupt onset of intensely itchy urticarial or papular lesions, often within abdominal

striae in the last month of pregnancy or immediate postpartum period. Rapid spread to the trunk and extremities is characteristic.
- Fine vesicles are present in up to 40% of cases, but no tense blisters.

Distribution

There is a curious tendency for first lesions to develop within abdominal striae, although this is certainly not universal. The face and mucosal surfaces are almost always spared.

Course

- Spontaneous resolution within days of delivery is the rule.
- Generally does not recur during subsequent gestations.
- No maternal risks or complication noted, except for an increased incidence of excessive weight gain or fetal twinning.

Laboratory Findings

- Laboratory investigations are normal.
- Histopathology is nonspecific and classically devoid of eosinophils. The presence of eosinophils, however, does not exclude PUPP.
- Direct and indirect immunofluorescence are negative or nonspecific. An increase in activated T cells within dermal infiltrates has led to speculation that PUPP may be a consequence of a delayed T-cell hypersensitivity to skin antigens.
- HLA typing shows no disease associations.

Differential Diagnosis

Because no definitive marker exists for PUPP, the diagnosis is clinical and by exclusion. As with HG, the differential is typically between incidental hives, viral exanthems, and HG. Immunofluorescence, though not indicated in all cases, is the key to distinguishing HG.

Treatment

Potent topical steroids and antihistamines may provide symptomatic support. Systemic steroids are quite helpful, although not invariably necessary.

Prurigo of Pregnancy

This group of rashes is less common than PUPP (estimated to occur in between 1:300 and 1:450 pregnancies) and by far the most confusing. Several variations have been reported. Confusion persists regarding entities reported without histopathology or routine laboratory investigations and prior to the advent of immunofluorescence. The unifying feature of this group is that there is no diagnostic clarity, only a similar clinical pattern. No doubt, this group will be subdivided with time.

Presentation and Characteristics

Clinical Appearance

- The classical presentation occurs during the second or third trimester with discrete or clustered scratch papules, predominantly on extensor surfaces. Lesions may or may not be follicular.
- There may be pustules, but not blisters.

Distribution

Generally on the extensor surfaces, sparing the face and mucosal surfaces.

Course

- Generally self-limited, the symptoms resolve over weeks to months post partum.
- No fetal or maternal risks have been reported.
- Recurrence during subsequent pregnancies is variable.

Laboratory Findings

- Liver function tests (by definition) are normal. Other laboratory findings have been inconsistently described.
- Histopathology is typically nonspecific. Whether inflammation tends to be follicular or not depends on whether poorly described variants are included in this group.
- Immunofluorescence is characteristically negative.

Differential Diagnosis

By definition, laboratory investigations and immunofluorescence are noncontributory. With no defining marker and only a nonspecific clinical pattern to unite the reported variants, there is little guidance to separate prurigo of pregnancy from atopy or diseases coincident to pregnancy.

Treatment

Treatment is symptomatic; no morbidity or mortality has been associated with this group.

Cholestasis of Pregnancy (Obstetric Cholestasis)

Jaundice occurs in approximately 1 in every 1,500 pregnancies. Cholestasis of pregnancy (CP) is the second most common cause of gestational jaundice, viral hepatitis being more common. CP accounts for approximately 20% of cases of obstetric jaundice, although the frequency depends on the demographics of the area.

The incidence of CP varies in different racial groups. It seems to be highest in Chile-Bolivia (6% to 27%) and Sweden (1% to 1.5%) and lowest among blacks and Asians. CP occurs in approximately 1:1,000 pregnancies in the United States. The defining features of CP are

- generalized pruritus, with or without jaundice, with no history of exposure to hepatitis or hepatotoxic drugs;
- the absence of primary lesions;
- elevated serum bile acids;
- disappearance of signs and symptoms following pregnancy; and
- recurrence during a subsequent gestation.

There is, however, a broad spectrum of clinical presentations.

CP is not really a primary *dermatosis* of pregnancy, because the defining feature is pruritus associated with cholestasis, but without dermatologic primary lesions. The literature on CP is unusually inconsistent.

Presentation and Characteristics

Clinical Appearance

- Classically presents during the last trimester of otherwise uneventful pregnancies. Onset as early as 8 weeks has been reported.
- Intense, generalized pruritus, worse at night and often worst on the palms and soles.
- Skin findings are all secondary.

Distribution

Symptoms are typically worse on the trunk, palms, and soles.

Course

- Symptoms may wax and wane, but persist throughout pregnancy.
- Up to 50% of patients may develop signs of hepatitis—dark urine, light-colored stools, or jaundice—within 2 weeks of presentation.

- Signs and symptoms disappear within weeks of delivery.
- Recurrences during subsequent gestations occur in 60% to 70% of cases. Recurrences are also common with use of oral contraceptives.
- Failure of pruritus to stop within days of delivery, or the persistence of elevated liver function tests, suggest underlying primary biliary cirrhosis.
- If intrahepatic cholestasis lasts for weeks, vitamin K absorption may be impaired, leading to a prolonged prothrombin time. Without exogenous vitamin K, fetal prothrombin activity may lead to an increased incidence of intracranial hemorrhage. The prothrombin time should monitored and intramuscular vitamin K administered as necessary.
- Meconium staining and premature labor occur with frequencies as high as 45%. Fetal distress and increased stillbirths are also reported, with mortality in some series as high as 13%.
- Most authors argue for increased fetal monitoring after 30 weeks, with delivery upon signs of meconium staining or fetal stress. Others argue for delivery at 38 weeks for mild symptoms, 36 weeks for severe cases.
- There appears to be a tendency for these women to develop cholelithiasis or gallbladder disease at increased rates later in life.

Laboratory Findings

- Hepatic ultrasonography is normal. Liver biopsy is not indicated.
- In those without jaundice, elevated serum bile acids may be the only identifiable laboratory abnormality (prurigo gravidarum). Conjugated (direct) bilirubin is increased, but rarely above 2 to 5 mg/dL. Alkaline phosphatase, GGT, and cholesterol are unreliable during pregnancy, but AST typically remains within 4 times normal, even in those with CP.

- Serum abnormalities confirm the presence or absence of disease. Whether or not serum levels correlate with disease severity is disputed.

Cause

- CP remains idiopathic and much of the existing literature is confusing and contradictory.
- Onset in association with a urinary tract infection has been reported in up to 50% of cases, although the causative relationship between the two is unclear.
- CP has been associated with autosomal dominant inheritance and the HLA-A31 haplotype, although these findings have been disputed.

Differential Diagnosis

Increased bile acid salts are the sine qua non and are typically 3 to 100 times normal.

Treatment

- Phototherapy, phenobarbital, and cholestyramine are the historical treatments and remain viable options.
- Ursodeoxycholic acid (15 mg/kg/d) is generally considered the treatment of choice. Its use appears to both control symptoms and decrease the risk of adverse fetal outcome(s).

Suggested Reading

Glanz A, Marschall HU, Mattsson LA. Intrahepatic cholestasis of pregnancy: Relationships between bile acid levels and fetal complication rates. Hepatology 2004;40:467–474.

Kroumpouzos G, Cohen LM. Dermatoses of pregnancy. J Am Acad Dermatol 2001;45:1–19.

CHAPTER 42

Where to Look for More Information About a Skin Disease

John C. Hall

"Doctor, I saw a patient yesterday who was diagnosed as having epidermolysis bullosa. I understand this is quite a rare condition. Where can I find the latest information on this subject?" This is the type of question frequently asked of a teaching dermatologist. A computer gives you references and some databases provide information about a dermatosis. But, assuming these are not readily available, there are other sources.

Print Resources

First, the inquiring physician or student should check out the Dictionary–Index of this book. Even for rare conditions, there is at least a definition of the disease. The Suggested Readings at the end of each chapter can also point one in the right direction for books or papers on a given subject.

Second, there are several comprehensive general texts on dermatology that include rare diseases. The following are suggested.

- Arndt KA, LeBoit DE, Robinson JK, Wintraub BU. Cutaneous medicine and surgery. Philadelphia, WB Saunders, 1996.
- Odum RB, James WD, Berger TG. Andrew's diseases of the skin: Clinical dermatology, ed 9. Philadelphia, WB Saunders, 2000.
- Demis DJ, Dahl M, Smith EB, Thiers BH. Clinical dermatology, 4 vols. Philadelphia, JB Lippincott (revised annually).
- Freedberg IM, Eisen AZ, Wolff K, et al. Fitzpatrick's dermatology in general medicine, ed 6, 2 vols. New York, McGraw-Hill, 2003.
- Champion RH, Burton JL, Burns DA, Breathnach SM. Rook/Wilkinson/Ebling textbook of

dermatology, ed 6, 4 vols. Cambridge, MA, Blackwell, 1998.

Online Resources

The National Library of Medicine, 8600 Rockville Pike, Bethesda, MD 20014, [www.nlm.nih.gov], has very good information on different medical sites. Other useful web sites include the following.

- Dermatology Slide Atlas at www.med.unc.edu/derm/atlas/welcome.htm
- A.B. Ackerman's Atlas Online at www.derm101.com
- Medical Dermatology at www.labordedermatology.com
- Internet Journal of Dermatology at www.ispub.com
- American Academy of Dermatology at www.aad.org
- Skin Cancer Foundation at www.skincancer.org
- British Association of Dermatologist (clinical practice guidelines) at www.bad.org.uk
- University of Iowa, Dermatology Dictionary. Dermpath Tutor at www.tray.dermatology.uiowa.edu/home
- The Journal of American Academy of Dermatology at www.eblue.org

The following journals are highly pertinent and are available online.

- *Acta Dermato-Venereologica,* 6 issues per year. Published by Taylor & Francis Group.
- *American Journal of Clinical Dermatology,* 6 issues a year. Published by Adis International.

- *American Journal of Contact Dermatitis,* W.B. Saunders. Although this journal is no longer published, you can continue to view the contents of this web site and you can order reprints from 2002 and earlier.
- *American Journal of Dermatopathology,* 6 issues a year. Official journal of the International Society of Dermatopathology.
- *Archives of Dermatology,* a monthly journal published by the American Medical Association, Chicago. It is indexed in both the June and December issues.
- *British Journal of Dermatology,* monthly. Published by Blackwell Synergy.
- *Clinics in Dermatology,* 6 issues a year. Published by Elsevier.
- *Cutis,* a monthly magazine for the general practitioner, published by Reed Medical Publishers.
- *Dermatologic Surgery,* published by Blackwell Synergy.
- *Dermatologic Therapy,* published by Blackwell Synergy.
- *Dermatology Online Journal,* Senior Editor, Barbara Burrall, MD, published by Arthur C. Huntley.
- *Internet Journal of Dermatology,* Editor-in-chief, Madeleine Duvic MD.
- *Journal of the American Academy of Dermatology,* a monthly journal, published by the American Academy of Dermatology.
- *Journal of Cutaneous Pathology,* 10 issues a year. Official Publication of The American Society of Dermatopathology. Published by Blackwell Synergy.
- *Journal of Dermatological Treatment,* 6 issues a year. Published by Taylor & Francis Group.
- *Journal of Drugs in Dermatology,* official publication of the International Society for Dermatologic Surgery.
- *Journal of Investigative Dermatology,* a monthly journal published on behalf of the Society for Investigative Dermatology, Blackwell Publishing.
- *Journal Watch Dermatology,* from the publishers of *The New England Journal of Medicine,* the Massachusetts Medical Society. It is published biweekly on the web and monthly in print.
- *Pediatric Dermatology,* bimonthly. Published by Blackwell Synergy.

DICTIONARY–INDEX

The purpose of the dictionary portion of this index is to define and classify some of the rarer dermatologic terms not covered in the text. Some very rare or unimportant terms have purposely been omitted, but undoubtedly some terms that are *not* rare and *are* important have also been omitted. Most of the histopathologic terms have been defined. Suggestions or corrections from the reader will be appreciated.

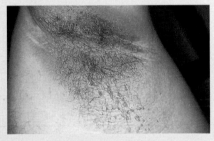

Pseudoacanthosis nigricans of axilla.

Page numbers followed by an "f" refer to figures.
Page numbers followed by a "t" refer to tables.

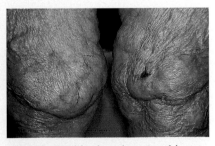

Acrodermatitis chronica atrophicans on legs.

Acrodermatitis enteropathica (*continued*) dermatitis, alopecia, and diarrhea. When zinc was added to pediatric formulas and to hyperalimentation regiments it became rare. Autosomal recessive.

Acrodermatitis, papular, of childhood. *See* Gianotti-Crosti syndrome

Acrodynia. Mercury poisoning usually in infants. Itching, painful swelling, pink, cold, clammy hands and feet with hemorrhagic puncta. Stomatitis and loss of teeth occur. Greater than 0.001 mg per liter merucury is found in the urine.

Acrokeratoelastoidosis. Different size symmetric horny glossy translucent papules on knuckles, thenar eminences, hypothenar eminences, dorsa and sides of fingers and margins of hands. May also involve tibia, anterior ankles, malleoli, Achilles' tendon, dorsal feet and dorsal toes.

Acrokeratosis, paraneoplastic (Bazex's syndrome). A specific sign of cancer of the upper respiratory and upper digestive tracts characterized by plum-colored acral skin lesions, paronychia, nail dysplasias, and keratoderma, 351t

Acrokeratosis verruciformis of Hopf. A rare disease affecting the dorsa of the hands and the feet characterized by flat warty papules. Probably hereditary. Differentiate from *flat warts* and from *epidermodysplasia verruciformis.*

Acromegaly. Hyperpituitary condition causing gross thickening of the skin with characteristic facies, enlarged hands, feet, digits, hyperhidrosis, hypertrichosis, and hyperpigmentation.

Acropustulosis of infancy. Tiny pustules or vesicles on the distal extremities that occur within the first year of life and are intensely pruritic. Spontaneous resolution usually occurs within the first 2 or 3 years of life, 394t, 395

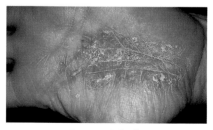

Acropustulosis.

Actinic dermatitis, chronic (Actinic reticuloid). Persistent erythema of face, hands, and other exposed areas. CD8+ cells infiltrate the skin due to sensitivity to UVA, UVB and even visible light. Especially in elderly men are associated with increased contact allergies. Strict UVA, UVB and visible light protection is difficult but beneficial. May become generalized and difficult clinically and histologically to tell from cutaneous T-cell lymphoma(mycosis fungoides). Contact dermatitis is a common association.

Actinic granuloma. *See* Annular elastotic giant cell granuloma

Actinic keratosis, 268t, 269t, 272f, 274t, 276–279, 277f, 278f, 285, 296, 366–367, 366f, 406f
  inflammation, 100t

Actinic prurigo. *See* Prurigo, actinic

Actinomycosis, 196t, 213–214

Active nevus, 289

Acute cutaneous lupus erythematosus (ACLE), 343, 345t

Acute hemorrhagic edema (Finkelstein disease, AHE). Benign cutaneous leukocytoclastic vasculitis in children under two years of age. Polycyclic plaques with dark neurotic center in a medallion, target or cockayde configuration sparing the trunk. Resolves in 1 to 2 weeks without sequelae and can be postinfectious.

Adaptive immunity, 106

Addison's disease, 341, 352

Adenoma, 297–298
  apocrine, 297–298

Adenoma sebaceum (Pringle's disease), 297, 361, 361f

Adenomas hamartomas, 297

Adhesion disorders, 377, 378t, 379f

Adiposis dolorosa (Dercum's disease). A lipoma-like disorder characterized by irregular and painful deposits of fat in the subcutaneous tissue of the trunk and limbs, more common in women than in men.

Adrenocorticotropic hormone, 95t

Adventitial dermis, 3

Aerosols, 38

AIDS. *See* Acquired immunodeficiency syndrome

Ainhum. Essentially a tropical disease of blacks that results in the amputation of a toe or toes because of constricting bands.

Albinism, 341, 388

Albright's hereditary osteodystrophy. Multiple areas of cutaneous ossification, skeletal abnormalities, abnormalities of the parathyroid gland, mental retardation, and shortening of the metacarpal bones.

Albright's syndrome. Large hyperpigmented macules, precocious puberty in females, and polyostotic fibrous dysplasia. The macules have a jagged border like the coast of Maine, unlike café-au-lait macules that usually have a smooth, or coast of California, border, 341

Aldara. *See* Imiquimod

Alkaptonuria. *See* Ochronosis

Allergic contact dermatitis (ACD), 110–111, 394t, 400, 401f

Allergic granulomatosis (Churg-Strauss syndrome). The combination of transitory pulmonary infiltrations of Loffler's syndrome, asthma, blood eosinophilia, and nodular purpuric or erythema multiforme-like skin lesions. Target organs beside skin and lung include kidney, upper respiratory tract, and central nervous system, 130

Allergy. An altered state of reactivity by a first exposure to antigen and made manifest by subsequent specific exposures, 76–104
  atopic eczema as, 83–91, 84f–88f, 89t
  contact dermatitis as, 76–83, 77f–80f
  cosmetic, 9, 23f, 74
  drug eruptions as, 91–104, 93f, 94f, 95t–99t, 99f, 100t–103t, 410–411, 413f
  food, 10, 89
  history taking for, 30
  nummular eczema as, 91, 92f
  occupational dermatoses as, 83
  sun. *See* Photodermatoses
  tests for, 9, 74

Allergy diet (Rowe), 10

Allopurinol (Zyloprim), 95t

Alopecia. From the Greek *alopekia,* meaning "hair loss.", 100t, 310–318, 311t, 313t, 314f–316f
  androgenetic pattern, 311
  areata, 41, 111–112, 313–315, 314f, 394t, 401, 402f
  central centrifugal cicatricial, 316–317
  cicatricial, 315f, 316–318
  cicatrisata, 200
  congenital triangular alopecia. Probably under reported, idiopathic, triangular-shaped temporal area of hair loss. Present at birth or in the first year of life that can be bilateral. (See Congenital triangular alopecia).
  drugs causing, 313t
  lymphocytic cicatricial, 316–317
  male-pattern, 406f
  moth eaten scalp, 216
  neutrophilic cicatricial, 317–318

cutaneous amyloidosis is a rare condition that can be suspected clinically but should be proven by histologic examination. Amyloid is a protein-carbohydrate complex, which on histologic section assumes a diagnostic stain when treated with certain chemicals. Several biochemical varieties have been delineated. Amyloidosis can be systemic or localized.

localized amyloidosis (lichen amyloidosis). The skin only is involved. Clinically, this dermatosis appears as a patch of lichenified papules seen most commonly on the anterior tibial area of the legs. These pruritic lesions can be differentiated from lichen simplex chronicus or hypertrophic lichen planus by biopsy. Some authors feel the amyloid deposits are due to keratinocyte breakdown products caused by scratching and lichen amyloidosis is, therefore, a variant of lichen simplex chronicus.

primary systemic amyloidosis. This peculiar and serious form of amyloidosis commonly involves the skin along with the tongue, the heart, and the musculature of the viscera. The skin lesions appear as transparent-looking, yellowish papules or nodules, which are occasionally hemorrhagic. Commonly (40%) "pinch purpura" which is ecchymosis due to minor trauma. This form is familial.

secondary amyloidosis. Secondary amyloid deposits are very rare in the skin but are less rare in the liver, the spleen, and the kidney, where they occur as a result of certain chronic infectious diseases, and in association with multiple myeloma.

Anetoderma. *See* Atrophies of the skin, macular atrophy

Angioedema, acquired. May be associated with urticaria (*see* Chap 12), other illnesses especially B-cell lymphoproliferative disease (AAE-I) or an autoantibody directed against the C1 inhibitor molecule (AAE-II), 100t

Angioedema, hereditary. Rare autosomal dominant form of angioedema that may be associated with respiratory and gastrointestinal symptoms. Low level or dysfunctional inhibitor of the first component of complement is the cause.

Angioendotheliomatosis, malignant (intravascular large cell lymphoma). Usually fatal B cell intravascular lymphoma in skin (lower dermal and subcutaneous blood vessels) and central nervous system. Erythematous telangiectatic plaques or nodules especially on lower extremities.

Angiofibromas. Asymptomatic skin-colored or pinkish-brown asymptomatic telangiectatic papules usually symmetrically scattered over central face. When multiple they have been considered pathognomonic for tuberous sclerosis but have been reported with multiple endocrine neoplasia type 1 (MEN1), 394t, 397

Angiohistiocytoma, multinucleate cell. *See* Multinucleate cell angiohistiocytoma

Angioimmunoblastic lymphadenopathy with dysproteinemia. Fever, night sweats, hepatosplenomegaly and generalized lymphadenopathy. Fifty percent with skin findings that are most often a transient morbilliform eruption. Plaques, purpura and urticarial lesions also occur. It is a subtype of T-cell lymphoma, which may be primary or, according to some authors, triggered by a drug allergy or viral infection.

Angiolymphoid hyperplasia with eosinophilia (Kimura's disease). A rare benign condition, usually seen on the face, characterized by a solitary or, less frequently, multiple dermal or subcutaneous nodules. There is a blood eosinophilia and there are eosinophils in the histologic infiltrate. Some consider Kimura's disease to be the systemic form only with deeper, larger lesions. It has been associated with human herpes virus 8.

Angioma serpiginosum. Characterized by multiple telangiectases, which may start from a congenital vascular nevus but that often arise spontaneously. This rare vascular condition is to be differentiated from *Schamberg's disease*, *Majocchi's disease*, and *pigmented purpuric dermatitis of Gougerot and Blum*.

Angioma, targetoid hemosiderotic. Solitary benign tumor in adults on trunk or extremities. Violaceous papule with ecchymotic evanescent ring. It may be caused by trauma.

Angioma, tufted. *See* Tufted angioma (Progressive capillary hemangioma or Nakagawa's angioblastoma). Rare vascular tumor usually on trunk, slow growing with a tendency to resolve. Usually developed within the first year of life but not present at birth. One third are tender and form dusky reddish-blue subcutaneous plaques or nodules that may be annular with depression resembling a "doughnut." Surrounding skin may be hyperhidrotic or have increased vellus hairs. It can be associated with Kasabach-Merritt syndrome.

Angiosarcoma. Malignancy of vascular tissue usually seen on the face and scalp of elderly male patients, or at the site of chronic lymphedema when it is referred to as Stewart-Treves syndrome.

Anhidrosis. The partial or complete absence of sweating, seen in ichthyosis, extensive psoriasis, scleroderma, prickly heat, vitamin A deficiency, one form of ectodermal dysplasia and other diseases. Partial anhidrosis is produced by many antiperspirants

Anhidrotic asthenia, tropical. Described in the South Pacific and in the desert in World War II. Soldiers showed increased sweating of neck and face and anhidrosis (lack of sweating)

Acrodermatitis chronica atrophicans. A moderately rare idiopathic atrophy in older adults, particularly women, characterized by the presence of thickened skin at the onset, with ulnar bands on the forearm, changing into atrophy of the legs below the knee and of the forearms. In the early stages this is to be differentiated from scleroderma. High doses of penicillin may be effective. Late stage of Lyme disease.

Atrophie blanche (segmental hyalinizing vasculitis). A form of cutaneous atrophy characterized by scar-like plaques with a border of telangiectasis and hyperpigmentation that cover large areas of the legs and the ankles, mainly of middle-aged or older women. May ulcerate and biopsy shows vasculitis.

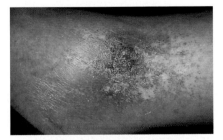

Atrophie blanche on ankle.

Atrophoderma, idiopathic, of Pasini and Pierini. Similar to morphea (localized scleroderma) but without induration. The round or irregular depressed atrophic areas are asymptomatic and appear mainly on the trunk of young females.

Folliculitis ulerythematosa reticulata. A very rare reticulated atrophic condition localized to the cheeks of the face; seen mainly in young adults.

Hemiatrophy. May be localized to one side of the face or may cover the entire half of the body. Vascular and neurogenic etiologies have been proposed, but most cases appear to be a form of *localized scleroderma.*

Lichen sclerosus et atrophicus (kraurosis vulvae, kraurosis penis, and *balanitis xerotica obliterans).* An uncommon atrophic process, mainly of women, which begins as a small whitish lesion that contains a central hyperkeratotic pinpoint-sized dell. These 0.5-cm or less whitish macules commonly coalesce to form whitish atrophic plaques. The most common localizations are on the neck, shoulders, arms, axillae, vulva, and perineum. Many consider kraurosis vulvae, kraurosis penis, and balanitis xerotica obliterans to be variants of this condition. Can be very pruritic and 5% risk of associated squamous cell carcinoma when occuring in adult female genitalia.

Macular atrophy (Anetoderma of Jadassohn). A very rare condition characterized by the appearance of circumscribed reddish macules that develop an atrophic center that progresses toward the edge of the lesion, seen mainly on the extremities. May be seen after acne, varicella, and other inflammatory skin diseases.

Poikiloderma atrophicans vasculare (Jacobi). This rare atrophic process of adults is characterized by the development of patches of telangiectasis, atrophy, and mottled pigmentation on any area of the body. This resembles chronic radiodermatitis clinically and may be associated with dermatomyositis, lupus erythematosis or scleroderma. May precede the development of a lymphoma and some generalized cases are already mycosis fungoides or cutaneous T-cell lymphoma(CTCL).

Secondary atrophy. From inflammatory diseases such as syphilis, chronic discoid lupus erythematosus, leprosy, tuberculosis, scleroderma, etc.

Ulerythema ophryogenes. A rare atrophic dermatitis that affects the outer part of the eyebrows, resulting in redness, scaling, and permanent loss of the involved hair.

Noninflammatory

Linear atrophy, striae albicantes or *distensae stretch marks.* On abdomen, thighs, and breasts associated with pregnancy, Cushing's disease, obesity, systemic and topical corticosteroids adolescence, and rapid weight gain.

Macular atrophy (anetoderma of Schweninger-Buzzi). Characterized by the presence of small, oval, whitish depressions or slightly elevated papules, which can be pressed back into the underlying tissue. Associated with antiphospholipid antibodies and thrombotic events.

Secondary atrophy. From sunlight, x-radiation, injury, and nerve diseases.

Senile atrophy. Often associated with senile pruritus senile purpura, and winter itch in elderly.

Congenital atrophies. Associated with other congenital ectodermal defects.

Atrophoderma of Moulin. Hyperpigmented, linear atrophoderma which follows lines of Blaschko beginning during childhood or adolescence. Usually proceeding inflammation.

Atypical cutaneous lymphoproliferative disorder (ACLD). Widespread, pruritic papules and plaques, often hyperpigmented (rarely hypopigmented) seen in the later stages of HIV infection. The pathology mimics cutaneous T-cell lymphoma (CTCL) but is usually composed of CD8(+) cells and only rarely progresses to true CTCL.

Autoerythrocyte sensitization syndrome (Gardner-Diamond syndrome, psychogenic purpura). Bizarre, tender ecchymotic lesions mainly in young females. May be associated with psychological disturbance. Skin lesions reproduced with intradermal injection of whole blood or red blood cell fractions.

Autohemotherapy. A form of nonspecific protein therapy, administered by removing 10 mL of venous blood from the arm and then immediately injecting that blood intramuscularly into the

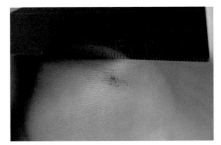

vesicles with eosinophilic infiltrate, generalized, pruritus and seen in association with radiation therapy mainly for cervical cancer. It spares palms, soles and mucous membranes.

Eosinophilic ulcer of the oral mucosa. Uncommon, self-limited ulcer that may be initiated by trauma. Histopathology is usually characteristic. One-third are painful and the commonest location of the ulcer is tongue, buccal mucosa and lip.

Epidermal nevus. Usually benign overgrowth of epidermal tissue. Can develop into squamous cell carcinoma. Rarely associated with underlying bone, central nervous system, eye or kidney abnormalities (epidermal nevus syndrome), 389, 390t, 392f

Epidermal nevus, inflammatory linear verrucous (ILVEN). Rare verrucous usually unilateral, acquired disorder along Blaschko's lines. Appears during the first few months of life and is pruritic and inflammatory.

Epidermal tumors, 268t, 295–297

Epidermis, 3–4

Epidermodysplasia verruciformis. A rare, apparently hereditary disease manifested by papulosquamous and warty lesions present at birth with no site of predilection. The prognosis for life is poor because of the eventual development of squamous cell carcinomas from the lesions. Numerous human papilloma viruses (HPV) have been found. HPV types 5 & 8 are especially associated with malignant transformation.

Epidermolysis bullosa, 179–180, 377, 378t, 379f, 388, 390f, 390t

Epidermolysis bullosa acquisita, 180

Epidermolysis bullosa nevi. Melanocytic nevi that have so far proven to be benign. Can occur at sites of previous blisters with a scalloped edge to match the blister border. Clinically the lesions are often large with clinical criteria of malignant melanoma. Junctional and dystrophic epidermolysis bullosa are the most commonly associated, 24

Epidermophytid. A dermatophytid due to *Epidermophyton* infection. *See also* Id reaction

Epidermophytosis. A fungus infection due to *Epidermophyton*

Epiloia. A triad of mental deficiency, epilepsy, and adenoma sebaceum. *See* Adenoma sebaceum; Tuberous sclerosis

Epithelioma, 296, 298–299, 298f, 299f
  apocrine, 298
  calcifying, 299
  cuniculatum. *See* Verrucous carcinoma
  eccrine, 299
  hair, 298–299

Epitheliomas, 281–285, 282f, 284f, 285f

Epstein-Barr virus (EBV), 237, 237f

e-PTFE implants. *See* Expanded polytetrafluoroethylene facial implants

Epulis. This term refers to any growth involving the gums., giant. A solitary neoplasm or granuloma from the periosteum of the jaw bone in the gingival area.

Erosio interdigitalis blastomycetica. Erosion and whitish maceration signifying a candidal and gram(-) bacterial infection of the webs between the fingers or toes.

Erosive adenomatosis of the nipple. Benign neoplastic conditions usually seen in middle-aged women that mimic Paget's disease clinically and adenocarcinoma histologically. Mastectomies have been unnecessarily done for this condition.

Eruptive melanocytic nevi. Simultaneous abrupt onset of numerous nevi acquired after immunosuppression. There is increased concern about melanoma in these patients.

Eruptive vellus hair cysts. Pediatric age group with 1-4mm flesh colored or reddish-brown papules with central hyperkeratosis or umbilication. Especially anterior chest and abdomen. There may be 20-200. Punch biopsy, acne surgery or aspirations shows a serpentine array of vellus hairs.

Erysipelas, 196t, 203, 203f

Erysipeloid. A chancre-type infection on the hand occurring at the site of accidental inoculation with the organism *Erysipelothrix rhusiopathiae,* seen in butchers, veterinarians, and fishermen. A localized form runs its course in 2 to 4 weeks. A generalized form develops a diffuse eruption with occasional constitutional symp-

toms such as arthritis. A very rare systemic form exhibits a skin eruption, joint pains, and endocarditis.

Erythema, 100t
  dyschromicum perstans. *See* Ashy dermatosis

Erythema ab igne. A marmoraceous-appearing redness that follows the prolonged application to the skin of radiant heat, such as from a heating pad or pretibial areas from sitting in front of a fireplace.

Erythema chronicum migrans, 128

Erythema elevatum diutinum. A persistent nodular, symmetrical eruption usually seen in middle-aged men with a rather characteristic histologic picture. This may be a deeper form of *granuloma annulare.*

Erythema gyratum repens, 351t

Erythema induratum, 129

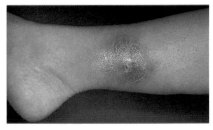

Erythema induratum.

Erythema infectiosum, 233

Erythema multiforme (EM), 24, 111, 127–128, 336f, 394t, 398
  bullosum, 182–183, 183f

Erythema nodosum, 128–130, 137

Erythema nodosum leprosum. Painful red or purple nodules usually on extremities with severe constitutional symptoms in lepromatous leprosy. It represents an immune complex vasculitis. Thalidomide, clofazimine, and prednisone have been used as therapy.

Erythema, palmar. Redness of the palms of the hands, which may be due to heredity, pulmonary disease, liver disease, rheumatoid arthritis, or pregnancy.

Erythema perstans. Over a dozen entities have been described that fit into this

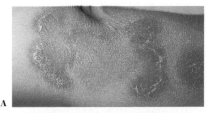

Erythema perstans on elbow
(*Drs. H. Shair and L. Grayson*).

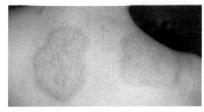

Erythema perstans on back.

Erythema perstans (*continued*)
persistent group of diseases that resemble persistent erythema multiforme. The following entities are included in this group: *erythema annulare centrifugum (Darier's) often idiopathic but may be associated with many underlying illnesses; erythema chronicum migrans (Lipschutz),* which may be due to a tick bite, as in Lyme disease; *erythema gyratum perstans (Fox); erythema figuratum perstans (Wende)* associated with scarlet fever; and *erythema gyratum repens (Gammel)* almost always associated with underlying cancer and the skin has appearance of grain of wood, 128

Erythema toxicum neonatorum. An evanescent skin eruption in newborns usually occurring within 48 hours after birth and lasting about 3 days; consists of erythema, papules, macules, and occasional pustules.

Erythermalgia. *See* Erythromelalgia

Erythrasma, 203–204

Erythroderma
bullous congenital ichthyosiform, 374t
ichthyosiform, T cell. *see* Sézary syndrome

Erythrodermia desquamativa. Term for Leiner's disease

Erythrokeratodermia progressive symmetrica (progressive symmetric erythrokeratodermia). Rare autosomal dominant persistent hyperkeratotic erythematous plaques especially head, extremities and buttocks. It appears during the first year of life and progressive for a few years and then may remit or remain stationary. Fifty percent with involvement of palms and soles.

Erythrokeratodermia variabilis. Rare, chronic, autosomal dominant usually developing months after birth. Red to brown patches that change from minutes to hours to days. Also variable keratotic brownish plaques and keratoderma of palms and soles may occur.

Erythromelalgia or erythermalgia. A rare disorder of hands and feet most common in middle age; characterized by swelling, redness, burning pain that is activated by exertion or heat and is refractory to treatment.

Erythromelanosis follicularis faciei. Hyperpigmentation, follicular plugging, and well demarcated erythema on the face especially in men.

Erythropoietic protoporphyria, 368t, 371

Erythrose pigmentaire peribuccale. A rare condition of middle-aged women, characterized by diffuse brownish red pigmentation about the mouth, the chin, and the neck with or without a slight burning sensation.

ESFA. *See* Eccrine syringofibroadenoma

Espundia, 428

Essential pruritis, 118–119

Excisions, 61, 61f

Excoriation, 16

Exfoliative dermatitis, 100t, 184–186, 186f, 414
primary, 184–185
secondary, 185–186, 186f

Exostosis, subungual. *See* Subungual

Expanded polytetrafluoroethylene facial implants (e-PTFE implants), 52–53, 53f

External otitis, 121–122

Eye makeup, 70–71

Eyelids, 19

Fabry's disease, 358–359

Factitial dermatitis, 190–191, 190f, 191f, 419

Fall dermatoses, 24

FAMI. *See* Fat autograft muscle injection

Familial benign chronic pemphigus, 180

Fanconi syndrome, 386t

Fanconi's syndrome, 341

Fasciitis, nodular. Painful, tender, rapidly growing, soft-tissue mass usually on an extremity and usually less than 3cm. Reactive, inflammatory, benign and can be excised or possibly treated by intralesional corticosteroids. Histopathathological examination may lead to an erroneous diagnosis of a malignancy.

Fat autograft muscle injection (FAMI), 49–51, 50f

Fat necrosis of the newborn. Rare indurated, well demarcated subcutaneous nodules and plaques over arms, legs, cheeks, buttocks or trunk within the first few weeks of life. Usually occurs following a complicated pregnancy and may be associated with hypercalcemia. Usually resolves without sequela.

Fat necrosis, subcutaneous. *See* Subcutaneous fat necrosis

Fat necrosis, subcutaneous, with pancreatic disease. Histologic picture is quite characteristic.

Fat tissue tumors, 300

Fatal granulomatous disease of childhood. A very rare, X-linked disease of mainly males characterized by eczematous lesions in infancy with progressive chronic granulomatous bacterial infections.

Favre-Racouchet's syndrome. The term for multiple comedones on the high cheek and temple areas in older persons due to chronic sun exposure, 406, 410f

Feldene, 97t

Fiberglass dermatitis. Irritant contact dermatitis with itching papules, erythema, vesicles, desquamation and excoriations. Dorsal hands, fingers and forearms present mainly in workers using reinforcement filling in printed circuit boards. One of the commonest occupational dermatoses.

Fibroblasts, 3

Fibrokeratoma, acquired digital. Tumor occurring in adults on fingers or toes; mimics a rudimentary supernumerary digit but without nerve tissue.

Fibroma, recurrent infantile digital. Fibrous nodules that occur at birth or sometimes during childhood on fingers and toes; may spontaneously involute and then recur.

Fibromas, pedunculated, 273–274, 274f

Fibrosarcoma, 299

Fibroxanthoma, atypical. Relatively uncommon, malignant (metastasis is rare), raised nodular lesion that occurs most often on the head and neck at chronically sun-exposed or irradiated sites. Treated with Mohs surgery to attempt to avoid frequent local recurrence.

Filariasis, 429–430

Filiform, 25

Filoviruses, 443t

Finger pebbles. Fine asymptomatic flesh colored grouped micropapules on the dorsum of fingers associated with diabetes mellitus.

Fissures, 16

Flagellate erythema. Erythematous centripetal linear streaks (zebra-like stripe eruption, flagellate erythema) on trunk and proximal extremities in a centripetal distribution. Seen in association with systemic bleomycin therapy and dermatomyositis.

Flagyl, 97t

Flea bites, 172, 433, 434f

Flow cytometry, 13

Fluconazole therapy, 264

Flukes. *See* Trematodes dermatosis

Fluorinated corticosteroids, 40

Fluorouracil preparations, 39

Foams, 38

Focal dermal hypoplasia (Goltz syndrome). X-linked dominant syndrome showing cribriform atrophy with increase or decrease pigment often along Blaschko lines. Eye, skeletal, teeth, nail and soft tissue abnormalities may occur.

Folliculitis, eosinophilic pustular. Recurrent extremely pruritic crops of sterile pustules. Has a characteristic histologic appearance and is seen most often in association with HIV-positive patients.

Folliculitis, hot tub. A bacterial folliculitis with inflammatory nodules caused by *Pseudomonas aeruginosa* in people exposed to poorly chlorinated hot tubs, jacuzzis, whirlpools, and swimming pools.

Folliculitis, perforating, of the nose. A folliculitis of the stiff hairs of the nasal mucocutaneous junction that penetrates deeply through to the external nasal skin. Unless the basic pathology is understood and corrected by plucking the involved stiff hair, the condition cannot be cured. The external papule can simulate a skin cancer.

Foreign body granuloma. *See also* Granuloma, foreign body
Foshay test. A 48-hour intradermal test that, if positive, indicates that the person has or has had *tularemia*.

Fox-Fordyce disease. A rare, intensely pruritic, chronic papular dermatosis of the axillae and the pubic area in women. The intense itching is due to the closure of the apocrine gland pore with rupture of the duct and escape of the apocrine sweat into the surrounding epidermis. Treatment is difficult.

Frambesia. *See* Yaws
Frey's syndrome. Auriculotemporal nerve syndrome where gustatory stimuli cause facial flushing or sweating in the distribution of the auriculotemporal nerve. Usually due to trauma to the parotid gland in adults.

Frostbite. Exposure to cold can cause pathologic changes in the skin that are related to the severity of the exposure but vary with the susceptibility of the person. Other terms in use that refer to cold injuries under varying conditions include *trench foot, immersion foot, pernio,* and *chilblains.*

Futcher's line. *See* Voigt-Futcher line

Gangosa. A severe ulcerative and mutilating form of yaws that affects the palate, pharynx, and nasal tissues.

Gangrene. symmetrical peripheral. A rare syndrome associated with a multitude of underlying medical problems. Disseminated intravascular coagulation occurs in most cases. Probably synonymous with purpura fulminans.

Gardner's syndrome. An autosomal dominant trait with osteomas, fibrous and fatty tumors, epidermoid inclusion cysts of the skin, and multiple gastrointestinal polyps, 386f

General paresis. A psychosis due to syphilitic meningoencephalitis.

Genital melanotic macule. Benign, hyperpigmented, asymptomatic, well-demarcated macule seen in the genitalia of men and women. It's not associated with underlying illness and histologically looks like a lentigo.

Gentian violet. A dye that destroys gram-positive bacteria and some fungi.

Gianotti-Crosti syndrome. (papular acrodermatitis of childhood, *see* Chap. 33). Characterized by acute onset of symmetrical, red or flesh-colored, flat-topped papules, usually 2 to 3 mm in diameter, mainly on the face and limbs. Nonpruritic, they last about 3 weeks. The cause is a virus, sometimes of the hepatitis type.

Giant cell fibromas. Uncommon, benign, oral cavity, asymptomatic, solitary papule usually less than 1cm and probably a reactive process to trauma or inflammation.

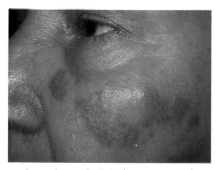

Granuloma faciale (*Dr. J. DeSpain*).

Jacquet's diaper dermatitis. Granulomatous
          erosive, diaper dermatitis in school
age children with chronic urinary
and/or fecal incontinence. May
mimic condyloma acuminatum.
Janeway nodes. Palmar, plantar, palmar fingers
          and plantar toes with painless, irreg-
          ular, hemorrhagic, nonblanchable
          papules seen with acute bacterial
          endocarditis.
Jarisch-Herxheimer reaction. *See* Herxheimer
          reaction
Jellyfish, 430
Jessner's syndrome (lymphocytic infiltrate of
          Jessner). Benign lymphocytic infil-
          tration of the skin, mainly of the
          face, resembling deep chronic dis-
          coid lupus erythematosus.

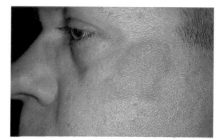

**Jessner's benign lymphocytic
infiltration of the skin.**

Job's syndrome (HIES). Hyperimmunoglobu-
          lin E, recurrent infections. Rare, con-
          genital.
Jogger's nipples. Painful erosions of nipples in
          runners, especially braless females,
          and when hard, irritating clothing is
          worn, 450t, 452
Junctional Epidermolysis Bullosa-Pyloric Atre-
          sia syndrome. Rare autosomal reces-
          sive with atresia of gastric antrum or
          pylorus and bullous disease of skin
          and oral mucosa.
Junctional nevus, 289, 290f
Jüngling's disease. *Osteitis fibrosa cystica* of the
          small long bones, particularly of the
          fingers, due to sarcoidosis.
Juvenile idiopathic arthritis, 110t
Juvenile xanthogranuloma, 394t, 398
Juxta-articular nodes. Syphilitic gummatous
          tumors occurring in the corium or
          subcutaneous layer of the skin in the
          region of the joints.

Kaposiform hemangioendothelioma. Usually
          seen on the trunk and develops at
          birth or in neonates in the first few
          months of life with approximately
          25% mortality rate due to tumor in-
          filtration or Kasabach-Merritt syn-
          drome. Destructive bone changes are
          not uncommon. Treatment is for as
other infantile hemangiomas. Trans-
          catheter embolization and surgical
          excision may be required.
Kaposi's sarcoma, 241, 242f, 300–301, 301f
Kasabach-Merritt syndrome. Rare syndrome
          of thrombocytopenia, bleeding and
          petechiae and association with rapid
          enlarging tufted angioma or Kaposi-
          form hemangioendothelioma.
Kassowitz-Diday's law. The observation that
          successive children of a syphilitic
          mother will become progressively
          less infected with syphilis or not be
          infected at all.
Kathon CG, 69
Kawasaki disease, 41. *See also* Mucocutaneous
          lymph node syndrome
Kawasaki's syndrome, 349
Keloid, 41, 286, 286f, 299
     treatment of. Intralesional corticosteroids,
          585-nm pulsed dye laser, 30 second
          liquid nitrogen cryosurgery and sili-
          con gel sheets for 12 to 24 hours
          each day for at least 2 months.
     Keloids, 16, 18f
Keratin, 4, 5f
Keratinization disorders, 373–377, 374t–375t,
          376f, 377f
Keratinocytes, 3
Keratoacanthoma, 285, 285f, 296
Keratoacanthoma centrifugum marginatum. A
          rare variant of keratoacanthoma that
          shows progressive peripheral growth
          with coincident central healing.
Keratoconjuntivitis sicca, 335
Keratoderma blennorrhagicum. A rare chronic
          inflammatory dermatosis with horny
          pustular crusted lesions mainly on
          the palms and the soles; occurs in
          conjunction with gonorrheal infec-
          tion of the genital tract and Reiter's
          syndrome.
Keratoderma climacterium. Circumscribed
          hyperkeratotic lesions of the palms
          and the soles of women of the
          menopausal age. These lesions
          resemble psoriasis, and the majority
          of cases are considered to be this
          disease.
Keratoderma, epidermolytic palmoplantar
          (EPPK of Vörner). Diffuse, yellow-
          ish, hyperkeratotic, thickening of
          palms and soles. Familiar or spo-
          radic and has a characteristic shape,
          and erythematous line of demarca-
          tion. May be hyperhidrotic and
          rarely with blisters. Autosomal dom-
          inant variant called Unna-Thost has
          a slightly different histopathology.
Keratohyalin granules, 3
Keratolytics, 32

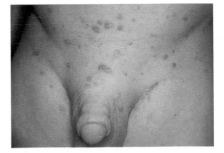

Letterer-Siwe disease of lower abdomen in child.

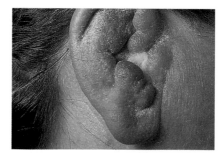

Lymphedema (elephantiasis nostras) of ear (*Dr. M. Feldaker*).

Meyerson's phenomenon (*continued*)
squamous cell carcinomas, and dermatofibroma associated with the appearance of these tumors. Affects healthy individuals, is rare, and has no proven etiology. The tumors stop forming after the inflammation dissipates.

MHP. *See* Monosymptomatic hypochondriacal psychosis

Microcystic adnexal carcinoma. Locally aggressive adnexal malignancy. Often recurs after radiation or surgery. Mainly central face with a slow growing cystic papule or plaque. May occur after radiation therapy and infiltration deeply into surrounding structures. Difficult diagnosis but histopathology is diagnostic, 299

Mid-dermal elastolysis. Rare acquired disease well-circumscribed fine wrinkling and/or papular protrusions especially trunk, neck and arms. Especially middle-aged women after prolonged artificial or natural ultraviolet exposure. Histopathological exam is diagnostic with loss of elastic tissue in the mid-dermis.

Migratory panniculitis, 130

Milia, 18, 275, 275f, 388, 390t

Miliaria, 7, 24, 440–441, 441f

Military dermatoses, 24

Milker's nodules. A viral disease contracted from infected udders of cows. The lesions, usually on the hands, consist of brown-red or purple firm nodules that subside in 4 to 6 weeks, conferring immunity.

Minimal erythema dose, 364

Minocycline, 97t

Minocycline hyperpigmentation, 341

Mitochondrial DNA syndromes. A group of genetic diseases that may appear at any age. Growth retardation, myopathy, seizures, renal failure, eye disease and occasionally skin disease. Symmetrical cervical lipomas and poikiloderma are the commonest skin manifestations. Defects of mitochondrial DNA can be acquired and be related to aging and many diseases.

Moeller's glossitis, 335

Mole. *See* Nevus

Molluscum contagiosum, 291, 394t, 395, 457

Mondor disease. Thrombophlebitis as subcutaneous veins on anterolateral thoracoabdominal wall. Palpable, visible, tender, painful cords in the mammary areas from the axilla to the subcostal

margin. Three times more common in women. It is usually benign and self-limited but underlying conditions especially breast cancer must be ruled out. Inciting events including trauma, surgery infection, increased physicial activity and pendulous breasts.

Mongolian spots, 302, 389, 390t, 392f

Monilethrix, 384t

Monoclonal antibodies. Specific antibodies produced from a hybrid cell. This hybrid cell results from the fusion of nuclear material from two cells. Used for therapy for cancer, psoriasis any many other diseases.

Monosymptomatic hypochondriacal psychosis (MHP), 189–190, 189f

Morbilliform, 26

Morphea, 346t

Morphine, 98t

Mosaic "fungus." Not a fungus but an artifact commonly found in KOH slide preparations taken from the feet and the hands. They consist of beaded lines along outlining epidermal cells.

Motor nerves, 5

Mucinosis. When fibroblasts produce an excess amount of acid mucopolysaccharides (mucin), they may replace the connective tissue elements. This occurs in myxedema and localized pretibial myxedema. *See also* Myxedema, localized

follicular (alopecia mucinosa). This rare disease is characterized by one or more symptomatic, well-circumscribed, indurated, slightly erythematous plaques with loss of hair. The most common site is the face. The plaques involute spontaneously after several months. Some cases are associated with a T-cell lymphoma.

papular. A rare cutaneous fibromucinous disease with a monoclonal serum protein of cathodal mobility. Clinically seen are localized or generalized papules, plaques, or nodules.

mucinosis, reticular erythematous (REM). Erythematous papules and plaques mainly on chest of middle-aged women. Worsens with sun exposure. Characteristic mucin and lymphocytic infiltrate around vessels and follicles.

Muckle-Wells syndrome. Rare autosomal dominant with urticaria-like eruptions in infancy associated with progressive perceptive deafness, limb pain, periodic fever, malaise, and amyloid nephropathy.

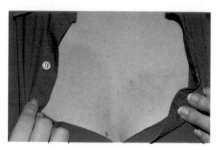

Reticular erythematous mucinosis (REM).

Mucocutaneous lymph node syndrome. (Kawasaki's disease). A self-limited febrile illness seen mainly in children, with conjunctivitis, dryness and redness of lips, reddening of palms and soles with later characteristic digital skin desquamation, polymorphous exanthema of the trunk, and swelling of cervical lymph nodes. May be associated with coronary artery aneurysms, 349

Mucormycosis. Nodules and ulcerations caused by *Mucor* or *Rhizopus* fungi in patients that are uremic, diabetic, or otherwise immunocompromised. May also occur under adhesive tape.

Mucous membrane disease, 332–336, 333f–336f, 414
aphthous stomatitis as, 332–333, 333f
Fordyce's disease with, 333–334
geographic tongue as, 332, 333f
herpes simplex with, 333–334
leukoplakia of, 335
mucosal lesions with, 334, 334f
rare, 334–336, 334f–336f

Muir-Torre syndrome. Rare genodermatosis (autosomal dominant) of sebaceous neoplasms (adenomas, especially sebaceous adenoma, epitheliomas, carcinomas) and visceral cancer (especially genitourinary and gastrointestinal) with prolonged survival.

Mulluscum contagiosum virus, 230–231, 231f

Multicentric reticulohistocytosis. Rare condition of reddish or yellow papules on the dorsal hands (especially nail folds and distal interphalangeal joints), ears, and bridge of nose. Associated with arthritis mutilans, and one fourth of patients have an underlying cancer. The histiocytic infiltrate is characteristic on pathology and may involve internal organs.

Multinucleate cell angiohistiocytoma. Rare red-brown grouped papules especially in middle-aged and elderly

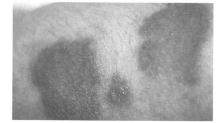

Neutrophilic acute febrile dermatosis (Sweet's syndrome) (*Dr. J. DeSpain*).

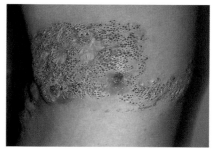

Nevus comedonicus on abdomen.

systemic infection. The cutaneous lesions of the subcutaneous tissue and bones are clinically similar to maduromycosis.

Nodes. Heberden's. Sometimes tender, firm bony outgrowth of the distal interphalangeal joints of the fingers of patients with osteoarthritis.

Nodes. Osler's. Transient, red, painful, nodules located on the palms and the soles in patients with chronic bacterial endocarditis.

Nodular chondrodermatitis of ear, 301

Nodular fasciitis. *See* Fasciitis, nodular

Nodular melanoma, 304

Nodular panniculitis, 129

Nodular vasculitis, 129

Nodules, 15, 17f, 394t, 395–398, 397f

Nodules, weathering of the ear. Asymptomatic fairly common, multiple, white smooth nodules along the free margin of the helix seen mainly in elderly males with marked sun damage.

Nonbullous congenital ichthyosiform erythroderma, 374t, 376f

Nonmelanin pigmentations, 341

Nonmelanoma skin cancer, 367–368

Nonsteroidal anti-inflammatory agents, 365

Nonthrombocytopenic purpura, 133

North American blastomycosis, 265–266, 265f

Notalgia paresthetica, 124. *See also* Pruritic hereditary localized patch on back

Nummular eczema, 21f, 24, 91, 92f, 102t, 406f, 410, 412f

Obliterans, arteriosclerosis. A degenerative change mainly in the arteries of the extremities; most commonly seen in elderly men. Leg ulcers and gangrene can result from these vascular changes.

Obliterans, thromboangiitis. *Buerger's disease* is an obliterative disease of the arteries and the veins that occurs almost exclusively in young men. It mainly involves the extremities and produces tissue ischemia, ulcers, and gangrene.

Obstetric cholestasis, 460t, 462–463

Occipital Horn syndrome, 383

Occlusive dressing therapy, 132

Occlusive folliculitis, 454–455, 454f

Occupational dermatoses, 83

Ochronosis. A rare hereditary metabolic disorder characterized by a brownish or blackish pigmentation of cartilages, ligaments, tendons, and intima of the large blood vessels due to the deposit of a polymer of homogentisic

acid. The urine in ochronosis turns black, particularly in the presence of alkali; hence the term *alkaptonuria*. *See also* pigmentary disorders. There is an exogenous form at the site of chronic topical hydroquinone application (see Chapter 9), 102t

Odors from the skin. *See* Lochman DS: Cutis 27:645, 1981

Ointments, 33, 35–38, 37t

Oleomas. Subcutaneous granulomas due to injection of sesame seed oil used for tissue augmentation or as a slow release substance for anabolic steroids. Usually in bodybuilders.

Olmsted's syndrome. Very rare; consists of congenital keratoderma of the palms and soles, onychodystrophy, constriction of digits, and periorofacial keratoses. Can be confused with acrodermatitis enteropathica.

Omenn's syndrome. Combined immunodeficiency. Rare, congenital. A type of severe combined immunodeficiency with lymphocytosis and leukocytosis with eosinophilia. Often fatal in childhood with a chronic skin eruption mimicking severe seborrhea, lymphadenopathy, hepatosplenomegaly, recurrent infections, fever, and failure to thrive. Humoral and cellular immunity are both defective, 114t, 400

Onchocerciasis, 430

Online resources, 464–465

Onycho-. A prefix from the Greek *onyx* meaning "nail."

Onychocryptosis, 326, 326f

Onychomycosis, 320–323, 322f, 323f

Ophiasis. Snake-like form of alopecia areata around the edges of the scalp. May be especially recalcitrant to therapy.

Optic atrophy. Atrophy of the optic nerve due to syphilitic involvement of the central nervous system of the tabetic type. Blindness is the end result.

Oral candidiasis, 261–262, 263f

Oral florid papillomatosis. *See* Verrucous carcinoma

Orf. A viral infection characterized by a vesicular and pustular eruption of the mouth and the lips of lambs. Sheep herders and veterinarians become inoculated on the hand and develop a primary-chancre type lesion.

Oriental sore, 427

Osler's disease, 300

Osler's nodes. Tender, erythematous, blanchable, oval, papules on palms, soles, palmar fingers and plantar toes associated with subacute bacterial endocarditis.

Osler-Weber-Rendu disease (Hereditary hemorrhagic telangiectasia). Begins in puberty. Progressive telangiectasias on lips, tongue, palate, nasal mucosa, palms, soles, fingers, nail beds, and throughout gastrointestinal tract. Pulmonary and intranial A-V malformations may occur. Epistaxis and bleeding from internal organs is problematic in this autosomal disease, 133

Osmidrosis. Malodorous apocrine gland sweating usually in an axillary location.

Osseous tumors, 301

Osteoma cutis, 301

Ostomy skin care. *See* Stomas

Pachonychia congenita, 384, 385f

Pachydactyly. Rare benign fibromatosis causing fusiform swelling of multiple fingers over the proximal interphalangeal joints or proximal phalanges.

Pachydermoperiostosis. Pachydermia, hypertrophic osteoarthropathy and finger clubbing are part of a rare genetic syndrome.

Pachyonychia congenita. A rare autosomal dominant condition with thickening of the palms and soles, thickening of the oral mucosa, and hyperkeratosis of the distal nail bed with accumulation of subungual debris.

Paederus dermatitis (Blister beetle dermatitis), 433–434, 435f

Paget's disease, 296–297, 351t

Palmar-plantar keratoderma, 373, 377f

Palmoplantar eccrine hidradenitis (PEH). Painful, erythematosus palmoplantar nodules in children with resolution after several days of bedrest. On biopsy, inflammation of neutrophils occur in and around eccrine glands and their ducts.

Panniculitis, 137

alpha-1-antitrypsin. A form of panniculitis associated with alpha-1-antitrypsin deficiency and severe panniculitis with ulceration. Clinical manifestations also include emphysema, hepatitis, xerosis, vasculitis, angioedema and panniculitis.

cold. Erythematous nodules mainly on the face in infants in association with cold exposure such as eating a popsicle. Usually dissipates spontaneously without sequelae.

histiocytic cytophagic. A chronic histiocytic disease of subcutaneous fat with fever, serositis, and purpura. The course may be fatal with pancytopenia due to

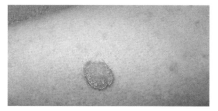

Porokeratosis of leg.

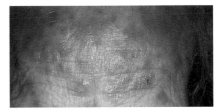

Pseudolymphoma of Spiegler-Fendt.

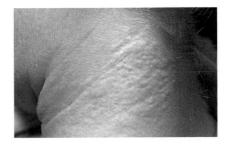

Pseudoxanthoma elasticum of neck.

Pyoderma gangrenosum, 354, 354f

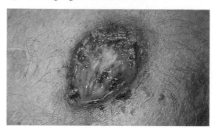

Pyoderma gangrenosum above nipple.